# MEDICAL TERMINOLOGY
## A Word-Building Approach

**6**th edition

## Jane Rice, RN, CMA-C

*Medical Assisting Program Director, Retired*
*Coosa Valley Technical College*
*Rome, Georgia*

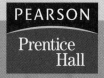

PEARSON

Prentice Hall

Upper Saddle River, New Jersey 07458

Library of Congress Cataloging-in-Publication Data

Rice, Jane.
    Medical terminology: A word-building approach / Jane Rice.—
6th ed.
        p.  ; cm.
        Includes index.
        ISBN–13: 978–0–13–222531–1
        ISBN–10: 0–13–222531–X
1. Medicine—Terminology.   2. Human anatomy—Terminology.   I. Title.
    [DNLM: 1. Medicine—Terminology—English.   2. Anato-
my—Terminology—English.   3. Terminology.   W 15
R496m 2008]
    R123.R523 2008
    610.1'4—dc22                                      2006036378

**Publisher:** Julie Levin Alexander
**Assistant to Publisher:** Regina Bruno
**Executive Editor:** Mark Cohen
**Associate Editor:** Melissa Kerian
**Editorial Assistant:** Nicole Ragonese
**Media Editor:** John J. Jordan
**Development Editors:** Elena Mauceri and Lynda Hatch
**Managing Production Editor:** Patrick Walsh
**Production Liaison:** Christina Zingone
**Production Editor:** Bruce Hobart, Pine Tree Composition
**Manufacturing Manager:** Ilene Sanford
**Manufacturing Buyer:** Pat Brown
**Design Coordinator/Cover Designer:** Mary Siener

**Interior Designer:** Anthony Gemmellaro
**Director of Marketing:** Karen Allman
**Executive Marketing Manager:** Katrin Beacom
**New Media Project Manager:** Stephen Hartner
**New Media Production:** Horus Development
**Composition:** Pine Tree Composition, Inc.
**Printer/Binder:** R.R. Donnelley & Sons
**Cover Printer:** Phoenix Color Corp.
**Cover Illustrator:** Robert Silvers, Runaway Technology.

Pearson Education Ltd., *London*
Pearson Education Australia Pty. Limited, *Sydney*
Pearson Education Singapore, Pte. Ltd.
Pearson Education North Asia Ltd., *Hong Kong*
Pearson Education Canada, Ltd., *Toronto*
Pearson Educación de Mexico, S.A. de C.V.
Pearson Education—Japan, *Tokyo*
Pearson Education Malaysia, Pte. Ltd.
Pearson Education, Upper Saddle River, New Jersey

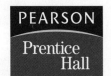

10 9 8 7 6 5 4 3
ISBN-13:978-0-13-222531-1
ISBN-10:0-13-222531-X

*In special memory
of my parents,
Warren Galileo
and Elizabeth Styles Justice,
and my sister,
Betty Sue Nelson.*

# CONTENTS IN BRIEF

# DETAILED CONTENTS

**CHAPTER 15**   **SPECIAL SENSES: THE EAR**                                                    **499**

**CHAPTER 16**   **SPECIAL SENSES: THE EYE**                                                    **529**

**CHAPTER 17**   **FEMALE REPRODUCTIVE SYSTEM**                                                 **563**

**CHAPTER 18** | **OBSTETRICS**   **599**

**CHAPTER 19** | **MALE REPRODUCTIVE SYSTEM**   **637**

This text has helped thousands of students over the years in successfully mastering the challenging yet exciting terminology of medicine. Its trademarks are twofold:

## 1. A word-building approach

A logical, simple system for learning medical vocabulary by building from word parts.

## 2. Accurate and complete coverage of human anatomy

Concise coverage of all major body structures and functions, organized by system. The sixth edition builds upon this framework and presents a dynamic learning system for the 21st Century. As you turn the pages to discover the features of this book, you will find an exciting blend of fresh ideas merged with proven methods.

## FRESH IDEAS

As we set out to create the sixth edition, we met with instructors and students from around the country and we spoke with countless additional manuscript reviewers who provided us with valuable feedback about how they teach and learn. We asked them to help us refine this learning system to best meet their needs. From this dialog we have emerged with a textbook that stands out in a number of important ways.

**Total instructional support package.** *Medical Terminology: A Word-Building Approach* now boasts an unparalleled collection of instructional resources to support educators of all kinds. These resources include video- and animation-enhanced PowerPoint lectures for each chapter that correlate to a customized lesson plan and lecture guide. For those instructors wishing to integrate Personal Response Systems ("clicker" technology) into their classrooms, these Power-Point lectures contain content that is compatible for a variety of systems. A 2,900-question test bank is also provided to adopters, offering a vast catalog of diverse questions all within an easy-to-use shell for building and customizing exams. Of course, all of these materials are also supported within online platforms such as Blackboard and WebCT. For more information about this complete set of resources please turn to page xxii.

**A design for today's visual learners.** Countless students and instructors have expressed the importance of instructive images and a vibrant, clear presentation of information. To this end, we have added over 150 images to this edition. Further, we have worked with a team of instructional designers to fine-tune the pedagogical clarity and overall aesthetic appeal of the book. These enhancements will provide readers with a visually engaging journey through this text.

**Important content added and refined.** Four new chapters have been added. These chapters are: Chapter 2 Suffixes, Chapter 3 Prefixes, Chapter 18 Obstetrics, and Chapter 22 Mental Health. All other chapters have been thoroughly updated and revised based on the valuable input of our educator advisory panel. We also added and refined several important features and so with this extensive revision *Medical Terminology: A Word-Building Approach* is now more accurate, complete, and user friendly than ever before.

## What's Changed At-A-Glance

This chart provides an at-a-glance summary of the changes and additions that we've made.

| Feature | Description |
| --- | --- |
| **Chapter 2 Suffixes**–*New!* | A new chapter that explores the many uses and nuances of suffixes used in a variety of medical terms. This lays an ideal foundation for the understanding of word building. |
| **Chapter 3 Prefixes**–*New!* | Another new chapter that reinforces the importance of word building. The many uses and meanings of prefixes are introduced here, followed by reinforcement exercises. |
| **Chapter 18 Obstetrics**–*New!* | A new chapter that addresses labor, delivery, and the postpartum period. It covers fertilization, prenatal care, drugs used during childbirth, and breastfeeding. |
| **Chapter 22 Mental Health**–*New!* | A new chapter that addresses mental health and mental disorders. It also presents an overview, symptoms, diagnosis, and treatment of mental illnesses. |
| **SOAP: Chart Note Analysis**–*New!* | An end-of-chapter capstone exercise that challenges readers to review, study, and think critically about "real word" case data of a patient's visit to a medical facility. ▼ |

### SOAP: Chart Note Analysis
A real-world case scenario that challenges readers to think critically.

---

**PATIENT:** Davis, Christopher     **DATE:** 01/15/2007
**DOB:** 11/24/2003   **AGE:** 3   **SEX:** Male
**INSURANCE:** Best Care Insurance

**Vital Signs:**
  T: 98.4 F
  P: 90
  R: 20
  BP: 85/60
  Ht: 3' 2"
  Wt: 36 lb
**Allergies:** penicillin
**Chief Complaint:** Waddling gait with increasing episodes of falling and apparent clumsiness. Activities of running and climbing very slowly in comparison to peers.

**S**  **Subjective:** Mother of 3 y/o white male states that she has noticed her son is beginning to appear "clumsy" with increasing episodes of falling. She has noticed that he looks like he is "waddling" when he walks. "He runs very slow, has trouble climbing playground equipment and trouble getting up off the floor. He isn't able to jump from a standing position, like his feet are glued to the floor. At times, he appears to be walking on his toes." She expresses concern that he did not learn to walk until after he was 18 months old, and that she is at risk for carrying the gene that causes muscular dystrophy.

**O**  **Objective:**
**General Appearance:** Pleasant child who exhibits no distress while sitting and playing on the floor. Noted difficulty rising from floor to standing position. Child used Gowers' maneuver to push himself upright.
**Lungs:** CTA
**Heart:** Normal rate and rhythm. No murmurs, gallops or rubs.
**Abd:** Bowel sounds all quadrants. Soft, no masses or tenderness.
**MS:** Abduction of arms to full 180° above head impaired, due to muscle weakness. Noted muscle weakness of bilateral lower extremities. No contractures with joint involvement. Calf muscles appear enlarged by connective tissue and fat. Upon palpation, felt "rubbery."
**Neuro:** Oriented to person and place. Reflexes intact.
**Skin:** Cool and moist, soft to touch. Noted generalized bruising at various stages on legs and arms.

**A**  **Assessment:** Duchenne Muscular Dystrophy (DMD)

**P**  **Plan:**
1. Schedule physical therapy to help delay permanent muscular contracture.
2. Recommend supportive measures such as splints and braces to minimize deformities and preserve mobility.
3. Recommend deep breathing exercises to help delay weakening of the muscles of respiration.
4. Suggest counseling and referral services as supportive measures for parent and child.
5. Provide the family with information on the Muscular Dystrophy Association, which is located 3561 E. Sunrise Drive, Tucson, AZ 85718. Telephone: 1-602-529-2000 or 1-800-572-1717. E-mail: mda@mdausa.org.

| Feature | Description |
|---|---|
| **Chapter 20 (Oncology) and 21 (Radiology and Nuclear Medicine)**–*Updated* | Now includes the newest information about treatments and technology. These new chapters have been reorganized for a better flow of information. |
| **Word Building Tables**–*Redesigned* | A more user-friendly approach to the **Building Your Medical Vocabulary** tables in each chapter. Several images have been added and are placed logically beside the words they describe within the table. We have also updated the content, improved presentation of the word parts and their definitions, deleted nonessential material, and added new information where appropriate. ▼ |
| **Over 150 New Illustrations and Photos** | An infusion of images brings the total to nearly 400 illustrations and photos that will highlight important areas of the text. ▼ |

**Word-Building Tables**
Logical at-a-glance summaries of all key terms.

| MEDICAL WORD | WORD PARTS (WHEN APPLICABLE) | | | DEFINITION |
|---|---|---|---|---|
| | Part | Type | Meaning | |
| **abrasion** (ă-brā′zhŭn) | ab- ras -ion | P R S | away from to scrape off process | Process of scraping away from a surface, such as skin or teeth, by friction. An abrasion may be the result of trauma, such as a "skinned knee" or from a therapy, such as dermabrasion of the skin for removal of scar tissue. It can also occur from the wearing down of a tooth from mastication (chewing). |
| **anesthetize** (ă-něs′thě-tīz) | an- esthet -ize | P R S | without, lack of feeling, sensation to make | To induce a loss of feeling or sensation with the administration of an anesthetic |
| **arousal** (a-rou′zel) | arous -al | R S | alertness, to rise pertaining to | Pertaining to a state of alertness |
| **asymmetrical** (ă-sĭ-mě′-trĭ-kăl) | a- symmetric -al | P R S | lack of, without symmetry pertaining to | Unequal in size or shape. Without proportion of the body or parts of the body; different in placement or arrangement about an axis. |
| **asystole** (ă-sĭs′tŏ-lē) | a- systole | P R | without contraction | Literally means *without contraction* of the heart; a life-threatening cardiac condition characterized by the absence of electrical and mechanical activity in the heart. |
| **comatose** (kō′mă-tōs) | comat -ose | R S | a deep sleep pertaining to | Pertaining to a state of deep sleep (coma) |
| **dysarthria** (dĭs-ăr′thrē-ă) | | | | Difficult articulatio from interference muscles of speech, age to a central or |
| **epithelium** (ěp″ĭ-thē′lē-ŭm) | epi- thel/i -um | P CF S | upon, above nipple tissue, structure | Structure that cov ternal organs of th of vessels, body ca gans. It is the laye outermost layer of layer of mucous a |

**New Illustrations and Photos**
An abundance of visual descriptions of important concepts, over 200 added to this edition.

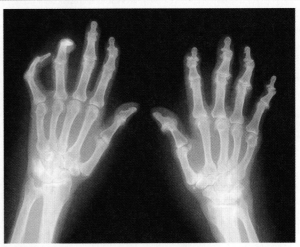

▶ **FIGURE 6–19** X-ray showing typical joint changes associated with osteoarthritis. (Source: Getty Images/Stone Allstock.)

# PROVEN METHODS

*Medical Terminology: A Word-Building Approach* employs a method that works. We've retained the elements that have made this book so popular.

## A Summary of Hallmark Features

| Feature | Description |
| --- | --- |
| **Chapter Outlines and Objectives** | Chapter-opening sections to help readers establish a game plan before they begin. |
| **Anatomically Precise Diagrams** | Visual references on nearly every page detailing anatomy and pathology concepts. |
| **Anatomy and Physiology Overview** | Essential coverage of the structure and function of the body with full-color art and tables. |
| **Life Span Considerations** | Boxed sections that provide interesting facts about the human body as it relates to the child and the older adult. ▼ |
| **Building Your Medical Vocabulary** | The foundation for learning medical terminology. By connecting various word parts in an organized sequence, thousands of words can be built and learned. The word list is alphabetized to demonstrate the variety of meanings created when common prefixes and suffixes are repeatedly applied to certain word roots and/or combining forms. A pronunciation guide follows each term. |
| **Drug Highlights** | Presents essential drug information that relates to the subject of the chapter. ▼ |

## LIFE SPAN CONSIDERATIONS

■ **THE CHILD**

Bone begins to develop during the second month of fetal life as cartilage cells enlarge, break down, disappear, and are replaced by bone-forming cells called **osteoblasts**. Most bones of the body are formed by this process, known as **endochondral ossification**. In this process, the bone cells deposit organic substances in the spaces vacated by cartilage to form bone matrix. As this process proceeds, blood vessels form within the bone and deposit salts such as calcium and phosphorus that serve to harden the developing bone.

The **epiphyseal plate** is the center for longitudinal bone growth in children. See Figure 6–9 ►. It is possible to determine the biological age of a child from the development of epiphyseal ossification centers as shown radiographically.

About three years after the onset of puberty, the ends of the long bones (**epiphyses**) knit securely to their shafts (**diaphysis**), and further growth can no longer take place.

The bones of children are more resilient than of adolescents and adults, tend to bend, and before breaking can become deformed. Fracture healing occurs more quickly in children because there is a rich blood supply to bones and their periosteum is thick and osteogenic activity is high.

**Calcium** is critical to the strength of bones. The daily recommendations of calcium by age group follow:

| | |
| --- | --- |
| 1 to 3 years | 500 mg |
| 4 to 8 years | 800 mg |
| 9 to 13 years | 1300 mg |
| 14 to 18 years | 1300 mg |

■ **THE OLDER ADULT**

Women build bone until about age 35 and then begin to lose about 1% of bone mass annually. Men usually start losing bone mass 10 to 20 years later. Most of the skeletal system changes that take place during the aging process involve changes in connective tissue. The

## DRUG HIGHLIGHTS

| | |
| --- | --- |
| **Anti-inflammatory agents** | Relieves the swelling, tenderness, redness, and pain of inflammation. Such agents can be classified as steroidal (corticosteroids) and nonsteroidal. |
| **Corticosteroids (Glucocorticoids)** | Steroid substance with potent anti-inflammatory effects *Examples: Depo-Medrol (methylprednisolone acetate), Aristocort (triamcinolone), Deltasone (prednisone), Haldrum (paramethasone acetate), and Delta-Cortef (prednisolone)* |
| **Nonsteroidal (NSAIDs)** | Agents used in the treatment of arthritis and related disorders *Examples: Bayer aspirin (acetylsalicylic acid), Motrin (ibuprofen), Feldene (piroxicam), Orudis (ketoprofen), and Naprosyn (naproxen)* |
| **Disease-modifying anti-rheumatic drugs (DMARDs)** | Can influence the course of the disease progression; therefore, their introduction in early rheumatoid arthritis is recommended to limit irreversible joint damage. *Examples: gold preparations Ridaura (auranofin) and Solganal (aurothioglucose); antimalarial Plaquenil Sulfate (hydroxychloroquine sulfate); a chelating agent Cuprimine (penicillamine) and the immunosuppressants Rheumatrex (methotrexate), Imuran (azathioprine), and Cytoxan (cyclophosphamide)* |
| **COX-2 inhibitors** | Cyclooxygenase (COX) is an enzyme involved in many aspects of normal cellular function and the inflammatory response. COX-2 is found in joints and other areas affected by inflammation as occurs with osteoarthritis and rheumatoid arthritis. Inhibition of COX-2 reduces the production of compounds associated with inflammation and pain. *Examples: Celebrex (celecoxib), and Mobic (meloxicam)* |
| **Antitumor necrosis factor (Anti-TNF) drugs** | These drugs have evolved out of the biotechnology industry and seem to slow, if not halt altogether, the destruction of the joints by disrupting the activity of tumor necrosis factor (TNF), a substance involved in the body's immune response. *Example: Enbrel (etanercept)* |
| **Agents used to treat gout** | Acute attacks of gout are treated with colchicine. Once the acute attack of gout has been controlled, drug therapy to control hyperuricemia can be initiated. *Example: Benemid (probenecid), Anturane (sulfinpyrazone), and Zyloprim (allopurinol)* |
| **Agents used to treat or prevent postmenopausal osteoporosis** | Include Fosamax (alendronate sodium) and Actonel (risedronate). Fosamax reduces the activity of the cells that cause bone loss and increases the amount of bone in most patients. Actonel inhibits osteoclast-mediated bone resorption and modulates bone metabolism. To receive the clinical benefits of either of these drugs the patient must be informed and follow the prescribed drug regimen. |

**Life Span Considerations**
Focus on the child and older adult

**Drug Highlights**
Essential pharmacology

| Feature | Description |
|---------|-------------|
| **Diagnostic and Laboratory Tests** | Provides a snapshot of current tests and procedures that are used in the physical assessment and diagnosis of certain conditions/diseases. |
| **Abbreviations** | Commonly used abbreviations, with their meanings, that are directly associated with the subject of the chapter. |
| **Pathology Spotlights** | An in-depth focus on selected diseases and conditions related to the chapter. These include current medical findings and interesting facts about various medical conditions. ▼ |
| **Pathology Checkpoint** | A concise checklist review of pathology-related terms that were covered in the chapter. |
| **Study and Review** | A self-paced study guide section featuring SOAP Chart Note Analysis questions and a variety of other study formats. It concludes with an illustrated preview of the vast student multimedia options. ▼ |

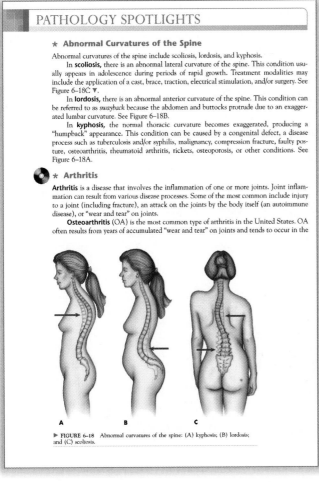

## PATHOLOGY SPOTLIGHTS

### ★ Abnormal Curvatures of the Spine

Abnormal curvatures of the spine include scoliosis, lordosis, and kyphosis.

In **scoliosis,** there is an abnormal lateral curvature of the spine. This condition usually appears in adolescence during periods of rapid growth. Treatment modalities may include the application of a cast, brace, traction, electrical stimulation, and/or surgery. See Figure 6–18C ▼.

In **lordosis,** there is an abnormal anterior curvature of the spine. This condition can be referred to as *swayback* because the abdomen and buttocks protrude due to an exaggerated lumbar curvature. See Figure 6–18B.

In **kyphosis,** the normal thoracic curvature becomes exaggerated, producing a "humpback" appearance. This condition can be caused by a congenital defect, a disease process such as tuberculosis and/or syphilis, malignancy, compression fracture, faulty posture, osteoarthritis, rheumatoid arthritis, rickets, osteoporosis, or other conditions. See Figure 6–18A.

### ★ Arthritis

**Arthritis** is a disease that involves the inflammation of one or more joints. Joint inflammation can result from various disease processes. Some of the most common include injury to a joint (including fracture), an attack on the joints by the body itself (an autoimmune disease), or "wear and tear" on joints.

**Osteoarthritis** (OA) is the most common type of arthritis in the United States. OA often results from years of accumulated "wear and tear" on joints and tends to occur in the

▶ FIGURE 6–18 Abnormal curvatures of the spine: (A) kyphosis; (B) lordosis; and (C) scoliosis.

**Pathology Spotlights**
Focus on selected diseases

## STUDY AND REVIEW

### Identifying Suffixes

*Underline the suffixes in the following medical words.*

1. cardiac
2. cephalad
3. enuresis
4. obstetrician
5. bronchiole
6. pustule
7. dentalgia
8. diabetes
9. hyperemesis
10. hemoptysis

### Defining Suffixes

*Give the meaning of the following suffixes.*

1. -asthenia _____
2. -ion _____
3. -itis _____
4. -malacia _____
5. -megaly _____
6. -pathy _____
7. -penia _____
8. -pepsia _____
9. -phobia _____
10. -rrhexis _____
11. -al _____
12. -ar _____
13. -ate _____
14. -ia _____
15. -ize _____
16. -oid _____
17. -or _____
18. -ose _____
19. -ous _____
20. -trophy _____
21. -um _____

### Spelling

*In the spaces provided, write the correct spelling of these misspelled terms:*

1. aurcle _____
2. bronchole _____
3. cardilogist _____
4. cephlad _____
5. cynaotic _____
6. embolsm _____
7. podatry _____
8. pustle _____

**Study and Review**
A variety of exercises for self quizzing

We are committed to providing students and instructors with exactly the tools they need to be successful in the classroom and beyond. Along these lines *Medical Terminology: A Word-Building Approach* is supported by the most complete and dynamic set of resources available today.

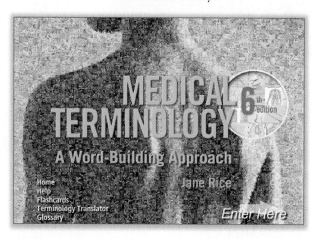

## Student CD-ROM

Every student text includes an interactive study guide on CD-ROM. Features include:

- **Custom Flashcard Generator**—allows students to create their own flashcards or study with a ready-made interactive version.
- **Audio Glossary**—provides definitions and audio pronunciations of each of the key terms presented in the text.
- **Terminology Translator**—contains the Spanish translations and audio pronunciations of over 5,000 medical terms.

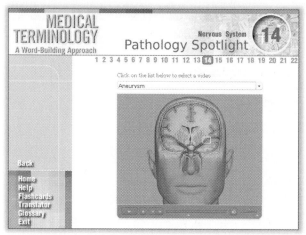

**Pathology Spotlights**—a set of videos that provides a mini-documentary profile of selected diseases presented within each chapter.

**12 different game modules**—provide students with a diverse and fun array of study tools.

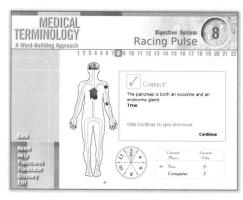

**Racing Pulse**

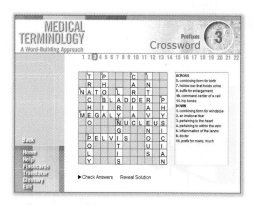

**Crossword**

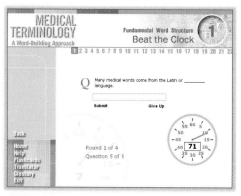

**Beat the Clock**

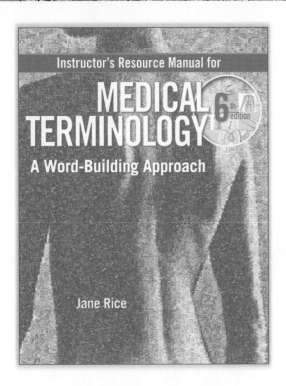

Instructor's Resource Manual for
# MEDICAL TERMINOLOGY 6th edition
## A Word-Building Approach
Jane Rice

## Instructor's Media Library

A multi-disc set containing all the electronic resources necessary to manage your course.

- The complete 2,900-question test bank that allows instructors to generate customized exams and quizzes.
- A comprehensive, turn-key lecture package in PowerPoint format containing discussion points, along with embedded color images from the textbook as well as bonus animations and videos to help infuse an extra spark into the classroom experience.
- PowerPoint content to support instructors who wish to use Personal Response Systems. For more information visit www.prenhall.com/prs.
- A complete image library that includes every photograph and illustration contained in the textbook.

## Instructor's Resource Manual

This manual contains a wealth of material to help faculty plan and manage the medical terminology course. It includes:

- *Medical Terminology Pearls of Wisdom,* a collection of best teaching practices shared by a national panel of master medical terminology educators.
- Step-by-step lectures, outlines, and daily lesson plans organized by learning objectives.
- A syllabus conversion guide to help instructors transition from a different text.
- A sample syllabus
- A complete 2,900-question test bank.

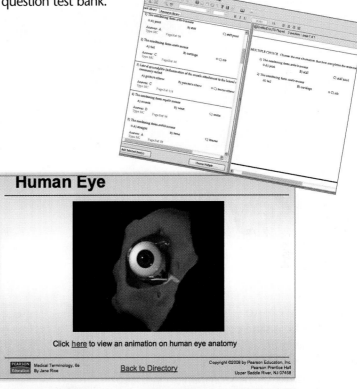

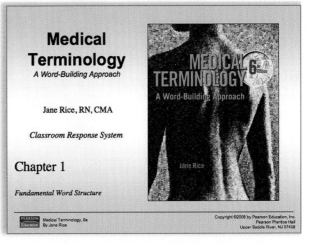

## Online Learning

No other medical terminology textbook has as full a selection of web-based resources as *Medical Terminology: A Word-Building Approach.* Whether you are looking for a basic Internet study experience, a robust, self-paced online course delivery system, or anything in between, we offer the solution that suits your needs.

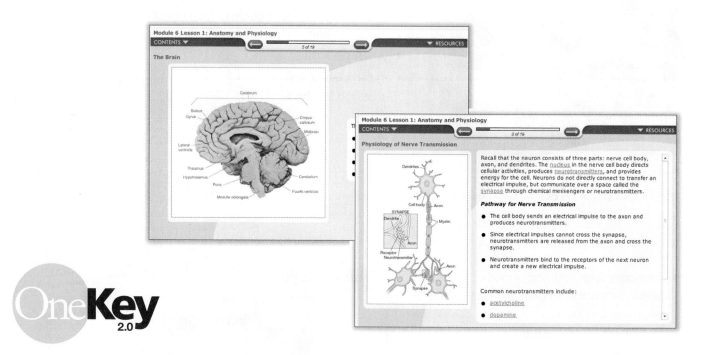

## Companion Website

Our most basic online option, this is a free-access website at **www.prenhall.com/rice** containing text-specific, interactive online workbook content. The Companion Website includes:

- Quizzes in multiple-choice, true/false, labeling, fill-in-the-blank, and essay formats. Instant feedback and rationales are provided.

- An audio glossary in which key terms are pronounced.

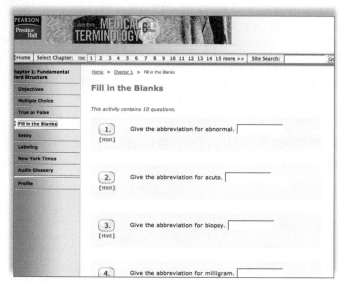

# ACKNOWLEDGMENTS

First, I would like to offer my warmest thanks to all of the individuals who have accepted *Medical Terminology: A Word-Building Approach* as their text. Over the past 22 years, I have been blessed with the gift of writing. It is my desire for this edition to make learning a wonderful experience for you, the learner and educator.

It has taken a "village" of people to create such a work of excellence. I want to express my gratitude to each person who worked so hard on this project and provided his or her unique talents to create and develop this edition. A sincere thank you to all the exceptional people at Prentice Hall Health. To Lynda Hatch—You were with me all the way. Through your guidance and excellent work, this sixth edition of my "dream" has reached a new dimension. To Elena Mauceri—You have been with me through many a revision, and I cherish your assistance and friendship. To Mark Cohen—It is really you who made this edition what it is. Your continual support of my work has proven to be the driving force in making an excellent book the best it can be. To Melissa Kerian—Your supervision of the ancillary components exceeds all expectations. To Carole Gooch, RN, MSN, ANP, Care Coordinator, Community Care Service Program, Northwest Georgia Public Health, who assisted me in creating the new SOAP: Chart Note Analysis feature—a special thank you.

Many individuals contributed to the improvements of this sixth edition. I extend to each of you my warmest appreciation:

Patrick Walsh                John Jordan
Mary Siener                  Karen Allman
Christina Zingone            Katrin Beacom
Nicole Ragonese              Amy Peltier

I would like to express my appreciation to the following people for their valuable contributions to the supplements:

## Student CD-ROM

**Pamela A. Eugene, BAS, RT (R)**
Associate Professor, Allied Health
Delgado Community College
New Orleans, Louisiana

**Trisha LaPointe, PharmD, BCPS**
Assistant Professor, Pharmacy Practice
Massachusetts College of Pharmacy
 and Health Sciences
Boston, Massachusetts

**Leesa Whicker, BA, CMA**
Program Chair, Medical Assisting
Central Piedmont Community College
Charlotte, North Carolina

**Kathy Zaiken, PharmD**
Assistant Professor, Pharmacy Practice
Director, MCPHS/Harvard Vanguard
 Medical Associates Pharmacy
 Practice Residency
Massachusetts College of Pharmacy
 and Health Sciences
Boston, Massachusetts

**Travis Seibold Sr., LLT, Phlb**
CEO, Seibold Media
Clinton, Utah

## Companion Web Site

**Pamela A. Eugene, BAS, RT (R)**
Associate Professor, Allied Health
Delgado Community College
New Orleans, Louisiana

**Jean M. Krueger-Watson, PhD**
Faculty, Health Occupations
Clark College
Vancouver, Washington

## Test Bank

**Susan Horn, AAS, CMA**
Coordinator, Medical Program
Indiana Business College
Lafayette, Indiana

**Jean M. Krueger-Watson, PhD**
Faculty, Health Occupations
   Department
Clark College
Vancouver, Washington

**Karen Perryman, BA, RT (R)(M), RDMS**
Adjunct Instructor, Health Sciences
Santa Rosa Junior College
Santa Rosa, California

## Personal Response Systems

**Jennifer Lamé, MPH, BS, RHIT**
Coding Certificate Program
   Coordinator
Southwest Wisconsin Technical
   College
Fennimore, Wisconsin

## Instructor's Resource Manual

**Donna Jeanne Pugh, BSN, RN**
Department Chair, Medical Programs
Florida Metropolitan University
Jacksonville, Florida

Portions of the Pathology Spotlights sections are from Discovery Communications (www.discovery.com) and Adam, Inc. We thank them for their contributions.

## Reviewers

I would also like to express my appreciation to the following reviewers for their valuable input:

**Lavonne Adams PhD, RN, CCRN**
Assistant Professor, Nursing
Texas Christian University
Fort Worth, Texas

**Patricia Anania-Firouzan, MSIS, RHIA**
Assistant Professor, Health Information
   Management
University of Pittsburgh
Pittsburgh, Pennsylvania

**Steve Arinder, BS, RRT**
Program Coordinator Respiratory Care
Chair Health Education
Meridian Community College
Meridian, Mississippi

**Louie Asuncion, MBA, HCA**
Assistant Professor, Health Occupations
Del Mar College
Corpus Christi, Texas

**Margaret Batson, RNC, MSN**
Instuctor, Nursing
San Joaquin Delta College
Stockton, California

**Molly Baxter, MS**
Instructor
Miller-Motte Technical College
Wilmington, North Carolina

**Jessie Y. Beecham, RN, MSN**
Nursing Faculty
El Centro College
Richardson, Texas

**Paul Bell, PhD, RHIA, CTR**
Associate Professor
School of Allied Health Sciences
East Carolina University
Greenville, North Carolina

**Sue Ellen Bice, MS, RHIA**
Professor, HIT & Allied Health
    Coordinator, Allied Health
Mohawk Valley Community College
Utica, New York

**Susan Whaley Boggs, RN, BSN, CNOR**
Program Coordinator, Surgical
    Technology
Piedmont Technical College
Greenwood, South Carolina

**Susan Boothe**
Instructor, Biology, Anatomy &
    Physiology
Alabama Southern Community
    College
Monroeville, Alabama

**Anne Boster, PT**
Instructor
Bishop State Community College
Mobile, Alabama

**Sue Boulden, BSN, CMA**
Medical Assisting Program Director
Mt Hood Community College
Gresham, Oregon

**Donna Broski, RN, MSN**
Assistant Professor, Health Careers
Cuyahoga Community College
Parma, Ohio

**Pam Byrd-Williams, MS**
Assistant Professor, Allied Health
Los Angeles Valley College
Valley Glen, California

**Donna J. Catron, RN, BSN, MEd**
Professional Nurse Educator
Jameson Memorial Hospital School of
    Nursing
New Castle, Pennsylvania

**Donnah Cole, RHIA**
Coordinator/Instructor, Medical
    Transcription
Asheville Buncombe Technical
    Community College
Asheville, North Carolina

**Michael Cook, MA, RRT**
Professor of Respiratory Therapy;
    Program Director, Industrial
    Technologies and Health Sciences
Mountain Empire Community College
Big Stone Gap, Virginia

**Lisa G. Countryman-Jones, BS,
    MT(ASCP), CLS**
ACCE Professor, Medical Laboratory
    Technology
Portland Community College
Portland, Oregon

**Donna Crapanzano, MPH, RPAC,
    CDE**
Clinical Assistant Professor
Stony Brook University
Stony Brook, New York

**Jeanne Christen, CLPlb, CLT, CLS**
Adjunct Faculty Chair, Health Care
    Core
Rio Salado College
Phoenix, Arizona

**Nadine Davis, RN, BSN**
Professor, Nursing
Golden West College
Huntington Beach, California

**Debra DelGenio, BBA, MBA**
Instructor, Business Office Technology
Augusta Technical College
Thomson, Georgia

**Antoinette Deshaies, RN, BSPA**
Adjunct Instructor
Glendale Community College
El Mirage, Arizona

**Mary Duffy**
Instructor, Medical Transcription
Career College of Northern Nevada
Reno, Nevada

**Shelba Durston, RN, MSN, CCRN**
Nursing Instructor
San Joaquin Delta College
Stockton, California

**Patricia Eighmey**
Merced College
Merced, California

**Wrennah L. Gabbert, RN, MSN, CPNP, FNP-C, PhD(c)**
Professional Specialist
Department of Nursing
Angelo State University
San Angelo, Texas

**Linda Galocy, RHIA, BS**
Clinical Coordinator
Indiana University Northwest
Gary, Indiana

**Toni J. Galvan, RN, MSN, CNS, CCRN, CEN**
Associate Professor, Nursing
Texas Tech University School
of Nursing
Lubbock, Texas

**Tammy T. Gant, RHIT, CMA, CAHI**
Program Director, Medical Assisting
Surry Community College
Dobson, North Carolina

**Mary Garcia, RN, BA**
Adjunct Instructor, Nursing
Wilbur Wright College
Chicago, Illinois

**Deb Gipson, BS, MT (ASCP)**
Instructor, Allied Health
Jackson State Community College
Jackson, Tennessee

**Rebecca Hageman, RHIAA, CCS**
Instructor, Health Information
Technology
Hutchinson Community College
Wichita, Kansas

**Beulah A. Hofmann, RN, MS**
Department of Nursing Director
Ivy Tech Community College
Greencastle, Indiana

**Edmond A. Hooker, MD**
Assistant Professor
Department of Health Services
Administration
Xavier University
Cincinnati, Ohio

**William J. Horton, BS, RHIA**
Adjunct Instructor
Hutchinson Community College
Hutchinson, Kansas

**Bud Hunton, MART(R), (QM)**
Health Care Educator
Sinclair Community College
Dayton, Ohio

**Trinity Ingram, MSN, RNC, PNP, CNS**
Instructor, Allied Health Online
Savannah Technical College
Savannah, Georgia

**Barbara Juarez, MSN, RN**
Nurse Educator, Nursing
Casper College
Casper, Wyoming

**Geri Kale-Smith, MS, CMA**
Coordinator, Medical Office
Administration Programs
Harper College
Palatine, Illinois

**Judy Kenshalo, BSN, PHN**
Instructor, Medical Assisting
Modesto Junior College
Modesto, California

**Peggy M. Krueger, MEd, BSN, RN, CMA**
Instructor, Medical Assisting
Linn Benton Community College
Albany, Oregon

**Jean M. Krueger-Watson, PhD**
Faculty, Health Occupations
Clark College
Vancouver, Washington

**Sandra A. Lehrke, RN, MS, CMA**
Medical Assistant Program Director
Anoka Technical College
Anoka, Minnesota

**Vivian Lilly, PhD, MBA, RN**
Dean of Health and Human Services
North Harris College
Houston, Texas

**Nancy Marks, AAS, MLT (ASCP), BA, MS**
Assistant Professor
Medical Office Assisting and Medical
    Laboratory Technology
Erie Community College
Williamsville, New York

**Rosaline Martinez-Culpepper, RN, MS**
Professor, Nursing
Chaffey College
Rancho Cucamonga, California

**Karen McCulloch, PT, PhD, NCS**
Associate Professor
University of North Carolina–Chapel
    Hill
Chapel Hill, North Carolina

**Michael McMinn, MA, RRT**
Professor, Health Sciences
Mott Community College
Swartz Creek, Michigan

**Sandra K. Mullins, MS Ed, ABD**
Associate Dean of Academics
Bluegrass Community and Technical
    College
Lexington, Kentucky

**Susan Kay Nelson, MSN, RN, APRN-BC**
Faculty Specialist II
Bronson Methodist School of Nursing
Western Michigan University
Kalamazoo, Michigan

**Linda J. Netzel, MA, OTR**
Professor; Academic Fieldwork
    Coordinator, Health and Human
    Services
Macomb Community College
Clinton Township, Michigan

**Erin Nixon, RN**
Adjunct Professor
Bakersfield College
Bakersfield, California

**Alice Noblin, RHIA, LHRM**
Instructor, Health Professions
University of Southern Florida
Orlando, Florida

**Kerry L. Openshaw, PhD**
Professor
Medical Professions Advisor
Bemidji State University
Bemidji, Minnesota

**Fred R. Pearson, PhD**
Professor of Public Health
Brigham Young University Idaho
Rexburg, Idaho

**Diane Peavy, RN, CPI, AHI, NCMA**
Director of Educational Services,
    Medical Assisting
Capps College
Foley, Alabama

**Roberta L. Pohlman, PhD**
Associate Professor
Department of Biological Science
Wright State University
Dayton, Ohio

**Mary Rahr, MS, RN, CMA**
Coordinator, New Clinic at NWTC
Northeast Wisconsin Technical
    College
Green Bay, Wisconsin

**Carol Reid, MS, RN**
Instructor
Century College
White Bear Lake, Minnesota

**Georgette Rosenfeld, MEd, RN, RRT**
Department Chair, Health Science
  Education
Indian River Community College
Fort Pierce, Florida

**Karen Roy, MS**
Chair, Department of Biology
Los Angeles Valley College
Valley Glen, California

**Kathleen Schaefer, RNC, MSN, MEd**
Assistant Professor; Chair, Associate
  Program in Nursing
Marymount University
Arlington, Virginia

**Nancy Schneider, MEd, BSN, RN, CIIM**
Instructor, Nursing
College of the Sequoias
Visalia, California

**Patricia L. Schrull, MSN, MBA, MEd RN**
Associate Professor, Program Director
Lorain County Community College
Elyria, Ohio

**Sally Schultz, MSN, RN**
Instructor, Nursing
Fox Valley Technical College
Appleton, Wisconsin

**Sarah L. Strang, BA, COT**
Certified Ophthalmic Technician
Lakeland Community College
Willoughby, Ohio

**Lenette Thompson**
Program Coordinator
Advisor; Dual Enrollment/ One-
  Plus-One Programs
Piedmont Technical College
Greenwood, South Carolina

**Margaret Trim, BS, MS**
Instructor/Coordinator, Biological
  Sciences
Central Ohio Technical College
Newark, Ohio

**Valeria Truitt, BS, MEd**
Adjunct Instructor, Medical Office
  Administration
Craven Community College
New Bern, North Carolina

**Linda Walter, RN, MSN**
Nursing Professor
Northwestern Michigan College
Traverse City, Michigan

**Frances M. Warrick, MS, RN**
Program Coordinator, Vocational
  Nursing
El Centro College
Dallas, Texas

**Debra Washington, CPC**
Instructor, Medical Transcription
South Suburban College
Harvey, Illinois

**Phyllis Watts, BA, MEd**
Professor, Business Health Services
  Management
Mott College
Flint, Michigan

**Bonnie Welniak, RN, MSN**
Assistant Professor, Nursing
Monroe County Community College
Monroe, Michigan

**Ellen F. Wirtz, RN, MN**
Director of Nursing
The University of Montana–Helena
  College of Technology
Helena, Montana

**Lori A. Woeste, EdD**
Assistant Professor
Department of Health Sciences
Illinois State University
Normal, Illinois

**Lisa Wright, MS, MT, SH, CMA**
Medical Assisting Program Coordinator
Chair, Medical Support Programs
  Department
Bristol Community College
Fall River, Massachusetts

# ABOUT THE AUTHOR

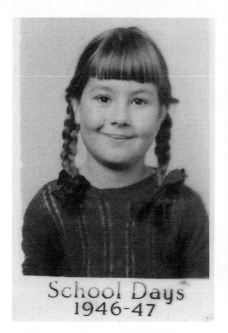

School Days
1946-47

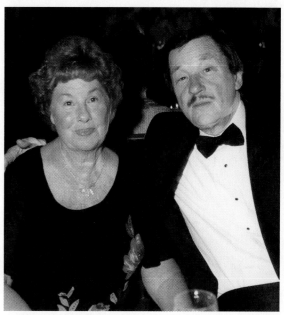

The year is 1947 and I am a little girl with brown hair that is braided into pigtails. I am very shy and afraid, for, you see, I am in the second grade and I cannot read. Not one little word. The teacher discovered this and made me sit on a tall metal stool in front of the classroom with a dunce cap on my head. Still to this day, I get very nervous when I have to get up in front of a crowd of people.

My mother taught me to read because back then, there were no special classes for children with learning disabilities. I did not learn "phonetics" but memorized everything. I still have trouble pronouncing words, but I can tell you all you want to know about a medical word.

After the death of two brothers, my father, and the impending death of my mother, I prayed for something else to do, something that would help take away the pain and the hurt. In 1982, my prayers were answered with a most precious gift: *Medical Terminology with Human Anatomy*, now titled *Medical Terminology: A Word-Building Approach*, which was first published in September 1985.

I owe so much to God and my best friend and husband, Charles Larry Rice. God continues to guide me in my writing. He provides me the knowledge and ability to organize, research, develop, and then to write. Larry, my husband of 41 years, is supportive and gives me the freedom to be an author. He is my love and hero. Also, I express my love to the flowers in my life: Melissa Rice-Noble, Doug Noble, and our grandchildren: Zachary, Benjamin, Jacob, Mary Katherine, and Elizabeth Ann.

Although I am now retired, I had a wonderful teaching career. I am forever beholden to the many wonderful students who taught me so much and touched my life with their unique qualities. I hope and pray that this sixth edition of *Medical Terminology: A Word-Building Approach* will enable you, the learner, to become the professional that you choose to be.

**Jane Rice, RN, CMA-C**

# Fundamental Word Structure

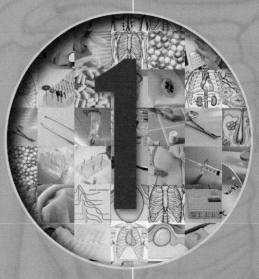

## ◼ OUTLINE

## ◼ OBJECTIVES

*On completion of this chapter, you will be able to:*

- Describe the fundamental elements that are used to build medical words.
- List three guidelines that will assist you with the building and spelling of medical words.
- Explain the use of abbreviations when writing and documenting data.
- Analyze, build, spell, and pronounce medical words.
- Identify and define selected abbreviations.
- Describe selected medical and surgical specialties, giving the scope of practice and the physician's title.
- Complete the Study and Review section.

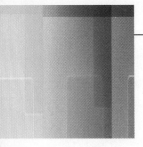

# Comprehension of Fundamental Word Structure

**Medical terminology** is the study of terms that are used in the art and science of medicine. It is a specialized language with its origin arising from the Greek influence on medicine. Hippocrates was a Greek physician who lived from 460 to 377 BC and whose vital role in medicine is still recognized today. He is called "The Father of Medicine" and is credited with establishing early ethical standards for physicians. Because of advances in scientific computerized technology, many new terms are coined daily; however, most of these terms are composed of word parts that have their origins in ancient Greek or Latin. Because of this foreign origin, it is necessary to learn the English translation of terms when learning the fundamentals of word structure.

## FUNDAMENTALS OF WORD STRUCTURE

The fundamental elements in medical terminology are the component parts used to build medical words. The abbreviations used for component parts in this text are *P* = **prefix**, *R* = **root**, *CF* = **combining form**, and *S* = **suffix**. The key to learning medical terminology is through a word-building technique used in this text. Combining forms and word roots are integrated into each chapter of the text, according to body system or specialty area. Suffixes and prefixes are presented in Chapters 2 and 3 and then will continue to be repeated throughout the text. To build your medical vocabulary, all you have to do is recall the word parts that you have learned and then link them with the new component parts presented in each chapter.

### Prefix

The term **prefix** means *to fix before* or *to fix to* the beginning of a word. A prefix can be a syllable or a group of syllables. Prefixes are united with or placed at the beginning of words to alter or modify their meanings or to create entirely new words. For example: the word **ex/cis/ion** means the process of cutting out; surgical removal. Note its component parts:

| | | |
|---|---|---|
| ex- | P or prefix meaning | out |
| cis | R or root meaning | to cut |
| -ion | S or suffix meaning | process |

### Word Root

A **root** is a word or word element from which other words are formed. It is the foundation of the word. The root conveys the central meaning of the word and forms the base to which prefixes and suffixes are attached for word modification.

For example: the word **mal/format/ion** means the process of being badly shaped; deformed. Note its component parts:

| | | |
|---|---|---|
| mal- | P or prefix meaning | bad |
| format | R or root meaning | a shaping |
| -ion | S or suffix meaning | process |

### Combining Form

A **combining form** is a word root to which a vowel has been added. A combining vowel (*a, e, i, o,* or *u*) links the root to the suffix or the word root to another root. The combining vowel does not have a meaning of its own. The vowel *o* is used more often than any other to make combining forms. Combining forms can be found at the beginning of a word or within the word.

For example: the word **chem/o/therapy** means treatment of disease by using chemical agents. Note the relationship of its component parts:

| | | |
|---|---|---|
| chem/o | CF or combining form meaning | chemical |
| -therapy | S or suffix meaning | treatment |

## Suffix

The term **suffix** means to fasten on, beneath, or under. A suffix can be a syllable or group of syllables united with or placed at the end of a word to alter or modify the meaning of the word or to create a new word. When you break down a word to understand it or when you give the meaning of the word or read its definition, you usually begin with the meaning of the suffix.

For example: the word *gastr/oma* means a **tumor** of the stomach and the word *gastr/itis* means **inflammation** of the stomach:

| | | |
|---|---|---|
| gastr | R or root meaning | stomach |
| -oma | S or suffix meaning | tumor |
| gastr | R or root meaning | stomach |
| -itis | S or suffix meaning | inflammation |

Word roots and combining forms, together with their definitions, are included in each chapter according to the cell, tissue, organ, system, or element they describe. This arrangement makes it possible for you to form associations between medical terms and the various body systems. To reinforce the learning process, this text provides you a general anatomy and physiology overview for each of the body systems that it includes.

## PRINCIPLES OF COMPONENT PARTS

As you learn definitions for prefixes, roots, combining forms, and suffixes, you will discover that some component parts have the same meanings as others. This occurs most often with words that relate to the organs of the body and the diseases that affect them. The existence of more than one component part for a particular meaning can be traced to differences in the Greek or Latin words from which they originated. Most of the terms for the body's organs originated from Latin words, whereas terms describing diseases that affect these organs have their origins in Greek.

Examples follow.

- **Uterus.** Latin word for one of the organs of the female reproductive system, the womb
- **Hyster.** Greek R (root) for womb
- **Hysterectomy.** Surgical excision of the womb from hyster R (root) meaning womb + -ectomy S (suffix) meaning surgical excision
- **Metr/i.** Greek CF (combining form) for uterus
- **Myometrium.** Muscular tissue of the uterus from my/o CF meaning muscle + metr/i CF meaning uterus + -um S meaning tissue

## IDENTIFICATION OF MEDICAL WORDS

When identifying medical words, you will learn to distinguish between and select the appropriate component parts for the meaning of the word. For example, the word **microscope** means an instrument for examining small objects. Note the following: *micro-* + *-scope; not -scope + micro-*. With the proper placement of component parts (P + S) the definition translates micro- = small and -scope = instrument for examining.

## SPELLING

Medical words of Greek origin are often difficult to spell because many of them begin with a silent letter or have a silent letter within the word. The following are examples of words that begin with silent letters:

| Silent Beginning | Pronounced | Medical Term | Pronunciation Guide |
|---|---|---|---|
| gn | n | **g**nathic | (năth´ĭk) |
| kn | n | **k**nuckle | (nŭk´ĕl) |
| mn | n | **m**nemonic | (nĭ-mōn´ĭk) |
| pn | n | **p**neumonia | (nū´-mō´nĭ-ă) |
| ps | s | **p**sychiatrist | (sī-kī´ă-trĭst) |
| pt | t | **p**tosis | (tō´sĭs) |

The following are examples of medical terms that contain silent letters within the word:

| Silent Letter | Medical Term | Pronunciation Guide |
|---|---|---|
| g | phle**g**m | (flĕm) |
| p | blepharo**p**tosis | (blĕf˝ă-rō-tō´ sis) |

Correct spelling is extremely important in medical terminology because the addition or omission of a single letter can change the meaning of a word to something entirely different. The following examples illustrate this point:

| Term/Letter Change | Meaning of Term | Term/Letter Change | Meaning of Term |
|---|---|---|---|
| a**b**duct | To lead **away** from the middle | ar**te**ritis | Inflammation of an **artery** |
| a**d**duct | To lead **toward** the middle | ar**th**ritis | Inflammation of a **joint** |

Following are some of the prefixes and suffixes that often contribute to spelling errors:

## Prefixes and Suffixes That Are Frequently Misspelled

| Prefix | Meaning | Suffix | Meaning |
|---|---|---|---|
| **ante-** | before, forward | **-poiesis** | formation |
| **anti-** | against | **-ptosis** | prolapse, drooping, sagging, falling down |
| **ecto-** | out, outside, outer | **-ptysis** | spitting |
| **endo-** | within, inner | **-rrhagia** | to burst forth, bursting forth |
| **hyper-** | above, beyond, excessive | **-rrhage** | to burst forth, bursting forth |
| **hypo-** | below, under, deficient | **-rrhaphy** | suture |
| **inter-** | between | **-rrhea** | flow, discharge |
| **intra-** | within | **-rrhexis** | rupture |
| **para-** | beside, alongside, abnormal | **-scope** | instrument for examining |
| **peri-** | around | **-scopy** | visual examination, to view, examine |
| **per-** | through | **-tome** | instrument to cut |
| **pre-** | before, in front of | **-tomy** | incision |
| **pro-** | before | **-tripsy** | crushing |
| **super-** | above, beyond | **-trophy** | nourishment, development |
| **supra-** | above, beyond | | |

Follow these guidelines for building and spelling of medical words.

1. If the suffix begins with a vowel, drop the combining vowel from the combining form and add the suffix. For example: gastr/*o* (*stomach*) + -oma (*tumor*) becomes gastroma when we drop the *o* from gastr*o*.

2. If the suffix begins with a consonant, keep the combining vowel and add the suffix to the combining form. For example: lip/*o* (*fat*) + -lysis (*destruction*) becomes lip*o*lysis and we keep the *o* on the combining form lip*o*.

3. Keep the combining vowel between two or more roots in a term. For example: electr*o* (*electricity*) + cardi*o* (*heart*) + -gram (*record*) becomes electr*o*cardi*o*gram and we keep the two combining vowels.

# FORMATION OF PLURAL ENDINGS

To change the following singular endings to plural endings, substitute the plural endings as illustrated:

| Singular Ending | Plural Ending | Singular Ending | Plural Ending |
| --- | --- | --- | --- |
| **a** as in burs**a** | to **ae** as in burs**ae** | **is** as in femor**is** | to **a** as in femor**a** |
| **ax** as in thor**ax** | to **aces** as in thor**aces** or **es** as in thorax**es** | **ix** as in append**ix** | to **ices** as in append**ices** |
| | | **nx** as in phala**nx** | to **ges** as in phalan**ges** |
| **en** as in foram**en** | to **ina** as in foram**ina** | **on** as in spermatozo**on** | to **a** as in spermatozo**a** |
| | | **um** as in ov**um** | to **a** as in ov**a** |
| **is** as in cris**is** | to **es** as in cris**es** | **us** as in nucle**us** | to **i** as in nucle**i** |
| **is** as in ir**is** | to **ides** as in ir**ides** | **y** as in arter**y** | to **i** and add **es** as in arter**ies** |

# USE OF ABBREVIATIONS

An **abbreviation** is a process of shortening a word or phrase into appropriate letters. It is used as a form of communication in writing and documenting data. More than a thousand medical abbreviations are in use today, and, however, more will be created as new treatments and procedures are developed. When using abbreviations caution must be exercised. Many have more than one meaning, such as **ER**, which means emergency room and endoplasmic reticulum, and **PA**, which means physician assistant, posteroanterior, and pernicious anemia. It is essential that you use or translate the correct meaning for the abbreviation being used. If there is any question about which abbreviation to use, it is best to spell out the word or phrase and not use an abbreviation.

The Institute for Safe Medication Practice (ISMP) and the Joint Commission on Accreditation of Healthcare Organizations (JCAHO) have developed a list of abbreviations considered to be dangerous because of the potential for misinterpretation. It is recommended that facilities using abbreviations for documentation keep a list of approved and unapproved abbreviations on hand and readily accessible. For more information on this list you can go to http://www.ismp.org and http://www.jointcommission.org.

In each chapter of this text, you will find selected abbreviations with their meanings. These abbreviations are in current use and are directly associated with the subject of the chapter. In the appendices, you will find an expanded alphabetical list of commonly used abbreviations and symbols. The abbreviations are presented using capital letters without periods except in those cases where lowercase letters and periods represent the norm or preferred method.

## PRONUNCIATION

Pronunciation of medical words may seem difficult; however, it is very important to pronounce medical words with the same or very similar sounds to convey their correct meanings. As in spelling, one mispronounced syllable can change the meaning of a medical word. This text uses a phonetically spelled pronunciation guide adapted from *Taber's Cyclopedic Medical Dictionary*, and you should practice speaking each term aloud when working with the various lists of medical terms or vocabulary words. Accent marks are used to indicate stress on certain syllables. A single accent mark (′) is called a *primary accent* and is used with the syllable that has the strongest stress. A double accent (″) is called a *secondary accent* and is given to syllables that are stressed less than primary syllables.

Diacritics are marks placed over or under vowels to indicate the long or short sound of the vowel. In this text, the macron (¯) shows the long sound of the vowel, the breve (˘) shows the short sound of the vowel, and the schwa (ə) indicates the uncolored, central vowel sound of most unstressed syllables [for example: antiseptic (an″ ti-sep′ tik) or diathermy (di′ ə-thĕr″ mĕ)].

# BUILDING YOUR MEDICAL VOCABULARY

This section provides the foundation for learning medical terminology. Review the following alphabetized word list. Note how common prefixes and suffixes are repeatedly applied to word roots and combining forms to create different meanings.

| | |
|---|---|
| **P** | Prefix |
| **R** | Root |
| **CF** | Combining form |
| **S** | Suffix |

| | |
|---|---|
| Pink words | Terms not built from word parts. |
| * | Indicates words covered in the Pathology Spotlights section. |
| ◉ | Check the CD-ROM for more information. |

| MEDICAL WORD | WORD PARTS (WHEN APPLICABLE) | | | DEFINITION |
|---|---|---|---|---|
| | **Part** | **Type** | **Meaning** | |
| **abate**<br>(ă-bāt′) | | | | To lessen, decrease, or cease |
| **abnormal (AB)**<br>(ăb-nōr′ măl) | ab-<br>norm<br>-al | P<br>R<br>S | away from<br>rule<br>pertaining to | Pertaining to away from the normal or rule |
| **abscess**<br>(ăb′ sĕs) | | | | Localized collection of pus, which may occur in any part of the body |
| **acute (ac)**<br>(ă-cūt′) | | | | Sudden, sharp, severe; a disease that has a sudden onset, severe symptoms, and a short course |
| **adhesion**<br>(ăd′ hē-zhŭn) | adhes<br>-ion | R<br>S | stuck to<br>process | Process of being stuck together |

| MEDICAL WORD | WORD PARTS (WHEN APPLICABLE) | | | DEFINITION |
|---|---|---|---|---|
| | Part | Type | Meaning | |
| **afferent**<br>(ăf′ ĕr ĕnt) | | | | Carrying impulses toward a center |
| **ambulatory (Amb)**<br>(ăm′ bŭ-lăh-tŏr″ ē) | | | | Condition of being able to walk, not confined to bed |
| **antidote**<br>(ăn′ tǐ-dōt) | | | | Substance given to counteract poisons and their effects |
| **antipyretic**<br>(ăn″ tǐ-pī-rĕt′ĭk) | anti-<br>pyret<br>-ic | P<br>R<br>S | against<br>fever<br>pertaining to | Pertaining to an agent that works against fever |
| **antiseptic**<br>(ăn″ tǐ-sĕp′ tǐk) | anti-<br>sept<br>-ic | P<br>R<br>S | against<br>putrefaction<br>pertaining to | Pertaining to an agent that works against sepsis; *putrefaction* |
| **antitussive**<br>(ăn″ tǐ-tǔs′ ǐv) | anti-<br>tuss<br>-ive | P<br>R<br>S | against<br>cough<br>nature of,<br>quality of | Pertaining to an agent that works against coughing |
| **apathy**<br>(ăp′ ă-thē) | | | | Condition in which one lacks feelings and emotions and is indifferent |
| **asepsis**<br>(ā-sĕp′ sǐs) | a-<br>-sepsis | P<br>S | without<br>decay | Without decay; *sterile,* free from all living microorganisms |
| **autoclave**<br>(ŏ′ tō-klāv) | | | | Apparatus used to sterilize articles by steam under pressure |
| **autonomy**<br>(ăw-tŏ′ nōm-ē)<br>(ŏ-tŏ′ nōmē) | auto-<br>nom<br>-y | P<br>R<br>S | self<br>law<br>condition | Condition of being self-governed; to function independently |
| **axillary (ax)**<br>(ăks′ ǐ-lār-ē) | axill<br>-ary | R<br>S | armpit<br>pertaining to | Pertaining to the armpit |
| **biopsy (Bx)**<br>(bī′ ŏp-sē) | bi(o)<br>-opsy | CF<br>S | life<br>to view | Surgical removal of a small piece of tissue for microscopic examination; used to determine a diagnosis of cancer or other disease processes in the body |
| **cachexia**<br>(kă-kĕks′ ǐ-ă) | cac-<br>-hexia | P<br>S | bad<br>condition | Condition of ill health, malnutrition, and wasting. It may occur in chronic diseases such as cancer and pulmonary tuberculosis. |
| **centigrade (C)**<br>(sĕn′ tǐ-grād) | centi-<br><br>-grade | P<br><br>S | one hundred,<br>one hundredth<br>a step | Having 100 steps or degrees, like the Celsius temperature scale; boiling point = 100°C and freezing point = 0°C |
| **centimeter (cm)**<br>(sĕn′ tǐ-mē-tĕr) | centi-<br><br>-meter | P<br><br>S | one hundred,<br>one hundredth<br>measure | Unit of measurement in the metric system; one hundredth of a meter |
| **centrifuge**<br>(sĕn′ trǐ-fūj) | centr/i<br>-fuge | CF<br>S | center<br>to flee | Device used in a laboratory to separate solids from liquids |
| **chemotherapy**<br>(kē″ mō-thĕr′ ă-pē) | chem/o<br>-therapy | CF<br>S | chemical<br>treatment | Treatment using chemical agents |

| MEDICAL WORD | WORD PARTS (WHEN APPLICABLE) | | | DEFINITION |
|---|---|---|---|---|
| | **Part** | **Type** | **Meaning** | |
| **chronic**<br>(krŏn ik) | | | | Pertaining to time; a disease that continues over a long time, showing little change in symptoms or course |
| **diagnosis (Dx)**<br>(dī" ăg-nō' sĭs) | dia-<br>-gnosis | P<br>S | through<br>knowledge | Determination of the cause and nature of a disease |
| **diaphoresis**<br>(dī" ă-fō-rē' sĭs) | dia-<br>-phoresis | P<br>S | through<br>to carry | To carry through sweat glands; *profuse sweating* |
| **disease**<br>(dĭ-zēz') | | | | Lack of ease; an abnormal condition of the body that presents a series of symptoms that sets it apart from normal or other abnormal body states |
| **disinfectant**<br>(dĭs" ĭn-fĕk' tănt) | dis-<br>infect<br>-ant | P<br>R<br>S | apart<br>to infect<br>forming | Chemical substance that can be applied to objects to destroy pathogenic microorganisms, such as bacteria |
| **efferent**<br>(ĕf' ĕr ĕnt) | | | | Carrying impulses away from a center |
| **empathy**<br>(ĕm' pă-thē) | | | | State of projecting one's own personality into the personality of another to understand the feelings, emotions, and behavior of the person |
| **epidemic**<br>(ĕp" i-dĕm' ik) | epi-<br>dem<br>-ic | P<br>R<br>S | upon<br>people<br>pertaining to | Pertaining to among people; the rapid, widespread occurrence of an infectious disease |
| **etiology**<br>(ē" tē-ŏl' ō-jē) | eti/o<br>-logy | CF<br>S | cause<br>study of | Study of the cause(s) of disease |
| **excision**<br>(ĕk-si' zhŭn) | ex-<br>cis<br>-ion | P<br>R<br>S | out<br>to cut<br>process | Process of cutting out, surgical removal |
| **febrile**<br>(fē' brĭl) | | | | Pertaining to fever |
| **gram (g)**<br>(grăm) | | | | Unit of weight in the metric system; a cubic centimeter or a milliliter of water is equal to the weight of a gram |
| **heterogeneous**<br>(hĕt" ĕr-ō-jē' nĭ-ŭs) | hetero-<br>gene<br><br>-ous | P<br>R<br><br>S | different<br>formation, produce<br>pertaining to | Pertaining to a different formation |
| **illness**<br>(ĭl'nĭs) | | | | State of being sick |
| **incision**<br>(ĭn-sĭzh'ŭn) | in-<br>cis<br>-ion | P<br>R<br>S | in, into<br>to cut<br>process | Process of cutting into |
| **kilogram (kg)**<br>(kĭl'ō-grăm) | kil/o<br>-gram | CF<br>S | a thousand<br>a weight | Unit of volume in the metric system; equal to 33.8 fl oz or 1.0567 qt |
| **liter (L)**<br>(lē'tĕr) | | | | Unit of weight in the metric system; *1000 g* |

| MEDICAL WORD | WORD PARTS (WHEN APPLICABLE) | | | DEFINITION |
|---|---|---|---|---|
| | Part | Type | Meaning | |
| **macroscopic**<br>(măk″ rō-skŏp ĭk) | macr/o<br>scop<br>-ic | CF<br>R<br>S | large<br>to examine<br>pertaining to | Pertaining to objects large enough to be examined by the naked eye |
| **malaise**<br>(mă-lāz′) | | | | Feeling of discomfort, uneasiness; often felt by a patient who has a chronic disease |
| **malformation**<br>(măl″ fōr-mā′shŭn) | mal-<br>format<br>-ion | P<br>R<br>S | bad<br>a shaping<br>process | Process of being badly shaped, deformed |
| **malignant**<br>(mă-lĭg′nănt) | malign<br>-ant | R<br>S | bad kind<br>forming | Bad wandering; pertaining to the spreading process of cancer from one area of the body to another area |
| **maximal**<br>(măks′ ĭ-măl) | maxim<br>-al | R<br>S | greatest<br>pertaining to | Pertaining to the greatest possible quantity, number, or degree |
| **microgram (mcg)**<br>(mī′ krō-grăm) | micro-<br>-gram | P<br>S | small<br>a weight | Unit of weight in the metric system; *0.001 mg* |
| **microorganism**<br>(mī″ krō-ōr′găn-ĭzm) | micro-<br>organ<br>-ism | P<br>R<br>S | small<br>organ<br>condition | Small living organisms that are not visible to the naked eye |
| **microscope**<br>(mī′ krō-skōp) | micro-<br>-scope | P<br>S | small<br>instrument<br>for examining | Instrument used to view small objects |
| **milligram (mg)**<br>(mĭl′ ĭ-grăm) | milli-<br>-gram | P<br>S | one-thousandth<br>a weight | Unit of weight in the metric system; *0.001 g* |
| **milliliter (mL)**<br>(mĭl′ ĭ-lē″ tĕr) | milli-<br>-liter | P<br>S | one-thousandth<br>liter | Unit of volume in the metric system; *0.001 L* |
| **minimal**<br>(mĭn′ ĭ-măl) | minim<br>-al | R<br>S | least<br>pertaining to | Pertaining to the least possible quantity, number, or degree |
| **multiform**<br>(mŭl′tĭ-form) | multi-<br>-form | P<br>S | many, much<br>shape | Occurring in or having many shapes |
| **necrosis**<br>(nĕ-krō′sis) | necr<br>-osis | R<br>S | death<br>condition (usually abnormal) | Condition of tissue death |
| **neopathy**<br>(nē-ŏp′ă-thē) | neo-<br>-pathy | P<br>S | new<br>disease | New disease |
| **oncology**<br>(ŏng-kŏl′ō-jē) | onc/o<br>-logy | CF<br>S | tumor<br>study of | Study of tumors |
| **pallor**<br>(păl′or) | | | | Paleness, a lack of color |
| **palmar**<br>(păl′mar) | palm<br>-ar | R<br>S | palm<br>pertaining to | Pertaining to the palm of the hand |
| **paracentesis**<br>(păr″ă-sĕn-tē′sĭs) | para-<br>-centesis | P<br>S | beside<br>surgical puncture | Surgical puncture of a body cavity for fluid removal |
| **prognosis**<br>(prŏg-nō′sĭs) | pro-<br>-gnosis | P<br>S | before<br>knowledge | Literally means prediction of the course of a disease and the recovery rate; *condition of foreknowledge* |

| MEDICAL WORD | WORD PARTS (WHEN APPLICABLE) | | | DEFINITION |
|---|---|---|---|---|
| | **Part** | **Type** | **Meaning** | |
| **prophylactic**<br>(prō-fi-lăk'tĭk) | prophylact<br>-ic | R<br>S | guarding<br>pertaining to | Pertaining to preventing or protecting against disease |
| **pyrogenic**<br>(pī″rō-jĕn' ĭk) | pyr/o<br>-genic | CF<br>S | heat, fire<br>formation, produce | Pertaining to the production of heat; *a fever* |
| **radiology**<br>(rā″dē-ŏl'ō-jē) | radi/o<br>-logy | CF<br>S | ray, x-ray<br>study of | Study of radioactive substances |
| **rapport**<br>(ră-pōr') | | | | Relationship of understanding between two individuals, especially between the patient and the physician |
| **syndrome**<br>(sĭn'drōm) | syn-<br>-drome | P<br>S | together, with<br>a course | Combination of signs and symptoms occurring together that characterize a specific disease |
| **thermometer**<br>(thĕr-mŏm'ĕ-tĕr) | therm/o<br>-meter | CF<br>S | hot, heat<br>instrument to measure | Instrument used to measure degree of heat |
| **topography**<br>(tō-pŏg'răh-fē) | top/o<br>-graphy | CF<br>S | place<br>recording | Description of a body part in relation to the anatomic region in which it is located |
| **triage**<br>(trē-ahzh') | | | | Sorting and classifying of injuries to determine priority of need and treatment |

# ABBREVIATIONS

| ABBREVIATION | MEANING | ABBREVIATION | MEANING |
|---|---|---|---|
| AB | abnormal | FP | family practice |
| ABMS | American Board of Medical Specialties | g | gram |
| | | GI | gastrointestinal |
| ac | acute | GYN | gynecology |
| Amb | ambulatory | kg | kilogram |
| ax | axillary | L | liter |
| Bx | biopsy | mcg | microgram |
| C | centigrade, Celsius | mg | milligram |
| cm | centimeter | mL | milliliter |
| CV | cardiovascular | Neuro | neurology |
| Derm | dermatology | OB | obstetrics |
| Dx | diagnosis | Orth | orthopedics |
| ENT | ear, nose, throat (otorhinolaryngology) | Path | pathology |
| | | Peds | pediatrics |
| FACP | Fellow of the American College of Physicians | Psych | psychiatry, psychology |
| FACS | Fellow of the American College of Surgeons | | |

# MEDICAL AND SURGICAL SPECIALTIES

Today, the practice of medicine involves many areas of specialization. The American Board of Medical Specialties (ABMS) was founded in 1933. This board established standards for and monitoring of specialty practice areas. A physician who has met standards beyond those of admission to licensure and has passed an examination in a specialty area becomes board certified. Various medical professional organizations establish their own standards and administer their own board certification examinations. Individuals successfully completing all requirements are called Fellows, such as Fellow of the American College of Surgeons (FACS) or Fellow of the American College of Physicians (FACP). Board certification may be required by a hospital for admission to the medical staff or for determination of a staff member's rank. See Table 1–1 for selected medical and surgical specialties and Table 1–2 for types of surgical specialties with description of practice.

## TABLE 1–1  Selected Medical and Surgical Specialties

| Specialty/Physician | Scope of Practice/Concentration | Word Parts |
|---|---|---|
| **Allergy/Immunology** <br> Allergist/Immunologist | Diseases of an allergic nature | immun/o—immune; log—study of; -ist—one who specializes |
| **Anesthesiology** <br> Anesthesiologist | Appropriate anesthesia for partial or complete loss of sensation | an—without; esthesi/o—feeling; log—study of; -ist—one who specializes |
| **Bariatrics** <br> Bariatrician | Prevention, control, and treatment of obesity | bar—weight/pressure; iatr—treatment; -ician—physician |
| **Cardiology** <br> Cardiologist | Diseases of the heart, arteries, veins, and capillaries | cardi/o—heart; log—study of; -ist—one who specializes |
| **Dermatology (Derm)** <br> Dermatologist | Diseases of the skin | dermat/o—skin; log—study of; -ist—one who specializes |
| **Endocrinology** <br> Endocrinologist | Diseases of the endocrine system (the glands and the hormones they secrete) | endo—within; crin/o—to secrete; log—study of; -ist—one who specializes |
| **Epidemiology** <br> Epidemiologist | Epidemic diseases | epi—upon; demi/o—people; log—study of; -ist—one who specializes |
| **Family Practice (FP)** <br> Family Practitioner | Care of members of the family regardless of age and/or sex | |
| **Gastroenterology** <br> Gastroenterologist | Diseases of the stomach and intestines | gastr/o—stomach; enter/o—intestine; log—study of; -ist— one who specializes |
| **Geriatrics** <br> Gerontologist | Study of aspects of aging | geront/o—old age; log—study of; -ist—one who specializes |
| **Gynecology (GYN)** <br> Gynecologist | Diseases of the female reproductive system | gynec/o—female; log—study of; -ist—one who specializes |
| **Hematology** <br> Hematologist | Diseases of the blood and blood-forming tissues | hemat/o—blood; log—study of; -ist—one who specializes |
| **Infectious Disease** | Diseases caused by the growth of pathogenic microorganisms within the body | |
| **Internal Medicine** <br> Internist | Diseases of internal origin not usually treated surgically | intern—within; -ist—one who specializes |
| **Nephrology** <br> Nephrologist | Diseases of the kidney and urinary system | nephr/o—kidney; log—study of; -ist—one who specializes |
| **Neurology (Neuro)** <br> Neurologist | Diseases of the nervous system | neur/o—nerve; log—study of; -ist—one who specializes |
| **Obstetrics (OB)** <br> Obstetrician | Treatment of the female during pregnancy, childbirth, and the postpartum | The Latin word element *obstetrix* means midwife. |
| **Oncology** <br> Oncologist | Study of tumors | onc/o—tumor; log—study of; -ist—one who specializes |

TABLE 1–1  **Selected Medical and Surgical Specialties (*cont.*)**

| Specialty/Physician | Scope of Practice/Concentration | Word Parts |
|---|---|---|
| **Ophthalmology**<br>Ophthalmologist | Diseases of the eye | ophthalm/o—eye; log—study of;<br>   -ist—one who specializes |
| **Orthopedic (Orth)**<br>**Surgery**<br>(*Orthopaedic*)<br>Orthopedist<br>(*Orthopaedist*) | Diseases and disorders involving<br>   locomotor structures of the body | orth/o—straight; ped—child;<br>   -ist—one who specializes |
| **Otorhinolaryngology**<br>**(ENT)**<br>Otorhinolaryngologist | Diseases of the ear, nose, and larynx | ot/o—ear; rhin/o—nose; laryng/o—larynx;<br>   log—study of; -ist—one who specializes |
| **Pathology (Path)**<br>Pathologist | Study of structural and functional<br>   changes in tissues and organs caused<br>   by disease | path/o—disease; log—study of;<br>   -ist—one who specializes |
| **Pediatrics (Peds)**<br>Pediatrician | Diseases of children | ped—child; iatr—treatment;<br>   -ician—physician |
| **Physical Medicine**<br>**and Rehabilitation**<br>Physiatrist | Treatment of disease by physical agents | phys—nature; iatr—treatment;<br>   -ist—one who specializes |
| **Proctology**<br>Proctologist | Diseases of the colon, rectum, and<br>   anus | proct/o—anus, rectum; log—study of; -ist—one<br>   who specializes |
| **Psychiatry (Psych)**<br>Psychiatrist | Diseases of the mind | psych/o—mind; iatr—treatment;<br>   -ist—one who specializes |
| **Pulmonary Disease**<br>Pulmonologist | Diseases of the lungs | pulmon/o—lung; log—study of;<br>   -ist—one who specializes |
| **Radiology**<br>Radiologist | Study of radioactive substances and<br>   their relationship to prevention, diag-<br>   nosis and treatment of disease | radi/o—x-ray; log—study of;<br>   -ist—one who specializes |
| **Rheumatology**<br>Rheumatologist | Rheumatic diseases | rheumat/o—rheumatism; log—study of; -ist—one<br>   who specializes |
| **Urology**<br>Urologist | Diseases of the urinary system | ur/o—urination; log—study of;<br>   -ist—one who specializes |

TABLE 1–2  **Types of Surgical Specialties with Description of Practice**

| Surgical Specialty | Description of Practice |
|---|---|

*Surgery* is defined as the branch of medicine dealing with manual and operative procedures for correction of deformities and defects, repair of injuries, and diagnosis and cure of certain diseases.

| | |
|---|---|
| **Cardiovascular (CV)** | Surgical repair and correction of cardiovascular dysfunctions |
| **Colon and Rectum** | Surgical repair and correction of colon and rectal dysfunctions |
| **Cosmetic, Reconstructive,**<br>**Plastic** | Surgical repair, reconstruction, revision, or change of the texture, configuration, or<br>   relationship of contiguous structures of any part of the human body |
| **General** | Surgical repair and correction of various body parts and/or organs |
| **Maxillofacial** | Surgical treatment of diseases, injuries, and defects of the human mouth and dental<br>   structures |
| **Neurologic** | Surgical repair and correction of neurologic dysfunctions |
| **Orthopedic (*Orthopaedic*)** | Surgical prevention and repair of musculoskeletal dysfunctions |
| **Thoracic** | Surgical repair and correction of organs within the rib cage |
| **Trauma** | Surgical repair and correction of traumatic injuries |
| **Vascular** | Surgical repair and correction of vascular (vessels) dysfunctions |

# STUDY AND REVIEW

## Word Parts

1. In the spaces provided, write the definition of these prefixes, roots, combining forms, and suffixes. Do not refer to the listings of medical words. Leave blank those words you cannot define.

2. After completing as many as you can, refer to the medical word listings to check your work. For each word missed or left blank, write the word and its definition several times on the margins of these pages or on a separate sheet of paper.

3. To maximize the learning process, it is to your advantage to do the following exercises as directed. To refer to the word-building section before completing these exercises invalidates the learning process.

## PREFIXES

*Give the definitions of the following prefixes.*

1. a- _____

2. ab- _____

3. anti- _____

4. auto- _____

5. cac- _____

6. centi- _____

7. dia- _____

8. hetero- _____

9. mal- _____

10. micro- _____

11. milli- _____

12. multi- _____

13. neo- _____

14. para- _____

15. pro- _____

16. syn- _____

17. dis- _____

18. epi- _____

19. ex- _____

20. in-_____

## ROOTS AND COMBINING FORMS

*Give the definitions of the following roots and combining forms.*

1. adhes _____

2. axill _____

3. centr/i _____

4. chem/o _____

5. format _____

6. gene _____

7. kil/o _____

8. macr/o _____

9. necr _____

10. nom _____

11. norm _____    12. onc/o _____

13. organ _____    14. pyret _____

15. pyr/o _____    16. radi/o _____

17. scop _____    18. sept _____

19. therm/o _____    20. top/o _____

21. tuss _____    22. infect _____

23. dem _____    24. eti/o _____

25. cis _____    26. malign _____

27. maxim _____    28. minim _____

29. palm _____    30. prophylact _____

## SUFFIXES

*Give the definitions of the following suffixes.*

1. -al _____    2. -ary _____

3. -centesis _____    4. -drome _____

5. -form _____    6. -fuge _____

7. -genic _____    8. -gnosis _____

9. -grade _____    10. -gram _____

11. -graphy _____    12. -hexia _____

13. -ic _____    14. -ion _____

15. -ism _____    16. -ive _____

17. -liter _____    18. -logy _____

19. -meter _____    20. -osis _____

21. -ous _____    22. -pathy _____

23. -phoresis _____    24. -scope _____

25. -sepsis _____    26. -therapy _____

27. -ar _____    28. -y _____

## Identifying Medical Terms

*In the spaces provided, write the medical terms for the following meanings.*

1. _____ Process of being stuck together

2. _____ Without decay

3. _____ Pertaining to the armpit

4. _____ Treatment using chemical agents

5. _____ Pertaining to a different formation

6. _____ Process of being badly shaped, deformed

7. _____ Instrument used to view small objects

8. _____ Occurring in or having many shapes

9. _____ New disease

10. _____ Study of tumors

## Spelling

*In the spaces provided, write the correct spelling of these misspelled terms.*

1. antseptic _____   2. autnomy _____

3. centmeter _____   4. diphoresis _____

5. miligram _____   6. necosis _____

7. parcentesis _____   8. radilogy _____

## Matching

*Select the appropriate lettered meaning for each of the following words.*

_____ 1. abate

_____ 2. antipyretic

_____ 3. cachexia

_____ 4. diagnosis

_____ 5. disease

_____ 6. etiology

_____ 7. illness

_____ 8. prognosis

_____ 9. prophylactic

_____ 10. triage

a. Lack of ease
b. State of being sick
c. Pertaining to protecting against disease
d. Pertaining to an agent that works against fever
e. Sorting and classifying injuries to determine priority of need and treatment
f. To lessen, decrease, or cease
g. Determination of the cause and nature of a disease
h. New disease
i. Prediction of the course of a disease and the recovery rate
j. Condition of ill health, malnutrition, and wasting
k. Study of the cause(s) of disease

## Abbreviations

*Place the correct word, phrase, or abbreviation in the space provided.*

1. AB _____

2. ax _____

3. biopsy _____

4. CV _____

5. Neuro _____

6. ear, nose, throat (otorhinolaryngology) _____

7. family practice _____

8. gram _____

9. GYN _____

10. Peds _____

# MULTIMEDIA PREVIEW

*Additional interactive resources and activities for this chapter can be found on the Companion Website. For videos, audio glossary, and review, access the accompanying CD-ROM in this book.*

## CD-ROM HIGHLIGHTS

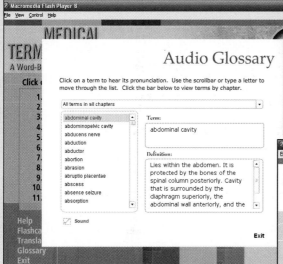

### AUDIO GLOSSARY/FLASHCARD GENERATOR

Practice your medical vocabulary and pronunciation at the same time. On this interactive feature each term is defined, spoken, and available in your personal flashcard library. Terms are listed alphabetically and by chapter.

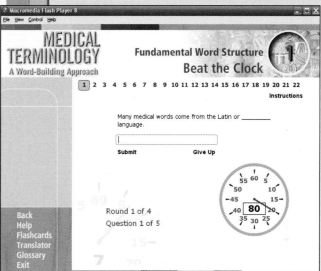

### BEAT THE CLOCK GAME

Challenge the clock by testing your medical terminology smarts against time. Click here for a game of knowledge, spelling, and speed. Can you correctly answer 20 questions before the final tick?

## WEBSITE HIGHLIGHTS—www.prenhall.com/rice

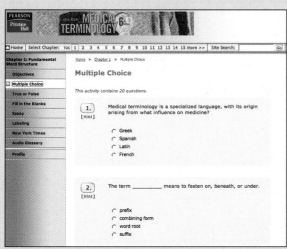

### MULTIPLE CHOICE QUIZ

Take advantage of the free-access on-line study guide that accompanies your textbook. You'll find a multiple choice quiz that provides instant feedback, allowing you to check your score and see what you got right or wrong. By clicking on this URL you'll also access links to download mp3 audio reviews, current news articles, and an audio glossary.

# Suffixes

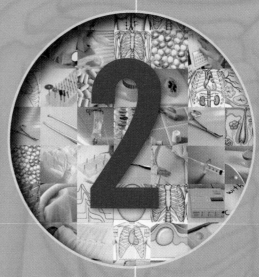

## ■ OBJECTIVES

*On completion of this chapter, you will be able to:*

- Recognize how suffixes are used when building medical words.
- Identify adjective, noun, and diminutive suffixes.
- Be aware of suffixes that have more than one meaning.
- Recognize suffixes that pertain to pathological conditions.
- Identify selected suffixes common to surgical and diagnostic procedures.
- Analyze, build, spell, and pronounce medical words.
- Complete the Study and Review section.

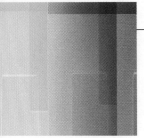

# Overview of Suffixes

The term **suffix** means to fasten on, beneath, or under. A suffix can be a syllable or group of syllables united with or placed at the end of a word to alter or modify the meaning of the word or to create a new word. A suffix is connected to a root or to a combining form to make new words. For example: the suffix *-ic* (which means pertaining to) can be combined with the root *gastr* (which means stomach) to make the medical word *gastr/ic* (pertaining to the stomach) or the suffix *-itis* (which means inflammation) can be combined with the root *gastr* to make another medical word *gastr/itis* (inflammation of the stomach).

A compound suffix is made up of more than one word component. It too is added to a root or a combining form to modify its meaning. For example, look at the suffix *-ectomy* (which means surgical excision). It is a combination of three word elements: *ec*, a prefix meaning out; *tom*, a root meaning to cut; and *-y*, a suffix meaning process. When the resulting suffix *-ectomy* is added to the root *gastr*, it forms the medical word *gastr/ectomy*, which means surgical excision of the stomach or literally *the process to cut out the stomach*.

Whenever you change the suffix, you alter the meaning of the word to which it is attached. For example, adding the suffix *-tomy* (incision) to the combining form *gastr/o* forms the medical word *gastr/o/tomy* (incision into the stomach). Notice that in the definition, the meaning associated with the suffix (incision) precedes the meaning associated with the combining form (stomach) to which it is attached. The term *gastr/o/tomy* means or can be read as incision into (the suffix) the stomach (the combining form).

Review the following guidelines, which were presented in Chapter 1. These will help you with the building and spelling of medical words:

1. If the suffix begins with a vowel, drop the combining vowel from the combining form and add the suffix. For example: gastr/o (*stomach*) + -oma (tumor) becomes gastroma when we drop the *o* from gastr*o*.
2. If the suffix begins with a consonant, keep the combining vowel and add the suffix to the combining form. For example, lip/o (*fat*) + -lysis (destruction) becomes lipolysis, and we keep the *o* on the combining form lip*o*.
3. Keep the combining vowel between two or more roots in a term. For example: electro (*electricity*) + cardio (*heart*) + -gram (*record*) becomes electrocardiogram, and we keep the combining vowels.

**Here is a helpful tip:** When giving the meaning of the word or reading its definition, you usually begin with the meaning of the suffix. Examples: gastr/**oma** is a **tumor** of the stomach; lip/o/**lysis** is the **destruction** of fat; electr/o/cardi/o/**gram** is a **record** of the electrical activity of the heart.

## GENERAL USE SUFFIXES

Listed in Table 2–1 is a collection of suffixes common to medical terminology. Note that all are preceded by a hyphen (-) to signify that they are to be linked to the end of a root or combining form. Example words are included for each suffix. To become familiar with the definition of these medical words, use the Index in the text to find their location. You will be learning each of these medical words as you progress through the chapters. Also, in the appendices, you will find a complete glossary of word parts to assist you in your understanding of medical terminology.

TABLE 2–1 **Selected Suffixes for General Use**

| Suffix | Meaning | Example Word |
|---|---|---|
| **-algesia** | condition of pain | an/*algesia* |
| **-ant** | forming | malign/*ant* |
| **-ase** | enzyme | amyl/*ase* |
| **-ate** | use, action | exud/*ate* |
| **-blast** | immature cell, germ cell | oste/o/*blast* |
| **-cide** | to kill | sperm/i/*cide* |
| **-crit** | to separate | hemat/o/*crit* |
| **-cuspid** | point | bi/*cuspid* |
| **-cyst** | bladder, sac | blast/o/*cyst* |
| **-cyte** | cell | neur/o/*cyte* |
| **-dipsia** | thirst | poly/*dipsia* |
| **-drome** | a course | syn/*drome* |
| **-er** | relating to, one who | radi/o/graph/*er* |
| **-gen** | formation, produce | muta/*gen* |
| **-genesis** | formation, produce | spermat/o/*genesis* |
| **-ide** | having a particular quality | radi/o/nucl/*ide* |
| **-ive** | nature of, quality of | un/respons/*ive* |
| **-liter** | liter | milli/*liter* |
| **-logy** | study of | gynec/o/*logy* |
| **-lymph** | clear fluid, serum, pale fluid | peri/*lymph* |
| **-or** | one who, a doer | turg/*or* |
| **-phil** | attraction | bas/o/*phil* |
| **-stasis** | control, stop, stand still | meta/*stasis* |
| **-therapy** | treatment | therm/o/*therapy* |
| **-thermy** | heat | hydro/*thermy* |
| **-um** | tissue, structure | epi/thel/i/*um* |
| **-uria** | urination, condition of urine | hemat/*uria* |

## GRAMMATICAL SUFFIXES

Grammatical suffixes are those that can be attached to a word root to form a part of speech, especially a noun or adjective, or to make a medical word singular or plural in its form. They are also used to indicate a diminutive form of a word that specifies a smaller version of the object indicated by the word root. You will find that many of these suffixes are the same as those used in the English language. See Tables 2–2 through 2–4.

TABLE 2–2 **Adjective Suffixes That Mean** *Pertaining To*

| Suffix | Word Analysis | Definition |
| --- | --- | --- |
| **-ac** | card/i/*ac* | Pertaining to the heart |
| **-ad** | cephal/*ad* | Pertaining to the head |
| **-al** | con/genit/*al* | Pertaining to presence at birth |
| **-ar** | muscul/*ar* | Pertaining to the muscles |
| **-ary** | integument/*ary* | Pertaining to the skin (a covering) |
| **-ic** | norm/o/cephal/*ic* | Pertaining to a normal appearance of the head as used in the objective description during a physical examination |
| **-ile** | pen/*ile* | Pertaining to the penis |
| **-ior** | anter/*ior* | Pertaining to a surface or part situated toward the front of the body |
| **-ose** | grandi/*ose* | Pertaining to a feeling of greatness |
| **-ous** | edemat/*ous* | Pertaining to an abnormal condition in which the body tissues contain an accumulation of fluid |
| **-tic** | cyan/o/*tic* | Pertaining to an abnormal condition of the skin and mucous membranes caused by oxygen deficiency in the blood |
| **-us** | de/cubit/*us* | Pertaining to a bedsore |
| **-y** | cardi/o/pulmonar/*y* | Pertaining to the heart and lungs |

TABLE 2–3 **Noun Suffixes That Mean** *Condition, Treatment,* **or** *Specialist*

| Suffix | Word Analysis | Definition |
| --- | --- | --- |
| **-esis** | enur/*esis* | Condition of involuntary emission of urine; bedwetting |
| **-ia** | a/lopec/*ia* | Condition of loss of hair; baldness |
| **-ism** | embol/*ism* | Condition in which a blood clot obstructs a blood vessel |
| **-iatry** | pod/*iatry* | Treatment of diseases and disorders of the foot |
| **-ician** | obstetr/*ician* | Physician who specializes in treating the female during pregnancy, childbirth, and the postpartum |
| **-ist** | cardi/o/log/*ist* | Physician who specializes in the study of the heart |
| **-osis** | hyper/hidr/*osis* | Condition of excessive sweating |
| **-y** | an/encephal/*y* | Congenital condition in which there is a lack of development of the brain |

TABLE 2–4 **Diminutive Suffixes That Mean** *Small* **or** *Minute*

| Suffix | Word Analysis | Definition |
| --- | --- | --- |
| **-cle** | aur/i/*cle* | Literally means *small ear* |
| **-icle** | ventr/*icle* | Literally means *little belly* |
| **-ole** | bronchi/*ole* | One of the smaller subdivisions of the bronchial tubes |
| **-ula** | mac/*ula* | Small spot or discolored area of the skin |
| **-ule** | pust/*ule* | Small, elevated, circumscribed lesion of the skin that is filled with pus |

## SUFFIXES THAT HAVE MORE THAN ONE MEANING

Some suffixes can have more than a single meaning, thereby making it a little more diffi-cult when defining the medical terms to which they are attached. An alphabetic listing of some of these suffixes is included in Table 2–5.

TABLE 2–5  **Selected Suffixes That Have More Than One Meaning**

| Suffix | Meanings |
| --- | --- |
| **-ate** | use, action, having the form of, possessing |
| **-blast** | immature cell, germ cell, embryonic cell |
| **-ectasis** | dilatation, dilation, distention, stretching, expansion |
| **-gen** | formation, produce |
| **-genesis** | formation, produce |
| **-genic** | formation, produce |
| **-gram** | a weight, mark, record |
| **-ive** | nature of, quality of |
| **-lymph** | serum, clear fluid, pale fluid |
| **-lysis** | destruction, separation, breakdown, loosening, dissolution |
| **-penia** | lack of, deficiency, abnormal reduction |
| **-plasm** | a thing formed, plasma |
| **-plegia** | stroke, paralysis, palsy |
| **-ptosis** | prolapse, drooping, falling down, sagging |
| **-rrhea** | flow, discharge |
| **-scopy** | to view, examine, visual examination |
| **-spasm** | tension, spasm, contraction |
| **-staxis** | dripping, trickling |
| **-trophy** | nourishment, development |
| **-y** | process, condition, pertaining to |

# SUFFIXES THAT PERTAIN TO PATHOLOGICAL CONDITIONS

Suffixes that carry meanings such as pain, weakness, swelling, softening, inflammation, and tumor are often combined with roots or combining forms to describe pathological conditions. The following is an alphabetic listing of some of the more frequently used suffixes associated with disease conditions and disorders. See Table 2–6.

TABLE 2–6  **Selected Suffixes That Pertain to Pathological Conditions**

| Suffix | Meaning | Pathological Condition |
|---|---|---|
| **-algia** | pain, ache | dent/*algia* |
| **-asthenia** | weakness | neur/*asthenia* |
| **-betes** | to go | dia/*betes* |
| **-cele** | hernia, tumor, swelling | cyst/o/*cele* |
| **-cusis** | hearing | presby/*cusis* |
| **-derma** | skin | xer/o/*derma* |
| **-dynia** | pain, ache | ot/o/*dynia* |
| **-ectasis** | dilation, distention | bronch/i/*ectasis* |
| **-edema** | swelling | papill/*edema* |
| **-emesis** | vomiting | hyper/*emesis* |
| **-ion** | process | in/fect/*ion* |
| **-itis** | inflammation | burs/*itis* |
| **-kinesis** | motion | hyper/*kinesis* |
| **-lepsy** | seizure | narc/o/*lepsy* |
| **-lexia** | diction, word, phrase | dys/*lexia* |
| **-malacia** | softening | oste/o/*malacia* |
| **-mania** | madness | pyro/*mania* |
| **-megaly** | enlargement, large | acr/o/*megaly* |
| **-mnesia** | memory | a/*mnesia* |
| **-noia** | mind | para/*noia* |
| **-oid** | resemble | ster/*oid* |
| **-oma** | tumor | carcin/*oma* |
| **-opia** | sight, vision | presby/*opia* |
| **-oxia** | oxygen | hyp/*oxia* |
| **-pathy** | disease, emotion | retin/o/*pathy* |
| **-penia** | deficiency | thromb/o/cyt/o/*penia* |
| **-pepsia** | to digest | dys/*pepsia* |
| **-phagia** | to eat, to swallow | a/*phagia* |
| **-phasia** | to speak, speech | dys/*phasia* |
| **-phobia** | fear | acr/o/*phobia* |
| **-plasia** | formation, produce | hyper/*plasia* |
| **-plasm** | a thing formed, plasma | neo/*plasm* |
| **-plegia** | paralysis, stroke | hemi/*plegia* |
| **-pnea** | breathing | sleep a/*pnea* |
| **-ptosis** | drooping, prolapse, sagging | blephar/o/*ptosis* |
| **-ptysis** | spitting | hem/o/*ptysis* |
| **-rrhage** | bursting forth | hem/o/*rrhage* |
| **-rrhea** | flow, discharge | rhin/o/*rrhea* |
| **-rrhexis** | rupture | hyster/o/*rrhexis* |
| **-spasm** | tension, spasm, contraction | my/o/*spasm* |
| **-trophy** | nourishment, development | hyper/*trophy* |

# SUFFIXES ASSOCIATED WITH SURGICAL AND DIAGNOSTIC PROCEDURES

Suffixes with meanings such as puncture, surgical excision, instrument to measure, and new opening are often combined with roots or combining forms to describe surgical and/or diagnostic procedures. See Table 2–7 for an alphabetic listing of some of the more frequently used suffixes associated with surgery and diagnosis.

TABLE 2–7   **Selected Suffixes Used in Surgical and Diagnostic Procedures**

| Suffix | Meaning | Example Word |
| --- | --- | --- |
| **-centesis** | surgical puncture | amni/o/*centesis* |
| **-clasis** | a break | oste/o/*clasis* |
| **-desis** | binding | arthr/o/*desis* |
| **-ectomy** | surgical excision, surgical removal, resection | vas/*ectomy* |
| **-gram** | a weight, mark, record | dactyl/o/*gram* |
| **-graph** | instrument for recording | radi/o/*graph* |
| **-graphy** | recording | mamm/o/*graphy* |
| **-ize** | to make, to treat or combine with | an/esthet/*ize* |
| **-lysis** | destruction, separation, breakdown, loosening | lip/o/*lysis* |
| **-meter** | instrument to measure, measure | audi/o/*meter* |
| **-metry** | measurment | pelvi/*metry* |
| **-opsy** | to view | bi/*opsy* |
| **-pexy** | surgical fixation | gastr/o/*pexy* |
| **-pheresis** | remove | plasma/*pheresis* |
| **-plasty** | surgical repair | rhin/o/*plasty* |
| **-rrhaphy** | suture | my/o/*rrhaphy* |
| **-scope** | instrument for examining | ophthalm/o/*scope* |
| **-scopy** | visual examination, to view, examine | lapar/o/*scopy* |
| **-stomy** | new opening | ile/o/*stomy* |
| **-tome** | instrument to cut | derma/*tome* |
| **-tomy** | incision | myring/o/*tomy* |
| **-tripsy** | crushing | lith/o/*tripsy* |

# BUILDING YOUR MEDICAL VOCABULARY

This section provides the foundation for learning medical terminology. Review the following alphabetized word list. Note how common prefixes and suffixes are repeatedly applied to word roots and combining forms to create different meanings.

| | |
|---|---|
| P | Prefix |
| R | Root |
| CF | Combining form |
| S | Suffix |

| | |
|---|---|
| Pink words | Terms not built from word parts. |
| * | Indicates words covered in the Pathology Spotlights section. |
| (CD icon) | Check the CD-ROM for more information. |

| MEDICAL WORD | WORD PARTS (WHEN APPLICABLE) | | | DEFINITION |
|---|---|---|---|---|
| | **Part** | **Type** | **Meaning** | |
| **abrasion**<br>(ă-brā′zhŭn) | ab-<br>ras<br>-ion | P<br>R<br>S | away from<br>to scrape off<br>process | Process of scraping away from a surface, such as skin or teeth, by friction. An abrasion may be the result of trauma, such as a "skinned knee" or from a therapy, such as dermabrasion of the skin for removal of scar tissue. It can also occur from the wearing down of a tooth from mastication (chewing). |
| **anesthetize**<br>(ă-nĕs′thĕ-tīz) | an-<br>esthet<br>-ize | P<br>R<br>S | without, lack of<br>feeling, sensation<br>to make | To induce a loss of feeling or sensation with the administration of an anesthetic |
| **arousal**<br>(a-rou′zel) | arous<br>-al | R<br>S | alertness, to rise<br>pertaining to | Pertaining to a state of alertness |
| **asymmetrical**<br>(ā-sĭ-mĕ′-trĭ-kăl) | a-<br>symmetric<br>-al | P<br>R<br>S | lack of, without<br>symmetry<br>pertaining to | Unequal in size or shape. Without proportion of the body or parts of the body; different in placement or arrangement about an axis. |
| **asystole**<br>(ă-sĭs′tō-lē) | a-<br>systole | P<br>R | without<br>contraction | Literally means *without contraction* of the heart; a life-threatening cardiac condition characterized by the absence of electrical and mechanical activity in the heart. |
| **comatose**<br>(kō′mă-tōs) | comat<br>-ose | R<br>S | a deep sleep<br>pertaining to | Pertaining to a state of deep sleep (coma) |
| **dysarthria**<br>(dĭs-ăr′thrē-ă) | | | | Difficult articulation of speech, resulting from interference in the control over the muscles of speech, usually caused by damage to a central or peripheral motor nerve |
| **epithelium**<br>(ĕp″ĭ-thē′lē-ŭm) | epi-<br>thel/i<br>-um | P<br>CF<br>S | upon, above<br>nipple<br>tissue, structure | Structure that covers the internal and external organs of the body and the lining of vessels, body cavities, glands, and organs. It is the layer of cells forming the outermost layer of the skin and the surface layer of mucous and serous membranes. |

| MEDICAL WORD | WORD PARTS (WHEN APPLICABLE) | | | DEFINITION |
|---|---|---|---|---|
| | **Part** | **Type** | **Meaning** | |
| **exogenous** (ĕks-ŏj′ĕ-nŭs) | ex (o)- gen -ous | P R S | out formation produce pertaining to | Pertaining to originating outside the body or an organ of the body or produced from external causes, such as a disease caused by a bacterial or viral agent foreign to the body |
| **grandiose** (grăn′dē-ōs) | grand/i -ose | CF S | great pertaining to | Pertaining to a feeling of *greatness.* In psychiatry, it refers to a person's unrealistic and exaggerated concept of self-worth, importance, wealth, and ability. |
| **gynecoid** (jĭn′ĕ-koyd) | gynec -oid | R S | female resemble | To resemble a female |
| **hypertrophy** (hī-pĕr′trŏ-fē) | hyper- -trophy | P S | excessive nourishment | Literally means *excessive nourishment;* the increase in the size of an organ, structure, or the body caused by an increase in the size of the cells rather than the number of cells; also called *overgrowth* |
| **infection** (ĭn-fĕk′shŭn) | infect -ion | R S | to infect process | Process whereby a pathogenic microorganism invades the body, reproduces, multiplies, and causes disease |
| **irregular** (ir-rĕg′ū-lăr) | ir- regul -ar | P R S | not rule pertaining to | Pertaining to not being regular |
| **nasolabial** (nā″zō-lā′bĭ-ăl) | nas/o labi -al | CF R S | nose lip pertaining to | Pertaining to the nose and lip |
| **palpate** (păl′pāt) | palp -ate | R S | touch use, action | To use the hands or fingers to examine by touch; to feel |
| **steroid** (stĕr′oyd) | ster -oid | R S | solid resemble | Literally means *resembling a solid substance;* applies to any one of a large group of substances chemically related to sterols |
| **trauma** (traw′mă) | | | | Physical injury or wound caused by external force, violence, or a toxic substance; also refers to psychological injury resulting from a severe emotional shock, which can cause disordered feelings and/or behavior |
| **turgor** (tur′jor) | turg -or | R S | swelling one who | Generally refers to the expected resiliency of the skin caused by the outward pressure of the cells and interstitial fluid. An evaluation of the skin turgor is an essential part of physical assessment. |

# STUDY AND REVIEW

## Identifying Suffixes

*Underline the suffixes in the following medical words.*

1. cardiac
2. cephalad
3. enuresis
4. obstetrician
5. bronchiole
6. pustule
7. dentalgia
8. diabetes
9. hyperemesis
10. hemoptysis

## Defining Suffixes

*Give the meaning of the following suffixes.*

1. -asthenia _____
2. -ion _____
3. -itis _____
4. -malacia _____
5. -megaly _____
6. -pathy _____
7. -penia _____
8. -pepsia _____
9. -phobia _____
10. -rrhexis _____
11. -al _____
12. -ar _____
13. -ate _____
14. -ia _____
15. -ize _____
16. -oid _____
17. -or _____
18. -ose _____
19. -ous _____
20. -trophy _____
21. -um _____

## Spelling

*In the spaces provided, write the correct spelling of these misspelled terms.*

1. aurcle _____
2. bronchole _____
3. cardilogist _____
4. cephlad _____
5. cynaotic _____
6. embolsm _____
7. podatry _____
8. pustle _____

## Using Suffixes to Build Medical Words

*Using a suffix from the following list, build the appropriate medical word.*

-al       -ior

-ar       -ile

-ary      -osis

-ia       -ula

-icle     -us

1.  Condition of excessive sweating              hyper/hidr/ _____

2.  Pertaining to muscles                        muscul/ _____

3.  Small spot or discolored area of the skin    mac/ _____

4.  Condition of loss of hair                    a/lopec/ _____

5.  Literally means *little belly*               ventr/ _____

6.  Pertaining to a bedsore                      de/cubit/_____

7.  Pertaining to the skin                       integument/ _____

8.  Pertaining to the penis                      pen/ _____

9.  Pertaining to present at birth               con/genit/ _____

10. Pertaining to toward the front of the body   anter/ _____

## Identifying Medical Terms

*In the spaces provided, write the medical terms for the following meanings.*

1.  _____ Process of scraping away from a surface

2.  _____ To induce a loss of feeling or sensation

3.  _____ Pertaining to a state of alertness

4.  _____ Unequal in size or shape

5.  _____ Literally means *without contraction*

6.  _____ Pertaining to a state of deep sleep

7.  _____ Difficult articulation of speech

8.  _____ Pertaining to a feeling of *greatness*

9.  _____ To resemble a female

10. _____ To use the hands or fingers to examine by touch

# MULTIMEDIA PREVIEW

*Additional interactive resources and activities for this chapter can be found on the Companion Website. For videos, audio glossary, and review, access the accompanying CD-ROM in this book.*

## CD-ROM HIGHLIGHTS

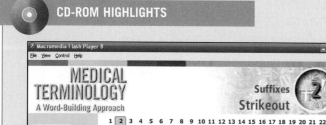

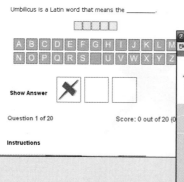

### STRIKEOUT!

Click on the alphabet tiles to fill in the empty squares in the word or phrase to complete the sentence. This game quizzes your vocabulary and spelling. But choose your letters carefully because three strikes and you're out!

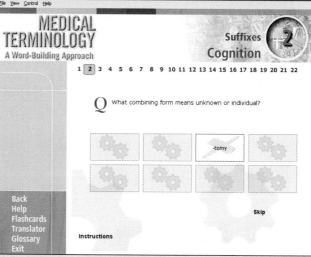

### COGNITION

Use your memory to make a match. This variation of the Concentration game will challenge you to study eight terms and then remember their location to complete a quiz. Click on each title that reveals the correct answers.

## WEBSITE HIGHLIGHTS—www.prenhall.com/rice

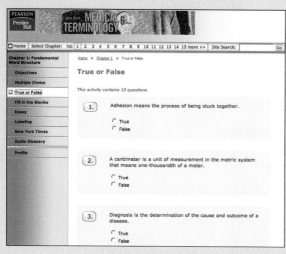

### TRUE/FALSE QUIZ

Take advantage of the free-access on-line study guide that accompanies your textbook. You'll find a true/false quiz that provides instant feedback, allowing you to check your score and see what you got right or wrong. By clicking on this URL you'll also access links to download mp3 audio reviews, current news articles, and an audio glossary.

# Prefixes

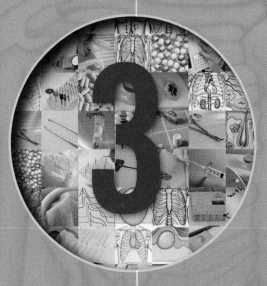

## OUTLINE

## OBJECTIVES

*On completion of this chapter, you will be able to:*

- Recognize how prefixes are used when building medical words.
- Identify prefixes that are commonly used in medical terminology.
- Be aware of prefixes that have more than one meaning.
- Recognize prefixes that pertain to position or placement.
- Identify selected prefixes that pertain to numbers and amounts.
- Analyze, build, spell, and pronounce medical words.
- Complete the Study and Review section.

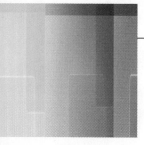

# Overview of Prefixes

The term **prefix** means *to fix before* or *to fix to the beginning* of a word. A prefix can be a syllable or a group of syllables. Prefixes are united with or placed at the beginning of words to alter or modify their meanings or to create entirely new words. For example, by adding the prefix *ab-* to the word *normal* the word **ab/norm/al** is created. As you know, there is a big difference between normal and abnormal. Ab/norm/al means pertaining to away from the norm. Remember that when giving the meaning of the word or reading its definition, you usually begin with the meaning of the suffix. Note the component parts of the word abnormal:

| | | |
|---|---|---|
| ab- | P or prefix meaning | away from |
| norm | R or root meaning | norm |
| -al | S or suffix meaning | pertaining to |

Not all medical words have a prefix, but when they do, the prefix will alter or modify the meaning of the word. For example, see the following list of medical words that were formed by uniting various prefixes with a single suffix (*-pnea*).

| Prefix | Suffix | Medical Word | Definition |
|---|---|---|---|
| **a-** (lack of) | -pnea (breathing) | *a*pnea | Lack of breathing |
| **brady-** (slow) | -pnea (breathing) | *brady*pnea | Slow breathing |
| **dys-** (difficult) | -pnea (breathing) | *dys*pnea | Difficult breathing |
| **eu-** (good, normal) | -pnea (breathing) | *eu*pnea | Good, normal breathing |
| **hyper-** (excessive) | -pnea (breathing) | *hyper*pnea | Excessive breathing |
| **hypo-** (deficient) | -pnea (breathing) | *hypo*pnea | Deficient breathing |
| **tachy-** (fast) | -pnea (breathing) | *tachy*pnea | Fast breathing |

## GENERAL USE PREFIXES

See Table 3–1 for a collection of prefixes that are commonly used in medical terminology. These prefixes can be linked with a word root or a suffix.

TABLE 3–1 **Selected Prefixes for General Use**

| Prefix | Meanings | Example Words |
|---|---|---|
| **a, an-** | no, without, lack of, apart | *a*/mnes/ia; *an*/algesia |
| **anti-, contra-** | against | *anti*/gen; *contra*/cept/ion |
| **auto-** | self | *auto*/trans/fus/ion |
| **brachy-** | short | *brachy*/card/ia |
| **brady-** | slow | *brady*/card/ia |
| **cac-, mal-** | bad | *cac*/hexia; *mal*/format/ion |
| **dia-** | through, between | *dia*/gnosis |
| **dys-** | bad, difficult, painful, abnormal | *dys*/meno/rrhea |
| **eu-** | good, normal | *eu*/pnea |
| **ex-, exo-** | out, away from | *ex*/cis/ion; *exo*/crine |
| **hetero-** | different | *hetero*/sexu/al |
| **homeo-** | similar, same, likeness, constant | *homeo*/stasis |
| **hydro-** | water | *hydro*/therapy |
| **micro-** | small | *micro*/cephal/us |
| **oligo-** | scanty, little | *oligo*/meno/rrhea |
| **pan-** | all | *pan*/cyto/penia |
| **pseudo-** | false | *pseudo*/cyesis |
| **sym-, syn-** | together, with | *sym*/physis; *syn*/cope |

## PREFIXES THAT HAVE MORE THAN ONE MEANING

Just like suffixes, many prefixes have more than one meaning. See Table 3–2. To be able to identify the correct meaning of the prefix, you will need to analyze the definition of the medical word. For example, in the medical word **dyspnea** (difficult breathing), *dys-* means difficult. Note that *dys-* also means bad, painful, or abnormal, but in dyspnea these meanings do not apply. As you learn the various component parts that are used to build medical words, you will acquire the knowledge to select and use the correct meaning for each word.

TABLE 3–2 **Selected Prefixes That Have More Than One Meaning**

| Prefix | Meanings | Prefix | Meanings |
|---|---|---|---|
| **a-, an-** | no, not, without, lack of, apart | **extra-** | outside, beyond |
| **ad-** | toward, near, to | **hyper-** | above, beyond, excessive |
| **bi-** | two, double | **hypo-** | below, under, deficient |
| **de-** | down, away from | **in-** | in, into, not |
| **di-** | two, double | **mega-** | large, great |
| **dia-** | through, between, complete | **meta-** | beyond, over, between, change |
| **dif-, dis-** | apart, free from, separate | **para-** | beside, alongside, abnormal |
| **dys-** | bad, difficult, painful, abnormal | **poly-** | many, much, excessive |
| **ec-, ecto-** | out, outside, outer | **post-** | after, behind |
| **end-, endo-** | within, inner | **pre-** | before, in front of |
| **ep-, epi-** | upon, over, above | **pro-** | before, in front of |
| **eu-** | good, normal | **super-** | upper, above |
| **ex-, exo-** | out, away from | **supra-** | above, beyond |

# PREFIXES THAT PERTAIN TO POSITION OR PLACEMENT

Prefixes that carry meanings such as *away from*, *toward*, *before*, *above*, and *below* are often combined with roots and suffixes to describe a position or placement. See Table 3–3 for an alphabetic listing of some of the more frequently used prefixes associated with position or placements.

**TABLE 3–3  Prefixes That Pertain to Position or Placement**

| Prefix | Meanings | Example Words |
|---|---|---|
| **ab-** | away from | *ab*/norm/al |
| **ad-** | toward, near, to | *ad*/duct/or |
| **ana-** | up, apart, backward | *ana*/phylaxis |
| **ante-** | before, forward | *ante*/partum |
| **cata-** | down | *cata*/bol/ism |
| **circum-, peri-** | around | *circum*/cis/ion; *peri*/cardi/um |
| **endo-** | within, inner | *endo*/card/itis |
| **epi-** | upon, above, over | *epi*/gastr/ic |
| **ex-** | out, away from | *ex*/cis/ion |
| **extra-** | outside, beyond | *extra*/corpore/al |
| **hyper-** | above, beyond, excessive | *hyper*/tens/ion |
| **hypo-** | below, under, deficient | *hypo*/tens/ion |
| **inter-** | between | *inter*/cost/al |
| **intra-** | within, into | *intra*/uter/ine |
| **meso-** | middle | *meso*/theli/oma |
| **para-** | beside, alongside | *para*/plegia |
| **retro-** | backward | *retro*/vers/ion |
| **sub-** | below, under, beneath | *sub*/lingu/al |
| **supra-** | above, beyond, superior | *supra*/ren/al |

# PREFIXES THAT PERTAIN TO NUMBERS AND AMOUNTS

Prefixes with meanings such as *both*, *ten*, *double*, *many*, *half*, and *none* are often combined with roots or suffixes to describe numbers or amounts. See Table 3–4 for an alphabetic list of some of the more frequently used prefixes associated with numbers and amounts.

**TABLE 3–4  Prefixes That Pertain to Numbers and Amounts**

| Prefix | Meanings | Example Words |
|---|---|---|
| **ambi-** | both | *ambi*/later/al |
| **bi-** | two, double | *bi*/later/al |
| **bin-** | twice, two | *bin*/ocul/ar |
| **centi-** | one hundredth | *centi*/meter |
| **deca-** | ten | *deca*/gram |
| **di(s)-** | two, apart | *dis*/locat/ion |
| **milli-** | one thousandth | *milli*/liter |
| **mono-** | one | *mono*/nucle/osis |
| **multi-** | many, much | *multi*/para |
| **nulli-** | none | *nulli*/para |
| **poly-** | many | *poly*/uria |
| **primi-** | first | *primi*/para |
| **quadri-** | four | *quadri*/plegia |
| **semi-, hemi-** | half | *semi*/lun/ar, *hemi*/plegia |
| **tri-** | three | *tri*/som/y |
| **uni-** | one | *uni*/later/al |

# BUILDING YOUR MEDICAL VOCABULARY

This section provides the foundation for learning medical terminology. Review the following alphabetized word list. Note how common prefixes and suffixes are repeatedly applied to word roots and combining forms to create different meanings.

| P | Prefix |
|---|---|
| R | Root |
| CF | Combining form |
| S | Suffix |

| Pink words | Terms not built from word parts. |
|---|---|
| * | Indicates words covered in the Pathology Spotlights section. |
| (CD-ROM icon) | Check the CD-ROM for more information. |

| MEDICAL WORD | WORD PARTS (WHEN APPLICABLE) | | | DEFINITION |
|---|---|---|---|---|
| | Part | Type | Meaning | |
| **afebrile**<br>(ă-fĕb′rĭl) | a-<br>febr<br>-ile | P<br>R<br>S | without<br>fever<br>pertaining to | Pertaining to without fever |
| **anicteric**<br>(ăn″ĭk-tĕr′ĭk) | an-<br>icter<br>-ic | P<br>R<br>S | without<br>jaundice<br>pertaining to | Pertaining to without jaundice (yellowish discoloration of the skin, whites of the eyes, mucous membranes and body fluids) |
| **arrest**<br>(ă-rĕst′) | | | | To stop, inhibit, restrain. A condition of being stopped, such as occurs in cardiac arrest when cardiac output and effective circulation stop. |
| **bifurcate**<br>(bī′fŭr-kāt) | bi-<br>furc<br>-ate | P<br>R<br>S | two<br>fork<br>use, action | Having two forks or two branches or two divisions; forked |
| **binary**<br>(bī′nār-ē) | bin-<br>-ary | P<br>S | twice<br>pertaining to | Pertaining to separating into two branches or composed of two elements |
| **concentration**<br>(kŏn-sĕn-trā′shŭn) | con-<br>centrat<br>-ion | P<br>R<br>S | with, together<br>center<br>process | In psychology, the process of being able to bring to the center one thought and focus on it, while excluding other thoughts |
| **decompensation**<br>(dē-kŏm-pen-sā′shŭn) | de-<br>compensat<br><br>-ion | P<br>R<br><br>S | down, away from<br>to make good again<br>process | Failure of a system. In cardiology—failure of the heart to maintain adequate circulation; in psychology—failure of the defense mechanism system that may occur during a relapsing of a mental condition. |
| **enucleate**<br>(ē-nū′klē-āt) | | | | Literally means *to remove the kernel of.* It is used to describe the removal of the eyeball surgically or to remove a cataract surgically. It also means to remove a part or a mass in its entirety. |

| MEDICAL WORD | WORD PARTS (WHEN APPLICABLE) | | | DEFINITION |
|---|---|---|---|---|
| | **Part** | **Type** | **Meaning** | |
| **extraocular**<br>(ĕks"tră-ŏk'ū-lăr) | extra-<br>ocul<br>-ar | P<br>R<br>S | outside<br>eye<br>pertaining to | Pertaining to outside the eye, as used in describing the extraocular eye muscles. These are the muscles that control eye movement and eye coordination. |
| **hyperactive**<br>(hī"pĕr-ăk'tĭv) | hyper-<br>act<br>-ive | P<br>R<br>S | excessive<br>act<br>nature of,<br>quality of | Nature or quality of excessive activity; this can refer to the entire organism or to a particular entity such as the thyroid, heart, or muscles. It may also describe an individual who exhibits constant overactivity. |
| **hypoplasia**<br>(hī"pō-plā'zē-ă) | hypo-<br>-plasia | P<br>S | under<br>formation | Underdevelopment of a tissue, organ, or body |
| **insomnia**<br>(ĭn-sŏm'nē-ah) | in-<br>somn<br>-ia | P<br>R<br>S | not<br>sleep<br>condition | Condition of not being able to sleep. People with insomnia can have difficulty falling asleep, wake up often during the night and have trouble going back to sleep, wake up too early in the morning, or experience unrefreshing sleep. |
| **intermediary**<br>(ĭn"tĕr-mē'dē-ār-ē) | inter<br>medi<br>-ary | P<br>R<br>S | between<br>toward the middle<br>pertaining to | Pertaining to situated between two bodies or occurring between two periods of time |
| **latent**<br>(lă'tē-nt) | | | | Lying hidden; quiet, not active |
| **lumen**<br>(lū'mĕn) | | | | Space within an artery, vein, intestine, or tube. It is also the hollow core of a hypodermic needle, which forms an oval-shaped opening when exposed at the beveled (flat, slanted surface) point. |
| **multifocal**<br>(mŭl"tĭ-fō'kăl) | multi-<br>foc<br>-al | P<br>R<br>S | many<br>focus<br>pertaining to | Pertaining to or arising from many locations |
| **occlusion**<br>(ŏ-kloo'zhŭn) | | | | Process of closing or state of being closed of a passage |
| **parasternal**<br>(păr-ă-stĕrn'ăl) | para-<br>stern<br><br>-al | P<br>R<br><br>S | beside<br>sternum,<br>breastbone<br>pertaining to | Pertaining to beside the sternum (breastbone) |
| **patent**<br>(pă'ĕnt) | | | | Wide open; freely open |
| **pericardial**<br>(pĕr-ĭ-kăr'dē-ăl) | peri-<br>cardi<br>-al | P<br>R<br>S | around<br>heart<br>pertaining to | Pertaining to the pericardium (sac surrounding the heart) |
| **polydactyly**<br>(pŏl"ē-dăk'tĭ-lē) | poly-<br>dactyl<br>-y | P<br>R<br>S | many<br>finger or toe<br>pertaining to | Pertaining to having more than the normal number of fingers and toes |

| MEDICAL WORD | WORD PARTS (WHEN APPLICABLE) | | | DEFINITION |
|---|---|---|---|---|
| | **Part** | **Type** | **Meaning** | |
| **premenstrual**<br>(prē-měn'stroo-ăl) | pre-<br>menstru<br><br>-al | P<br>R<br><br>S | before<br>to discharge<br>the menses<br>pertaining to | Pertaining to the time before the discharge of the menses |
| **react**<br>(rē-ăkt') | re-<br>-act | P<br>S | again<br>to act | Literally means *to act again;* respond to a stimulus; to participate in a chemical reaction |
| **regurgitation**<br>(rē-gŭr"jĭ-tā'shŭn) | re-<br>gurgitat<br>-ion | P<br>R<br>S | backward<br>to flood<br>process | Process of a backward flow of solids or foods from the stomach to the mouth or the backflow of blood through a defective heart valve |
| **sign**<br>(sīn) | | | | Any objective evidence of an illness or disordered function of the body. A sign can be seen, heard, measured, or felt by the examiner. |
| **subacute**<br>(sŭb"ă-kūt') | sub-<br>acute | P<br>R | below<br>sharp | Literally means *below sharp;* it describes a state between acute and chronic with some acute features. It is used to describe the course of a disease process or the healing process following tissue injury. |
| **superinfection**<br>(soo"pěr-ĭn-fěk'shŭn) | super-<br>infect<br>-ion | P<br>R<br>S | upper, above<br>infect<br>process | New infection caused by a different organism from one that caused the initial infection. It can occur from a harmful effect of an antibiotic, when there is an overgrowth of a resistant strain of bacteria, fungi, or yeast. |
| **symptom**<br>(sĭm'tŭm) | | | | Any perceptible change in the function of the body that indicates disease; can be classified as objective (signs), subjective (symptoms described by the patient), and cardinal (vital signs: temperature, pulse, respiration, blood pressure) |
| **unconscious**<br>(ŭn-kŏn'shŭs) | un<br>consci<br>-ous | R<br>R<br>S | not<br>aware<br>pertaining to | Pertaining to not being aware; lacking in awareness of one's environment |

# STUDY AND REVIEW

## Identifying Prefixes

*Underline the prefixes in the following medical words.*

1. apnea
2. bradypnea
3. dyspnea
4. eupnea
5. hyperpnea
6. hypopnea
7. tachypnea
8. binary
9. concentration
10. extraocular

## Defining Prefixes

*Give the meaning of the following prefixes.*

1. anti- _____
2. brachy- _____
3. dia- _____
4. hetero- _____
5. homeo- _____
6. hydro- _____
7. micro- _____
8. oligo- _____
9. pan- _____
10. pseudo- _____
11. a- _____
12. an- _____
13. bi- _____
14. bin- _____
15. con- _____
16. de- _____
17. extra- _____
18. hyper- _____
19. hypo- _____
20. in- _____
21. inter- _____
22. multi- _____
23. para- _____
24. peri- _____
25. poly- _____
26. pre- _____
27. re- _____
28. sub- _____
29. super- _____
30. un- _____

## Spelling

*In the spaces provided, write the correct spelling of these misspelled terms.*

1. biary _____
2. concenteration _____
3. oclusion _____
4. parsternal _____
5. pericardal _____
6. latnt _____
7. patnt _____
8. unconsious _____

## Using Prefixes to Build Medical Words

*Using a prefix from the following list, build the appropriate medical word.*

| | | | | |
|---|---|---|---|---|
| an- | de- | hyper- | multi- | sub- |
| bi- | hypo- | inter- | poly- | un- |

1. Pertaining to without jaundice      _____ icteric

2. Nature of excessive activity      _____ active

3. Pertaining to arising from many locations      _____ focal

4. Failure of a system      _____ compensation

5. Pertaining to situated between two bodies      _____ mediary

6. Having two forks      _____ furcate

7. Pertaining to having more than the normal number of fingers and toes      _____ dactyly

8. Underdevelopment of a tissue, organ, or body      _____ plasia

9. *Below sharp*      _____ acute

10. Pertaining to not being aware      _____ conscious

## Identifying Medical Terms

*In the spaces provided, write the medical terms for the following meanings.*

1. _____ Pertaining to without fever

2. _____ Pertaining to outside the eye

3. _____ Condition of not being able to sleep

4. _____ To stop, inhibit, restrain

5. _____ *To remove the kernel of*

6. _____ Space within an artery, vein, intestine, or tube

7. _____ Wide open

8. _____ *To act again*

9. _____ Any objective evidence of an illness

10. _____ Any perceptible change in the function of the body that indicates disease

# MULTIMEDIA PREVIEW

*Additional interactive resources and activities for this chapter can be found on the Companion Website. For videos, audio glossary, and review, access the accompanying CD-ROM in this book.*

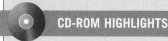 **CD-ROM HIGHLIGHTS**

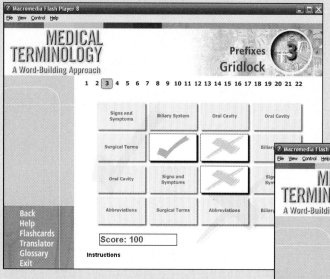

## GRIDLOCK GAME

Are you a *Jeopardy!* champ? Prove your quiz show smarts by clicking here to answer the medical terminology questions hidden beneath the tiles. Get them all right to clear the grid.

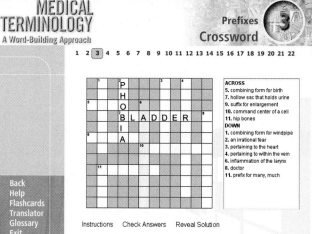

## CROSSWORD PUZZLE

Here is where learning and fun intersect! Simply use the clues to complete the puzzle grid. Whether you're a crossword wizard or only a novice, this activity will reinforce your understanding of key terms and concepts.

 **WEBSITE HIGHLIGHTS—www.prenhall.com/rice**

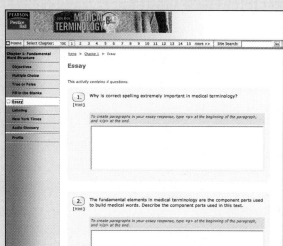

## ESSAY QUESTIONS

Click here and take advantage of the free-access on-line study guide that accompanies your textbook. You'll find a series of short answer essay questions that correspond to the concepts in this chapter. By clicking on this URL you'll also access links to download mp3 audio reviews, current news articles, and an audio glossary.

# Organization of the Body

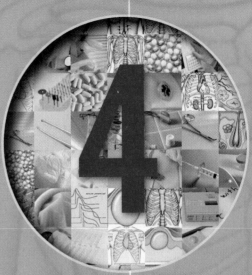

## ■ OUTLINE

## ■ OBJECTIVES

*On completion of this chapter, you will be able to:*

- Define terms that describe the body and its structural units.
- List the systems of the body and give the organs in each system.
- Define terms that are used to describe direction, planes, and cavities of the body.
- Understand word analysis as it relates to Head-to-Toe Assessment.
- Analyze, build, spell, and pronounce medical words.
- Comprehend the drugs highlighted in this chapter.
- Identify and define selected abbreviations.
- Describe a medical record.
- Define HIPAA.
- List and describe the general components of a patient's medical record.
- List and describe the four parts of the SOAP Chart Note record.
- Complete the Study and Review section.

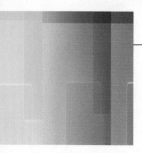

# Anatomy and Physiology Overview

This chapter introduces you to terms describing the body and its structural units. To aid you, these terms have been grouped into two major sections: The first offers an overview of the units that make up the human body, and the second covers terms used to describe anatomical positions and locations.

The human body is made up of atoms, molecules, organelles, cells, tissues, organs, and systems. See Figure 4–1 ▶. All of these parts normally function together in a unified and complex process known as **homeostasis** (a state of equilibrium that is maintained within the body's internal environment). This means that the body's fluid composition, its volume and characteristics, its temperature (T), blood pressure (BP), and the exchange of ($O_2$) and carbon dioxide ($CO_2$) remain within normal limits. By maintaining homeostasis, the cells of the body are in an environment that meets their needs and permits them to function normally under changing conditions. The body continually responds to changes in its environment, exchanges materials between its environment and its cells, metabolizes food, and excretes waste.

# HUMAN BODY: LEVELS OF ORGANIZATION

## Atoms

An **atom** is the smallest, basic chemical unit of matter. It consists of a nucleus that contains protons and neutrons and is surrounded by electrons. A **proton** is a positively charged particle; a **neutron** is neutral without an electrical charge. An **electron** is a negatively charged particle that revolves about the nucleus of an atom.

**Chemical elements** are made up of atoms, which can be classified on the basis of their atomic number into groups called elements. An **element** is a substance that cannot be separated into substances different from itself by ordinary chemical means. It is the basic component of which all matter is composed.

Principal elements found in the human body include aluminum, carbon, calcium, chlorine, cobalt, copper, fluorine, hydrogen, iodine, iron, manganese, magnesium, nitrogen, oxygen, phosphorus, potassium, sodium, sulfur, and zinc. Each of these elements plays an essential role in maintaining homeostasis. See Table 4–1.

### TABLE 4–1  Elements Found in the Human Body

| Symbol | Element | Symbol | Element |
|--------|---------|--------|---------|
| Al | Aluminum | Mn | Manganese |
| C | Carbon | Mg | Magnesium |
| Ca | Calcium | N | Nitrogen |
| Cl | Chlorine | O or $O_2$ | Oxygen |
| Co | Cobalt | P | Phosphorus |
| Cu | Copper | K | Potassium |
| F | Fluorine | Na | Sodium |
| H | Hydrogen | S | Sulfur |
| I | Iodine | Zn | Zinc |
| Fe | Iron | | |

LEVEL

EXAMPLES

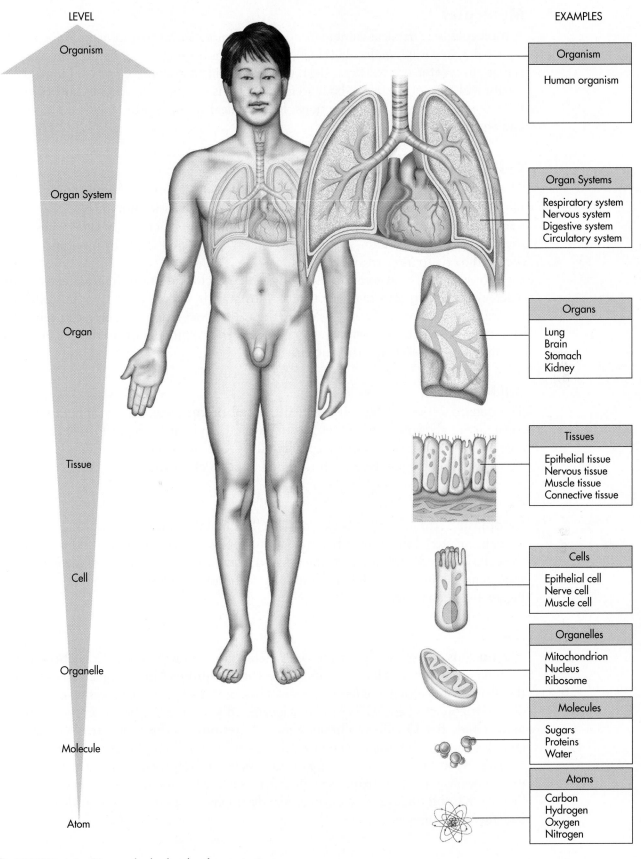

| Organism |
| Human organism |

| Organ Systems |
| Respiratory system<br>Nervous system<br>Digestive system<br>Circulatory system |

| Organs |
| Lung<br>Brain<br>Stomach<br>Kidney |

| Tissues |
| Epithelial tissue<br>Nervous tissue<br>Muscle tissue<br>Connective tissue |

| Cells |
| Epithelial cell<br>Nerve cell<br>Muscle cell |

| Organelles |
| Mitochondrion<br>Nucleus<br>Ribosome |

| Molecules |
| Sugars<br>Proteins<br>Water |

| Atoms |
| Carbon<br>Hydrogen<br>Oxygen<br>Nitrogen |

Organism

Organ System

Organ

Tissue

Cell

Organelle

Molecule

Atom

▶ FIGURE 4–1   Human body: levels of organization.

## Molecules

A **molecule** is a chemical combination of two or more atoms that form a specific chemical compound. In a water molecule ($H_2O$), oxygen forms polar covalent bonds with two hydrogen atoms. **Water** is a tasteless, clear, odorless liquid that makes up 65% of a male's body weight and 55% of a female's body weight. Water is the most important constituent of all body fluids, secretions, and excretions. It is an ideal transportation medium for inorganic and organic compounds.

## Cells

The body consists of trillions of cells working individually and with each other to sustain life. For the purposes of this book, **cells** are considered the basic building blocks for the various structures that together make up the human being. There are several types of cells, each specialized to perform specific functions. The size and shape of a cell are generally related directly to its function. See Figure 4–2 ▶.

For example, cells forming the skin overlap each other to form a protective barrier, whereas nerve cells are usually elongated with branches connecting to other cells for the transmission of sensory impulses. Despite these differences, however, cells can generally be said to have a number of common components. The common parts of the cell are the cell membrane, cytoplasm, and the nucleus.

### Cell Membrane

The outer covering of the cell is called the **cell membrane.** Cell membranes have the capability of allowing some substances to pass into and out of the cell while denying passage to other substances. This selectivity allows cells to receive nutrition and dispose of waste just as the human being eats food and disposes of waste.

### Cytoplasm

**Cytoplasm** is the substance between the cell membrane and the nuclear membrane. It is a jellylike material that is mostly water. The cytoplasm provides storage and work areas for the cell. The work and storage elements of the cell, called *organelles,* are the endoplasmic reticulum, ribosomes, Golgi apparatus, mitochondria, lysosomes, and centrioles. See Figure 4–3 ▶ and Table 4–2.

### Nucleus

The **nucleus** is responsible for the cell's metabolism, growth, and reproduction. It is the central portion of the cell that contains the **chromosomes** (microscopic bodies that carry the genes that determine hereditary characteristics). A single gene makes up each segment of deoxyribonucleic acid (DNA) and is located in a specific site on the chromosome. The human body has 23 pairs of chromosomes. A **genome** is the complete set of genes and chromosomes tucked inside each of the body's trillions of cells. Genes determine an individual's physical traits such as hair, skin, and eye color, body structure, and metabolic activity. They also control hereditary disorders such as cystic fibrosis, Down syndrome, hemophilia, Huntington's disease, muscular dystrophy, phenylketonuria, sickle cell anemia, and Tay-Sachs disease.

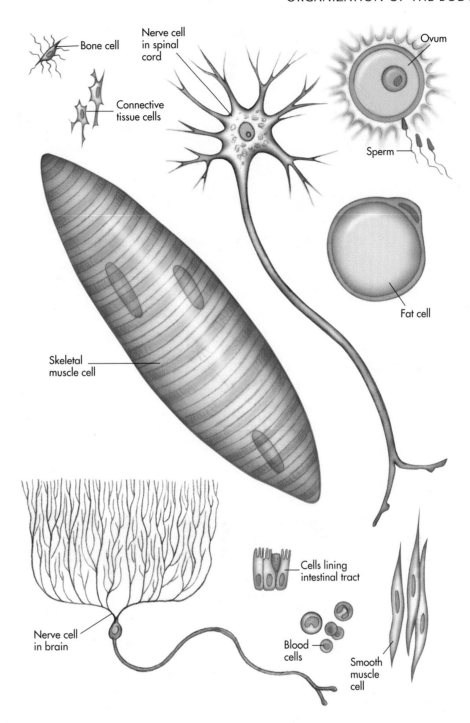

▶ **FIGURE 4–2**  Cells are the basic building blocks of the human body. They have many different shapes and vary in size and function. These examples show the range of forms and sizes with the dimensions they would have if magnified approximately 500 times.

## Stem Cells

**Stem cells** differ from other kinds of cells in the body. All stem cells have three general properties: They are capable of dividing and renewing themselves for long periods, they are unspecialized, and they can give rise to specialized cell types. Some primary sources of stem cells include embryos, adult tissues, and umbilical cord blood. An embryonic cell is an unspecialized cell that can turn itself into any type of tissue. It is derived primarily from

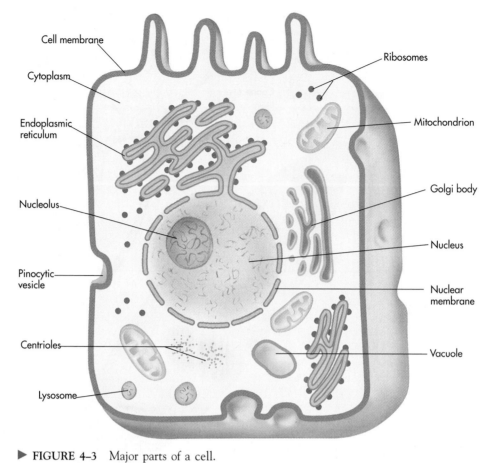

Cell membrane

Cytoplasm

Endoplasmic reticulum

Nucleolus

Pinocytic vesicle

Centrioles

Lysosome

Ribosomes

Mitochondrion

Golgi body

Nucleus

Nuclear membrane

Vacuole

▶ **FIGURE 4–3** Major parts of a cell.

## TABLE 4–2 **Major Cell Structures and Primary Functions**

| Cell Structures | Primary Functions |
| --- | --- |
| Cell membrane | Protects the cell; provides for communication via receptor proteins; surface proteins serve as positive identification tags; allows some substances to pass into and out of the cell while denying passage to other substances; this selectivity allows cells to receive nutrition and dispose of waste |
| Cytoplasm | Provides storage and work areas for the cell; the work and storage elements of the cell, called *organelles,* are the ribosomes, endoplasmic reticulum, Golgi apparatus, mitochondria, lysosomes, and centrioles |
| Ribosomes | Make enzymes and other proteins; nicknamed "protein factories" |
| Endoplasmic reticulum (ER) | Carries proteins and other substances through the cytoplasm |
| Golgi apparatus | Chemically processes the molecules from the endoplasmic reticulum and then packages them into vesicles; nicknamed "chemical processing and packaging center" |
| Mitochondria | Involved in cellular metabolism and respiration; provides the principle source of cellular energy and is the place where complex, energy-releasing chemical reactions occur continuously; nicknamed "power plants" |
| Lysosomes | Contain enzymes that can digest food compounds; nicknamed "digestive bags" |
| Centrioles | Play an important role in cell reproduction |
| Cilia | Hairlike processes that project from epithelial cells; help propel mucus, dust particles, and other foreign substances from the respiratory tract |
| Flagellum | "Tail" of the sperm that enables for the sperm to "swim" or move toward the ovum |
| Nucleus | Controls every *organelle* (little organ) in the cytoplasm; contains the genetic matter necessary for cell reproduction as well as control over activity within the cell's cytoplasm; responsible for the cell's metabolism, growth, and reproduction |

frozen **in vitro** (in glass, as in a test tube) fertilization embryos. An adult stem cell is a more specialized cell found in many kinds of tissue, such as bone marrow, skin, and the liver. An umbilical cord cell is a rich source of precursors of mature blood cells. It is obtained from cord blood at the time of birth. Research on stem cells is advancing knowledge about how an organism develops from a single cell and how healthy cells replace damaged cells in an adult organism. This promising area of science is also leading scientists to investigate the possibility of cell-based therapies to treat disease, which is often referred to as **regenerative** or **reparative medicine.**

## Tissues

A **tissue** is a grouping of similar cells that together perform specialized functions. There are four basic types of tissue in the body: **epithelial, connective, muscle,** and **nerve.** Each of the four basic tissues has several subtypes named for their shape, appearance, arrangement, or function. The following sections describe the four basic types of tissue.

### Epithelial Tissue

**Epithelial tissue** appears as sheetlike arrangements of cells, sometimes several layers thick, that form the outer layer of the skin, cover the surfaces of organs, line the walls of cavities, and form tubes, ducts, and portions of certain glands. The functions of epithelial tissues are protection, absorption, secretion, and excretion.

### Connective Tissue

The most widespread and abundant of the body tissues, **connective tissue** forms the supporting network for the organs of the body, sheaths the muscles, and connects muscles to bones and bones to joints. Bone is a dense form of connective tissue.

### Muscle Tissue

There are three types of **muscle tissue:** voluntary or striated, cardiac, and involuntary or smooth. Voluntary (striated) and involuntary (smooth) muscles are so described because of their appearance. Cardiac muscle is a specialized form of striated tissue under the control of the autonomic nervous system. Involuntary or smooth muscles are also controlled by this system. The voluntary or striated muscles are controlled by the person's will.

### Nerve Tissue

**Nerve tissue** consists of nerve cells (neurons) and supporting cells called *neuroglia*. It has the properties of excitability and conductivity and functions to control and coordinate the activities of the body.

## Organs

Tissues serving a common purpose or function make up structures called **organs,** which are specialized components of the body such as the brain, skin, or heart.

## Systems

A group of organs functioning together for a common purpose is called a **system.** The various body systems function in support of the body as a whole. See Figure 4–4 ▶ for the organ systems of the body.

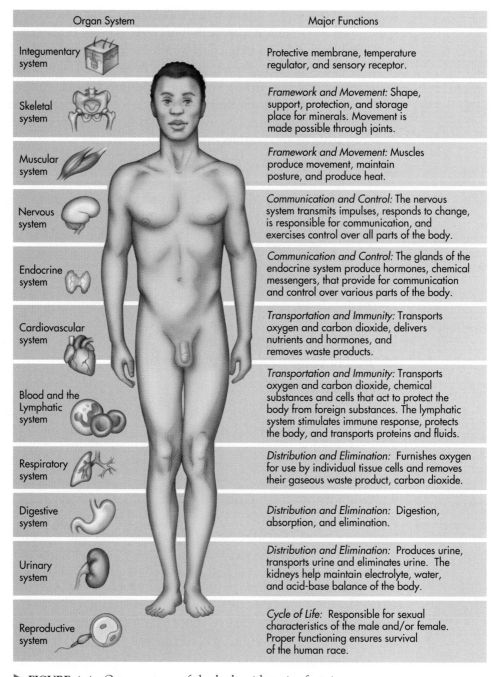

| Organ System | Major Functions |
|---|---|
| Integumentary system | Protective membrane, temperature regulator, and sensory receptor. |
| Skeletal system | *Framework and Movement:* Shape, support, protection, and storage place for minerals. Movement is made possible through joints. |
| Muscular system | *Framework and Movement:* Muscles produce movement, maintain posture, and produce heat. |
| Nervous system | *Communication and Control:* The nervous system transmits impulses, responds to change, is responsible for communication, and exercises control over all parts of the body. |
| Endocrine system | *Communication and Control:* The glands of the endocrine system produce hormones, chemical messengers, that provide for communication and control over various parts of the body. |
| Cardiovascular system | *Transportation and Immunity:* Transports oxygen and carbon dioxide, delivers nutrients and hormones, and removes waste products. |
| Blood and the Lymphatic system | *Transportation and Immunity:* Transports oxygen and carbon dioxide, chemical substances and cells that act to protect the body from foreign substances. The lymphatic system stimulates immune response, protects the body, and transports proteins and fluids. |
| Respiratory system | *Distribution and Elimination:* Furnishes oxygen for use by individual tissue cells and removes their gaseous waste product, carbon dioxide. |
| Digestive system | *Distribution and Elimination:* Digestion, absorption, and elimination. |
| Urinary system | *Distribution and Elimination:* Produces urine, transports urine and eliminates urine. The kidneys help maintain electrolyte, water, and acid-base balance of the body. |
| Reproductive system | *Cycle of Life:* Responsible for sexual characteristics of the male and/or female. Proper functioning ensures survival of the human race. |

▶ **FIGURE 4–4** Organ systems of the body with major functions.

## ANATOMICAL LOCATIONS AND POSITIONS

Four primary reference systems have been adopted to provide uniformity to the anatomical description of the body. These reference systems are **direction, planes, cavities,** and **structural unit.** The standard **anatomical position** for the body is erect, head facing forward, arms by the sides with palms to the front. Left and right are from the subject's point of view, not the examiner's.

### Direction

Directional and positional terms describe the location of organs or body parts in relationship to one another. They are used in describing physical assessment of a patient's presenting complaints and in pinpointing the location of a given sign or symptom.

The following terms are used to describe direction:

| Term | Description | Example |
| --- | --- | --- |
| Superior | Above, in an upward direction, toward the head | The head is superior to the neck of the body. |
| Anterior (ventral) | In front of or before, the front side of the body | The breasts are located on the anterior side of the body. |
| Posterior (dorsal) | Toward the back, back side of the body | The nape is the back of the neck and is located on the posterior side of the body. |
| Cephalic | Pertaining to the head | A cephalic presentation is one in which any part of the head of the fetus is presented during delivery. |
| Medial | Nearest the midline or middle | The umbilicus is a depressed point in the medial area of the abdomen. |
| Lateral | To the side, away from the middle | In the anatomical position, the arm is located on the lateral side of the body. |
| Proximal | Nearest the point of attachment or near the beginning of a structure | The proximal end of the humerus (upper bone of the arm) joins with part of the shoulder bone. |
| Distal | Away from the point of attachment or far from the beginning of a structure | The distal end of the humerus joins with part of the elbow. |

## Planes

The terms defined below are used to describe the imaginary planes that are depicted in Figure 4–5 ▶ as passing through the body and dividing it into various sections.

### Midsagittal Plane

The **midsagittal plane** vertically divides the body as it passes through the midline to form a **right half** and **left half.**

### Transverse or Horizontal Plane

A **transverse** or **horizontal plane** is any plane that divides the body into **superior** and **inferior** portions.

### Coronal or Frontal Plane

A **coronal plane** or **frontal plane** is any plane that divides the body at right angles to the midsagittal plane. The coronal plane divides the body into **anterior** (ventral) and **posterior** (dorsal) portions.

## Cavities

A **cavity** is a hollow space containing body organs. Body cavities are classified into two groups according to their location. On the front are the **ventral cavity** or **anterior cavity** and on the back are the **dorsal cavity** or **posterior cavity.** The various cavities found in the human body are depicted in Figure 4–6 ▶.

### Ventral Cavity

The **ventral cavity** is the hollow portion of the human torso extending from the neck to the pelvis and containing the heart and the organs of respiration, digestion, reproduction, and elimination. The ventral cavity can be subdivided into three distinct areas: thoracic, abdominal, and pelvic.

Thoracic Cavity.    The **thoracic cavity** is the area of the chest containing the heart and the lungs. Within this cavity, the space containing the **heart** is called the **pericardial** cavity and the spaces surrounding each **lung** are known as the **pleural** cavities. Other organs

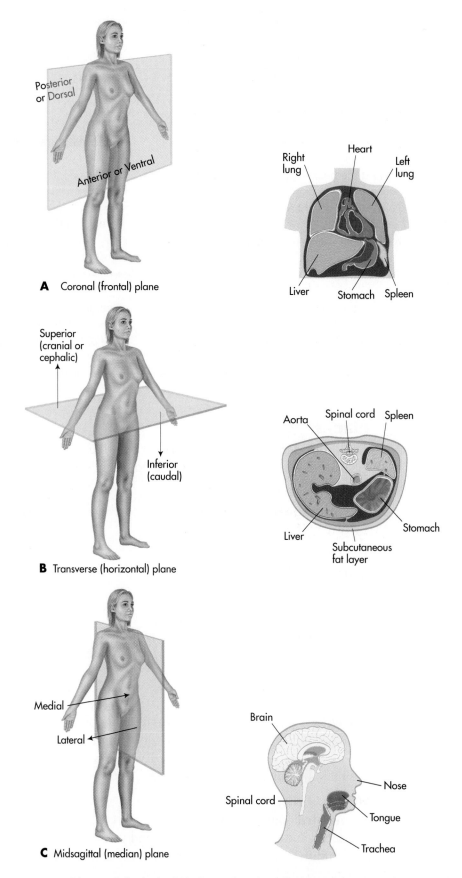

**A**   Coronal (frontal) plane

**B**   Transverse (horizontal) plane

**C**   Midsagittal (median) plane

▶ **FIGURE 4–5**   Planes of the body. (A) Coronal or frontal plane and a coronal view of the chest and stomach. (B) Transverse or horizontal plane and a cross-sectional view of the upper abdominal region. (C) Midsagittal or median plane and a sagittal view of the head.

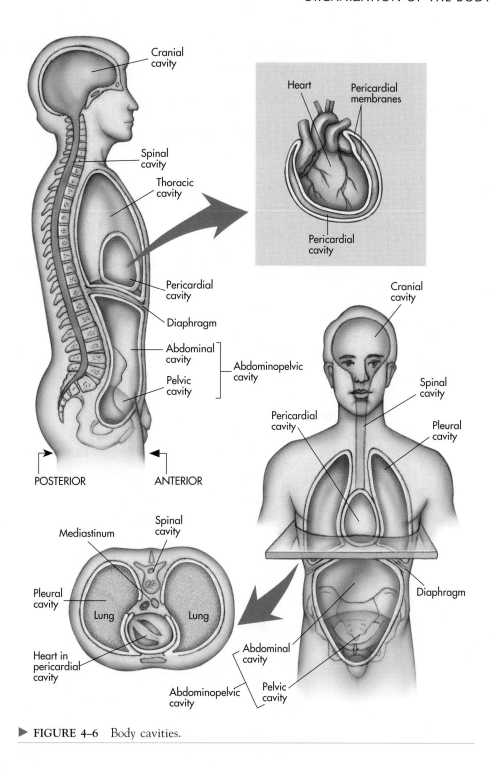

▶ **FIGURE 4–6**   Body cavities.

located in the thoracic cavity are the esophagus, trachea, thymus, and certain large blood and lymph vessels.

Abdominal Cavity.    The **abdominal cavity** is the space below the diaphragm, commonly referred to as the *belly*. It contains the stomach, intestines, and other organs of digestion.

Pelvic Cavity.    The **pelvic cavity** is the space formed by the bones of the pelvic area and contains the organs of reproduction and elimination.

### Dorsal Cavity

Containing the structures of the nervous system, the **dorsal cavity** is subdivided into the cranial cavity and the spinal cavity.

Cranial Cavity.    The **cranial cavity** is the space in the skull containing the brain.

Spinal Cavity.    The **spinal cavity** is the space within the bony spinal column that contains the spinal cord and spinal fluid.

### Abdominopelvic Cavity

The **abdominopelvic cavity** is the combination of the abdominal and pelvic cavities. It is divided into nine regions.

## Nine Regions of the Abdominopelvic Cavity

As a ready reference for locating visceral organs, anatomists divided the abdominopelvic cavity into nine regions (see Figure 4–7A ▼).

A tic-tac-toe pattern drawn across the abdominopelvic cavity delineates these regions:

**Right hypochondriac.** Upper right region at the level of the ninth rib cartilage
**Left hypochondriac.** Upper left region at the level of the ninth rib cartilage
**Epigastric.** Region over the stomach
**Right lumbar.** Right middle lateral region
**Left lumbar.** Left middle lateral region
**Umbilical.** In the center, between the right and left lumbar region; at the navel
**Right iliac (inguinal).** Right lower lateral region
**Left iliac (inguinal).** Left lower lateral region
**Hypogastric.** Lower middle region below the navel

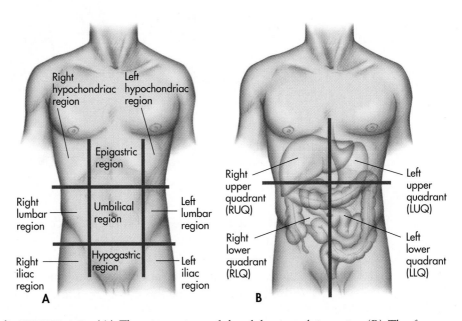

▶ **FIGURE 4–7**   (A) The nine regions of the abdominopelvic cavity. (B) The four regions of the abdomen that are referred to as *quadrants*.

## Abdomen Divided into Quadrants

The **abdomen** is divided into four corresponding regions that are used for descriptive and diagnostic purposes. By using these regions, one may describe the exact location of pain, a skin lesion, surgical incision, and/or abdominal tumor. The four **quadrants** (see Figure 4–7B) are as follows:

**Right upper (RUQ).** Contains the right lobe of the liver, gallbladder, part of the pancreas, and part of the small and large intestines

**Left upper (LUQ).** Contains the left lobe of the liver, stomach, spleen, part of the pancreas, and part of the small and large intestines

**Right lower (RLQ).** Contains part of the small and large intestines, appendix, right ovary, right fallopian tube, right ureter

**Left lower (LLQ).** Contains part of the small and large intestines, left ovary, left fallopian tube, left ureter

*Note:* Some organs, such as the urinary bladder and uterus, are located half in the right quadrant and half in the left quadrant. These organs are generally referred to as being in the *midline* of the body.

# HEAD-TO-TOE ASSESSMENT

The terminology associated with head-to-toe assessment can be useful when studying the organization of the body and in understanding information contained in a patient's medical record. The following body areas, along with their word parts and/or related terminology, are provided for your study.

| Body Area | Word Part(s) | Body Area | Word Part(s) |
|---|---|---|---|
| Abdomen (belly) | abdomin/o (ăb-dō′-mĭ-nō) | Finger | dactyl/o (dăk′-tĭ-lō) |
| Ankle (tarsus) | tars/o (tăr′sō) | Foot | pod/o (pŏd′ō) |
| Arm | brach/i (bră′-chĭ) | Gums | gingiv (gĭn-gĭv) |
| Back | poster (pŏs-tĕ-r) | Hand | manus; chir/o (mă-nūs; kĭ′rō) |
| Bones | oste/o (ŏs-tē-ō) | Head | cephal/o (sĕ-fă-lō) |
| Breast | mast; mamm/o (măst; măm′-ō) | Heart | cardi/o (kăr-dĭ-o) |
| Cheek | bucc/o (bŭk′-kō) | Hip | coxa (kŏk′-să) |
| Chest | thorac/o (thō-ră′-kō) | Leg | crur (crūr) |
| Ear | ot/o (ō-tō) | Liver | hepat/o (hĕ-pă-tō) |
| Elbow | cubital; olecran/o (cū-bĭ-tăl′; ō-lĕk′răn-ŏ) | Lungs | pulm/o; pulmon/o; pneum/o; pneumon/o (pūl-mō; pūl-mō-nō; nū″mō; nū-mōnō) |
| Eye | ophthalm/o; ocul/o; opt/o (ōp-thăl′-mō; ō-kū-lō; ōp-tō) | Mouth | or/o (ō-rō) |

| Body Area | Word Part(s) | Body Area | Word Part(s) |
|-----------|--------------|-----------|--------------|
| Muscles | muscul/o (mūs-cū-lō) | Stomach | gastr/o (găs'-trō) |
| Navel | umbilic; omphal/o (ŭm-bĭ-lĭ'-k; ŏm-făl-ō) | Teeth | dent (dĕnt') |
| Neck | cervic/o (sĕr'-vĭ-cō) | Temples | tempor (tĕm-pōr) |
| Nerves | neur/o (nū'-rō) | Thigh bone | femor/o (fĕ-mōr-ō) |
| Nose | rhin/o; nas/o (rĭ'-nō; nă'-sō) | Throat | pharyng/o (fă-rĭn'-jō) |
| Ribs | cost/o (cōs'-tō) | Thumb | pollex (pōl'-lĕx) |
| Side | later (lă-tĕr) | Tongue | lingu/o; gloss/o (lĭn-gū-ō; glōs-sō) |
| Skin | derm/a; dermat/o; derm/o; cutane/o (dĕr'-mă; dĕr'mă-tō; dĕr'mō; kū-tā'nō) | Wrist | carp/o (căr'-pō) |
| Skull | crani/o (kră'-nĭ-ō) | | |

# BUILDING YOUR MEDICAL VOCABULARY

This section provides the foundation for learning medical terminology. Review the following alphabetized word list. Note how common prefixes and suffixes are repeatedly applied to word roots and combining forms to create different meanings.

| | | | |
|---|---|---|---|
| **P** | Prefix | Pink words | Terms not built from word parts. |
| **R** | Root | | |
| **CF** | Combining form | * | Indicates words covered in the Pathology Spotlights section. |
| **S** | Suffix | | |
| | | 💿 | Check the CD-ROM for more information. |

| MEDICAL WORD | WORD PARTS (WHEN APPLICABLE) | | | DEFINITION |
|--------------|------|------|---------|------------|
| | **Part** | **Type** | **Meaning** | |
| **adipose** (ăd" ĭ-pōs) | adip | R | fat | Pertaining to fatty tissue throughout the body |
| | -ose | S | pertaining to | |
| **ambilateral** (ăm" bĭ-lăt' ĕr-ăl) | ambi- | P | both | Pertaining to both sides |
| | later | R | side | |
| | -al | S | pertaining to | |
| **anatomy** (ăn-ăt' ō-mē) | ana- | P | up; apart | Literally means *to cut up* or *to cut apart;* the study of the structure of an organism such as humans. A specialist in the field of anatomy can learn about the structure of the human body by cutting it apart. This process is called **dissection.** |
| | -tomy | S | incision | |

| MEDICAL WORD | WORD PARTS (WHEN APPLICABLE) | | | DEFINITION |
|---|---|---|---|---|
| | **Part** | **Type** | **Meaning** | |
| **android** (ăn' droyd) | andr -oid | R S | man resemble | To resemble man |
| **anterior** (an-tĕr' ē-ōr) | anter -ior | R S | toward the front pertaining to | Pertaining to a surface or part situated toward the front of the body |
| **apex** (ā' pĕks) | | | | Pointed end of a cone-shaped structure |
| **base** (bās) | | | | Lower part or foundation of a structure |
| **bilateral** (bī-lăt' ĕr-ăl) | bi- later -al | P R S | two side pertaining to | Pertaining to two sides |
| **biology** (bi-ŏl' ō-jē) | bi/o -logy | CF S | life study of | Study of life |
| **caudal** (kŏd' ăl) | caud -al | R S | tail pertaining to | Pertaining to the tail |
| **center** (sĕn' tĕr) | | | | Midpoint of a body or activity |
| **chromosome** (krō-mō-sōm) | chromo- -some | P S | color body | Microscopic bodies that carry the genes that determine hereditary characteristics |
| **cilia** (sĭl' ē-ă) | | | | Hairlike processes that project from epithelial cells; they help propel mucus, dust particles, and other foreign substances from the respiratory tract |
| **cranial** (krā-nē-ăl) | cran/i -al | CF S | cranium pertaining to | Pertaining to the cranium (the portion of the skull that contains the brain) |
| **cytology** (sī-tŏl' ō-jē) | cyt/o -logy | CF S | cell study of | Study of cells |
| **deep** | | | | Far down from the surface |
| **dehydrate** (dē-hī' drāt) | de- hydr -ate | P R S | down, away from water use, action | To remove water; to lose or be deprived of water from the body; to become dry |
| **diffusion** (di-fū' zhŭn) | dif- fus -ion | P R S | apart to pour process | Process in which parts of a substance move from areas of high concentration to areas of lower concentration |
| **distal** (dĭs' tăl) | dist  -al | R  S | away from the point of origin pertaining to | Farthest from the center or point of origin |
| **dorsal** (dōr' săl) | dors -al | R S | backward pertaining to | Pertaining to the back side of the body |
| **ectomorph** (ĕk' tō-morf) | ecto- -morph | P S | outside form, shape | Slender physical body form marked by predominance of tissue derived from the ectoderm (the outer layer of cells in the developing embryo) |

| MEDICAL WORD | WORD PARTS (WHEN APPLICABLE) | | | DEFINITION |
|---|---|---|---|---|
| | Part | Type | Meaning | |
| **endomorph**<br>(ĕn" dō-morf) | endo-<br>-morph | P<br>S | within<br>form, shape | Round physical body form marked by predominance of tissue derived from the endoderm (the inner layer of cells in the developing embryo) |
| **filtration**<br>(fĭl-trā' shŭn) | filtrat<br>-ion | R<br>S | to strain through<br>process | Process of filtering or straining particles from a solution |
| **gene**<br>(jēn) | | | | Hereditary unit that transmits and determines one's characteristics or hereditary traits |
| **histology**<br>(hĭs-tŏl' ō-jē) | hist/o<br>-logy | CF<br>S | tissue<br>study of | Study of tissue |
| **homeostasis**<br>(hō" mē-ō-stā' sĭs) | homeo-<br>-stasis | P<br>S | similar, same<br>control, stop, stand still | State of equilibrium maintained in the body's internal environment |
| **horizontal**<br>(hŏr'ă-zŏn' tăl) | horizont<br>-al | R<br>S | horizon<br>pertaining to | Pertaining to the horizon, of or near the horizon, lying flat, even, level |
| **human genome**<br>(hū' măn jē' nōm) | | | | Complete set of genes and chromosomes tucked inside each of the body's trillions of cells |
| **inferior**<br>(ĭn-fē' rē-or) | infer<br>-ior | R<br>S | below<br>pertaining to | Pertaining to below or in a downward direction |
| **inguinal**<br>(ĭng' gwĭ-năl) | inguin<br>-al | R<br>S | groin<br>pertaining to | Pertaining to the groin, of or near the groin |
| **internal**<br>(ĭn tĕr' nal) | intern<br>-al | R<br>S | within<br>pertaining to | Pertaining to within or the inside |
| **karyogenesis**<br>(kăr" i-ō-jĕn'ĕ- sĭs) | kary/o<br>-genesis | CF<br>S | cell's nucleus<br>formation, produce | Formation of a cell's nucleus |
| **lateral**<br>(lăt' ĕr-ăl) | later<br>-al | R<br>S | side<br>pertaining to | Pertaining to the side |
| **medial**<br>(mē' dē al) | medi<br>-al | R<br>S | toward the middle<br>pertaining to | Pertaining to the middle or midline |
| **mesomorph**<br>(mĕs' ō-morf) | meso-<br>-morph | P<br>S | middle<br>form, shape | Well-proportioned body form marked by predominance of tissue derived from the mesoderm (the middle layer of cells in the developing embryo) |
| **organic**<br>(or-găn' ĭk) | organ<br>-ic | R<br>S | organ<br>pertaining to | Pertaining to an organ or organs; pertaining to or derived from vegetable or animal forms of life |
| **pathology**<br>(pă-thŏl' ō-jē) | path/o<br>-logy | CF<br>S | disease<br>study of | Study of disease |
| **perfusion**<br>(pur-fū' zhŭn) | per-<br>fus<br>-ion | P<br>R<br>S | through<br>to pour<br>process | Process of pouring through |

| MEDICAL WORD | WORD PARTS (WHEN APPLICABLE) | | | DEFINITION |
|---|---|---|---|---|
| | **Part** | **Type** | **Meaning** | |
| **phenotype** (fē′ nō-tīp) | phen/o -type | CF S | to show type | Physical appearance or type of makeup of an individual |
| **physiology** (fiz″ i-ŏl′ ō-jē) | physi/o -logy | CF S | nature study of | Study of the nature of living organisms |
| **posterior** (pŏs-tē′ rĭ-ōr) | poster -ior | R S | behind, toward the back pertaining to | Pertaining to the back part of a structure; toward the back |
| **protoplasm** (prō-tō-plăzm) | proto- -plasm | P S | first a thing formed, plasma | Essential matter of a living cell |
| **proximal** (prŏk′ sĭm-ăl) | proxim -al | R S | near the point of origin pertaining to | Nearest the center or point of origin; nearest the point of attachment |
| **somatotrophic** (sō″ mă-tō-trŏf′ ĭk) | somat/o troph -ic | CF R S | body a turning pertaining to | Pertaining to stimulation of body growth |
| **superficial** (sū″ pĕr-fĭsh′ ăl) | superfic/i -al | CF S | near the surface pertaining to | Pertaining to the surface, on or near the surface |
| **superior** (sū-pēr′ rĭ-ōr) | super- -ior | P S | upper, above pertaining to | Pertaining to above or in an upward direction |
| **systemic** (sis-tĕm′ ĭk) | system -ic | R S | a composite whole pertaining to | Pertaining to the body as a whole |
| **topical** (tŏp′ ĭ-kăl) | topic -al | R S | place pertaining to | Pertaining to a place, definite locale |
| **unilateral** (ū″ nĭ-lăt′ ĕr-ăl) | uni- later -al | P R S | one side pertaining to | Pertaining to one side |
| **ventral** (vĕn′ trăl) | ventr -al | R S | near the belly side pertaining to | Pertaining to the front side of the body, abdomen, belly surface |
| **vertex** (vĕr′ tĕks) | | | | Top or highest point; top or crown of the head |
| **visceral** (vĭs′ ĕr-ăl) | viscer -al | R S | body organs pertaining to | Pertaining to body organs enclosed within a cavity, especially abdominal organs |

# DRUG HIGHLIGHTS

A **drug** is a medicinal substance that may alter or modify the functions of a living organism. There are thousands of drugs that are available as over-the-counter (OTC) medicines and do not require a prescription. A prescription is a written legal document that gives directions for compounding, dispensing, and administering a medication to a patient.

In general, there are five medical uses for drugs. These are: therapeutic, diagnostic, curative, replacement, and preventive or prophylactic.

**Therapeutic Use.** Used in the treatment of a disease or condition, such as an allergy, to relieve the symptoms or to sustain the patient until other measures are instituted.

**Diagnostic Use.** Certain drugs are used in conjunction with radiology to allow the physician to pinpoint the location of a disease process.

**Curative Use.** Certain drugs, such as antibiotics, kill or remove the causative agent of a disease.

**Replacement Use.** Certain drugs, such as hormones and vitamins, are used to replace substances normally found in the body.

**Preventive or Prophylactic Use.** Certain drugs, such as immunizing agents, are used to ward off or lessen the severity of a disease.

| | |
|---|---|
| **Drug names** | Most drugs may be cited by their chemical, generic, and trade or brand (proprietary) name. The *chemical name* is usually the formula that denotes the composition of the drug. It is made up of letters and numbers that represent the drug's molecular structure. The *generic name* is the drug's official name and is descriptive of its chemical structure and is written in lowercase letters. A generic drug can be manufactured by more than one pharmaceutical company. When this is the case, each company markets the drug under its own unique trade or brand name. A *trade or brand name (proprietary)* is registered by the US Patent Office as well as approved by the US Food and Drug Administration (FDA). A trade or brand name is capitalized. |
| | *Example: Chemical name: 4-hydroxyl-2-methyl-N-2-pyridinyl-2H-1, 2-benzothiazine-3-carboxamide 1, 1-dioxide* |
| | *Generic name: piroxicam* |
| | *Trade or Brand name: Feldene (Nonsterioidal anti-inflammatory drug)* |
| **Undesirable actions of drugs** | Most drugs have the potential for causing an action other than their intended action. For example, antibiotics that are administered orally may disrupt the normal bacterial flora of the gastrointestinal tract and cause gastric discomfort. This type of reaction is known as a *side effect*. An *adverse reaction* is an unfavorable or harmful unintended action of a drug. For example, the adverse reaction of Demerol may be lightheadedness, dizziness, sedation, nausea, and sweating. A *drug interaction* can occur when one drug potentiates (increases the action) or diminishes the action of another drug. Drugs can also interact with foods, alcohol, tobacco, and other substances. |
| **Medication order and dosage** | The *medication order* is given for a specific patient and denotes the name of the drug, the dosage, the form of the drug, the time for or frequency of administration, and the route by which the drug is to be given. |
| | The *dosage* is the amount of medicine that is prescribed for administration. The form of the drug can be liquid, solid, semisolid, tablet, capsule, transdermal therapeutic patch, etc. |
| | The *route of administration* can be by mouth, by injection, into the eye(s), ear(s), nostril(s), rectum, vagina, etc. It is important for the patient to know when and how to take a medication. |

# ABBREVIATIONS

| ABBREVIATION | MEANING | ABBREVIATION | MEANING |
|---|---|---|---|
| abd | abdomen, abdominal | HIPAA | Health Insurance Portability and Accountability Act of 1996 |
| A&P | anatomy and physiology | | |
| AP | anteroposterior | Ht | height |
| BP | blood pressure | Hx | history |
| CC | chief complaint | LAT, lat | lateral |
| CNS | central nervous system | LLQ | left lower quadrant |
| $CO_2$ | carbon dioxide | LUQ | left upper quadrant |
| CV | cardiovascular | O or $O_2$ | oxygen |
| DMD | Duchenne Muscular Dystrophy | OTC | over-the-counter (drugs) |
| DNA | deoxyribonucleic acid | PA | posteroanterior |
| DOB | date of birth | PE | physical examination |
| Dx | diagnosis | PHI | protected health information |
| ENT | ear, nose, throat (otorhinolaryngology) | resp | respiratory |
| | | RLQ | right lower quadrant |
| ER | endoplasmic reticulum (as used in this chapter); also means emergency room | RUQ | right upper quadrant |
| | | SS | Social Security |
| | | Sx | symptom |
| GI | gastrointestinal | T | temperature |
| $H_2O$ | water | TPR | temperature, pulse, respiration |
| HCT | hematocrit | Wt | weight |
| HHS | Health and Human Services | y/o | year(s) old |

# THE MEDICAL RECORD

The **medical record** is a written transcript of information about a patient and his or her health care. This record contains the observations, medical or surgical interventions, and treatment outcomes provided during hospitalization or a visit to a doctor's office. It includes information that the patient provides concerning his or her symptoms (Sx) and medical history, results of examinations, reports of x-rays and laboratory tests, diagnoses, and treatment plans.

This information is compiled and used by doctors, nurses, and other medical professionals to ensure that the patient receives quality health care. The physical medical record belongs to the health care provider, but the information in it belongs to the patient. The medical record serves as the following:

Basis for planning care and treatment
Means by which doctors, nurses, and others caring for the patient can communicate
Legal document describing the care the patient received
Means by which the patient or insurance company can verify that services billed were actually provided

In addition to information about physical health, these records may include information about family relationships, sexual behavior, substance abuse, and even private thoughts and feelings. This information is often keyed to a Social Security (SS) number and may be easily accessible to others because of a lack of consistent privacy protection in the use of Social Security numbers.

Information from medical records could influence one's credit, admission to educational institutions, and employment. It could also affect a person's ability to get health insurance or the rates paid for coverage. More important, having others know intimate details about a person's life can mean a loss of dignity and autonomy.

Over a decade ago, Congress called on the Department of Health and Human Services (HHS) to issue patient privacy protections as part of the Health Insurance Portability and Accountability Act (HIPAA), which was passed in 1996. HIPAA is a set of rules that doctors, hospitals, and other health care providers must follow to help ensure that all medical records, medical billing, and patient accounts meet certain consistent standards with regard to documentation, handling, and privacy. In addition, HIPAA requires that all patients be able to access their own medical records, correct errors or omissions, and be informed about how personal information is shared or used and about privacy procedures.

HIPAA also includes provisions designed to encourage electronic transactions and requires safeguards to protect the security and confidentiality of health information. It covers health plans, health care clearinghouses, and those health care providers who conduct certain financial and administrative transactions (e.g., enrollment, billing, and eligibility verification) electronically.

Under HIPAA Privacy Rule (45 CFR Parts 160 and 164), protected health information (PHI) is defined very broadly. PHI includes individually identifiable health information related to the past, present, or future physical or mental health or condition, the provision of health care to an individual, or the past, present, or future payment for the provision of health care to an individual. Even the fact that an individual received medical care is protected information under the regulation.

The Privacy Rule establishes a federal mandate for individual rights in health information, imposes restrictions on uses and disclosures of individually identifiable health information, and provides for civil and criminal penalties for violations. The complementary Security Rule includes standards for protection of health information in electronic form. For more information go to http://www.hhs.gov/ocr/hipaa.

## Types and Components of a Medical Record

There are various types of medical records. They can be kept on paper, **microfilm** (photographs of records in a reduced size), or **microfiche** (sheets of microfilm), or in electronic form. A patient's medical record is often referred to as a *chart* or *file*. The general components of a patient's medical record include the following:

**Patient Information Form.** Document that is filled out by the patient on the first visit to the physician's office and then updated as necessary, providing data that relates directly to the patient including last name, first name, gender, date of birth (DOB), marital status, street address, city, state, zip code, telephone number, Social Security number, employment status, address and phone number of employer, name and contact information for the person who is responsible for the patient's bill, and vital information concerning who should be contacted in case of an emergency

**Medical History (Hx).** Document describing past and current history of all medical conditions experienced by the patient

**Physical Examination (PE).** Record that includes a current head-to-toe assessment of the patient's physical condition

**Consent Form.** Signed document by the patient or legal guardian giving permission for treatment

**Informed Consent Form.** Signed document by the patient or legal guardian that explains the purpose, risks, and benefits of a procedure and serves as proof that the patient was properly informed before undergoing a procedure

**Physician's Orders.** Record of the prescribed care, medications, tests, and treatments for a given patient

**Nurse's Notes.** Record of a patient's care that includes vital signs, particularly temperature, pulse, and respiration (TPR) and blood pressure (BP), and treatments, procedures, and patient's responses to such care. See Figure 4–8 ▼.

**Physician's Progress Notes.** Documentation given by the physician regarding the patient's condition, results of the physician's examination, summary of test results, plan of treatment, and updating of data as appropriate (assessment and diagnosis (Dx))

**Consultation Reports.** Documentation given by specialists whom the physician has asked to evaluate the patient

**Ancillary/Miscellaneous Reports.** Documentation of procedures or therapies provided during a patient's care, such as physical therapy, respiratory therapy, or chemotherapy

**Diagnostic Tests/Laboratory Reports.** Documents providing the results of all diagnostic and laboratory tests performed on the patient

**Operative Report.** Documentation from the surgeon detailing the operation, including the preoperative and postoperative diagnosis, specific details of the surgical procedure, how well the patient tolerated the procedure, and any complications that occurred

**Anesthesiology Report.** Documentation from the attending anesthesiologist or anesthetist that includes a detailed account of anesthesia during surgery, which drugs were used, dose and time given, patient response, monitoring of vital signs, how well the patient tolerated the anesthesia, and any complications that occurred

**Pathology Report.** Documentation from the pathologist regarding the findings or results of samples taken from the patient, such as bone marrow, blood, or tissue

**Discharge Summary (also called Clinical Resumé, Clinical Summary, or Discharge Abstract).** Outline summary of the patient's hospital care, including date of admission, diagnosis, course of treatment and patient's response(s), results of tests, final diagnosis, follow-up plans, and date of discharge

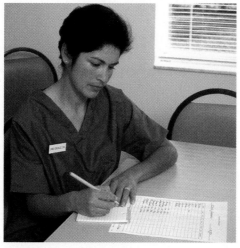

FIGURE 4–8 Nurse's notes.

## SOAP: Chart Note

**SOAP—subjective, objective, assessment, plan**—chart notes are written to improve communication among those caring for the patient. It is a method of displaying patient data in a concise, organized format. The four parts of a SOAP chart note follow:

1. **Subjective.** Symptoms that the subject (patient) feels and describes to the health care professional. These symptoms arise within the individual and are not perceptible to an observer. Examples include pain, nausea, dizziness, tightness in the chest, lump in the throat, weakness of the legs, and "butterflies" in the stomach. The health care professional can see the physical reaction of the patient to the symptom but not the actual symptom. Subjective symptoms can be verbally expressed by a parent or a significant other. For instance, "He runs very slow, has trouble climbing playground equipment and trouble getting up off the floor" or "She is so tired she can't get out of bed some mornings." Also included in the subjective section are any allergies as reported by the patient and the patient's chief complaint (CC).

2. **Objective.** Symptoms that can be observed, such as those that are seen, felt, smelled, heard, or measured. Included in the objective analysis are the vital signs (TPR and BP), data relating to the physical examination (PE) such as height (Ht), weight (Wt), general appearance, condition of the lungs, heart, abdomen, musculoskeletal and nervous systems, and the skin. The results of laboratory and diagnostic tests may also be included. It is common practice for the nurse or other medical professional assisting the physician to record the patient's vital signs, allergies, and chief complaint at the top of the chart.

3. **Assessment.** Includes the diagnosis of the patient's condition.

4. **Plan.** Includes the management and treatment regimen for the patient; may include laboratory tests, radiological tests, physical therapy, diet therapy, medications, medical and surgical interventions, patient referrals such as counseling and finding a support group, patient teaching, and follow-up directions.

A SOAP chart note should express current patient data, including the date of the visit, patient's name, date of birth, age, sex, and insurance carrier's name. See page 63 for an example of a SOAP: Chart Note.

# SOAP: Chart Note Example

**PATIENT:** Davis, Christopher                                            **DATE:** 01/15/2007
**DOB:** 11/24/2003        **AGE:** 3        **SEX:** Male
**INSURANCE:** Best Care Insurance

**Vital Signs:**
  **T:** 98.4 F
  **P:** 90
  **R:** 20
  **BP:** 85/60
  **Ht:** 3' 2"
  **Wt:** 36 lb
**Allergies:** penicillin
**Chief Complaint:** Waddling gait with increasing episodes of falling and apparent clumsiness. Activities of running and climbing very slowly in comparison to peers.

**S** | **Subjective:** Mother of 3 y/o white male states that she has noticed her son is beginning to appear "clumsy" with increasing episodes of falling. She has noticed that he looks like he is "waddling" when he walks. "He runs very slow, has trouble climbing playground equipment and trouble getting up off the floor. He isn't able to jump from a standing position, like his feet are glued to the floor. At times, he appears to be walking on his toes." She expresses concern that he did not learn to walk until after he was 18 months old, and that she is at risk for carrying the gene that causes muscular dystrophy.

**O** | **Objective:**
**General Appearance:** Pleasant child who exhibits no distress while sitting and playing on the floor. Noted difficulty rising from floor to standing position. Child used Gowers' maneuver to push himself upright.
**Lungs:** CTA
**Heart:** Normal rate and rhythm. No murmurs, gallops or rubs.
**Abd:** Bowel sounds all quadrants. Soft, no masses or tenderness.
**MS:** Abduction of arms to full 180° above head impaired, due to muscle weakness. Noted muscle weakness of bilateral lower extremities. No contractures with joint involvement. Calf muscles appear enlarged by connective tissue and fat. Upon palpation, felt "rubbery."
**Neuro:** Oriented to person and place. Reflexes intact.
**Skin:** Cool and moist, soft to touch. Noted generalized bruising at various stages on legs and arms.

**A** | **Assessment:** Duchenne Muscular Dystrophy (DMD)

**P** | **Plan:**
1. Schedule physical therapy to help delay permanent muscular contracture.
2. Recommend supportive measures such as splints and braces to minimize deformities and preserve mobility.
3. Recommend deep breathing exercises to help delay weakening of the muscles of respiration.
4. Suggest counseling and referral services as supportive measures for parent and child.
5. Provide the family with information on the Muscular Dystrophy Association, which is located 3561 E. Sunrise Drive, Tucson, AZ 85718. Telephone: 1-602-529-2000 or 1-800-572-1717. E-mail: mda@mdausa.org.

# STUDY AND REVIEW

## Anatomy and Physiology

*Write your answers to the following questions. Do not refer to the text.*

1. The _____ consist of millions of _____ working individually and with each other to _____ life.

2. The outer covering of the cell is known as the _____, which has the capability of allowing some substances to pass into and out of the cell.

3. The common parts of the cell are the _____, _____, and _____.

4. Three functions of the cell's nucleus are _____ _____, and _____.

5. An _____ is an unspecialized cell that can turn itself into any type of tissue.

6. List the four functions of epithelial tissue.

   a. _____   b. _____

   c. _____   d. _____

7. _____ tissue is the most widespread and abundant of the four body tissues.

8. Name the three types of muscle tissue.

   a. _____   b. _____   c. _____

9. Two properties of nerve tissue are _____ and _____.

10. Define *organ*. _____.

11. Define *body system*. _____.

12. Name the organ systems listed in this text.

   a. _____   b. _____

   c. _____   d. _____

   e. _____   f. _____

   g. _____   h. _____

   i. _____   j. _____

   k. _____

13. Define the following directional terms.

    a. superior _____      b. anterior _____

    c. posterior _____      d. cephalic _____

    e. medial _____      f. lateral _____

    g. proximal _____      h. distal _____

14. The _____ _____ vertically divides the body. It passes through the midline to form a right and left half.

15. The _____ plane is any plane that divides the body into superior and inferior portions.

16. The _____ plane is any plane that divides the body at right angles to the plane described in Question 14.

17. List the three distinct cavities that are located in the ventral cavity.

    a. _____     b. _____     c. _____

18. Name the two distinct cavities located in the dorsal cavity.

    a. _____     b. _____

## Word Parts

1. In the spaces provided, write the definition of these prefixes, roots, combining forms, and suffixes. Do not refer to the listings of medical words. Leave blank those words you cannot define.

2. After completing as many as you can, refer to the medical word listings to check your work. For each word missed or left blank, write the word and its definition several times on the margins of these pages or on a separate sheet of paper.

3. To maximize the learning process, it is to your advantage to do the following exercises as directed. To refer to the word-building section before completing these exercises invalidates the learning process.

## PREFIXES

*Give the definitions of the following prefixes.*

1. ambi- _____      2. ana- _____

3. bi- _____      4. chromo- _____

5. de- _____      6. dif- _____

7. ecto- _____     8. endo- _____

9. homeo- _____     10. meso- _____

11. per- _____     12. proto- _____

13. uni- _____     14. super- _____


## ROOTS AND COMBINING FORMS

*Give the definitions of the following roots and combining forms.*

1. adip _____     2. andr _____

3. bi/o _____     4. caud _____

5. cyt _____     6. cyt/o _____

7. fus _____     8. hist/o _____

9. hydr _____     10. kary/o _____

11. later _____     12. path/o _____

13. physi/o _____     14. pin/o _____

15. somat/o _____     16. topic _____

17. troph _____     18. viscer _____

19. anter _____     20. cran/i _____

21. dist _____     22. dors _____

23. filtrat _____     24. horizont _____

25. infer _____     26. inguin _____

27. intern _____     28. later _____

29. medi _____     30. organ _____

31. phen/o _____     32. poster _____

33. proxim _____     34. superfic/i _____

35. system _____     36. ventr _____


## SUFFIXES

*Give the definitions for the following suffixes.*

1. -al _____     2. -ate _____

3. -genesis _____     4. -ic _____

5. -ion _____

6. -logy _____

7. -morph _____

8. -oid _____

9. -ose _____

10. -plasm _____

11. -some _____

12. -stasis _____

13. -tomy _____

14. -ior _____

15. -ad _____

16. -type _____

## Identifying Medical Terms

*In the spaces provided, write the medical terms for the following meanings.*

1. _____ To resemble man

2. _____ Pertaining to two sides

3. _____ Study of cells

4. _____ Slender physical body form

5. _____ Formation of a cell's nucleus

6. _____ Pertaining to the stimulation of body growth

7. _____ Pertaining to one side

## Spelling

*In the spaces provided, write the correct spelling of these misspelled terms.*

1. adpose _____

2. caual _____

3. cytlogy _____

4. difusion _____

5. histlogy _____

6. mesmorph _____

7. prefusion _____

8. proxmal _____

9. somattrophic _____

10. unlateral _____

## Matching

*Select the appropriate lettered meaning for each of the following words.*

_____ 1. ambilateral

_____ 2. anatomy

_____ 3. atom

_____ 4. chromosome

_____ 5. cilia

_____ 6. homeostasis

_____ 7. human genome

_____ 8. phenotype

_____ 9. physiology

_____ 10. vertex

a. Hairlike processes that project from epithelial cells
b. Top or highest point
c. Pertaining to both sides
d. Study of the structure of an organism such as a human
e. Smallest, basic chemical unit of matter
f. Microscopic bodies that carry the genes that determine hereditary characteristics
g. Complete set of genes and chromosomes
h. Physical appearance or type of makeup of an individual
i. State of equilibrium maintained in the body's internal environment
j. Study of the nature of living organism
k. Study of disease

## Abbreviations

*Place the correct word, phrase, or abbreviation in the space provided.*

1. abdomen _____

2. A&P _____

3. CNS _____

4. cardiovascular _____

5. gastrointestinal _____

6. LAT, lat _____

7. resp _____

8. ER _____

9. AP _____

10. PA _____

## SOAP: Chart Note Exercise

*Write your answers to the following questions.*

1. Describe *medical record.* _____

_____

2. Define *HIPAA*. _____

3. List 15 general components of a patient's medical record.

   a. _____      b. _____

   c. _____      d. _____

   e. _____      f. _____

   g. _____      h. _____

   i. _____      j. _____

   k. _____      l. _____

   m. _____      n. _____

   o. _____

4. List the four parts of the SOAP chart note record.

   a. _____

   b. _____

   c. _____

   d. _____

5. Assessment includes the _____ of the patient's condition.

6. The _____ includes the management and treatment regimen for the patient.

# MULTIMEDIA PREVIEW

*Additional interactive resources and activities for this chapter can be found on the Companion Website. For videos, audio glossary, and review, access the accompanying CD-ROM in this book.*

## CD-ROM HIGHLIGHTS

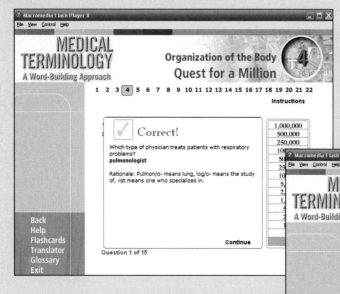

### QUEST FOR A MILLION

Who wants to win a million points? If it's you, then click on this game to begin your challenge. If you correctly answer 15 questions in a row, then you're a winner. But be very careful, because one wrong response will take you back down to zero.

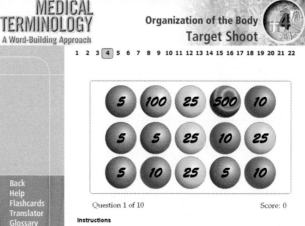

### TARGET SHOOTING

Here's a game that requires a quick mind and an even faster finger! As colored balls flash on your screen, click on the highest point values to reveal a question. A correct answer earns the points. How high can you score?

## WEBSITE HIGHLIGHTS—www.prenhall.com/rice

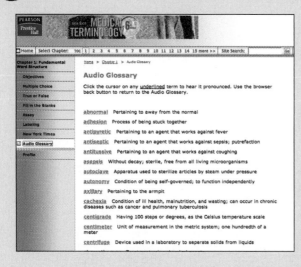

### AUDIO GLOSSARY

Click here and take advantage of the free-access on-line study guide that accompanies your textbook. You'll find an audio glossary with definitions and audio pronunciations for every term in the book. By clicking on this URL you'll also access a variety of quizzes with instant feedback, links to download mp3 audio reviews, and current news articles.

# Integumentary System

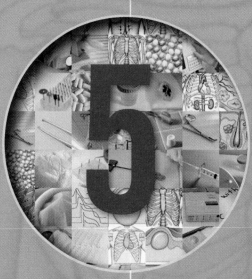

## OUTLINE

## OBJECTIVES

*On completion of this chapter, you will be able to:*

- Describe the integumentary system and its accessory structures.
- List the functions of the skin.
- Describe skin differences of the child and the older adult.
- Analyze, build, spell, and pronounce medical words.
- Comprehend the drugs highlighted in this chapter.
- Describe diagnostic and laboratory tests related to the integumentary system.
- Identify and define selected abbreviations.
- Describe each of the conditions presented in the Pathology Spotlights.
- Review the Pathology Checkpoint.
- Complete the Study and Review section and the Chart Note Analysis.

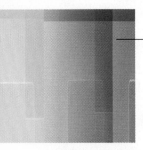

# Anatomy and Physiology Overview

The integumentary system is composed of the skin and its accessory structures: hair, nails, sebaceous glands, and sweat glands (see the following table). This overview of the anatomy and physiology of the skin offers a general description of the integumentary system as an aid to those learning the terminology associated with its functions.

## Integumentary System

| Organ/Structure | Primary Functions |
| --- | --- |
| Skin | Protection, regulation, sensation and secretion |
| Epidermis | Outer protective covering of the body |
| *Stratum corneum* | Forms protective covering for the body |
| *Stratum lucidum* | Translucent layer that is frequently absent and not seen in thinner skin |
| *Stratum granulosum* | Acts in the keratinization process, its cells become hard or horny |
| *Stratum germinativum* | Regenerates the epidermis |
| Dermis | Nourishes the epidermis, provides strength and supports blood vessels |
| *Papillae* | Produce ridges that are one's fingerprints |
| Subcutaneous tissue | Support, nourishes, insulates, and cushions the skin |
| Hair | Provides sensation and some protection for the head. Hair around the eyes, in the nose, and in the ears filters out foreign particles. |
| Nails | Protects ends of fingers and toes |
| Sebaceous (oil) glands | Lubricates the hair and skin |
| Sudoriferous (sweat) glands | Secretes sweat or perspiration, which helps to cool the body by evaporation. Sweat also rids the body of waste. |

# FUNCTIONS OF THE SKIN

The **skin** is the external covering of the body. In an average adult, it covers more than 3,000 square inches of surface area, weighs more than 6 pounds, and is the largest organ in the body. The skin is well supplied with blood vessels and nerves and has four main functions: protection, regulation, sensation, and secretion.

## Protection

The skin serves as a protective membrane against invasion by bacteria and other potentially harmful agents that could try to penetrate into deeper tissues. It also protects against mechanical injury of delicate cells located beneath its epidermis or outer covering. The skin also serves to inhibit excessive loss of water and electrolytes and provides a reservoir for storing food and water. The skin guards the body against excessive exposure to the sun's ultraviolet rays by producing a protective pigmentation, and it helps to produce the body's supply of vitamin D.

## Regulation

The skin serves to raise or lower body temperature as necessary. When the body needs to lose heat, the blood vessels in the skin dilate, bringing more blood to the surface for cooling by **radiation.** At the same time, the sweat glands are secreting more sweat for cooling by means of **evaporation.** Conversely, when the body needs to conserve heat, the reflex actions of the nervous system cause the skin's blood vessels to constrict, thereby allowing more heat-carrying blood to circulate to the muscles and vital organs.

## Sensation

The skin contains millions of microscopic nerve endings that act as **sensory receptors** for pain, touch, heat, cold, and pressure. When stimulation occurs, nerve impulses are sent to the cerebral cortex of the brain. The nerve endings in the skin are specialized according to the type of sensory information transmitted and, once this information reaches the brain, it triggers any necessary response. For example, touching a hot surface with the hand causes the brain to recognize the senses of **touch, heat,** and **pain** and results in the immediate removal of the hand from the hot surface.

## Secretion

The skin contains millions of sweat glands, which secrete **perspiration** or **sweat,** and **sebaceous glands,** which secrete **oil** (sebum) for lubrication. Perspiration is largely water with a small amount of salt and other chemical compounds. This secretion, when left to accumulate, causes body odor, especially where it is trapped among hairs in the axillary region. **Sebum,** is an oily secretion that acts to protect the body from dehydration and possible absorption of harmful substances.

# LAYERS OF THE SKIN

The skin is essentially composed of two layers, the epidermis and the dermis.

## The Epidermis

The **epidermis** can be divided into four strata: the stratum corneum, the stratum lucidum, the stratum granulosum, and the stratum germinativum. See Figure 5–1 ▶ for the locations of these strata within the epidermis.

### Stratum Corneum

The **stratum corneum** is the outermost, horny layer, consisting of dead cells filled with a protein substance called **keratin.** It forms the protective covering for the body, and its thickness varies with the use made of the particular body part. Because of the pressure on their surfaces during use, the soles of the feet and palms of the hands have thicker layers of stratum corneum than do the eyelids or the forehead.

### Stratum Lucidum

The **stratum lucidum** is a translucent layer lying directly beneath the stratum corneum. It is frequently absent and is not seen in thinner skin. Cells in this layer are also dead or dying.

### Stratum Granulosum

The **stratum granulosum** consists of several layers of living cells that are in the process of becoming a part of the previously mentioned strata. Its cells are active in the **keratinization** process, during which they lose their nuclei and become hard or horny.

### Stratum Germinativum

The **stratum germinativum** is composed of several layers of living cells capable of **mitosis,** or cell division. Sometimes called the **mucosum** or **malpighii,** the stratum germinativum is the innermost layer and is responsible for the regeneration of the epidermis. Damage to this layer, as in severe burns, necessitates the use of skin grafts. **Melanin,** the pigment that gives color to the skin, is formed in this layer. The more abundant the melanin, the darker the color of the skin.

## Dermis

Sometimes called the **corium** or **true skin,** the **dermis** is composed of connective tissue containing lymphatics, nerves and nerve endings, blood vessels, sebaceous and sweat

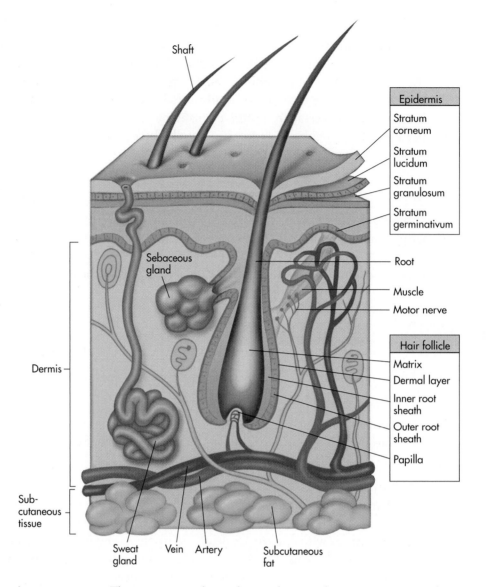

▶ **FIGURE 5–1** The integument: the epidermis, dermis, subcutaneous tissue, and its appendages.

glands, elastic fibers, and hair follicles. It is divided into two layers: the **upper layer** or **papillary layer** and the **lower layer** or **reticular layer.** The papillary layer is arranged into parallel rows of microscopic structures called **papillae,** which produce the ridges of the skin that are one's fingerprints or footprints. The reticular layer is composed of white fibrous tissue that supports the blood vessels. The dermis is attached to underlying structures by the **subcutaneous tissue.** This tissue supports, nourishes, insulates, and cushions the skin.

## ACCESSORY STRUCTURES OF THE SKIN

The hair, nails, sebaceous glands, and sweat glands are the accessory structures of the skin.

### Hair

A **hair** is a thin, threadlike structure formed by a group of cells that develop within a hair **follicle** or **socket.** Each hair is composed of a **shaft,** which is the visible portion, and a **root,** which is embedded within the follicle. At the base of each follicle is a loop of capillaries enclosed within connective tissue called the **hair papilla.** The **pilomotor muscle** attaches to the side of each follicle. When the skin is cooled or the individual has an emotional reaction, the skin often forms **"gooseflesh"** as a result of contraction by these muscles. Hair is distributed over the whole body with the exception of the palms of the hands and soles of the feet. It is thicker on the scalp and thinner on the other parts of the body. Hair around the eyes, in the nose, and in the ears serves to filter out foreign particles. The color of a person's hair is a product of genetic background and is determined by the amount of pigmentation within the hair shaft. Hair grows at approximately 0.5 inch a month, and its growth is not affected by cutting.

## Nails

**Fingernails** and **toenails** are horny cell structures of the epidermis and are composed of hard keratin. A nail consists of a **body**, a **root**, and a **matrix** or **nailbed** (Figure 5–2 ▼). The crescent-shaped white area of the nail is the **lunula.** Nail growth may vary with age, disease, and hormone deficiency. Average growth is 1 mm per week, and a lost fingernail usually regenerates in 3½ to 5½ months. A lost toenail may require 6 to 8 months for regeneration.

## Sebaceous (oil) Glands

The oil-secreting glands of the skin are called **sebaceous glands.** They have tiny ducts that open into the hair follicles, and their secretion, **sebum,** lubricates the hair as well as the skin. The amount of secretion is controlled by the endocrine system and varies with age, puberty, and pregnancy.

## Sudoriferous (sweat) Glands

Approximately 2 million **sweat glands** (coiled, tubular glands) are distributed over the entire surface of the body with the exception of the margin of the lips, glans penis, and the inner surface of the prepuce. They are more numerous on the palms of the hands, soles of the feet, forehead, and axillae. Sweat glands secrete sweat or perspiration, which helps to cool the body by evaporation. Sweat also rids the body of waste through the pores of the skin. Left to accumulate, sweat becomes odorous by the action of bacteria. The body loses about 0.5 L of fluid per day through sweat.

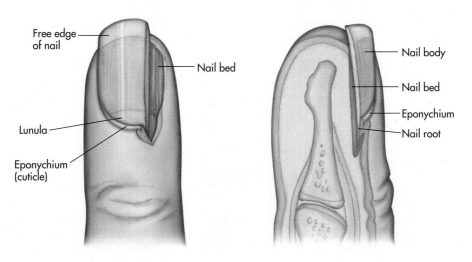

▶ **FIGURE 5–2** The fingernail, an appendage of the integument.

# LIFE SPAN CONSIDERATIONS

## ■ THE CHILD

**Vernix caseosa,** a cheeselike substance, covers the fetus until birth. At first, the fetal skin is transparent and blood vessels are clearly visible. In about 13 to 16 weeks, downy lanugo hair begins to develop, especially on the head. At 21 to 24 weeks, the skin is reddish and wrinkled and has little subcutaneous fat. At birth, the subcutaneous glands are developed, and the skin is smooth and pink. Preterm and term newborns have less subcutaneous fat than adults; therefore, they are more sensitive to heat and cold. Babies can blister easily.

Skin conditions can be acute or chronic, local or systemic, and some are congenital, such as strawberry nevi and Mongolian spots. Certain children's skin conditions are associated with age, such as milia in babies and acne in adolescents. **Milia** are white pinhead-size papules occurring on the face, and sometimes the trunk, of a newborn. They usually disappear in several weeks. **Acne** is an inflammatory condition of the sebaceous glands and the hair follicles (**pimples**). See Figure 5–3 ▼.

Skin infections in children generally produce systemic symptoms, such as fever and malaise. Sebaceous glands do not produce sebum until about 8 to 10 years of age; therefore, a child's skin is more dry and chaps easily.

The hair of the child will vary according to race, texture, quality, and distribution. A newborn could have no hair on its head or a head covered with hair. Hair can become dry and brittle, due to improper nutrition. During a severe illness, hair loss and color change can occur.

## ■ THE OLDER ADULT

With increasing years beyond reproductive maturity, the body begins the process of aging. By the year 2030, one in five people in the United States will be at least 65 years old. The process of aging varies with each individual. Aging is not a disease but a sequence of events regulated by complex processes.

As a person ages, the skin becomes looser as the dermal papilla grows less dense. Collagen and elastic fibers of the upper dermis decrease and skin loses its elastic tone and wrinkles more easily. Skin conditions are common in the older adult. Dryness (**xerosis**) and itching (**pruritus**) are common. Premalignant and malignant skin lesions increase with aging. Carcinomas appear frequently on the nose, eyelid, or cheek. **Basal cell carcinomas (BCC)** account for 80 percent of the skin cancers seen in the older adult. See Figure 5–4 ▼. These cancers are generally slow growing but should be surgically removed as soon as possible.

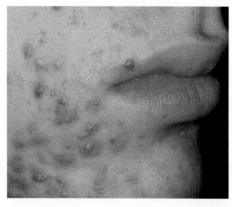

▶ **FIGURE 5–3** Acne. (Courtesy of Jason L. Smith, MD)

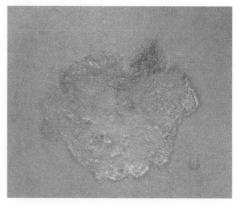

▶ **FIGURE 5–4** Basal cell carcinoma. (Courtesy of Jason L. Smith, MD)

By age 50, approximately half of all people have some gray hair. Scalp hair thins in women and men. The hair becomes dry and often brittle. Older women may have an increase in facial hair. Men may have an increase in hair of the nares (nostrils), eyebrows, or helix of the ear. In addition to the changes in the skin and hair, nails flatten and become discolored, dry, and brittle.

# BUILDING YOUR MEDICAL VOCABULARY

This section provides the foundation for learning medical terminology. Review the following alphabetized word list. Note how common prefixes and suffixes are repeatedly applied to word roots and combining forms to create different meanings.

| | |
|---|---|
| P | Prefix |
| R | Root |
| CF | Combining form |
| S | Suffix |

| | |
|---|---|
| Pink words | Terms not built from word parts. |
| * | Indicates words covered in the Pathology Spotlights section. |
| 💿 | Check the CD-ROM for more information. |

| MEDICAL WORD | WORD PARTS (WHEN APPLICABLE) | | | DEFINITION |
|---|---|---|---|---|
| | Part | Type | Meaning | |
| **acne**<br>(ăk′ nē) | | | | Inflammatory condition of the sebaceous glands and the hair follicles; *pimples*. See Figure 5–3 on page 76. |
| **acrochordon**<br>(ăk″ rō-kor′ dŏn) | acr/o<br>chord<br>-on | CF<br>R<br>S | extremity<br>cord<br>pertaining to | Small outgrowth of epidermal and dermal tissue; *skin tags* |
| **actinic dermatitis**<br>(ăk-tĭn′ ĭk dĕr″ mă-tī′ tĭs) | actin<br>-ic<br>dermat<br>-itis | R<br>S<br>R<br>S | ray<br>pertaining to<br>skin<br>inflammation | Inflammation of the skin caused by exposure to radiant energy, such as x-rays, ultraviolet light, and sunlight. See Figure 5–5 ▼. |

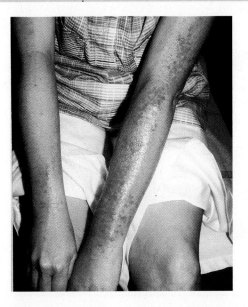

▶ **FIGURE 5–5**  Photodermatitis. (Courtesy of Jason L. Smith, MD)

| MEDICAL WORD | WORD PARTS (WHEN APPLICABLE) | | | DEFINITION |
|---|---|---|---|---|
| | Part | Type | Meaning | |
| **albinism**<br>(ăl′ bĭn-ĭsm) | albin<br>-ism | R<br>S | white<br>condition | Absence of pigment in the skin, hair, and eyes |
| **alopecia**<br>(al″ ō-pē′ shĭ-ă) | a-<br>lopec<br>-ia | P<br>R<br>S | without, lack of<br>fox mange<br>condition | Loss of hair, baldness; *alopecia areata* is loss of hair in defined patches usually involving the scalp. See Figure 5–6 ▼. Male pattern alopecia begins in the frontal area and proceeds until only a horseshoe area of the hair remains in the back and temples. See Figure 5–7 ▼. |
| **anhidrosis**<br>(ăn″ hī-drō′ sĭs) | an-<br>hidr<br>-osis | P<br>R<br>S | without, lack of<br>sweat<br>condition<br>(usually abnormal) | Condition in which there is a lack or complete absence of sweating |
| **autograft**<br>(ŏ-tō-grăft) | auto-<br>-graft | P<br>S | self<br>pencil, grafting knife | Graft taken from one part of the patient's body and transferred to another part |
| **avulsion**<br>(ă-vŭlshŭn) | a-<br>vuls<br>-ion | P<br>R<br>S | away from<br>to pull<br>process | Process of forcibly tearing off a part or structure of the body, such as a finger or toe |
| **basal cell carcinoma (BCC)**<br>(bā′ săl sel kăr″ sĭ-nō″ mă) | | | | Epithelial malignant tumor of the skin that rarely metastasizes. It usually begins as a small, shiny papule and enlarges to form a whitish border around a central depression. See Figure 5–4 on page 76. |
| **bite** | | | | Injury in which a part of the skin is torn by an insect, animal, or human, resulting in an abrasion, puncture, or laceration. See Figures 5–8 ▶, 5–9 ▶ and 5–10 ▶. |
| **boil** | | | | Acute, painful nodule formed in the subcutaneous layers of the skin, gland, or hair follicle; most often caused by the invasion of staphylococci; *furuncle* |

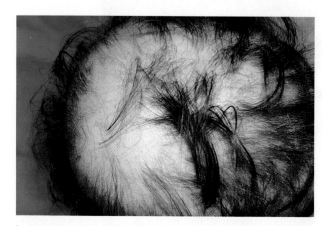

▶ **FIGURE 5–6**   Alopecia areata. (Courtesy of Jason L. Smith, MD)

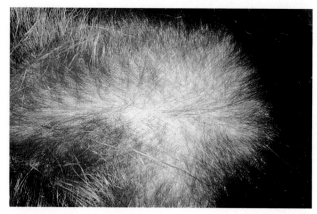

▶ **FIGURE 5–7**   Male pattern alopecia. (Courtesy of Jason L. Smith, MD)

| MEDICAL WORD | WORD PARTS (WHEN APPLICABLE) | | | DEFINITION |
|---|---|---|---|---|
| | Part | Type | Meaning | |
| **bulla**<br>(bŭl′ lă) | | | | Larger blister; *a bleb*. See Figure 5–11 ▼. |
| **burn** | | | | Injury to tissue caused by heat, fire, chemical agents, electricity, lightning, or radiation; classified according to degree or depth of skin damage. See Figure 5–12 ▼. ✱ See Pathology Spotlight: Burns on page 96. |
| **callus**<br>(kăl′ ŭs) | | | | Hardened skin |

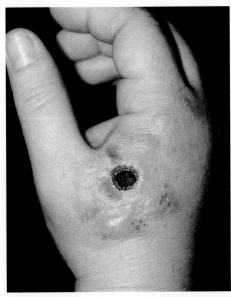

▶ FIGURE 5–8    Brown recluse spider bites. (Courtesy of Jason L. Smith, MD)

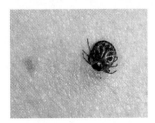

▶ FIGURE 5–9    Tick bite. (Courtesy of Jason L. Smith, MD)

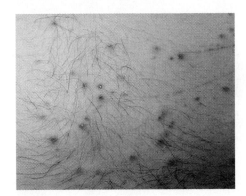

▶ FIGURE 5–10    Flea bites. (Courtesy of Jason L. Smith, MD)

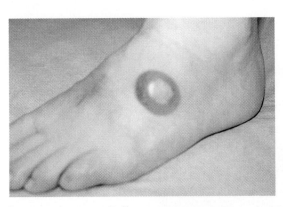

▶ FIGURE 5–11    Bulla. (Courtesy of Jason L. Smith, MD)

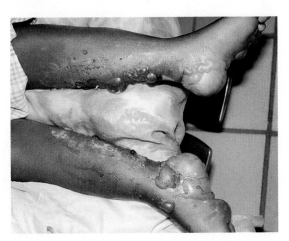

▶ FIGURE 5–12    Burn, second degree. (Courtesy of Jason L. Smith, MD)

| MEDICAL WORD | WORD PARTS (WHEN APPLICABLE) | | | DEFINITION |
|---|---|---|---|---|
| | Part | Type | Meaning | |
| **candidiasis**<br>(kǎn″ dǐ-dī′ ǎ-sǐs) | | | | Infection of the skin or mucous membranes with any species of *Candida* but chiefly *Candida albicans. Candida* is a genus of yeasts and was formerly called *Monilia.* See Figure 5–13 ▼. |
| **carbuncle**<br>(kǎr′ bǔng″ kl) | | | | Infection of the subcutaneous tissue, usually composed of a cluster of boils. See Figure 5–14 ▼. |
| **causalgia**<br>(kǒ-sǎl′ jǐ-ǎ) | caus<br>-algia | R<br>S | heat<br>pain | Intense burning pain associated with trophic skin changes in the hand or foot after trauma to the part |
| **cellulitis**<br>(sěl-ū-lī′ tǐs) | cellul<br>-itis | R<br>S | little cell<br>inflammation | Inflammation of cellular or connective tissue. See Figure 5–15 ▼. |
| **cicatrix**<br>(sǐk′ ǎ-trǐks) | | | | Scar left after the healing of a wound |

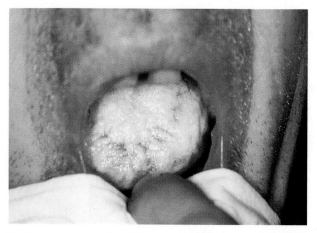

▶ **FIGURE 5–13** Candidiasis. (Courtesy of Jason L. Smith, MD)

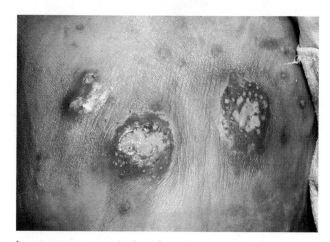

▶ **FIGURE 5–14** Carbuncles. (Courtesy of Jason L. Smith, MD)

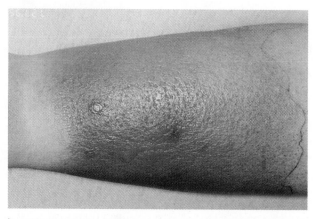

▶ **FIGURE 5–15** Cellulitis. (Courtesy of Jason L. Smith, MD)

| MEDICAL WORD | WORD PARTS (WHEN APPLICABLE) | | | DEFINITION |
|---|---|---|---|---|
| | Part | Type | Meaning | |
| **comedo** (kŏm′ ē-dō) | | | | Blackhead |
| **corn** (korn) (ko(e)rn) | | | | Horny induration and thickening of the skin on the toes caused by ill-fitting shoes |
| **cryosurgery** (krī″ ō-sĕr′ jĕr-ē) | | | | Technique of using subfreezing temperature (usually with liquid nitrogen) to produce well-demarcated areas of cell injury and destruction |
| **cutaneous** (kū-tā′ nē-ŭs) | cutane -ous | R S | skin pertaining to | Pertaining to the skin |
| **cyst** (sĭst) | | | | Closed sac that contains fluid, semifluid, or solid material |
| **debridement** (da-brē-mōn) | | | | Removal of foreign material or damaged or dead tissue, especially in a wound. It is used to promote healing and to prevent infection. |
| **decubitus (decub)** (dē-kū′ bĭ-tŭs) | de- cubit -us | P R S | down to lie pertaining to | Literally means *a lying down;* a bedsore. ✱ See Pathology Spotlight: Decubitus Ulcer on page 93. |
| **dehiscence** (dē-hĭs′ ĕns) | | | | Separation or bursting open of a surgical wound. See Figure 5–16 ▼. |
| **dermabrasion** (dĕrm′ ă-brā″zhŭn) | | | | Surgical procedure to remove acne scars, nevi, tattoos, or fine wrinkles on the skin by using sandpaper, wire brushes, or other abrasive materials on an anesthetized epidermis |
| **dermatitis** (dĕr″ mă-ti′ tĭs) | dermat -itis | R S | skin inflammation | Inflammation of the skin. See Figure 5–17 ▼. |

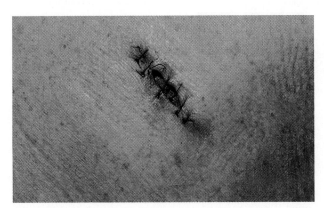

▶ **FIGURE 5–16** Wound dehiscence, back. (Courtesy of Jason L. Smith, MD)

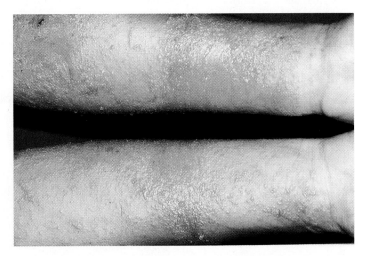

▶ **FIGURE 5–17** Dermatitis; poison ivy. (Courtesy of Jason L. Smith, MD)

| MEDICAL WORD | WORD PARTS (WHEN APPLICABLE) | | | DEFINITION |
|---|---|---|---|---|
| | Part | Type | Meaning | |
| **dermatologist** <br>(dĕr′ mah-tol′ŏ-jĭst) | dermat/o <br>log <br>-ist | CF <br>R <br>S | skin <br>study of <br>one who specializes | Physician who specializes in the study of the skin |
| **dermatology (Derm)** <br>(dĕr″ mah-tol′ ŏ-jē) | dermat/o <br>-logy | CF <br>S | skin <br>study of | Study of the skin |
| **dermatome** <br>(dĕr″ mah-tōm) | derm/a <br>-tome | CF <br>S | skin <br>instrument to cut | Instrument used to cut the skin for grafting |
| **dermomycosis** <br>(dĕr′ mō-mī-kō′ sĭs) | derm/o <br>myc <br>-osis | CF <br>R <br>S | skin <br>fungus <br>condition (usually abnormal) | Skin condition caused by a fungus |
| **ecchymosis** <br>(ĕk-ĭ-mō′ sĭs) | ec- <br>chym <br>-osis | P <br>R <br>S | out <br>juice <br>condition (usually abnormal) | Condition in which the blood seeps into the skin causing discolorations ranging from blue-black to greenish yellow |
| **eczema** <br>(ĕk′ zĕ-mă) | | | | Inflammatory skin disease of the epidermis. ✱ See Pathology Spotlight: Eczema on page 93. |
| **erythema** <br>(ĕr″ ĭ-thē′ mă) | | | | Redness of the skin; may be caused by capillary congestion, inflammation, heat, sunlight, or cold temperature. *Erythema infectiosum* is known as Fifth disease, a mild, moderately contagious disease caused by the human parvovirus B-19. It is most commonly seen in school-age children and is thought to be spread via respiratory secretions from infected persons. See Figure 5–18 ▼. |
| **erythroderma** <br>(ĕ-rĭth″ rō-dĕr′-mă) | erythr/o <br>-derma | CF <br>S | red <br>skin | Abnormal redness of the skin occurring over widespread areas of the body. |
| **eschar** <br>(ĕs′ kăr) | | | | Slough, scab |

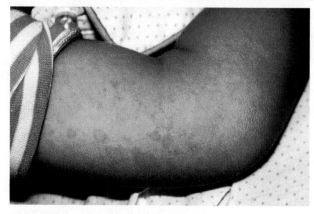

▶ FIGURE 5–18  Erythema infectiosum (Fifth disease). (Courtesy of Jason L. Smith, MD)

| MEDICAL WORD | WORD PARTS (WHEN APPLICABLE) | | | DEFINITION |
|---|---|---|---|---|
| | **Part** | **Type** | **Meaning** | |
| **excoriation** (ĕks-kō" rē-ā' shŭn) | ex- coriat -ion | P R S | out corium process | Abrasion of the epidermis by scratching, trauma, chemicals, burns, etc. |
| **exudate** (ĕks' ū-dāt) | | | | Production of pus or serum |
| **folliculitis** (fō-lĭk" ū-lī' tĭs) | follicul -itis | R S | little bag inflammation | Inflammation of a follicle or follicles. See Figure 5–19 ▼. |
| **gangrene** (găng'grēn) | | | | Literally means *an eating sore*. It is a necrosis, or death, of tissue or bone that usually results from a deficient or absent blood supply to the area. |
| **herpes simplex** (hĕr' pēz sĭm' plĕks) | | | | An inflammatory skin disease caused by a herpes virus (Type I); *cold sore or fever blister*. See Figure 5–20 ▼. |
| **hidradenitis** (hī-drăd-ĕ-nī' tĭs) | hidr aden -itis | R R S | sweat gland inflammation | Inflammation of the sweat glands |
| **hives** (hīvz) | | | | Eruption of itching and burning swellings on the skin; *urticaria*. See Figure 5–21 ▶. |
| **hyperhidrosis** (hī" pĕr-hī-drō' sĭs) | hyper- hidr -osis | P R S | excessive sweat condition (usually abnormal) | Condition of excessive sweating |
| **hypodermic** (hī" pō-dĕr' mĭk) | hypo- derm -ic | P R S | under skin pertaining to | Pertaining to under the skin or inserted under the skin, as a hypodermic injection |

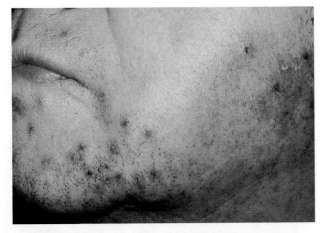

▶ **FIGURE 5–19** Staphylococcal folliculitis. (Courtesy of Jason L. Smith, MD)

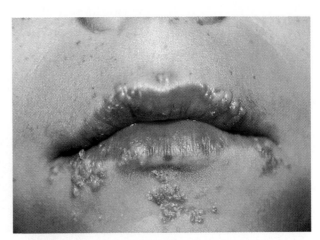

▶ **FIGURE 5–20** Herpes labialis. (Courtesy of Jason L. Smith, MD)

| MEDICAL WORD | WORD PARTS (WHEN APPLICABLE) | | | DEFINITION |
|---|---|---|---|---|
| | **Part** | **Type** | **Meaning** | |
| **icteric**<br>(ik-tĕr′ ik) | icter<br>-ic | R<br>S | jaundice<br>pertaining to | Pertaining to jaundice |
| **impetigo**<br>(ĭm″ pĕ-tī′ gō) | | | | Skin infection marked by vesicles or bullae; usually caused by streptococci or staphylococci. See Figure 5–22 ▼. |
| **integumentary**<br>(ĭn-tĕg″ ū-mĕn′ tă-rē) | integument<br>-ary | R<br>S | a covering<br>pertaining to | Covering; the skin, consisting of the dermis and the epidermis |
| **intradermal (ID)**<br>(in″ trăh-dĕr′ măl) | intra-<br>derm<br>-al | P<br>R<br>S | within<br>skin<br>pertaining to | Pertaining to within the skin, as an intradermal injection |
| **jaundice**<br>(jawn′ dĭs) | jaund<br>-ic(e) | R<br>S | yellow<br>pertaining to | Yellow; a symptom of a disease in which there is excessive bile in the blood; the skin, whites of the eyes, and mucous membranes are yellow; *icterus* |
| **keloid**<br>(kē′ lŏyd) | kel<br>-oid | R<br>S | tumor<br>resemble | Overgrowth of scar tissue caused by excessive collagen formation. See Figure 5–23 ▼. |
| **lentigo**<br>(lĕn-tī′ gō) | | | | A flat, brownish spot on the skin sometimes caused by exposure to the sun and weather; *freckle* |

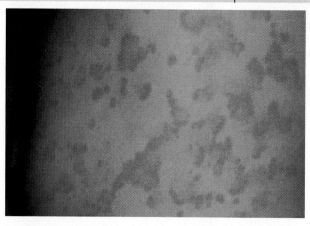

▶ **FIGURE 5–21** Urticaria (hives). (Courtesy of Jason L. Smith, MD)

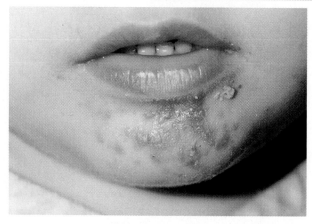

▶ **FIGURE 5–22** Impetigo. (Courtesy of Jason L. Smith, MD)

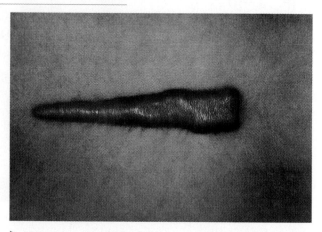

▶ **FIGURE 5–23** Keloid. (Courtesy of Jason L. Smith, MD)

| MEDICAL WORD | WORD PARTS (WHEN APPLICABLE) | | | DEFINITION |
|---|---|---|---|---|
| | Part | Type | Meaning | |
| **leukoderma**<br>(lū″ kō-děr′ mă) | leuk/o<br>-derma | CF<br>S | white<br>skin | Localized loss of pigmentation of the skin |
| **leukoplakia**<br>(lū″ kō-plā′ kē-ă) | leuk/o<br>plak<br>-ia | CF<br>R<br>S | white<br>plate<br>condition | White spots or patches formed on the mucous membrane of the tongue or cheek; the spots are smooth, hard, and irregular in shape and can become malignant |
| **lupus**<br>(lū′ pŭs) | | | | Originally used to describe a destructive type of skin lesion; current usage of the word is usually in combination with the words *vulgaris* or *erythematosus: lupus vulgaris* or *lupus erythematosus* |
| **melanocarcinoma**<br>(měl″ ă-nō-kar″ sĭn-ō′ mă) | melan/o<br>carcin<br>-oma | CF<br>R<br>S | black<br>cancer<br>tumor | Cancerous tumor that has black pigmentation |
| **melanoma**<br>(měl″ ă-nō′ mă) | melan<br>-oma | R<br>S | black<br>tumor | Malignant black mole or tumor. ✳ See in Pathology Spotlight: Skin Cancer on page 95 and Figure 5–40. |
| **miliaria**<br>(mĭl-ē-ā′ rē-ă) | miliar<br>-ia | R<br>S | millet (tiny)<br>condition | Called *prickly heat;* commonly seen in newborns and/or infants. It is caused by excessive body warmth. There is retention of sweat in the sweat glands, which have become blocked or inflamed, and then rupture or leak into the skin. *Miliaria* appears as a rash with tiny pinhead sized papules, vesicles, and/or pustules. See Figure 5–24 ▼. |
| **mole**<br>(mōl) | | | | Pigmented, elevated spot above the surface of the skin; a *nevus.* See Figure 5–25 ▼. |
| **onychitis**<br>(ŏn″ ĭ-kī′ tĭs) | onych<br>-itis | R<br>S | nail<br>inflammation | Inflammation of the nail |

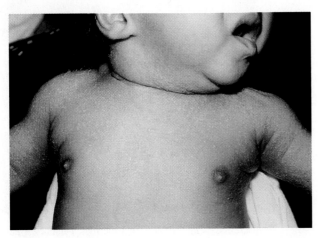

▶ FIGURE 5–24   Miliaria. (Courtesy of Jason L. Smith, MD)

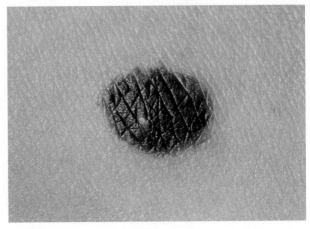

▶ FIGURE 5–25   Nevus (mole). (Courtesy of Jason L. Smith, MD)

| MEDICAL WORD | WORD PARTS (WHEN APPLICABLE) | | | DEFINITION |
|---|---|---|---|---|
| | Part | Type | Meaning | |
| **onychomycosis**<br>(ŏn″ ĭ-kō-mī-kō′ sĭs) | onych/o<br>myc<br>-osis | CF<br>R<br>S | nail<br>fungus<br>condition (usually<br>abnormal) | Condition of the nail caused by a fungus.<br>See Figure 5–26 ▼. |
| **pachyderma**<br>(păk-ē-der′ mă) | pachy<br>-derma | R<br>S | thick<br>skin | Thick skin |
| **paronychia**<br>(păr″ ō-nĭk′ ĭ-ă) | par-<br>onych<br>-ia | P<br>R<br>S | around<br>nail<br>condition | Infectious condition of the marginal<br>structures around the nail |
| **pediculosis**<br>(pĕ-dĭk″ ū-lō′ sĭs) | pedicul<br>-osis | R<br>S | a louse<br>condition<br>(usually abnormal) | Condition of infestation with lice. See<br>Figure 5–27 ▼. |
| **petechiae**<br>(pē-tē′ kĭ-ē) | | | | Small, pinpoint, purplish hemorrhagic<br>spots on the skin |
| **pruritus**<br>(proo-rī′ tŭs) | prurit<br>-us | R<br>S | itching<br>pertaining to | Severe itching |
| **psoriasis**<br>(sō-rī′ ă-sĭs) | | | | Chronic skin disease characterized by pink<br>or dull-red lesions surmounted by silvery<br>scaling. ✳ See Pathology Spotlight:<br>Psoriasis on page 94 and Figure 5–39. |
| **purpura**<br>(pur′ pū-ra) | | | | Purplish discoloration of the skin caused<br>by extravasation of blood into the tissues.<br>See Figure 5–28 ▶. |
| **rhytidoplasty**<br>(rĭt′ ĭ-dō-plăs″ tē) | rhytid/o<br>-plasty | CF<br>S | wrinkle<br>surgical repair | Plastic surgery for the removal of wrinkles |
| **roseola**<br>(rō-zē′ ō-lă) | | | | Any rose-colored rash marked by *maculae*<br>or red spots on the skin. See Figure<br>5–29 ▶. |

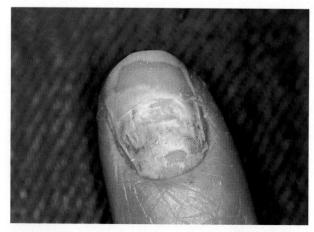

▶ **FIGURE 5–26**   Onychomycosis. (Courtesy of Jason L. Smith, MD)

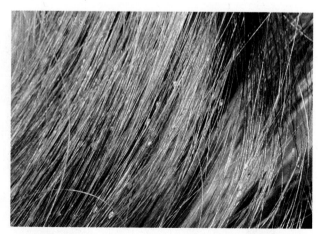

▶ **FIGURE 5–27**   Pediculosis capitis. (Courtesy of Jason L. Smith, MD)

| MEDICAL WORD | WORD PARTS (WHEN APPLICABLE) | | | DEFINITION |
|---|---|---|---|---|
| | Part | Type | Meaning | |
| **rubella** (roo-bĕl′ lă) | | | | Systemic disease caused by a virus and characterized by a rash and fever; also called *German measles* and *three-day measles* |
| **rubeola** (roo-bē′ ō-lă) | | | | Contagious disease characterized by fever, inflammation of the mucous membranes, and rose-colored spots on the skin; also called *measles* |
| **scabies** (skā′ bēz) or (skā′ bĭ-ēz) | | | | Contagious skin disease characterized by papules, vesicles, pustules, burrows, and intense itching; it is caused by the itch mite and is also called *the itch*. See Figure 5–30 ▼. |
| **scar** | | | | Mark left by the healing process of a wound, sore, or injury |
| **scleroderma** (skli rō-dĕr′ mă) | scler/o -derma | CF S | hard skin | Chronic condition with hardening of the skin and other connective tissues of the body |

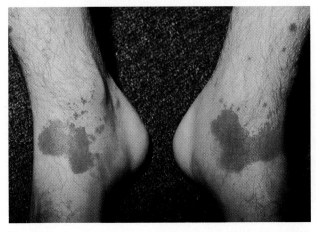

▶ **FIGURE 5–28**  Purpura. (Courtesy of Jason L. Smith, MD)

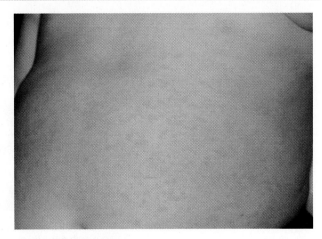

▶ **FIGURE 5–29**  Roseola. (Courtesy of Jason L. Smith, MD)

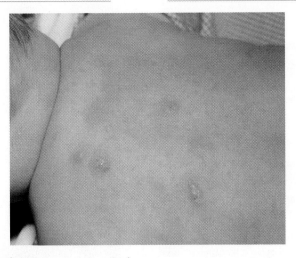

▶ **FIGURE 5–30**  Scabies. (Courtesy of Jason L. Smith, MD)

| MEDICAL WORD | WORD PARTS (WHEN APPLICABLE) | | | DEFINITION |
|---|---|---|---|---|
| | Part | Type | Meaning | |
| **seborrhea**<br>(sĕb″ or-ē′ ă) | seb/o<br>-rrhea | CF<br>S | oil<br>flow | Excessive flow of oil from the sebaceous glands |
| **sebum**<br>(sē′ bŭm) | | | | Fatty or oily secretion produced by the sebaceous glands |
| **senile keratosis**<br>(sĕn′ ĭl kĕr″ ă-tō′ sĭs) | senile<br>kerat<br>-osis | R<br>R<br>S | old<br>horn<br>condition<br>(usually abnormal) | Condition occurring in older people wherein there is dry skin and localized scaling caused by excessive exposure to the sun. See Figure 5–31 ▼. |
| **squamous cell carcinoma (SCC)**<br>(skwā′ mŭs sel kăr sĭ-nō′ mă) | | | | Malignant tumor of squamous epithelial tissue. See Figure 5–32 ▼. |
| **striae (plural)**<br>(strī′ ē) | | | | Streaks or lines on the breasts, thighs, abdomen, or buttocks caused by weakening of elastic tissue. See Figure 5–33 ▼. |

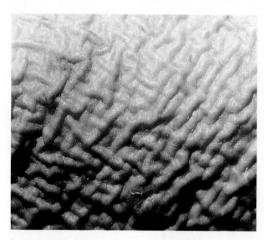

▶ **FIGURE 5–31**  Photoaging solar elastosis; senile keratosis. (Courtesy of Jason L. Smith, MD)

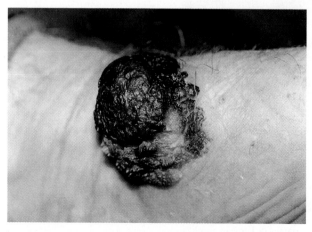

▶ **FIGURE 5–32**  Squamous cell carcinoma. (Courtesy of Jason L. Smith, MD)

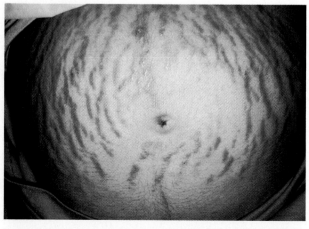

▶ **FIGURE 5–33**  Striae. (Courtesy of Jason L. Smith, MD)

| MEDICAL WORD | WORD PARTS (WHEN APPLICABLE) | | | DEFINITION |
|---|---|---|---|---|
| | Part | Type | Meaning | |
| **subcutaneous** **(Sub-Q, sub Q)** (sŭb kū-tā′ nē-ŭs) | sub- cutane -ous | P R S | below skin pertaining to | Pertaining to below the skin, as a subcutaneous injection |
| **subungual** (sŭb-ŭng′ gwăl) | sub- ungu -al | P R S | below nail pertaining to | Pertaining to below the nail |
| **taut** (tŏt) | | | | Tight, firm; to pull or draw tight a surface, such as the skin |
| **telangiectasia** (tĕl-ăn″ jē-ĕk-tā′ zē-ă) | tel ang/i -ectasia | R CF S | end, distant vessel dilatation | Dilatation of small blood vessels that may appear as a *birthmark* |
| **thermanesthesia** (thĕrm″ ăn-ĕs-thē′ zē-ă) | therm an- -esthesia | R P S | hot, heat without, lack of sensation | Inability to distinguish between the sensations of heat and cold |
| **tinea** (tĭn′ ē-ă) | | | | Contagious skin diseases affecting both humans and domestic animals, caused by certain fungi, and marked by the localized appearance of discolored, scaly patches on the skin; also called *ringworm*. See Figure 5–34 ▼. |
| **trichomycosis** (trĭk″ō-mi-kō′ sĭs) | trich/o myc -osis | CF R S | hair fungus condition (usually abnormal) | Fungal condition of the hair |
| **ulcer** (ŭl′ sĕr) | | | | Open lesion or sore of the epidermis or mucous membrane. See Figure 5–35 ▼. |

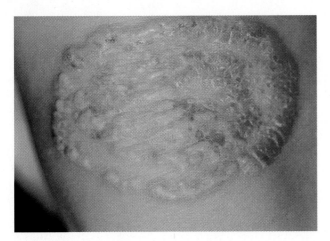

▶ **FIGURE 5–34**   Tinea corporis. (Courtesy of Jason L. Smith, MD)

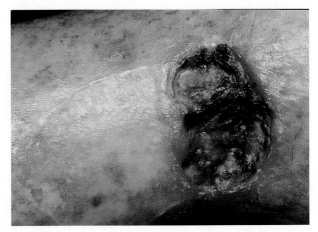

▶ **FIGURE 5–35**   Leg ulcer radiation site. (Courtesy of Jason L. Smith, MD)

| MEDICAL WORD | WORD PARTS (WHEN APPLICABLE) | | | DEFINITION |
|---|---|---|---|---|
| | Part | Type | Meaning | |
| **varicella**<br>(văr″i-sĕl′ ă) | | | | Contagious viral disease characterized by fever, headache, and a crop of red spots that become macules, papules, vesicles, and crusts; also called *chickenpox.* See Figure 5–36 ▼. |
| **vitiligo**<br>(vĭt″ ĭl-ĭ′ gō) | | | | Skin condition characterized by milk-white patches surrounded by areas of normal pigmentation |
| **wart** | | | | Elevation of viral origin on the epidermis; *verruca.* A plantar wart, known as *verruca plantaris,* occurs on a pressure-bearing area, especially the sole of the foot. See Figure 5–37 ▼. |
| **wound**<br>(woond) | | | | Injury to soft tissue caused by trauma; generally classified as open or closed |
| **xanthoderma**<br>(zăn″ thō-dĕr′ mă) | xanth/o<br>-derma | CF<br>S | yellow<br>skin | Yellow skin |
| **xanthoma**<br>(zăn-thō′ mă) | xanth<br>-oma | R<br>S | yellow<br>tumor | Yellow tumor |
| **xeroderma**<br>(zē″ rō-dĕr′ mă) | xer/o<br>-derma | CF<br>S | dry<br>skin | Dry skin |
| **xerosis**<br>(zē-rō′ sĭs) | xer<br>-osis | R<br>S | dry<br>condition<br>(usually abnormal) | Abnormal dryness of skin, mucous membranes, or the conjunctiva |

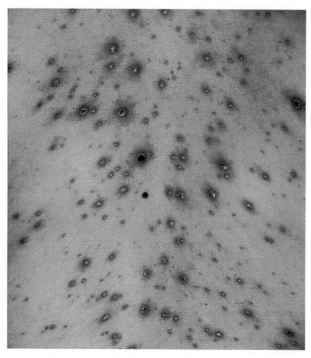

▶ **FIGURE 5–36** Varicella (chickenpox). (Courtesy of Jason L. Smith, MD)

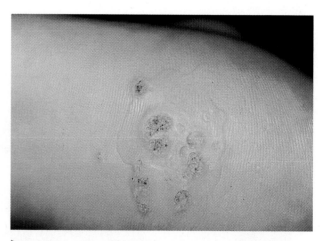

▶ **FIGURE 5–37** Plantar wart. (Courtesy of Jason L. Smith, MD)

# DRUG HIGHLIGHTS

| | |
|---|---|
| **Emollients** | Substances that are generally oily in nature. These substances are used for dry skin caused by aging, excessive bathing, and psoriasis.<br><br>*Examples: Dermassage and Desitin* |
| **Keratolytics** | Agents that cause or promote loosening of horny (keratin) layers of the skin. These agents may be used for acne, warts, psoriasis, corns, calluses, and fungal infections.<br><br>*Examples: Duofilm, Keralyt, and Compound W* |
| **Local anesthetic agents** | Agents that inhibit the conduction of nerve impulses from sensory nerves and thereby reduce pain and discomfort. These agents may be used topically to reduce discomfort associated with insect bites, burns, and poison ivy.<br><br>*Examples: Solarcaine, Xylocaine, and Dyclone* |
| **Antihistamine agents** | Agents that act to prevent the action of histamine. Used to help relieve symptoms, such as itching, in allergic responses and contact dermatitis.<br><br>*Example: diphenhydramine (Benadryl)* |
| **Antipruritic agents** | Agents that prevent or relieve itching.<br><br>*Examples: Topical—PBZ (tripelennamine HCl); Oral—Benadryl (diphenhydramine HCl) and Atarax (hydroxyzine HCl)* |
| **Antibiotic agents** | Agents that destroy or stop the growth of microorganisms. These agents are used to prevent infection associated with minor skin abrasions and to treat superficial skin infections and acne. Several antibiotic agents are combined in a single product to take advantage of the different antimicrobial spectrum of each drug.<br><br>*Examples: Neosporin, Polysporin, and Mycitracin* |
| **Antifungal agents** | Agents that destroy or inhibit the growth of fungi and yeast. These agents are used to treat fungus and/or yeast infection of the skin, nails, and scalp.<br><br>*Examples: Fungizone (amphotericin B), Lotrimin (clotrimazole) and Lamisil (terbinafine)* |
| **Antiviral agents** | Agents that combat specific viral diseases. Zovirax (acyclovir) is used in the treatment of herpes simplex virus types 1 and 2, varicella-zoster, Epstein-Barr, and cytomegalovirus. *Relenza (zanamivir)* has antiviral activity against influenza A and B viruses. |
| **Anti-inflammatory agents** | Agents used to relieve the swelling, tenderness, redness, and pain of inflammation. Topically applied corticosteroids are used in the treatment of dermatitis and psoriasis.<br><br>*Examples: Hydrocortisone, Decadron (dexamethasone), and Temovate (clobetasol propionate)*<br><br>Oral corticosteroids are used in the treatment of contact dermatitis, such as in poison ivy, when the symptoms are severe.<br><br>*Example: Sterapred (prednisone) 12-day unipak* |
| **Antiseptic agents** | Agents that prevent or inhibit the growth of pathogens. Antiseptics are generally applied to the surface of living tissue.<br><br>*Examples: Isopropyl alcohol and Zephrian (benzalkonium chloride)* |

| Other drugs | *Retin-A (tretinoin)* is available as a cream, gel, or liquid. It is used in the treatment of acne vulgaris. |
|---|---|
| | *Rogaine (minoxidil)* is available as a topical solution to stimulate hair growth. It was first approved as a treatment of male pattern baldness. |
| | *Botulinum Toxin Type A (Botox Cosmetic)* is approved by the FDA to temporarily improve the appearance of moderate to severe frown lines between the eyebrows (glabellar lines). Small doses of a sterile, purified botulinum toxin are injected into the affected muscles and block the release of the chemical acetylcholine that would otherwise signal the muscle to contract. The toxin thus temporarily paralyzes or weakens the injected muscle. |

# DIAGNOSTIC AND LAB TESTS

| TEST | DESCRIPTION |
|---|---|
| **Tuberculosis skin tests** (tū-bĕr″ kū-lō′ sĭs) | Performed to identify the presence of the *Tubercle bacilli*. The tine, Heaf, or Mantoux test are used. The tine and Heaf tests are intradermal tests performed using a sterile, disposable, multiple-puncture lancet. The tuberculin is on metal tines that are pressed into the skin. A hardened raised area at the test site 48 to 72 hours later indicates the presence of the pathogens in the blood.<br><br>In the Mantoux test 0.1 mL of purified protein derivative (PPD) tuberculin is intradermally injected. Test results are read 48 to 72 hours after administration. |
| **Scratch (epicutaneous) or prick test** (skrăch) | Involves the placement of a suspected allergen in the uppermost layers of the epidermis. One technique used is to place a drop of the allergen on the skin of the forearm or back. Pass a sterile lancet or needle through the drop, and prick the skin no deeper than the uppermost layers of the epidermis. Redness or swelling at the scratch site within 10 minutes indicates allergy to the substance. This indicates that the test result is positive. If no reaction occurs, the test result is negative. |
| **Sweat test (chloride)** (swĕt) | Performed on sweat to determine the level of chloride concentration on the skin. In **cystic fibrosis**, there is an increase in skin chloride. |
| **Tzanck test** (tsănk) | Microscopic examination of a small piece of tissue that has been surgically scraped from a pustule. The specimen is placed on a slide and stained, and the type of viral infection can be identified. |
| **Wound culture** (woond) | Performed on wound exudate to determine the presence of microorganisms. An effective antibiotic can be prescribed for identified microbes. |
| **Biopsy (skin)** (bī′ ŏp-sē) | Excision and micropic examination of any skin lesion that exhibits signs or characteristics of malignancy to establish a diagnosis. Usually only a small piece of living tissue is needed for examination. |

# ABBREVIATIONS

| ABBREVIATION | MEANING | ABBREVIATION | MEANING |
|---|---|---|---|
| BCC | basal cell carcinoma | SG | skin graft |
| Bx | biopsy | SLE | systemic lupus erythematosus |
| decub | decubitus | | |
| Derm | dermatology | SCC | squamous cell carcinoma |
| FB | foreign body | staph | staphylococcus |
| FUO | fever of undetermined origin | STD | skin test done |
| | | strep | streptococcus |
| HCl | hydrochloric acid | STSG | split thickness skin graft |
| Hx | history | Sub-Q, sub Q | subcutaneous |
| ID | intradermal | TIMs | topical immunomodulators |
| I&D | incision and drainage | | |
| NPUAP | National Pressure Ulcer Advisory Panel | ung | ointment |
| | | UV | ultraviolet |
| PUVA | psoralen-ultraviolet light | | |

# PATHOLOGY SPOTLIGHTS

## ✱ Decubitus Ulcer

Also known as a *bedsore* or *pressure ulcer*, a **decubitus ulcer** is an area of skin and tissue that becomes injured or broken down. See the Skin Signs section on page 96, as well as Figure 5–41. The literal meaning of the word *decubitus* is a *lying down*. This meaning points to what causes a decubitus (pressure) ulcer: When a person is in a sitting or lying position for too long without shifting his or her weight, the constant pressure against the tissue causes a decreased blood supply to that area. Without a blood supply, the affected tissue dies. The most common places for pressure ulcers are over bony prominences such as elbows, heels, hips, ankles, shoulders, the back, and the back of the head.

The National Pressure Ulcer Advisory Panel (NPUAP) created a system for evaluating pressure sores (see Figure 5–38 ▶), which is based on a staging system from Stage I (earliest signs) to Stage IV (worst):

**Stage I.** A reddened area on the skin that, when pressed, is "non-blanchable" (does not turn white). This indicates that a pressure ulcer is starting to develop.

**Stage II.** The skin blisters or forms an open sore. The area around the sore may be red and irritated.

**Stage III.** The skin breakdown now looks like a crater in which there is damage to the tissue below the skin.

**Stage IV.** The pressure ulcer has become so deep that there is damage to the muscle and bone, sometimes to the tendons and joints.

## ✱ Eczema

**Eczema,** which is also called *atopic* or *contact dermatitis*, is a chronic skin disorder characterized by scaly and itching rashes. People with eczema often have a family history of eczema, or allergic conditions such as asthma and hay fever. Eczema is most common in infants, and at least half of those cases clear by age 3. In adults, it is generally a chronic condition.

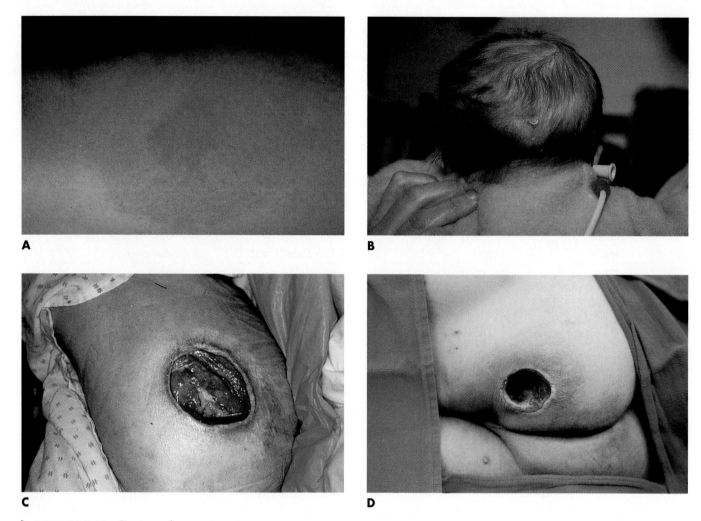

A

B

C

D

▶ **FIGURE 5–38**　Pressure ulcer staging. (Courtesy of Sandra Quigley, Children's Hospital, Boston, MA)

Treatment depends on the appearance or stage of the lesions. For example, acute "weeping" lesions, dry scaly lesions, or chronic dry, thickened lesions are each treated differently. Weeping lesions may be treated with moisturizers, mild soaps, or wet dressings. Less severe cases and dry, scaly lesions may be treated with mild anti-itch lotions or low-potency topical corticosteroids. Chronic thickened areas may be treated with ointments or creams that contain tar compounds, medium to very high potency corticosteroids, and lubricating ingredients. In severe cases, systemic corticosteroids may be prescribed to reduce inflammation. The most promising treatment for eczema is a new class of non-steroidal skin medications called *topical immunomodulators* (TIMs).

## ✱ Psoriasis

**Psoriasis** is a common skin condition that is characterized by frequent episodes of redness, itching, and thick, dry, scales on the skin (see Figure 5–39 ▶). It is a very common condition that affects approximately 3 million Americans. The condition may affect people of any age, but it most commonly begins between ages 15 and 35. It is believed to be an inherited disorder related to an inflammatory response in which the immune system targets the body's own cells. Normally, it takes about a month for new skin cells to move up from the lower layers to the surface. In psoriasis, this process takes only a few days, resulting in a buildup of dead skin cells and formation of thick scales. It can be seen most commonly on the trunk, elbows, knees, scalp, skin folds, or fingernails, but it can affect any (or all) parts of the skin.

Treatment varies with the extent and severity of the disorder. Psoriasis lesions that cover all or most of the body can require hospitalization and be acutely painful. In such

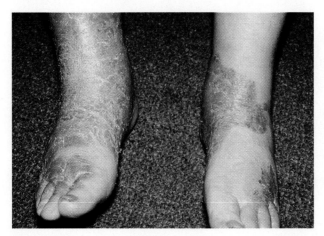

▶ **FIGURE 5–39**   Psoriasis, lower extremities. (Courtesy of Jason L. Smith, MD)

severe cases, the body loses vast quantities of fluid and is susceptible to severe secondary infections that can become systemic, involve internal organs, and even progress to septic shock and death. Treatment includes analgesics, sedation, intravenous fluids, retinoids (such as Retin-A), and antibiotics (such as cyclosporine). Mild cases are usually treated at home with topical medications such as prescription or nonprescription dandruff shampoos, cortisone or other corticosteroids, and antifungal medications.

Nonpharmacologic treatments include moderate exposure to sunlight or phototherapy. In **phototherapy,** the skin is sensitized by the application of coal tar ointment or by taking oral medications that cause the skin to become sensitive to light. The person is then exposed to ultraviolet light.

## ✳ Skin Cancer

**Skin cancer** is a disease in which malignant cells are found in the epidermis, which contains three kinds of cells: flat, scaly cells on the surface called *squamous cells;* round cells called *basal cells*, and cells called *melanocytes*, which give the skin its color.

The most common sign of skin cancer is a change in the skin, such as a growth or a sore that will not heal. Sometimes there may be a small lump. This lump can be smooth, shiny and waxy looking, or it can be red or reddish brown. Skin cancer may also appear as a flat red spot that is rough or scaly. Not all changes in the skin are cancer, but it is very important to have a dermatologist evaluate any change that occurs in one's skin.

Cancer that develops in the pigment cells is called **melanoma**. See Figure 5–40 ▶. It usually occurs in adults but is occasionally found in children and adolescents. Melanoma strikes more than 50,000 Americans annually and causes an estimated 7,800 deaths.

Often the first sign of melanoma is change in the size, shape, or color of a mole. The **ABCDs** of melanoma describe the changes that can occur in a mole using the letters:

**A**—asymmetry; the shape of one half does not match the other.

**B**—border; the edges are ragged, notched, or blurred.

**C**—color; is uneven. Shades of black, brown, or tan are present. Areas of white, red, or blue may be seen.

**D**—diameter; there is a change in size.

Melanoma is a more serious type of cancer than basal cell or squamous cell cancers. Like most cancers, melanoma is best treated when it is found early. It can metastasize quickly to other parts of the body through the lymphatic system or through the blood.

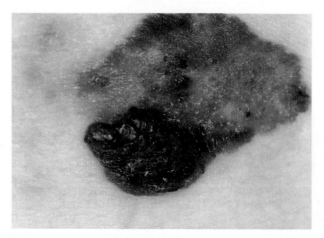

▶ **FIGURE 5–40**    Melanoma, forearm. (Courtesy of Jason L. Smith, MD)

## ✳ Skin Signs

**Skin signs** are objective evidence of an illness or disorder. They can be seen, measured, or felt. They may be described as lesions that are circumscribed areas of pathologically altered tissue. Types of skin signs are shown and described in Figure 5–41 ▶.

## ✳ Burns

**Burns** are classified according to degree or depth of skin damage. The three classifications are first degree, second degree and third degree. See Figure 5–42 ▶. A **first-degree burn** (superficial) occurs when only the outer layer of the skin (epidermis) is burned. The skin is usually red, with some degree of swelling and pain. A **second-degree burn** (partial thickness) occurs when the second layer of skin (dermis) is also burned. Blisters develop, and the skin takes on an intensely reddened, splotchy appearance. Second-degree burns produce severe pain and swelling. A **third-degree burn** (full thickness) involves all three layers of skin (epidermis, dermis, and fat layer), usually destroying the sweat glands, hair follicles, and nerve endings as well. Areas involved are generally charred black or appear dry and white. Because the nerve endings have been burned, the person does not usually feel pain.

Treatment varies with the degree of burn. For minor burns, including second-degree burns limited to an area no larger than 2 to 3 inches in diameter, the following action is recommended:

- Cool the burn. Hold the burned area under cold running water or immerse the burn in cold water or cool it with cold compresses. Cooling the burn reduces swelling by conducting heat away from the skin. Do not put ice on the burn.
- Cover the burn with a clean gauze bandage. Bandaging keeps air off the burned skin, reduces pain, and protects blistered skin.

For second-degree burns over 2 to 3 inches and third-degree burns, call for emergency assistance (dial 911). Until an emergency unit arrives, you may follow these steps:

1. Do not remove burned clothing. However, do make sure the victim is no longer in contact with smoldering materials or exposed to smoke or heat.
2. Do not immerse severe large burns in cold water. Doing so could cause shock.
3. Check for signs of circulation (breathing, coughing, or movement). If there is no breathing or other sign of circulation, begin cardiopulmonary resuscitation (CPR).

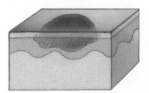

A macule is a discolored spot on the skin; freckle

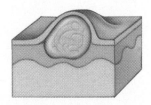

A pustule is a small, elevated, circumscribed lesion of the skin that is filled with pus; varicella (chickenpox)

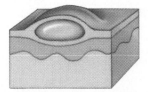

A wheal is a localized, evanescent elevation of the skin that is often accompanied by itching; urticaria

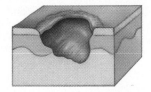

An erosion or ulcer is an eating or gnawing away of tissue; decubitus ulcer

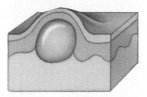

A papule is a solid, circumscribed, elevated area on the skin; pimple

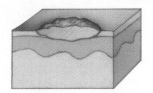

A crust is a dry, serous or seropurulent, brown, yellow, red, or green exudation that is seen in secondary lesions; eczema

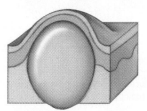

A nodule is a larger papule; acne vulgaris

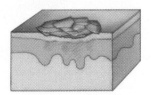

A scale is a thin, dry flake of cornified epithelial cells; psoriasis

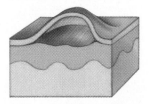

A vesicle is a small fluid filled sac; blister. A bulla is a large vesicle.

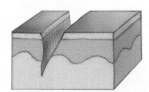

A fissure is a crack-like sore or slit that extends through the epidermis into the dermis; athlete's foot

▶ FIGURE 5–41 Skin signs are objective evidence of an illness or disorder. They can be seen, measured, or felt.

**4.** Cover the area of the burn. Use a cool, moist, sterile bandage; clean, moist cloth; or moist towels.

The **Rule of Nines** is a method of estimating the extent of burns received by a patient. It is expressed as a percentage of body surface area. In this method, the body is divided into sections of 9%, or multiples of 9%, or divisions of 9%. Accurate estimation of the extent of a burn is very important because it is used to determine the amount and type of IV fluids administered to the patient. These fluids are used to replace fluid loss and to help correct electrolyte imbalance due to tissue damage. See Figure 5–43 ▶.

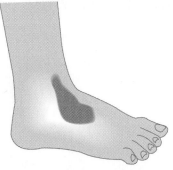

**Superficial Partial Thickness (first degree)** Damages only outer layer of skin; burn is painful and red; heals in a few days (e.g., sunburn)

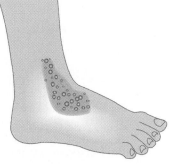

**Partial Thickness (second degree)** Involves epidermis and upper layers of dermis; may have sparing of sweat glands and sebaceous glands; heals in 10–14 days

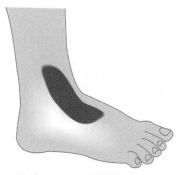

**Full Thickness (third degree)** Involves all of epidermis and dermis; may also involve underlying tissue; nerve ending usually destroyed; requires skin grafting

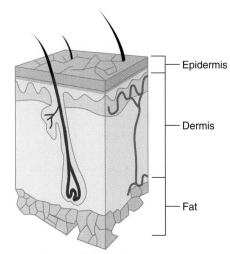

Epidermis

Dermis

Fat

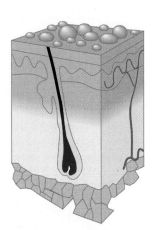

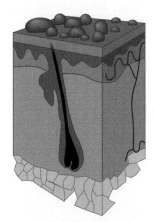

Erythema, blanches on pressure, no bullae, peeling after a few days due to premature cell death

Blisters or bullae, erythema, blanches on pressure, pain and sensativity to cold air, minimal scar formation

Skin may appear brown, black, deep cherry red, white to gray, waxy or translucent, usually no pain injured area may appear sunken

▶ **FIGURE 5–42** Characteristics of burns by depth of thermal injury.

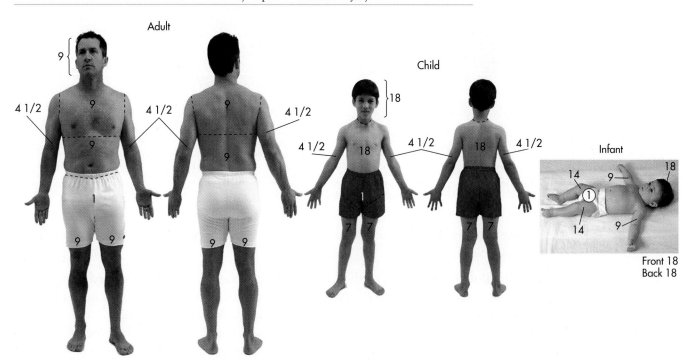

▶ **FIGURE 5–43** Rule of Nines for burns (all numbers are percent of body surface).

# ✓ PATHOLOGY CHECKPOINT

*Following is a concise list of the pathology-related terms that you have seen in the chapter. Review this checklist to make sure that you are familiar with the meaning of each term before moving to the next section.*

## Conditions and Symptoms ✱

- ❏ acne
- ❏ acrochordon
- ❏ actinic dermatitis
- ❏ albinism
- ❏ alopecia
- ❏ anhidrosis
- ❏ avulsion
- ❏ basal cell carcinoma
- ❏ bite
- ❏ boil
- ❏ bulla
- ❏ burns
- ❏ callus
- ❏ candidiasis
- ❏ carbuncle
- ❏ causalgia
- ❏ cellulites
- ❏ cicatrix
- ❏ comedo
- ❏ corn
- ❏ cyst
- ❏ decubitus
- ❏ dehiscence
- ❏ dermatitis
- ❏ dermomycosis
- ❏ ecchymosis
- ❏ eczema
- ❏ erythema
- ❏ erythroderma
- ❏ eschar
- ❏ excoriation

- ❏ exudate
- ❏ folliculitis
- ❏ gangrene
- ❏ herpes simplex
- ❏ hidradenitis
- ❏ hives
- ❏ hyperhydrosis
- ❏ icteric
- ❏ impetigo
- ❏ jaundice
- ❏ keloid
- ❏ lentigo
- ❏ leukoderma
- ❏ leukoplakia
- ❏ lupus
- ❏ melanocarcinoma
- ❏ melanoma
- ❏ miliaria
- ❏ mole
- ❏ onychitis
- ❏ onychomycosis
- ❏ pachyderma
- ❏ paronychia
- ❏ pediculosis
- ❏ petechiae
- ❏ pruritus
- ❏ psoriasis
- ❏ purpura
- ❏ roseola
- ❏ rubella
- ❏ rubeola
- ❏ scabies

- ❏ scar
- ❏ scleroderma
- ❏ seborrhea
- ❏ senile keratosis
- ❏ squamous cell carcinoma
- ❏ striae
- ❏ telangiectasia
- ❏ thermanesthesia
- ❏ tinea
- ❏ trichomycosis
- ❏ ulcer
- ❏ varicella
- ❏ vitiligo
- ❏ wart
- ❏ wound
- ❏ xanthoderma
- ❏ xanthoma
- ❏ xeroderma
- ❏ xerosis

## Diagnosis and Treatment ✱

- ❏ autograft
- ❏ cryosurgery
- ❏ debridement
- ❏ dermabrasion
- ❏ dermatome
- ❏ hypodermic (injection)
- ❏ intradermal (injection)
- ❏ subcutaneous (injection)
- ❏ subungual
- ❏ rhytidoplasty

# STUDY AND REVIEW

## Anatomy and Physiology

*Write your answers to the following questions. Do not refer to the text.*

1. Name the primary organ of the integumentary system. _____

2. Name the four accessory structures of the integumentary system.

   a. _____     b. _____

   c. _____     d. _____

3. State the four main functions of the skin.

   a. _____     b. _____

   c. _____     d. _____

4. The skin is essentially composed of two layers, the _____ and

   the _____.

5. Name the four strata of the epidermis.

   a. _____     b. _____

   c. _____     d. _____

6. _____ is a protein substance found in the dead cells of the epidermis.

7. _____ is a pigment that gives color to the skin.

8. The _____ is known as the *corium* or *true skin*.

9. Name the two layers of the part of the skin described in question 8.

   a. _____     b. _____

10. The crescent-shaped white area of the nail is the _____.

## Word Parts

1. In the spaces provided, write the definition of these prefixes, roots, combining forms, and suffixes. Do not refer to the listings of medical words. Leave blank those words you cannot define.

2. After completing as many as you can, refer to the medical word listings to check your work. For each word missed or left blank, write the word and its definition several times on the margins of these pages or on a separate sheet of paper.

3. To maximize the learning process, it is to your advantage to do the following exercises as directed. To refer to the word-building section before completing these exercises invalidates the learning process.

## PREFIXES

*Give the definitions of the following prefixes.*

1. a-, an- _____
2. auto- _____
3. ec- _____
4. de- _____
5. ex- _____
6. hyper- _____
7. hypo- _____
8. intra- _____
9. par- _____
10. sub- _____

## ROOTS AND COMBINING FORMS

*Give the definitions of the following roots and combining forms.*

1. acr/o _____
2. actin _____
3. aden _____
4. albin _____
5. carcin _____
6. caus _____
7. chym _____
8. coriat _____
9. cutane _____
10. derm _____
11. derm/a _____
12. dermat _____
13. dermat/o _____
14. derm/o _____
15. lopec _____
16. erythr/o _____
17. hidr _____
18. icter _____
19. kel _____
20. kerat _____
21. leuk/o _____
22. log _____
23. melan _____
24. melan/o _____
25. myc _____
26. onych _____
27. cellul _____
28. onych/o _____
29. pachy _____
30. pedicul _____
31. chord _____
32. rhytid/o _____
33. scler/o _____
34. seb/o _____
35. senile _____
36. therm _____
37. vuls _____
38. trich/o _____

39. ungu _____

40. xanth/o _____

41. xer/o _____

42. cubit _____

43. follicul _____

44. integument _____

45. jaund _____

46. plak _____

47. miliar _____

48. prurit _____

49. tel _____

50. ang/i _____

## SUFFIXES

*Give the definitions of the following suffixes.*

1. -al _____

2. -algia _____

3. -on _____

4. -us _____

5. -derma _____

6. -ary _____

7. -esthesia _____

8. -graft _____

9. -ia _____

10. -ic _____

11. -ion _____

12. -ism _____

13. -ist _____

14. -itis _____

15. -logy _____

16. -ectasia _____

17. -oid _____

18. -oma _____

19. -osis _____

20. -ous _____

21. -plasty _____

22. -rrhea _____

23. -tome _____

## Identifying Medical Terms

*In the spaces provided, write the medical terms for the following meanings.*

1. _____ Inflammation of the skin caused by exposure to actinic rays

2. _____ Pertaining to the skin

3. _____ Inflammation of the skin

4. _____ Study of the skin

5. _____ Severe itching

6. _____ Condition of excessive sweating

7. _____ Pertaining to under the skin

8. _____ Pertaining to jaundice

9. _____ Inflammation of the nail

10. _____ Thick skin

11. _____ Inability to distinguish between the sensations of heat and cold

12. _____ Yellow skin

## Spelling

*In the spaces provided, write the correct spelling of these misspelled terms.*

1. caualgia _____

2. dermomcosis _____

3. echymosis _____

4. exoriation _____

5. hyprhidrosis _____

6. melnoma _____

7. onychomyosis _____

8. rhytdoplasty _____

9. sleroderma _____

10. sebrrhea _____

## Matching

*Select the appropriate lettered meaning for each of the following words.*

_____ 1. acne

_____ 2. alopecia

_____ 3. cicatrix

_____ 4. comedo

_____ 5. decubitus

_____ 6. dehiscence

_____ 7. exudate

_____ 8. leukoplakia

_____ 9. petechiae

_____ 10. pruritus

a. Small, pinpoint, purplish hemorrhagic spots on the skin

b. Production of pus or serum

c. Severe itching

d. Inflammatory condition of the sebaceous gland and the hair follicles

e. Scar left after the healing of a wound

f. Loss of hair, baldness

g. White spots or patches formed on the mucous membrane of the tongue or cheek

h. Blackhead

i. Separation or bursting open of a surgical wound

j. Bedsore

k. Slough, scab

## Abbreviations

*Place the correct word, phrase, or abbreviation in the space provided.*

1. fever of undetermined origin _____

2. topical immunomodulators _____

3. Hx_____

4. incision and drainage _____

5. skin graft _____

6. ID _____

7. temperature _____

8. ultraviolet _____

9. FB _____

10. PUVA _____

## Diagnostic and Laboratory Tests

*Select the best answer to each multiple choice question. Circle the letter of your choice.*

1. An intradermal test performed using a sterile, disposable, multiple puncture lancet is:
   a. sweat test
   b. Mantoux test
   c. tine test
   d. Tzanck test

2. A test done on wound exudate to determine the presence of microorganisms is:
   a. sweat test
   b. biopsy
   c. Tzanck test
   d. wound culture

3. A microscopic examination of a small piece of tissue that has been surgically scraped from a pustule is:
   a. Tzanck test
   b. sweat test
   c. biopsy
   d. wound culture

4. Tests performed to identify the presence of the *Tubercle bacilli* include the:
   a. tine, Heaf, and sweat
   b. tine, Heaf, and Mantoux
   c. tine, Tzanck, and Mantoux
   d. tine, Mantoux, and sweat

5. The _____ test used to determine the level of chloride concentration on the skin is:
   a. sweat
   b. Tzanck
   c. tine
   d. Mantoux

# PRACTICAL APPLICATION

## S O A P : Chart Note Analysis

*This exercise will make you aware of information, abbreviations, and medical terminology typically found in a dermatology patient's chart note.*

### Abbreviations Key

| | | | |
|---|---|---|---|
| bid | twice a day | PO | orally, by mouth |
| BP | blood pressure | q | every |
| CTA | clear to auscultation | qid | four times a day |
| DOB | date of birth | R | respiration |
| F | Fahrenheit | SOAP | subjective, objective, assessment, plan |
| HEENT | head, eyes, ears, nose, throat | T | temperature |
| Ht | height | Tab | tablet |
| JVD | jugular vein distention | tid | three times a day |
| lb | pound | TM | tympanic membrane |
| mg | milligram | WNL | within normal limits |
| NKDA | no known drug allergies | Wt | weight |
| P | pulse | y/o | year(s) old |

*Read the following chart note and then answer the questions that follow.*

**PATIENT:** Gonzalez, Jose L.                                              **DATE:** 05/13/07
**DOB:** 03/13/1965        **AGE:** 42        **SEX:** Male
**INSURANCE:** Excel Healthcare

    **Vital Signs:**
        T: 98.6F
        P: 72
        R: 18
        BP: 132/88
        Ht: 5′ 8″
        Wt: 155 lb

**Allergies:** NKDA

**Chief Complaint:** Moderate to severe pruritus with small vesicles bilaterally on hands, forearms, and ankles. Erythroderma with moderate to severe edema of surrounding tissue.

**S** **Subjective:** 42 y/o Hispanic male presents with complaints of rash and small blisters on hands, forearms, and ankles × 2 days. Patient stated he had been working in the wooded area of his yard last weekend, clipping a vine from a tree. Voiced complaints of "itching like crazy" for the past 2 days.

**O** **Objective:**
**General Appearance:** The patient appeared to be anxious about his present state. His overall health appeared to be WNL.
**HEENT:** (head) normocephalic, (eyes) conjunctiva clear, sclera white, no lesions, (ears) TM normal with landmarks intact, (nose) no discharge, (throat) mucosa pink, no lesions or exudate

**Neck:** No bruits or JVD, full range of motion, no pain, trachea midline

**Lungs:** CTA

**Heart:** Normal rate and rhythm

**Skin:** Vesicular lesions with erythematous base in linear distribution are noted on hands and forearms bilaterally. Also noted on ankles bilaterally.

**A**  **Assessment:** Contact Dermatitis, Poison Ivy

**P**  **Plan:**

1. Patient is treated for contact dermatitis, poison ivy. Treatment regimen includes an antihistamine agent: loratadine (Claritin) 10mg 1 Tab PO q 12 hours for itching; Temovate 0.05% cream—corticosteroid therapy, apply to affected area bid and Sterapred 12 day unipak—take as directed.
2. Inform patient that antibiotic therapy can be prescribed if secondary infection occurs.
3. Recommend tub soaks with colloidal oatmeal (Aveeno).
4. Instruct to apply cold, wet compresses tid or qid × 20 minutes while vesicles present to relieve itching.
5. Suggest that Calamine lotion may be helpful especially with exudative inflammation to assist with drying.

**FYI:** To help prevent contact dermatitis with poison ivy, teach the patient how to recognize and avoid poison ivy. One form of poison ivy is a low plant. It is usually found in groups of many plants and looks like weeds growing from 6 to 30 inches high. The other form is a "hairy" vine that grows up a tree. Each form has stems with 3 leaves. See Figure 5–44 ▼. There is an old saying people should remember: "Leaflets three, let it be." Inform the patient when working outside to wear clothing that covers arms and legs. If in contact with poison ivy, oak, or sumac, wash skin immediately with soap and water to remove oleoresin within 15 minutes of exposure. Also, wash all clothing including gloves, jackets, shoes, and shoestrings as soon as possible. Oleoresin, the extract of the plant, can be active for 6 months on surfaces such as clothing.

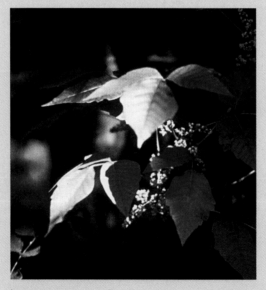

▶ **FIGURE 5–44**  Poison ivy. (Source: Pearson Education/PH College)

## Chart Note Questions
*Place the correct answer in the space provided.*

1. What is the abbreviation for twice a day? _____

2. When the patient states, "itching like crazy," the medical term you would note in his chart is:

   _____

3. The chart notes that small blisters appear on the forearms. What is the medical term for blisters?

   _____

4. A person who is sensitive to poison ivy may develop what condition? _____

5. Claritin is a/an _____ used to relieve itching.

6. Prevention is a key concept in today's health care delivery system. List four preventive measures that this patient could use to help and/or prevent his condition.

   _____        _____

   _____        _____

7. What is the medical term for redness of the skin? _____

8. What medical term do you use to chart "moderate to severe swelling of surrounding tissue"?

   _____

9. List three nonprescriptive measures patients can use to relieve itching:

   _____

   _____

   _____

10. How long can Oleoresin remain active before contacting and becoming reactive with human skin?

   _____

# MULTIMEDIA PREVIEW

*Additional interactive resources and activities for this chapter can be found on the Companion Website. For videos, audio glossary, and review, access the accompanying CD-ROM in this book.*

 **CD-ROM HIGHLIGHTS**

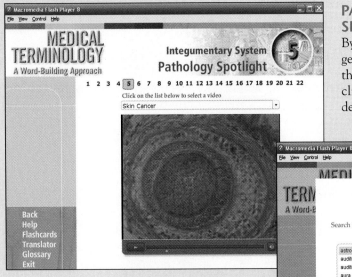

## PATHOLOGY SPOTLIGHT— SKIN CANCER

By viewing concepts in moving, living color, you'll get a fuller picture of the pathologies presented in this chapter. Earlier we discussed skin cancer. Now click on this feature to watch a video that describes this condition in more detail.

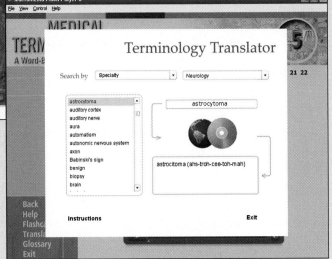

## TERMINOLOGY TRANSLATOR

Say it in Spanish! We've translated over 5,000 medical terms and you can see how they're spelled and pronounced. Clicking on this feature is a great way to practice communicating medical information in a new language. ¡*Vamos!*

 **WEBSITE HIGHLIGHTS—www.prenhall.com/rice**

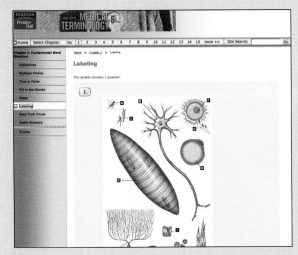

## LABELING EXERCISE

Click here and take advantage of the free-access online study guide that accompanies your textbook. You'll find a labeling question that corresponds to a picture in this chapter. By clicking on this URL you'll also access links to download mp3 audio reviews, current news articles, and an audio glossary.

# Skeletal System

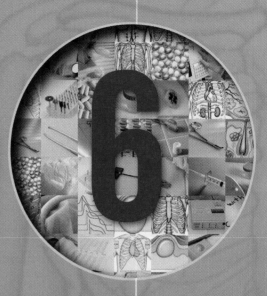

## ■ OUTLINE

## ■ OBJECTIVES

*On completion of this chapter, you will be able to:*

- Describe the skeletal system.
- Describe various types of body movement.
- Describe the vertebral column.
- Identify abnormal curvatures of the spine.
- Describe the differences in the pelvis of a male and female.
- Describe various types of fractures.
- Describe skeletal differences of the child and the older adult.
- Analyze, build, spell, and pronounce medical words.
- Comprehend the drugs highlighted in this chapter.
- Describe diagnostic and laboratory tests related to the skeletal system.
- Identify and define selected abbreviations.
- Describe each of the conditions presented in the Pathology Spotlights.
- Review the Pathology Checkpoint.
- Complete the Study and Review section and the Chart Note Analysis.

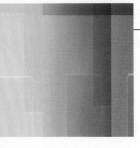

# Anatomy and Physiology Overview

The skeletal system is composed of 206 bones that, with **cartilage, tendons,** and **ligaments,** make up the **framework** or skeleton of the body. The skeleton can be divided into two main groups of bones: the **axial skeleton** consisting of 80 bones and the **appendicular skeleton** with the remaining 126 bones. The principal bones of the axial skeleton are the skull, spine, ribs, and sternum. The shoulder girdle, arms, and hands and the pelvic girdle, legs, and feet are the primary bones of the appendicular skeleton. See Figure 6–1 ▼ for an anterior and posterior view of the skeleton.

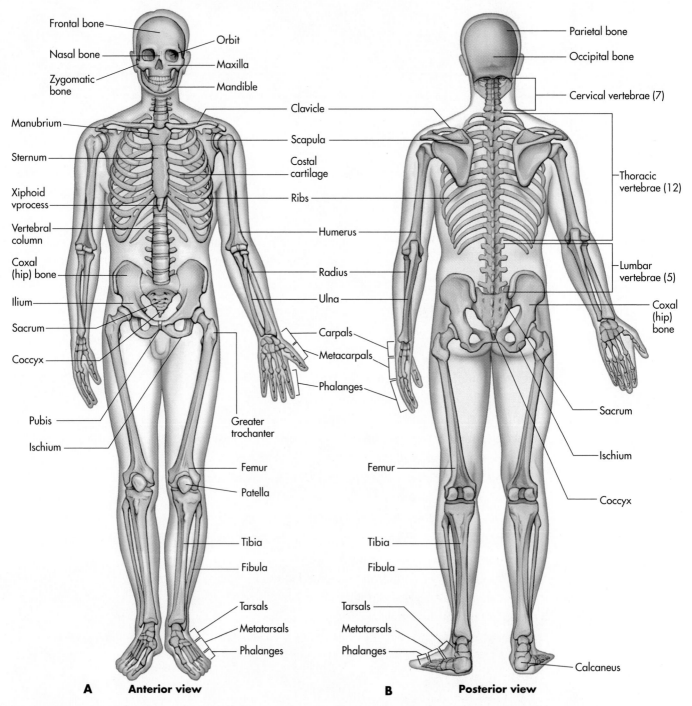

**A**   **Anterior view**   **B**   **Posterior view**

▶ **FIGURE 6–1**   The anterior and posterior human skeleton.

## Skeletal System

| Organ/Structure | Primary Functions |
|---|---|
| Bones | • Provide shape, support, protection, and the framework of the body<br>• Serve as a storage place for mineral salts, calcium, and phosphorus<br>• Play an important role in the formation of blood cells<br>• Provide areas for the attachment of skeletal muscles<br>• Help make movement possible |
| Cartilages | • Form the major portion of the embryonic skeleton and part of the skeleton in adults |
| Tendons | • Attach muscles to bones; consist of connective tissue |
| Ligaments (lig) | • Connect the articular ends of bones, binding them together and facilitating or limiting motion; attach bone to bone<br>• Connect cartilage and other structures<br>• Serve to support or attach fascia |

# BONES

The **bones** are the primary organs of the skeletal system and are composed of about 50% water and 50% solid matter. The solid matter in bone is a calcified, rigid substance known as **osseous tissue.**

## Classification of Bones

Bones are classified according to their shapes. See Figure 6–2 ▶. Table 6–1 classifies the bones and gives an example of each type.

TABLE 6–1  **Classifications of Bone**

| Shape | Example of This Classification |
|---|---|
| Flat | Ribs, scapula (shoulder blade), parts of the pelvic girdle, bones of the skull |
| Long | Tibia (shin bone), femur (thigh bone), humerus, radius |
| Short | Carpals, tarsals |
| Irregular | Vertebrae, ossicles of the ear |
| Sesamoid | Patella (kneecap) |
| Sutural or Wormian | Between the flat bones of the skull |

## Functions of Bones

The following are the main functions of bones:

1. Provide shape, support, and the framework of the body.
2. Provide protection for internal organs.
3. Serve as a storage place for mineral salts, calcium, and phosphorus.
4. Play an important role in **hematopoiesis** (the formation of blood cells), which normally takes place in the bone marrow.
5. Provide areas for the attachment of skeletal muscles.
6. Help to make movement possible through **articulation.**

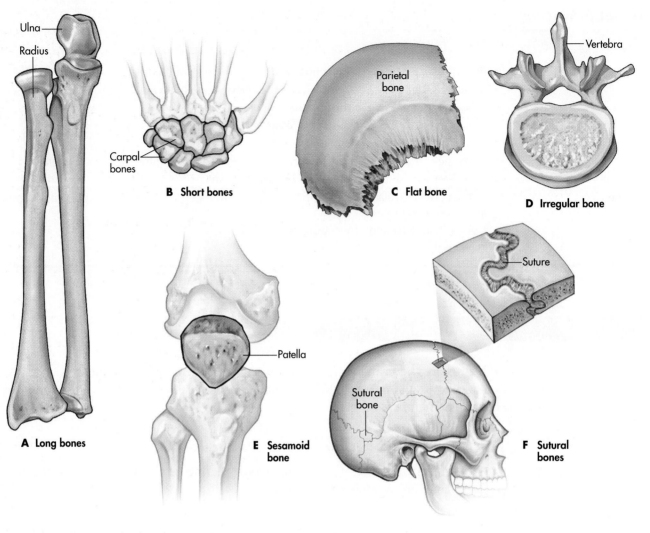

Ulna
Radius
Carpal bones
**B  Short bones**
Parietal bone
**C  Flat bone**
Vertebra
**D  Irregular bone**
Patella
**E  Sesamoid bone**
Suture
Sutural bone
**F  Sutural bones**
**A  Long bones**

▶ **FIGURE 6–2**  Classification of bones by shape.

## Structure of a Long Bone

Long bones, such as the tibia, femur, humerus, or radius, have most of the features found in all bones. These features are shown in Figure 6–3 ▶.

**Epiphysis.** The ends of a developing bone.

**Diaphysis.** The shaft of a long bone.

**Periosteum.** The membrane that forms the covering of bones except at their articular surfaces.

**Compact bone.** The dense, hard layer of bone tissue.

**Medullary canal.** A narrow space or cavity throughout the length of the diaphysis.

**Endosteum.** A tough, connective tissue membrane lining the medullary canal and containing the bone marrow.

**Cancellous or spongy bone.** The reticular tissue that makes up most of the volume of bone.

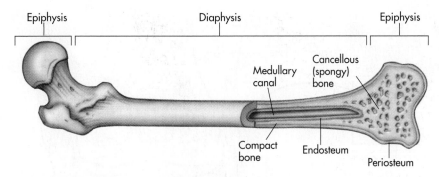

▶ **FIGURE 6–3** Features found in a long bone.

## Bone Markings

Certain commonly used terms describe the **markings of bones.** These markings are listed so you can better understand their role in joining bones together, providing areas for muscle attachments, and serving as a passageway for blood vessels, ligaments, and nerves. See Table 6–2.

### TABLE 6–2 Bone Markings

| Marking | Description of the Bone Structure |
| --- | --- |
| Condyle | Rounded projection that enters into the formation of a joint, articulation |
| Crest | Ridge on a bone |
| Fissure | Slitlike opening between two bones |
| Foramen | Opening in the bone for blood vessels, ligaments, and nerves |
| Fossa | Shallow depression in or on a bone |
| Head | Rounded end of a bone |
| Meatus | Tubelike passage or canal |
| Process | Enlargement or protrusion of a bone |
| Sinus | Air cavity within certain bones |
| Spine | Pointed, sharp, slender process |
| Sulcus | Groove, furrow, depression, or fissure |
| Trochanter | Either of the two bony projections below the neck of the femur |
| Tubercle | Small, rounded process |
| Tuberosity | Large, rounded process |

## JOINTS AND MOVEMENT

A **joint** (jt) is an articulation, a place where two or more bones connect. See Figure 6–4 ▶. The manner in which bones connect determines the type of movement allowed at the joint. Joints are classified as follows:

**Synarthrosis.** Does not permit movement. The bones are in close contact with each other, but there is no joint cavity. An example is a *cranial suture.*

**Amphiarthrosis.** Permits very slight movement. An example of this type of joint is a *vertebra.*

**Diarthrosis.** Allows free movement in a variety of directions. Examples of this type of joint are the *knee, hip, elbow, wrist,* and *foot.*

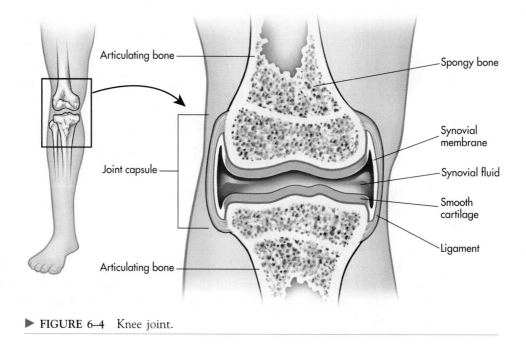

▶ **FIGURE 6–4**   Knee joint.

The following terms describe types of body movement that occur at the **diarthrotic joints** (see Figure 6–5 ▶):

**Abduction.** Moving a body part away from the middle.
**Adduction.** Moving a body part toward the middle.
**Circumduction.** Moving a body part in a circular motion.
**Dorsiflexion.** Bending a body part backward.
**Eversion.** Turning outward.
**Extension.** Straightening a flexed limb.
**Flexion.** Bending a limb.
**Inversion.** Turning inward.
**Pronation.** Lying prone (face downward); also turning the palm downward.
**Protraction.** Moving a body part forward.
**Retraction.** Moving a body part backward.
**Rotation.** Moving a body part around a central axis.
**Supination.** Lying supine (face upward); also turning the palm or foot upward.

# VERTEBRAL COLUMN

The **vertebral column** is composed of a series of separate bones (**vertebrae**) connected in such a way to form four spinal curves. These curves have been identified as the cervical, thoracic, lumbar, and sacral. The *cervical curve* consists of the first 7 vertebrae, the *thoracic curve* consists of the next 12 vertebrae, the *lumbar curve* consists of the next 5 vertebrae, and the *sacral curve* consists of the sacrum and coccyx (tailbone) (see Figure 6–6 ▶).

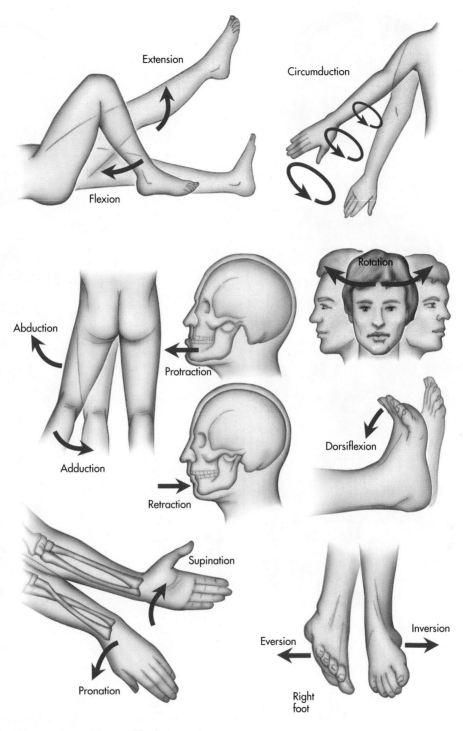

▶ **FIGURE 6–5** Types of body movements.

It is known that a curved structure has more strength than a straight structure. The spinal curves of the human body are most important because they help support the weight of the body and provide the balance that is necessary to walk on two feet. Young children who are beginning to walk often have a pot-bellied stance because of a lumbar lordosis. This posture usually disappears around five years of age. After six years of age, the spine

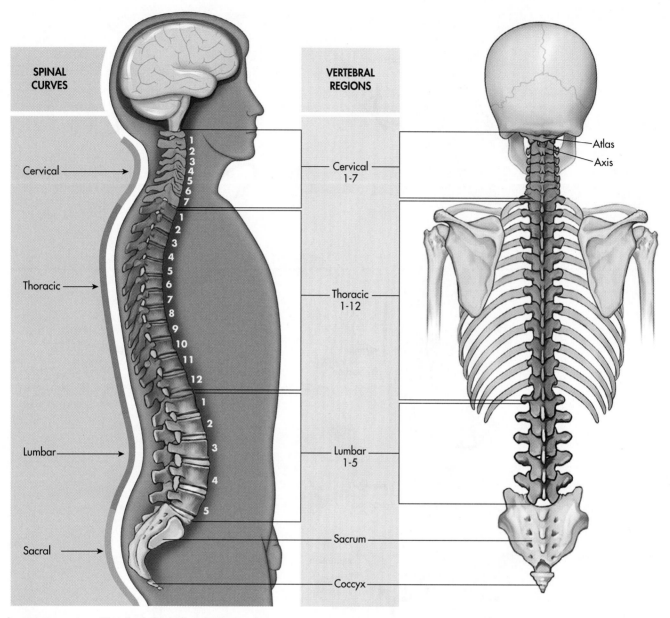

SPINAL
CURVES

Cervical

Thoracic

Lumbar

Sacral

1
2
3
4
5
6
7

1
2
3
4
5
6
7
8
9
10
11
12

1
2
3
4
5

VERTEBRAL
REGIONS

Cervical
1-7

Thoracic
1-12

Lumbar
1-5

Sacrum

Coccyx

Atlas
Axis

▶ **FIGURE 6–6**   Vertebral (spinal) column.

has normal thoracic convex (arched; curved evenly) and lumbar concave (rounded; hollowed out) curves. See Figure 6–7 ▶ for the normal development of posture and spinal curves.

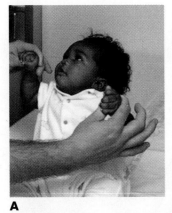
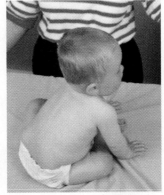
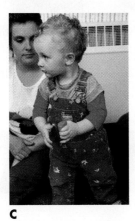
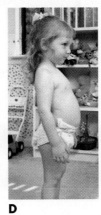
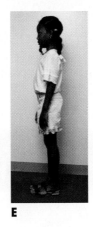

◀ **FIGURE 6–7** Normal development of posture and spinal curves. (A) Infant 2–3 months: Holds head erect when held upright; thoracic kyphosis when sitting. (B) 6–8 months: Sits without support; spine is straight. (C) 10–15 months: Walks independently; straight spine. (D) Toddler: Protruding abdomen; lumbar lordosis. (E) School-age child: Height of shoulders and hips is level; balanced thoracic convex and lumbar concave curves.

## ANATOMICAL DIFFERENCES IN THE PELVIS OF A MALE AND FEMALE

The **pelvis** is the lower portion of the trunk of the body. It forms a basin bound anteriorly and laterally by the hip bones and posteriorly by the sacrum and coccyx.

The bony pelvis is formed by the sacrum, the coccyx, and the bones that form the hip and pubic arch, the ilium, pubis, and ischium. These bones are separate in the child but become fused in adulthood.

### Male Pelvis

The **male pelvis** is shaped like a *funnel*, forming a narrower outlet than the female. It is heavier and stronger than the female pelvis; therefore, it is more suited for lifting and running. The normal male pelvis is the **android** (resembling a male) type. See Figure 6–8A ▶.

### Female Pelvis

The **female pelvis** is shaped like a *basin*. It can be oval to round, and it is wider than the male pelvis. The female pelvis is constructed to accommodate the fetus during pregnancy and to facilitate its downward passage through the pelvic cavity in childbirth. In general, the female pelvis is broader and lighter than the male pelvis. The most common female pelvis is the **gynecoid** (resembling the female) type. See Figure 6–8B.

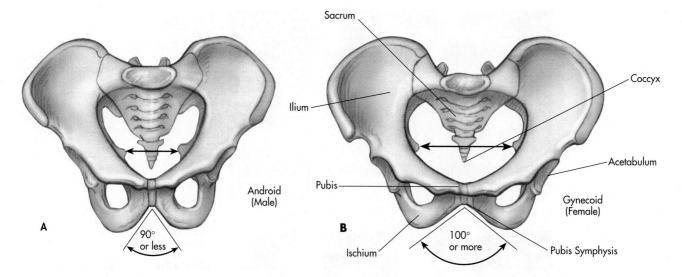

▶ **FIGURE 6–8** (A) The male pelvis (android)is shaped like a funnel, forming a narrower outlet than the female. (B) The female pelvis (gynecoid) is shaped like a basin.

# LIFE SPAN CONSIDERATIONS

## ■ THE CHILD

Bone begins to develop during the second month of fetal life as cartilage cells enlarge, break down, disappear, and are replaced by bone-forming cells called **osteoblasts.** Most bones of the body are formed by this process, known as **endochondral ossification.** In this process, the bone cells deposit organic substances in the spaces vacated by cartilage to form bone matrix. As this process proceeds, blood vessels form within the bone and deposit salts such as calcium and phosphorus that serve to harden the developing bone.

The **epiphyseal plate** is the center for longitudinal bone growth in children. See Figure 6–9 ▶. It is possible to determine the biological age of a child from the development of epiphyseal ossification centers as shown radiographically.

About three years after the onset of puberty, the ends of the long bones (**epiphyses**) knit securely to their shafts (**diaphysis**), and further growth can no longer take place.

The bones of children are more resilient than of adolescents and adults, tend to bend, and before breaking can become deformed. Fracture healing occurs more quickly in children because there is a rich blood supply to bones and their periosteum is thick and osteogenic activity is high.

**Calcium** is critical to the strength of bones. The daily recommendations of calcium by age group follow:

| | |
|---|---|
| 1 to 3 years | 500 mg |
| 4 to 8 years | 800 mg |
| 9 to 13 years | 1300 mg |
| 14 to 18 years | 1300 mg |

## ■ THE OLDER ADULT

Women build bone until about age 35 and then begin to lose about 1% of bone mass annually. Men usually start losing bone mass 10 to 20 years later. Most of the skeletal system changes that take place during the aging process involve changes in connective tissue. The

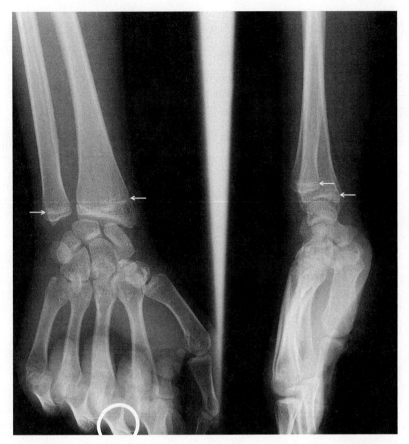

▶ FIGURE 6–9   Epiphyseal plate (arrows). (Courtesy of Teresa Resch)

loss of bone mass and bone strength are due to the loss of bone mineral content during later life. Calcium salts can be deposited in the matrix, and the cartilage becomes hard and brittle.

Age-related **osteoporosis,** loss of bone mass, is often seen in older women and men. Other changes that could occur involve the joints because there is diminished viscosity of the synovial fluid, degeneration of collagen and elastin cells, outgrowth of cartilaginous clusters in response to continuous wear and tear, and formation of scar tissues and calcification in the joint capsules.

Low levels of calcium can make people more susceptible to osteoporosis and stress fractures, especially those that are commonly seen in the older adult. Bone healing in the older adult is slower and impaired because osteoblasts are less able to use calcium to restructure bone tissue. The National Academy of Sciences suggests that people 51 and older consume 1200 mg of calcium per day to help strengthen their bones.

# BUILDING YOUR MEDICAL VOCABULARY

This section provides the foundation for learning medical terminology. Review the following alphabetized word list. Note how common prefixes and suffixes are repeatedly applied to word roots and combining forms to create different meanings.

| | |
|---|---|
| **P** | Prefix |
| **R** | Root |
| **CF** | Combining form |
| **S** | Suffix |

| | |
|---|---|
| Pink words | Terms not built from word parts. |
| * | Indicates words covered in the Pathology Spotlights section. |
| 💿 | Check the CD-ROM for more information. |

| MEDICAL WORD | Part | Type | Meaning | DEFINITION |
|---|---|---|---|---|
| **acetabulum**<br>(ăs″ ĕ-tăb′ ū-lŭm) | acetabul<br><br>-um | R<br><br>S | acetabulum, hip socket, structure, tissue | Cup-shaped socket of the hipbone into which the thighbone fits |
| **achondroplasia**<br>(ă-kŏn″ drō-plā′ sĭ-ă) | a-<br>chondr/o<br>-plasia | P<br>CF<br>S | without<br>cartilage<br>formation | Defect in the formation of cartilage at the epiphyses of long bones |
| **acroarthritis**<br>(ăk″rō-ăr-thrī′ tĭs) | acr/o<br>arthr<br>-itis | CF<br>R<br>S | extremity<br>joint<br>inflammation | Inflammation of the joints of the hands or feet |
| **acromion**<br>(ă-krō′ mĭ-ŏn) | acr<br>-omion | R<br>S | extremity, point<br>shoulder | Projection of the spine of the scapula that forms the point of the shoulder and articulates with the clavicle |
| **ankylosis**<br>(ăng″ kĭ-lō′ sĭs) | ankyl<br><br>-osis | R<br><br>S | stiffening, crooked<br>condition (usually abnormal) | Condition of stiffening of a joint |
| **arthralgia**<br>(ăr-thrăl′ jĭ-ă) | arthr<br>-algia | R<br>S | joint<br>pain | Pain in a joint |
| **arthritis**<br>(ăr-thrī′tĭs)<br> | arthr<br>-itis | R<br>S | joint<br>inflammation | Inflammation of a joint. ✳ See Pathology Spotlight: Arthritis on page 133. |
| **arthrocentesis**<br>(ăr″ thrō-sĕn-tē′ sĭs) | arthr/o<br>-centesis | CF<br>S | joint<br>surgical puncture | Surgical puncture of a joint for removal of fluid |
| **arthroplasty**<br>(ăr″ thrō-plăs′ tē) | arthr/o<br>-plasty | CF<br>S | joint<br>surgical repair | Surgical repair of a joint |
| **arthroscope**<br>(ăr-thrŏs′ kōp) | arthr/o<br>-scope | CF<br>S | joint<br>instrument for examining | Instrument used to examine the interior of a joint |
| **bone marrow transplant**<br>(bōn măr′ ō trăns′ plant) | | | | Surgical process of transferring bone marrow from a donor to a patient |

| MEDICAL WORD | WORD PARTS (WHEN APPLICABLE) | | | DEFINITION |
|---|---|---|---|---|
| | Part | Type | Meaning | |
| **bursa**<br>(bŭr′ sah) | | | | Padlike sac between muscles, tendons, and bones that is lined with synovial membrane and contains a fluid, *synovia* |
| **bursitis**<br>(bŭr-sī′ tĭs) | burs<br>-itis | R<br>S | a pouch<br>inflammation | Inflammation of a bursa |
| **calcaneal**<br>(kăl-kā′ nē-ăl) | calcan/e<br>-al | CF<br>S | heel bone<br>pertaining to | Pertaining to the heel bone |
| **calcium (Ca)**<br>(kăl′ sĭ-ŭm) | | | | Mineral that is essential for bone growth, teeth development, blood coagulation, and many other functions |
| **carpal**<br>(kär′ pəl) | carp<br>-al | R<br>S | wrist<br>pertaining to | Pertaining to the wrist bones. There are two rows of four bones in the wrist for a total of eight wrist bones. |
| **carpal tunnel syndrome**<br>(kär′ pĕl tŭn′ ĕl sĭn′ drōm) | | | | Condition caused by compression of the median nerve by the carpal ligament; symptoms: soreness, tenderness, weakness, pain, tingling, and numbness at the wrist. ✱ See Pathology Spotlight: Carpal Tunnel Syndrome on page 134 and Figure 6–22. |
| **cartilage**<br>(kär′ tĭ-lĭj) | cartil<br>-age | R<br>S | gristle<br>related to | Specialized type of fibrous connective tissue found at the ends of bone; forms the major portions of the embryonic skeleton before birth |
| **cast**<br>(kăst) | | | | Type of material made of plaster of paris, sodium silicate, starch, or dextrin used to immobilize a fractured bone, a dislocation, or a sprain. See Figure 6–10 ▼. |

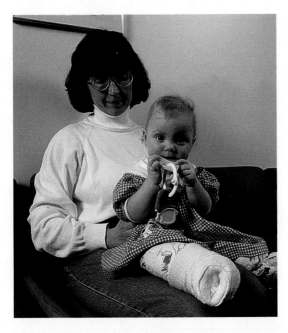

◄ **FIGURE 6–10**   This girl has a long leg cast, which was applied after surgery to correct her clubfoot.

| MEDICAL WORD | WORD PARTS (WHEN APPLICABLE) | | | DEFINITION |
|---|---|---|---|---|
| | Part | Type | Meaning | |
| **chondral**<br>(kŏn' drăl) | chondr<br>-al | R<br>S | cartilage<br>pertaining to | Pertaining to cartilage |
| **chondrocostal**<br>(kŏn" drō-kŏs' tăl) | chondr/o<br>cost<br>-al | CF<br>R<br>S | cartilage<br>rib<br>pertaining to | Pertaining to the rib cartilage |
| **clavicular**<br>(klă-vĭk' ū-lăr) | clavicul<br><br><br>-ar | R<br><br><br>S | clavicle, collar<br>bone<br><br>pertaining to | Pertaining to the clavicle (*collar bone*) |
| **coccygeal**<br>(kŏk-sĭj' ĭ-ăl) | coccyg/e<br>-al | CF<br>S | coccyx, tailbone<br>pertaining to | Pertaining to the coccyx (*tailbone*) |
| **coccygodynia**<br>(kŏk-sĭ-gō-dĭn' ĭ-ă) | coccyg/o<br>-dynia | CF<br>S | coccyx, tailbone<br>pain | Pain in the coccyx (*tailbone*) |
| **collagen**<br>(kŏl'ă-jĕn) | coll/a<br>-gen | CF<br>S | glue<br>formation,<br>produce | Fibrous insoluble protein found in the connective tissue, skin, ligaments, and cartilage |
| **connective**<br>(kə' nĕk' tĭv) | connect<br>-ive | R<br>S | to bind together<br>nature of | Pertaining to connecting or binding together |
| **costal**<br>(käst' əl) | cost<br>-al | R<br>S | rib<br>pertaining to | Pertaining to the rib |
| **costosternal**<br>(kŏs" tō-stěr' năl) | cost/o<br>stern<br>-al | CF<br>R<br>S | rib<br>sternum<br>pertaining to | Pertaining to a rib and the sternum |
| **craniectomy**<br>(krā" nĭ-ěk' tŏ-mē) | crani/(o)<br>-ectomy | CF<br>S | skull<br>surgical excision | Surgical excision of a portion of the skull. *Note that the suffix begins with a vowel, drop the (o) from the combining form and add –ectomy to form craniectomy.* |
| **craniotomy**<br>(krā" nĭ-ŏt' ō-mē) | crani/o<br>-tomy | CF<br>S | skull<br>incision | Incision into the skull |
| **dactylic**<br>(dăk' tĭl' ĭk) | dactyl<br>-ic | R<br>S | finger or toe<br>pertaining to | Pertaining to the finger or toe |
| **dactylogram**<br>(dăk-til'ə grăm) | dactyl/o<br>-gram | CF<br>S | finger or toe<br>mark, record | Fingerprint |
| **dislocation**<br>(dĭs" lō-kā' shŭn) | dis-<br>locat<br>-ion | P<br>R<br>S | apart<br>to place<br>process | Displacement of a bone from a joint |
| **femoral**<br>(fěm' ŏr-ăl) | femor<br>-al | R<br>S | femur<br>pertaining to | Pertaining to the femur; the *thigh bone,* the longest bone in the body |
| **fibular**<br>(fĭb' ū-lăr) | fibul<br>-ar | R<br>S | fibula<br>pertaining to | Pertaining to the fibula; the *smaller of the two lower leg bones* |
| **fixation**<br>(fĭks-ā' shŭn) | fixat<br>-ion | R<br>S | fastened<br>process | Process of holding or fastening in a fixed position; making rigid, immobilizing |
| **flatfoot**<br>(flăt fut) | | | | Abnormal flatness of the sole and arch of the foot; also known as *pes planus* |

| MEDICAL WORD | WORD PARTS (WHEN APPLICABLE) | | | DEFINITION |
|---|---|---|---|---|
| | **Part** | **Type** | **Meaning** | |
| **genu valgum** (jē′ nū văl gŭm) | | | | Knock-knee. See Figure 6–11A ▼. |
| **genu varum** (jē′ nū vā′ rŭm) | | | | Bowleg. See Figure 6–11B ▼. |
| **gout** (gowt) | | | | Hereditary metabolic disease that is a form of acute arthritis; usually begins in the knee or foot but can affect any joint. ✳ See Pathology Spotlight: Arthritis on page 140 and Figure 6–20. |
| **hallux** (hăl″ ŭks) | | | | Big or great toe |
| **hammertoe** (hăm′ er-tō) | | | | Acquired flexion deformity of the interphalangeal joint. See Figure 6–12 ▼. |
| **humeral** (hū′ měr-ăl) | humer -al | R S | humerus pertaining to | Pertaining to the humerus (*upper arm bone*) |
| **hydrarthrosis** (hi″ drăr-thrō′ sĭs) | hydr- arthr -osis | P R S | water joint condition (usually abnormal) | Accumulation of watery fluid in the cavity of a joint |
| **iliac** (ĭl′ ē-ăk) | ili -ac | R S | ilium pertaining to | Pertaining to the ilium |
| **iliosacral** (ĭl″ ĭ-ō-sā′ krăl) | ili/o sacr -al | CF R S | ilium sacrum pertaining to | Pertaining to the ilium and the sacrum |

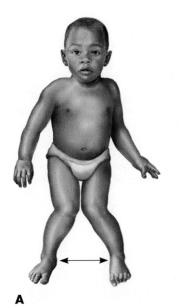
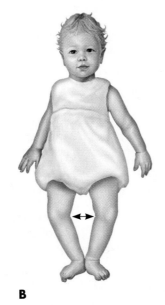

**A**   **B**

▶ FIGURE 6–11   (A) Genu valgum, or knock-knee. Note that the ankles are far apart when the knees are together. (B) Genu varum, or bowleg. The legs are bowed so that the knees are far apart as the child stands.

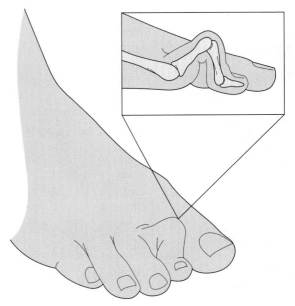

▶ FIGURE 6–12   Hammertoe.

| MEDICAL WORD | WORD PARTS (WHEN APPLICABLE) | | | DEFINITION |
|---|---|---|---|---|
| | **Part** | **Type** | **Meaning** | |
| **intercostal**<br>(ĭn" tēr-kŏs' tăl) | inter<br>cost<br>-al | R<br>R<br>S | between<br>rib<br>pertaining to | Pertaining to between the ribs |
| **ischial**<br>(ĭs' kĭ-al) | isch/i<br>-al | CF<br>S | ischium, hip<br>pertaining to | Pertaining to the ischium, hip |
| **ischialgia**<br>(ĭs" kĭ-ăl' jĭ-ă) | isch/i<br>-algia | CF<br>S | ischium, hip<br>pain | Pain in the ischium, hip |
| **kyphosis**<br>(kī-fō' sĭs) | kyph<br>-osis | R<br>S | a hump<br>condition<br>(usually abnormal) | Humpback. ✱ See Pathology Spotlight: Abnormal Curvatures of the Spine on page 133 and Figure 6–18A. |
| **laminectomy**<br>(lăm" ĭ-nĕk' tō-mē) | lamin<br><br>-ectomy | R<br><br>S | lamina (thin plate)<br>surgical excision | Surgical excision of a vertebral posterior arch |
| **ligament (lig)**<br>(lĭg' ă-mĕnt) | | | | Band of fibrous connective tissue that connects bones, cartilages, and other structures; also serves as a place for the attachment of fascia |
| **lordosis**<br>(lŏr-dō' sĭs) | lord<br><br>-osis | R<br><br>S | bending, curve, swayback<br>condition (usually abnormal) | Abnormal anterior curvature of the lumbar spine (*swayback*). ✱ See Pathology Spotlight: Abnormal Curvatures of the Spine on page 133 and Figure 6–18B. |
| **lumbar**<br>(lŭm' băr) | lumb<br>-ar | R<br>S | loin, lower back<br>pertaining to | Pertaining to the loins (*lower back*) |
| **lumbodynia**<br>(lŭm" bō-dĭn' ĭ-ă) | lumb/o<br>-dynia | CF<br>S | loin, lower back<br>pain | Pain in the loins (*lower back*) |
| **mandibular**<br>(măn-dĭb' ū-lăr) | mandibul<br>-ar | R<br>S | lower jawbone<br>pertaining to | Pertaining to the lower jawbone |
| **maxillary**<br>(măk' sĭ-lĕr" ē) | maxill<br>-ary | R<br>S | jawbone<br>pertaining to | Pertaining to the upper jawbone |
| **meniscus**<br>(mĕn-ĭs' kŭs) | menisc<br>-us | R<br>S | crescent<br>structure | Crescent-shaped interarticular fibrocartilage structure found in certain joints, especially the lateral and medial *menisci* (semilunar cartilages) of the knee joint |
| **metacarpals**<br>(mĕt" ă-kär' pəl) | meta-<br>carp<br>-al | P<br>R<br>S | beyond<br>wrist<br>pertaining to | Pertaining to the bones of the hand. There are five radiating bones in the fingers. |
| **metacarpectomy**<br>(mĕt" ă-kär-pĕk' tō-mē) | meta-<br>carp<br>-ectomy | P<br>R<br>S | beyond<br>wrist<br>surgical excision | Surgical excision of one or more bones of the hand |
| **myelitis**<br>(mī-ĕ-li' tĭs) | myel<br>-itis | R<br>S | bone marrow<br>inflammation | Inflammation of the bone marrow |
| **myeloma**<br>(mī-ē-lō' mă) | myel<br>-oma | R<br>S | bone marrow<br>tumor | Tumor of the bone marrow |

| MEDICAL WORD | WORD PARTS (WHEN APPLICABLE) | | | DEFINITION |
|---|---|---|---|---|
| | **Part** | **Type** | **Meaning** | |
| **myelopoiesis**<br>(mī′ ĕl-ō-poy-ē′ sĭs) | myel/o<br>-poiesis | CF<br>S | bone marrow<br>formation | Formation of bone marrow |
| **olecranal**<br>(ō-lĕk′ răn-ăl) | olecran<br>-al | R<br>S | elbow<br>pertaining to | Pertaining to the elbow |
| **orthopedics**<br>(or″thō-pē′ dĭks) | | | | Branch of medicine concerned with diseases and disorders involving locomotor structures of the body |
| **orthopedist**<br>((or″thō-pē′dĭst) | | | | Physician who specializes in orthopedics |
| **osteoarthritis (OA)**<br>(ŏs″tē-ō-ăr-thrī′ tĭs) | oste/o<br>arthr<br>-itis | CF<br>R<br>S | bone<br>joint<br>inflammation | Inflammation of the bone and joint.<br>✱ See Pathology Spotlight: Arthritis on page 133 and Figure 6–19. |
| **osteoblast**<br>(ŏs′ tē-ō-blăst″) | oste/o<br>-blast | CF<br>S | bone<br>immature cell,<br>germ cell | Bone-forming cell |
| **osteocarcinoma**<br>(ŏs″tē-ō-kăr″sĭn-ō mă) | oste/o<br>carcin<br>-oma | CF<br>R<br>S | bone<br>cancer<br>tumor | Cancerous tumor of a bone; new growth of epithelial tissue |
| **osteochondritis**<br>(ŏs″tē-ō-kŏn-drī′ tĭs) | oste/o<br>chondr<br>-itis | CF<br>R<br>S | bone<br>cartilage<br>inflammation | Inflammation of the bone and cartilage |
| **osteogenesis**<br>(ŏs″ tē-ō-jĕn′ ĕ-sĭs) | oste/o<br>-genesis | CF<br>S | bone<br>formation,<br>produce | Formation of bone |
| **osteomalacia**<br>(ŏs″tē-ō-măl-ā′ shĭ-ă) | oste/o<br>-malacia | CF<br>S | bone<br>softening | Softening of the bones |
| **osteomyelitis**<br>(ŏs″tē-ō-mī″ ĕl-ī′ tĭs) | oste/o<br>myel<br>-itis | CF<br>R<br>S | bone<br>bone marrow<br>inflammation | Inflammation of the bone marrow. See Figure 6–13 ▼. |
| **osteopenia**<br>(ŏs″tē-ō-pē′ nĭ-ă) | oste/o<br>-penia | CF<br>S | bone<br>deficiency | Deficiency of bone tissue, regardless of the cause |

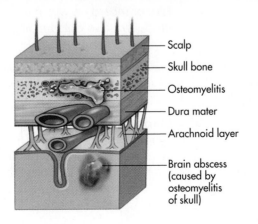
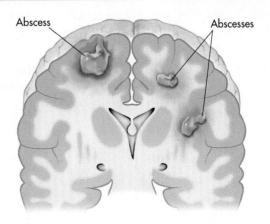

▶ FIGURE 6–13 Abscess of the brain due to osteomyelitis.

| MEDICAL WORD | WORD PARTS (WHEN APPLICABLE) | | | DEFINITION |
|---|---|---|---|---|
| | **Part** | **Type** | **Meaning** | |
| **osteoporosis**<br>(ŏs″tē-ō-por-ō′ sĭs) | oste/o<br>por<br>-osis | CF<br>R<br>S | bone<br>a passage<br>condition (usu-<br>ally abnormal) | Condition that results in reduction of bone mass. ✱ See Pathology Spotlight: Osteoporosis on page 138 and Figure 6–25. |
| **osteosarcoma**<br>(ŏs″tē-ō-săr-kō′ mă) | oste/o<br>sarc<br>-oma | CF<br>R<br>S | bone<br>flesh<br>tumor | Malignant tumor of the bone; cancer arising from connective tissue |
| **osteotome**<br>(ŏs′ tē-ō-tōm″) | oste/o<br>-tome | CF<br>S | bone<br>instrument to cut | Instrument used for cutting bone |
| **patellar**<br>(pă-tĕl′ ăr) | patell<br>-ar | R<br>S | kneecap<br>pertaining to | Pertaining to the patella; the *kneecap* |
| **pedal**<br>(pĕd′l) | ped<br>-al | R<br>S | foot<br>pertaining to | Pertaining to the foot |
| **periosteoedema**<br>(pĕr″ĭ-ŏs″tē-ō-ĕ-dē′ mă) | peri-<br>oste/o<br>-edema | P<br>CF<br>S | around<br>bone<br>swelling | Swelling around a bone |
| **phalangeal**<br>(fā-lăn′ jē-ăl) | phalang/e<br><br>-al | CF<br><br>S | phalanges<br>(finger/toe bones)<br>pertaining to | Pertaining to the bones of the fingers and the toes |
| **phosphorus (P)**<br>(fŏs′ fō-rŭs) | phos<br>phor<br>-us | R<br>R<br>S | light<br>carrying<br>pertaining to | Mineral that is essential in bone formation, muscle contraction, and many other functions |
| **polyarthritis**<br>(pŏl″ē-ăr-thrī′ tĭs) | poly-<br>arthr<br>-itis | P<br>R<br>S | many, much<br>joint<br>inflammation | Inflammation of more than one joint |
| **rachigraph**<br>(rā′ kĭ-grăf) | rach/i<br>-graph | CF<br>S | spine<br>instrument for<br>recording | Instrument used to measure the curvature of the spine |
| **radial**<br>(rā′ dĭ-ăl) | rad/i<br>-al | CF<br>S | radius<br>pertaining to | Pertaining to the radius (lateral lower arm bone in line with the thumb). *A radial pulse can be found on the thumb side of the arm.* |
| **radiograph**<br>(rā′ dĭ-ō-grăf) | radi/o<br>-graph | CF<br>S | x-ray<br>record, instrument<br>for recording | Film or record on which an x-ray image is produced; also called *radiogram* |
| **reduction**<br>(rē-dŭk′ shŭn) | re-<br>duct<br>-ion | P<br>R<br>S | back<br>to lead<br>process | Manipulative or surgical procedure used to correct a fracture or hernia |
| **rheumatoid arthritis (RA)**<br>(roo′ mă-toyd ăr-thrī′ tĭs) | rheumat<br>-oid<br>arthr<br>-itis | R<br>S<br>R<br>S | discharge<br>resemble<br>joint<br>inflammation | Chronic systemic disease characterized by inflammation of the joints, stiffness, pain, and swelling that results in crippling deformities. See Figure 6–14 ▶. ✱ See Pathology Spotlight: Arthritis on page 135 and Figure 6–21. |

| MEDICAL WORD | WORD PARTS (WHEN APPLICABLE) | | | DEFINITION |
|---|---|---|---|---|
| | Part | Type | Meaning | |
| **rickets**<br>(rĭk′ ĕts) | | | | Deficiency condition in children primarily caused by a lack of vitamin D; can also result from inadequate intake or excessive loss of calcium |
| **scapular**<br>(skăp′ ū-lăr) | scapul<br>-ar | R<br>S | shoulder blade<br>pertaining to | Pertaining to the shoulder blade |
| **scoliosis**<br>(skō″lĭ-ō′ sĭs) | scoli<br>-osis | R<br>S | curvature<br>condition (usually abnormal) | Condition of lateral curvature of the spine. The characteristic signs include asymmetry of the trunk, uneven shoulders and hips, a one-sided rib hump, and a prominent scapula. See Figure 6–15 ▼. ✷ See Pathology Spotlight: Abnormal Curvature of the Spine on page 133 and Figure 6–18C. |

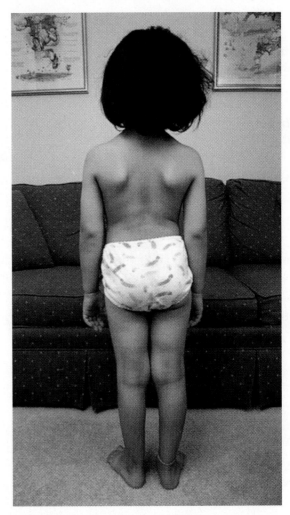

▶ **FIGURE 6–15**  Does this child have legs of different lengths or scoliosis? Look at the level of the iliac crests and shoulders to see if they are level. See the more prominent crease at the waist on the right side? This child could have scoliosis.

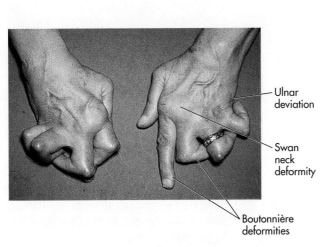

—Ulnar deviation

—Swan neck deformity

Boutonnière deformities

▶ **FIGURE 6–14**  Typical hand deformities associated with rheumatoid arthritis. (Reprinted with permission of Photo Researchers, Inc.)

| MEDICAL WORD | WORD PARTS (WHEN APPLICABLE) | | | DEFINITION |
|---|---|---|---|---|
| | **Part** | **Type** | **Meaning** | |
| **spinal**<br>(spī′ năl) | spin<br>-al | R<br>S | spine<br>pertaining to | Pertaining to the spine |
| **splint**<br>(splĭnt) | | | | Appliance used for fixation, support, and rest of an injured body part |
| **spondylitis**<br>(spŏn-dĭl-ī′ tĭs) | spondyl<br>-itis | R<br>S | vertebra<br>inflammation | Inflammation of one or more vertebrae |
| **sprain**<br>(sprān) | | | | Twisting a joint that causes pain and disability |
| **spur**<br>(spər) | | | | Sharp or pointed projection, as on a bone |
| **sternal**<br>(stēr′ năl) | stern<br><br>-al | R<br><br>S | sternum,<br>breastbone<br>pertaining to | Pertaining to the sternum (*breastbone*) |
| **sternotomy**<br>(stĕr-nŏt′ ō-mē) | stern/o<br><br>-tomy | CF<br><br>S | sternum,<br>breastbone<br>incision | Surgical incision of the sternum (*breastbone*) |
| **subclavicular**<br>(sŭb″klă-vĭk′ ū-lăr) | sub-<br>clavicul<br><br>-ar | P<br>R<br><br>S | under, beneath<br>clavicle,<br>collar bone<br>pertaining to | Pertaining to beneath the clavicle (*collar bone*) |
| **subcostal**<br>(sŭb-kŏs′ tăl) | sub-<br>cost<br>-al | P<br>R<br>S | under, beneath<br>rib<br>pertaining to | Pertaining to beneath the ribs |
| **submaxilla**<br>(sŭb″măk-sĭl′ ă) | sub-<br>maxilla | P<br>R | under, beneath<br>jaw | Below the jaw or mandible |
| **symphysis**<br>(sĭm′ fĭ-sĭs) | sym-<br>-physis | P<br>S | together<br>growth | State of growing together |
| **tendonitis**<br>(tĕn′ dŭ-nī tĭs) | tendon<br>-itis | R<br>S | tendon<br>inflammation | Inflammation of a tendon |
| **tennis elbow**<br>(tĕn′ ĭs ĕl′ bō) | | | | Chronic condition characterized by pain caused by excessive pronation and supination activities of the forearm; usually caused by strain, as in playing tennis |
| **tibial**<br>(tĭb′ ĭ-ăl) | tibi<br>-al | R<br>S | tibia<br>pertaining to | Pertaining to the tibia; the *shin bone*. Larger of the two bones of the lower leg. |
| **traction (Tx)**<br>(trăk′ shŭn) | tract<br>-ion | R<br>S | to draw<br>process | Process of drawing or pulling on bones or muscles to relieve displacement and facilitate healing. See Figure 6–16 ▶. |
| **ulnar**<br>(ŭl′ năr) | uln<br>-ar | R<br>S | ulna, elbow<br>pertaining to | Pertaining to the ulna (medial lower arm bone), or to the nerve or artery named from it. *The ulna is located on the little finger side of the arm.* |

| MEDICAL WORD | WORD PARTS (WHEN APPLICABLE) | | | DEFINITION |
|---|---|---|---|---|
| | Part | Type | Meaning | |
| **ulnocarpal** (ŭl"nō-kăr' păl) | uln/o carp -al | CF R S | ulna, elbow wrist pertaining to | Pertaining to the ulna side of the wrist |
| **vertebral** (vĕr' tĕ-brăl) | vertebr -al | R S | vertebra pertaining to | Pertaining to a vertebra |
| **vertebrosternal** (vĕr"tĕ-brō-ster' năl) | vertebr/o stern -al | CF R S | vertebra sternum pertaining to | Pertaining to a vertebra and the sternum |
| **xiphoid** (zĭf' oyd) | xiph -oid | R S | sword resemble | Literally means *resembling a sword.* The xiphoid process is the lowest portion of the sternum; a sword-shaped cartilaginous process supported by bone. |

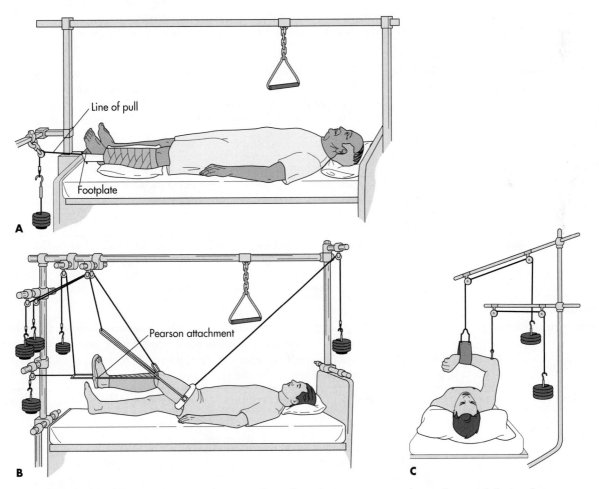

▶ **FIGURE 6–16**  Traction is the application of a pulling force to maintain bone alignment during fracture healing. Different fractures require different types of traction. (A) Skin traction (also called *straight traction*) such as Buck's traction shown here, is often used for hip fractures. (B) Balanced suspension traction is commonly used for fractures of the femur. (C) Skeletal traction, in which the pulling force is applied directly to the bone, may be used to treat fractures of the humerus.

# DRUG HIGHLIGHTS

| | |
|---|---|
| **Anti-inflammatory agents** | Relieves the swelling, tenderness, redness, and pain of inflammation. Such agents can be classified as steroidal (corticosteroids) and nonsteroidal. |
| **Corticosteroids** | Steroid substance with potent anti-inflammatory effects |
| **(Glucocorticoids)** | *Examples: Depo-Medrol (methylprednisolone acetate), Aristocort (triamcinolone), Deltasone (prednisone), and Delta-Cortef (prednisolone)* |
| **Nonsteroidal** | Agents used in the treatment of arthritis and related disorders |
| **(NSAIDs)** | *Examples: Bayer aspirin (acetylsalicylic acid), Motrin (ibuprofen), Feldene (piroxicam), Orudis (ketoprofen), and Naprosyn (naproxen)* |
| **Disease-modifying anti-rheumatic drugs (DMARDs)** | Can influence the course of the disease progression; therefore, their introduction in early rheumatoid arthritis is recommended to limit irreversible joint damage. |
| | *Examples: gold preparations Ridaura (auranofin) and Solganol (aurothioglucose); antimalarial Plaquenil Sulfate (hydroxychloroquine sulfate); a chelating agent Cuprimine (penicillamine) and the immunosuppressants Rheumatrex (methotrexate), Imuran (azathioprine), and Cytoxan (cyclophosphamide)* |
| **COX-2 inhibitors** | Cyclooxygenase (COX) is an enzyme involved in many aspects of normal cellular function and in the inflammatory response. COX-2 is found in joints and other areas affected by inflammation as occurs with osteoarthritis and rheumatoid arthritis. Inhibition of COX-2 reduces the production of compounds associated with inflammation and pain. |
| | *Examples: Celebrex (celecoxib), and Mobic (meloxicam)* |
| **Antitumor necrosis factor (Anti-TNF) drugs** | These drugs have evolved out of the biotechnology industry and seem to slow, if not halt altogether, the destruction of the joints by disrupting the activity of tumor necrosis factor (TNF), a substance involved in the body's immune response. |
| | *Example: Enbrel (etanercept)* |
| **Agents used to treat gout** | Acute attacks of gout are treated with colchicine. Once the acute attack of gout has been controlled, drug therapy to control hyperuricemia can be initiated. |
| | *Example: Benemid (probenecid), Anturane (sulfinpyrazone), and Zyloprim (allopurinol)* |
| **Agents used to treat or prevent postmenopausal osteoporosis** | Include *Fosamax (alendronate sodium) and Actonel (risedronate)*<br>Fosamax reduces the activity of the cells that cause bone loss and increases the amount of bone in most patients. Actonel inhibits osteoclast-mediated bone resorption and modulates bone metabolism. To receive the clinical benefits of either of these drugs the patient must be informed and follow the prescribed drug regimen. |
| **Analgesics** | Agents that relieve pain without causing loss of consciousness. They are classified as narcotic or non-narcotic. |
| **Narcotic** | *Examples: Demerol (meperidine HCl) and morphine sulfate* |
| **Non-narcotic** | *Examples: Tylenol (acetaminophen), aspirin, ibuprofen (Advil, Motrin, Nuprin), and Naprosyn (naproxen)* |

# DIAGNOSTIC AND LAB TESTS

| TEST | DESCRIPTION |
|------|-------------|
| **Arthrography** (ăr-thrŏg′ ră-fē) | Diagnostic examination of a joint (usually the knee) in which air and then a radiopaque contrast medium are injected into the joint space, x-rays are taken, and internal injuries of the meniscus, cartilage, and ligaments can be seen if present. |
| **Arthroscopy** (ăr-thrŏs′ kō-pē) | Process of examining internal structures of a joint via an arthroscope; usually done after an arthrography and before joint surgery. |
| **Goniometry** (gō″ nē-ŏm′ ĕt-rē) | Measurement of joint movements, especially range of motion (ROM) and angles via a goniometer. See Figure 6–17 ▼. |
| **Photon absorptiometry** (fō′ tŏn ăb-sorp′ shē-ŏm′ ĕt-rĕ) | Bone scan that uses a low beam of radiation to measure bone-mineral density and bone loss in the lumbar vertebrae; useful in monitoring osteoporosis. |
| **Thermography** (thĕr-mŏg′ ră-fē) | Process of recording heat patterns of the body's surface; can be used to investigate the pathophysiology of rheumatoid arthritis. |
| **X-ray** (ĕks′ rā) | Examination of bones using an electromagnetic wave of high energy produced by the collision of a beam of electrons with a target in a vacuum tube; used to identify fractures and pathologic conditions of the bones and joints such as rheumatoid arthritis, spondylitis, and tumors. |
| **Alkaline phosphatase blood test** (ăl′ kă-līn fŏs′ fă-tās) | Blood test to determine the level of alkaline phosphatase; increased level in osteoblastic bone tumors, rickets, osteomalacia, and during fracture healing. |
| **Antinuclear antibodies (ANA)** (ăn″ tĭ-nū′ klē-ăr ăn′ tĭ-bŏd″ ēs) | Present in a variety of immunologic diseases; positive result can indicate rheumatoid arthritis. |

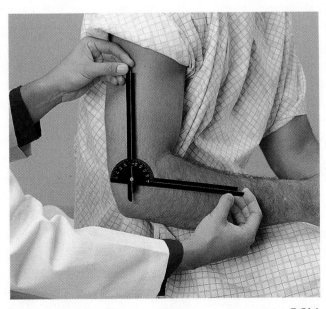

▶ **FIGURE 6–17** Using a goniometer to measure joint ROM.

| | |
|---|---|
| **Bone mineral density test (BMD)** (bōn mī-nĕ′răl dĕn-sī′ty) | Test used to measure bone mass or bone mineral density. Several different machines measure bone density. Peripheral machines measure density in the finger, wrist, kneecap, shin bone, and heel. Central machines measure density in the hip, spine, and total body. |
| **Calcium (Ca) blood test** (kăl′ sē-ŭm) | Calcium level of the blood can be increased in metastatic bone cancer, acute osteoporosis, prolonged immobilization, and during fracture healing; can be decreased in osteomalacia and rickets. |
| **C-Reactive protein blood test (CRP)** (sē-rē-ăk″ tĭv prō′ tē-in) | Positive result can indicate rheumatoid arthritis, acute inflammatory change, and widespread metastasis. |
| **Phosphorus (P) blood test** (fŏs′ fō-rŭs) | Phosphorus level of the blood can be increased in osteoporosis and fracture healing. |
| **Serum rheumatoid factor (RF)** (sē′ rŭm roo′ mă-toyd făk′ tŏr) | Immunoglobulin present in the serum of 50% to 95% of adults with rheumatoid arthritis. |
| **Uric acid blood test** (ū′ rĭk ăs′ ĭd) | Uric acid is increased in gout, arthritis, multiple myeloma, and rheumatism. |

# ABBREVIATIONS

| ABBREVIATION | MEANING | ABBREVIATION | MEANING |
|---|---|---|---|
| ACL | anterior cruciate ligament | LLCC | long leg cylinder cast |
| ANA | antinuclear antibodies | NSAIDs | nonsteroidal anti-inflammatory drugs |
| AP | anteroposterior | | |
| BMD | bone mineral density (test) | OA | osteoarthritis |
| C 1 | cervical vertebra, first | ORTHO | orthopedics, orthopaedics |
| C 2 | cervical vertebra, second | P | phosphorus |
| C 3 | cervical vertebra, third | PCL | posterior cruciate ligament |
| Ca | calcium | PEMFs | pulsing electromagnetic fields |
| CDH | congenital dislocation of hip | PWB | partial weight bearing |
| CRP | C-reactive protein blood test | RA | rheumatoid arthritis |
| DJD | degenerative joint disease | RF | rheumatoid factor |
| DMARDs | disease-modifying antirheumatic drugs | ROM | range of motion |
| | | SAC | short arm cast |
| Fx | fracture | SLC | short leg cast |
| JRA | juvenile rheumatoid arthritis | SPECT | single photon emission computed tomography |
| jt | joint | | |
| KJ | knee jerk | T 1 | thoracic vertebra, first |
| L 1 | lumbar vertebra, first | T 2 | thoracic vertebra, second |
| L 2 | lumbar vertebra, second | T 3 | thoracic vertebra, third |
| L 3 | lumbar vertebra, third | TMJ | temporomandibular joint |
| LAC | long arm cast | TNF | tumor necrosis factor |
| lig | ligament | Tx | traction |
| LLC | long leg cast | | |

# PATHOLOGY SPOTLIGHTS

## ✱ Abnormal Curvatures of the Spine

Abnormal curvatures of the spine include scoliosis, lordosis, and kyphosis.

In **scoliosis,** there is an abnormal lateral curvature of the spine. This condition usually appears in adolescence during periods of rapid growth. Treatment modalities may include the application of a cast, brace, traction, electrical stimulation, and/or surgery. See Figure 6–18C ▼.

In **lordosis,** there is an abnormal anterior curvature of the lumbar spine. This condition can be referred to as *swayback* because the abdomen and buttocks protrude due to an exaggerated lumbar curvature. See Figure 6–18B.

In **kyphosis,** the normal thoracic curvature becomes exaggerated, producing a "humpback" appearance. This condition can be caused by a congenital defect, a disease process such as tuberculosis and/or syphilis, malignancy, compression fracture, faulty posture, osteoarthritis, rheumatoid arthritis, rickets, osteoporosis, or other conditions. See Figure 6–18A.

 ## ✱ Arthritis

**Arthritis** is a disease that involves the inflammation of one or more joints. Joint inflammation can result from various disease processes. Some of the most common include injury to a joint (including fracture), an attack on the joints by the body itself (an autoimmune disease), or "wear and tear" on joints.

**Osteoarthritis** (OA) is the most common type of arthritis in the United States. OA often results from years of accumulated "wear and tear" on joints and tends to occur in the

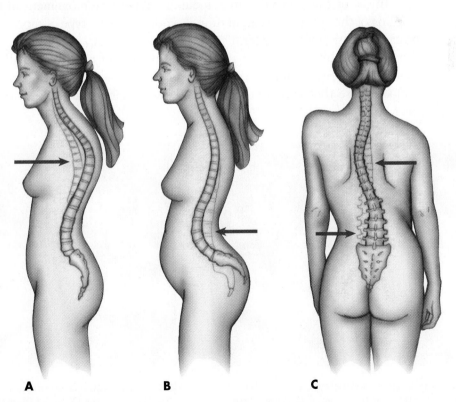

▶ **FIGURE 6–18** Abnormal curvatures of the spine: (A) kyphosis; (B) lordosis; and (C) scoliosis.

older adult in hips, knees, and finger joints. See Figure 6–19 ▼. In people over 55 years of age, women are more likely to suffer from osteoarthritis. Obesity, a history of trauma, and various genetic and metabolic diseases also increase the risk of osteoarthritis.

**Gout** is a hereditary metabolic disease caused by hyperuricemia, excessive amounts of uric acid in the blood, and deposits of urates of sodium (uric acid crystals) in and around the joints. It is a form of acute arthritis and is marked by joint inflammation. Seen most often in men over 40 years of age, it usually begins in the knee or foot. See Figure 6–20 ▼.

**Rheumatoid arthritis** (RA) is a chronic autoimmune disease characterized by inflammation of the joints, stiffness, pain, and swelling that results in crippling deformities. It also affects many of the body's organs and systems. See Figure 6–21 ▶.

Other autoimmune disorders, such as lupus, and scleroderma, can cause arthritis as well. In these diseases, the immune system attacks the joints.

About 37 million people in the United States, almost 1 in 7 people, have some form of arthritis. Symptoms can include joint pain and swelling, morning stiffness, warmth around a joint, redness of the skin around a joint, and reduced ability to move a joint.

Arthritis treatment varies, depending on the particular type, how severe the disease is, which joints are affected, the degree to which the patient is affected, and the person's age, occupation, and daily activities. Treatment usually consists of exercise, heat or cold treatments, methods to protect the joints, various medications, and possibly surgery.

## ＊ Carpal Tunnel Syndrome

Bounded by bones and ligaments, the **carpal tunnel** is a narrow passageway about as big around as a person's thumb and located on the palm side of the wrist. This tunnel protects a main nerve to the hand and nine tendons that bend the fingers. When pressure is put on the median nerve, it produces the numbness, pain and, eventually, hand weakness that characterize carpal tunnel syndrome. See Figure 6–22 ▶.

Injury or trauma to the area, including repetitive movement of the wrists, can cause swelling of the tissues and carpal tunnel syndrome. This type of repetitive-action injury can be caused by sports such as tennis and racquetball or can occur during sewing, keyboarding, driving, assembly-line work, painting, writing, use of tools (especially hand tools or tools that vibrate), or similar activities. Some of the jobs associated with carpal tunnel syndrome include those that involve data entry or use of vibrating tools, mining, and professional musicians.

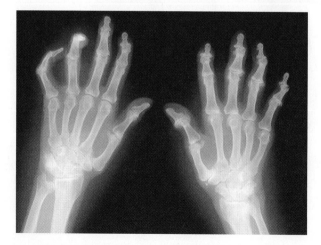

▶ **FIGURE 6–19**   X-ray showing typical joint changes associated with osteoarthritis. (Source: Getty Images/Stone Allstock.)

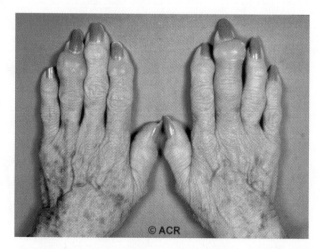

▶ **FIGURE 6–20**   Gout of the finger joint. (Source: © 1972–2004 American College of Rheumatology Clinical Slide Collection. Used with permission.)

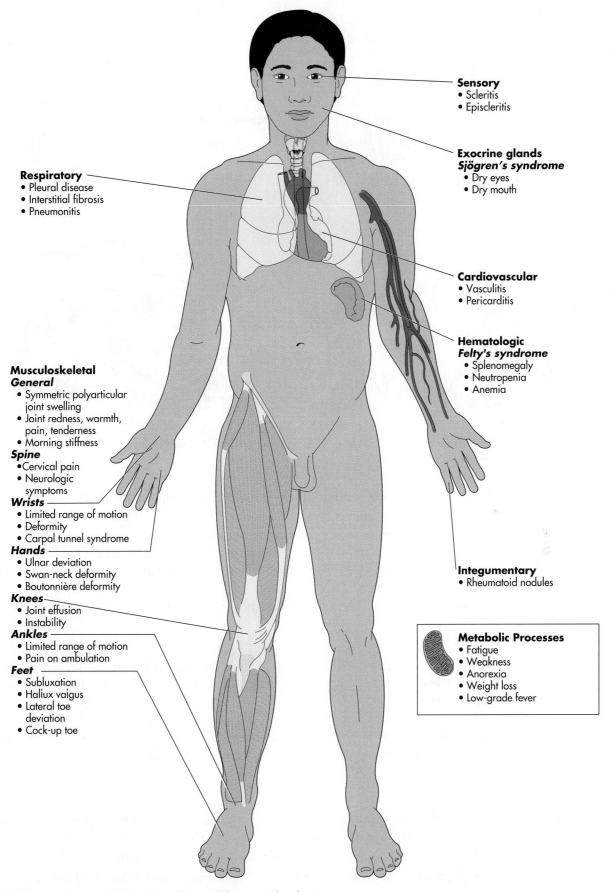

**Sensory**
• Scleritis
• Episcleritis

**Exocrine glands**
*Sjögren's syndrome*
• Dry eyes
• Dry mouth

**Respiratory**
• Pleural disease
• Interstitial fibrosis
• Pneumonitis

**Cardiovascular**
• Vasculitis
• Pericarditis

**Hematologic**
*Felty's syndrome*
• Splenomegaly
• Neutropenia
• Anemia

**Musculoskeletal**
*General*
• Symmetric polyarticular joint swelling
• Joint redness, warmth, pain, tenderness
• Morning stiffness
*Spine*
• Cervical pain
• Neurologic symptoms
*Wrists*
• Limited range of motion
• Deformity
• Carpal tunnel syndrome
*Hands*
• Ulnar deviation
• Swan-neck deformity
• Boutonnière deformity
*Knees*
• Joint effusion
• Instability
*Ankles*
• Limited range of motion
• Pain on ambulation
*Feet*
• Subluxation
• Haliux vaigus
• Lateral toe deviation
• Cock-up toe

**Integumentary**
• Rheumatoid nodules

**Metabolic Processes**
• Fatigue
• Weakness
• Anorexia
• Weight loss
• Low-grade fever

▶ **FIGURE 6–21**   Multisystem effects of rheumatoid arthritis.

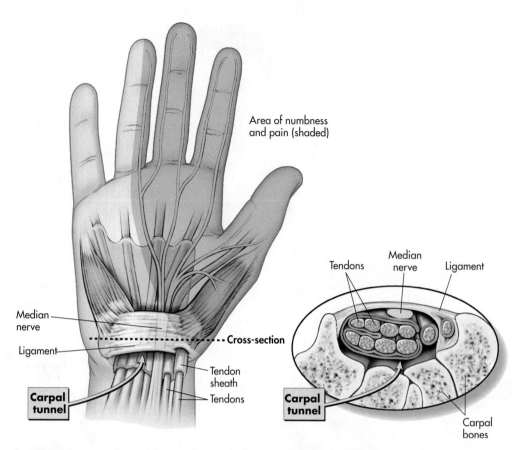

▶ **FIGURE 6–22**  Cross-section of wrist showing tendons and nerves involved in carpal tunnel syndrome.

Treatment can include having the patient wear night splints for the wrist for several weeks. If unsuccessful, the splints are worn during the day and hot or cold compresses can be added. Other types of treatment include modifications in the work area.

Medications used in the treatment of carpal tunnel syndrome include NSAIDs such as ibuprofen or naproxen. The carpal tunnel may also be injected with corticosteroids. Surgery, called *carpal tunnel release*, can help those with carpal tunnel syndrome. In severe cases, electromyography or nerve conduction studies are used to follow the recovery of the nerve.

## ✳ **Fractures**

**Fractures** (Fx) are classified according to their external appearance, the site of the fracture, and the nature of the crack or break in the bone. Important fracture types are indicated in Figure 6–23 ▶.

Many fractures fall into more than one category. For example, Colles' fracture is a transverse fracture, but depending on the injury, it can also be a comminuted fracture that can be either open or closed. The following list provides a summary of the types of fractures:

- **Closed,** or **simple,** fractures do not involve a break in the skin; they are completely internal.
- **Open,** or **compound,** fractures are more dangerous because the fracture projects through the skin and there is a possibility of infection or hemorrhage. See Figure 6–24 ▶.
- **Comminuted** fractures shatter the affected part into a multitude of bony fragments.
- **Transverse** fractures break the shaft of a bone across its longitudinal axis.
- **Greenstick** fractures usually occur in children whose long bones have not fully ossified; only one side of the shaft is broken, and the other is bent (like a greenstick).

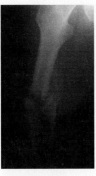

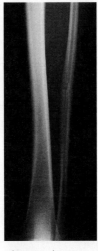

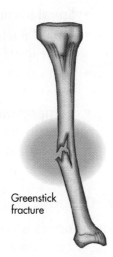

Femur, AP view, comminuted fracture

Tibia, simple, transverse fracture

Greenstick fracture

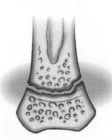

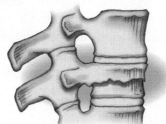

Pott's fracture—dislocation

Compression fracture

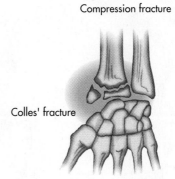

Epiphyseal plate fracture

Colles' fracture

▶ **FIGURE 6–23**    Various types of fractures.

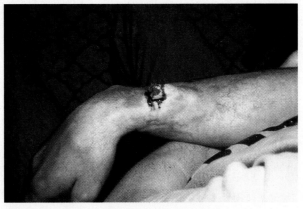

▶ **FIGURE 6–24**    Open fracture of the wrist. (Source: Pearson Education/PH College)

- **Spiral** fractures produced by twisting stresses are spread along the length of a bone.
- **Colles'** fracture is often the result of reaching out to cushion a fall; there is a break in the distal portion of the radius.
- **Pott's** fracture occurs at the ankle and affects both bones of the lower leg (fibula and tibia).
- **Compression** fractures occur in vertebrae subjected to extreme stresses, as when one falls and lands on his or her bottom.
- **Epiphyseal** fractures usually occur where the matrix is undergoing calcification and chondrocytes (cartilage cells) are dying; this type of fracture is seen in children.

## ∗ Osteoporosis

**Osteoporosis** is a condition characterized by the progressive loss of bone density and thinning of bone tissue. See Figure 6–25 ▼. Osteoporosis occurs when the body fails to form enough new bone or when too much old bone is reabsorbed by the body, or both. Osteoporosis frequently occurs when there is not enough calcium in the diet. The body then uses calcium stored in bones, weakening them and making them vulnerable to breaking. Sufficient intake of vitamin D is also important for calcium absorption.

Osteoporosis affects more than 25 million Americans, most of them women 50 to 70 years of age. Each year, the disease leads to 1.4 million bone fractures, including more than 500,000 vertebral fractures, 300,000 hip fractures, and 200,000 wrist fractures.

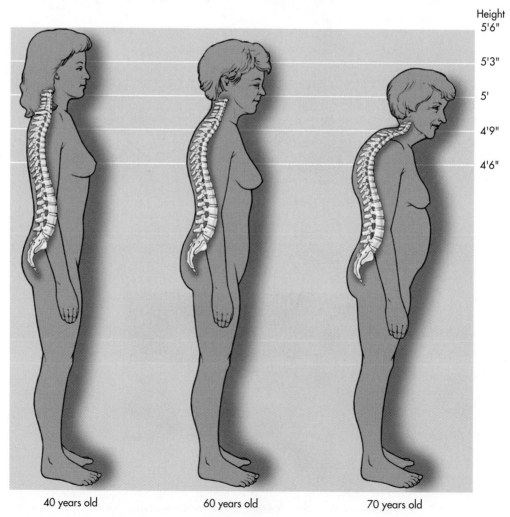

| | | Height |
|---|---|---|
| | | 5'6" |
| | | 5'3" |
| | | 5' |
| | | 4'9" |
| | | 4'6" |

40 years old        60 years old        70 years old

▶ **FIGURE 6–25**  Spinal changes caused by osteoporosis.

Some risk factors are involved in developing osteoporosis:

- Family history of osteoporosis.
- Lack of exercise, especially weight-bearing exercise, which stimulates bone growth.
- Thin, small frame.
- Never been pregnant.
- Early menopause (before 45 years).
- Tendency to fractures and loss of height in recent years.
- Avoidance of dairy products as a child.
- Use of cigarettes and alcoholic beverages.
- Diet high in salt, caffeine, or fat.
- Insufficient intake of vitamin D.

Tests such as bone mineral density (BMD) testing are most frequently used for diagnosis and evaluation of osteoporosis. The result of the test is called a *T-score*. A patient is considered osteoporotic if the bone mass is at least 20% below normal. A score of $-2.5$ or less is considered high risk, a score of $-1.0$ to $-2.5$ is considered medium risk, and a score of $-1.0$ or greater is low risk.

Treatments for osteoporosis focus on slowing down or stopping bone loss, preventing bone fractures by minimizing the risk of falls, and controlling pain associated with the disease.

# ✓ PATHOLOGY CHECKPOINT

*Following is a concise list of the pathology-related terms that you have seen in the chapter. Review this checklist to make sure that you are familiar with the meaning of each term before moving to the next section.*

## Conditions and Symptoms ✱

- ❑ achondroplasia
- ❑ acroarthritis
- ❑ ankylosis
- ❑ arthralgia
- ❑ arthritis
- ❑ bursitis
- ❑ carpal tunnel syndrome
- ❑ coccygodynia
- ❑ dislocation
- ❑ flatfoot
- ❑ fractures
- ❑ genu valgum
- ❑ genu varum
- ❑ gout
- ❑ hammertoe
- ❑ hydrarthrosis
- ❑ ischialgia
- ❑ kyphosis
- ❑ lordosis
- ❑ lumbodynia
- ❑ myelitis
- ❑ myeloma
- ❑ osteoarthritis
- ❑ osteocarcinoma
- ❑ osteochondritis
- ❑ osteomalacia
- ❑ osteomyelitis
- ❑ osteopenia
- ❑ osteoporosis
- ❑ osteosarcoma
- ❑ periosteoedema
- ❑ polyarthritis
- ❑ rheumatoid arthritis
- ❑ rickets
- ❑ scoliosis
- ❑ spondylitis
- ❑ sprain
- ❑ spur
- ❑ tendonitis
- ❑ tennis elbow

## Diagnosis and Treatment ✱

- ❑ arthrocentesis
- ❑ arthroplasty
- ❑ arthroscope
- ❑ bone mineral density test
- ❑ bone marrow transplant
- ❑ cast
- ❑ craniectomy
- ❑ craniotomy
- ❑ fixation
- ❑ laminectomy
- ❑ metacarpectomy
- ❑ osteotome
- ❑ rachigraph
- ❑ radiograph
- ❑ reduction
- ❑ splint
- ❑ sternotomy
- ❑ traction

# STUDY AND REVIEW

## Anatomy and Physiology

*Write your answers to the following questions. Do not refer to the text.*

1. The skeletal system is composed of _____ bones.

2. Name the two main divisions of the skeletal system.

   a. _____        b. _____

3. Name five classifications of bone and give an example of each.

   a. _____ Example _____

   b. _____ Example _____

   c. _____ Example _____

   d. _____ Example _____

   e. _____ Example _____

4. State the six main functions of the skeletal system.

   a. _____        b. _____

   c. _____        d. _____

   e. _____        f. _____

5. Define the following features of a long bone.

   a. Epiphysis _____

   b. Diaphysis _____

   c. Periosteum _____

   d. Compact bone _____

   e. Medullary canal _____

   f. Endosteum _____

   g. Cancellous or spongy bone _____

6. Match the term in the left column with its definition from the right. Place the
   correct number from the right column in the space provided in the left column.

_____ 1. Meatus

_____ 2. Head

_____ 3. Tuberosity

_____ 4. Process

_____ 5. Condyle

_____ 6. Tubercle

_____ 7. Crest

_____ 8. Trochanter

_____ 9. Sinus

_____ 10. Fissure

_____ 11. Fossa

_____ 12. Spine

_____ 13. Foramen

_____ 14. Sulcus

a. Air cavity within certain bones
b. Shallow depression in or on a bone
c. Pointed, sharp, slender process
d. Large, rounded process
e. Groove, furrow, depression, or fissure
f. Tubelike passage or canal
g. Opening in the bone for blood vessels, ligaments, and nerves
h. Rounded projection that enters into the formation of a joint, articulation
i. Ridge on a bone
j. Small, rounded process
k. Rounded end of a bone
l. Slitlike opening between two bones
m. Enlargement or protrusion of a bone
n. Either of the two bony projections below the neck of the femur

7. Name the three classifications of joints.

a. _____        b. _____

c. _____

8. _____ is moving a body part away from the middle.

9. Adduction is _____.

10. _____ is moving a body part in a circular motion.

11. Dorsiflexion is _____.

12. _____ is turning outward.

13. Extension is _____.

14. _____ is bending a limb.

15. Inversion is _____.

16. _____ is lying face downward.

17. Protraction is _____.

18. _____ is moving a body part backward.

19. Rotation is _____.

20. _____ is lying face upward.

## Word Parts

1. In the spaces provided, write the definition of these prefixes, roots, combining forms, and suffixes. Do not refer to the listings of medical words. Leave blank those words you cannot define.

2. After completing as many as you can, refer to the medical word listings to check your work. For each word missed or left blank, write the word and its definition several times on the margins of these pages or on a separate sheet of paper.

3. To maximize the learning process, it is to your advantage to do the following exercises as directed. To refer to the word-building section before completing these exercises invalidates the learning process.

## PREFIXES

*Give the definitions of the following prefixes.*

1. a- _____

2. dis- _____

3. hydr- _____

4. inter- _____

5. meta- _____

6. peri- _____

7. poly- _____

8. sub- _____

9. sym- _____

10. re- _____

## ROOTS AND COMBINING FORMS

*Give the definitions of the following roots and combining forms.*

1. acetabul _____

2. cartil _____

3. acr _____

4. acr/o _____

5. ankyl _____

6. arthr _____

7. arthr/o _____

8. burs _____

9. calcan/e _____

10. locat _____

11. carcin _____

12. carp _____

13. carp/o _____

14. chondr _____

15. chondr/o _____

16. clavicul _____

17. fixat _____

18. coccyg/e _____

19. coccyg/o _____

20. coll/a _____

21. duct _____

22. connect _____

23. cost _____

24. cost/o _____

25. menisc _____

26. phos _____

27. crani/(o) _____

28. crani/o _____

29. dactyl _____

30. dactyl/o _____

31. femor _____

32. phor _____

33. fibul _____

34. radi/o _____

35. humer _____

36. ili _____

37. ili/o _____

38. isch/i _____

39. kyph _____

40. lamin _____

41. lord _____

42. lumb _____

43. lumb/o _____

44. mandibul _____

45. maxill _____

46. maxilla _____

47. myel _____

48. myel/o _____

49. rheumat _____

50. olecran _____

51. oste/o _____

52. patell _____

53. tract _____

54. ped _____

55. phalang/e _____

56. por _____

57. rachi _____

58. radi _____

59. sacr _____

60. sarc _____

61. scapul _____

62. scoli _____

63. scoli/o _____

64. spin _____

65. spondyl _____

66. stern _____

67. stern/o _____

68. tenon _____

69. tibi _____

70. uln _____

71. uln/o _____

72. vertebr _____

73. vertebr/o _____

74. xiph _____

## SUFFIXES

*Give the definitions of the following suffixes.*

1. -ac _____

2. -al _____

3. -algia _____

4. -ar _____

5. -ary _____

6. -blast _____

7. -centesis _____

8. -age _____

9. -ion _____

10. -dynia _____

11. -ectomy _____

12. -edema _____

13. -gen _____     14. -genesis _____

15. -gram _____     16. -graph _____

17. -ic _____     18. -itis _____

19. -ive _____     20. -scope _____

21. -malacia _____     22. -us _____

23. -oid _____     24. -oma _____

25. -omion _____     26. -osis _____

27. -penia _____     28. -physis _____

29. -plasia _____     30. -plasty _____

31. -poiesis _____     32. -tome _____

33. -tomy _____     34. -um _____

## Identifying Medical Terms

*In the spaces provided, write the medical terms for the following meanings.*

1. _____ Inflammation of the joints of the hands or feet

2. _____ Condition of stiffening of a joint

3. _____ Inflammation of a joint

4. _____ Pertaining to the heel bone

5. _____ Pertaining to cartilage

6. _____ Pain in the coccyx

7. _____ Pertaining to the rib

8. _____ Surgical excision of a portion of the skull

9. _____ Pertaining to the finger or toe

10. _____ Condition of fluid in a joint

11. _____ Pertaining to between the ribs

12. _____ Pain in the hip

13. _____ Pertaining to the loins

14. _____ Tumor of the bone marrow

15. _____ Inflammation of the joint and bone

16. _____ Inflammation of the bone marrow

17. _____ Lack of bone tissue

18. _____ Pertaining to the foot

19. _____ Resembling a sword

## Spelling

*In the spaces provided, write the correct spelling of these misspelled terms.*

1. acrmoin _____

2. arthrscope _____

3. buritis _____

4. chondblast _____

5. conective _____

6. cranplasty _____

7. dislocaton _____

8. ischal _____

9. melyitis _____

10. ostchonditis _____

11. phosphous _____

12. patelar _____

13. phalangal _____

14. rachgraph _____

15. scolosis _____

16. spondlitis _____

17. symphsis _____

18. tenonis _____

19. ulncarpal _____

20. vertbral _____

## Matching

*Select the appropriate lettered meaning for each of the following words.*

_____ 1. arthroscope

_____ 2. carpal tunnel syndrome

_____ 3. fixation

_____ 4. gout

_____ 5. hammertoe

_____ 6. kyphosis

_____ 7. metacarpal

_____ 8. rickets

_____ 9. tennis elbow

_____ 10. ulnar

a. Deficiency condition in children primarily caused by a lack of vitamin D

b. Acquired flexion deformity of the interphalangeal joint

c. Hereditary metabolic disease that is a form of acute arthritis

d. Chronic condition characterized by pain that is caused by excessive pronation and supination activities of the forearm

e. Making rigid, immobilizing

f. Pertaining to the elbow

g. Pertaining to the bones of the hand

h. Humpback

i. Instrument used to examine the interior of a joint

j. Condition caused by compression of the median nerve by the carpal ligament

k. Pertaining to the knee

## Abbreviations

*Place the correct word, phrase, or abbreviation in the space provided.*

1. congenital dislocation of hip _____

2. degenerative joint disease _____

3. LLC _____

4. OA _____

5. pulsing electromagnetic fields _____

6. RA _____

7. single photon emission computed tomography _____

8. T1 _____

9. TMJ _____

10. traction _____

## Diagnostic and Laboratory Test

*Select the best answer to each multiple choice question. Circle the letter of your choice.*

1. _____ is a diagnostic examination of a joint in which air and then a radiopaque contrast medium are injected into the joint space, x-rays are taken, and internal injuries of the meniscus, cartilage, and ligaments may be seen, if present.
   a. Arthroscopy
   b. Goniometry
   c. Arthrography
   d. Thermography

2. The process of recording heat patterns of the body's surface is:
   a. arthrography
   b. arthroscopy
   c. goniometry
   d. thermography

3. _____ is increased in gout, arthritis, multiple myeloma, and rheumatism.
   a. Calcium
   b. Phosphorus
   c. Uric acid
   d. Alkaline phosphatase

4. _____ level of the blood can be increased in osteoporosis and fracture healing.
   a. Antinuclear antibodies
   b. Phosphorus
   c. Uric acid
   d. Alkaline phosphatase

5. _____ is/are present in a variety of immunologic diseases.
   a. Alkaline phosphatase
   b. Antinuclear antibodies
   c. C-Reactive protein
   d. Uric acid

# PRACTICAL APPLICATION

## S O A P : Chart Note Analysis

*This exercise will make you aware of information, abbreviations, and medical terminology typically found in an orthopedic patient's chart note.*

### Abbreviations Key

| | | | | |
|---|---|---|---|---|
| Abd | abdomen | | Neuro | neurology |
| BMI | body mass index | | NKDA | no known drug allergies |
| BP | blood pressure | | P | pulse |
| CTA | clear to auscultation | | R | respiration |
| DEXA | dual-energy x-ray absorptiometry | | SOAP | subjective, objective, assessment |
| DOB | date of birth | | | plan |
| F | Fahrenheit | | T | temperature |
| GYN | gynecology | | Tab | tablet |
| Ht | height | | VS | vital signs |
| lb | pound | | WNL | within normal limits |
| LMP | last menstrual period | | Wt | weight |
| mg | milligram | | y/o | year(s) old |
| MS | musculoskeletal | | | |

*Read the following chart note and then answer the questions that follow.*

**PATIENT:** Casey, Florence                                                        **DATE:** 6/10/07
**DOB:** 12/29/1944        **AGE:** 62        **SEX:** Female
**INSURANCE:** 21st Century Health Company

**Vital Signs:**
T: 98.4 F
P: 72
R: 18
BP: 128/80
Ht: 5' 1"
Wt: 142 lb

**Allergies:** NKDA

**Chief Complaint:** Loss of height, kyphosis, and lumbodynia.

**S**  **Subjective:** 62 y/o female presents with complaints that her back "hurts all the time." She has noticed she is becoming shorter and developing a "humpback." Patient states her LMP was approximately seventeen years ago at age 45 and that her height "has always been 5 feet 3 inches."

**O**  **Objective:**
**General Appearance:** Small frame, overweight, white female with noted humpback, backward head tilt and slight flexion of hip and knees. Appears to experience mild pain in lower back during movements.
**Lungs:** CTA
**Heart:** Normal rate and rhythm. No murmurs, gallops, or rubs.

**Abd:** Bowel sounds in all 4 quadrants. No masses or tenderness.

**MS:** Dorsal kyphosis and cervical lordosis, shortening of the trunk and comparatively long extremities, no tenderness upon spinal palpation.

**Neuro:** Alert and oriented × 3. Reflexes intact.

**Skin:** Warm and dry to touch. No breakdown noted.

**GYN:** LMP was 17 years ago.

**A**    **Assessment:** Osteoporosis

**P**    Plan:

1. Schedule DEXA to measure bone density, confirm diagnosis, predict future risk of fractures, and assist in monitoring changes in medical condition and response to medication. **Note:** A bone density test should be scheduled every 2 years for evaluation of effectiveness of treatment.
2. Actonel (risedronate sodium) 5mg Tab 1 PO daily
3. Begin regular exercise program 3 to 5 days weekly for at least 30 minutes each day. Weight-bearing exercise such as walking and dancing are recommended.
4. Follow a diet rich in calcium, phosphorus, magnesium, and vitamins A, C, D and the B-complex vitamins. Good sources of vitamin A are dairy products, fish liver oils, animal liver, green and yellow vegetables. Good sources of vitamin D are ultraviolet rays, dairy products, and commercial foods that contain supplemental vitamin D (milk and cereals). Good Sources of vitamin C are citrus fruits, tomatoes, melons, fresh berries, raw vegetables, and sweet potatoes. Good sources of the B-complex vitamins are organ meats, dried beans, poultry, eggs, yeast, fish, whole grains, and dark-green vegetables. Good sources of calcium are dairy products, beans, cauliflower, egg yolk, molasses, leafy green vegetables, tofu, sardines, clams, and oysters. Good sources of phosphorus are dairy products, eggs, fish, poultry, meats, dried peas and beans, whole grain cereals, and nuts. Good sources of magnesium are whole grain cereals, fruits, milk, nuts, vegetables, seafood, and meats.
5. Take a supplement of calcium with Vitamin D daily.
6. Inform the patient of the National Osteoporosis Foundation's telephone number, 1-202-223-2226, and the organization's web site at www.nof.org.

 **FYI:** With normal aging, individuals can lose 1.0 to 1.5 inches in height. In asymptomatic women, loss of more than 1.5 inches in height can be related to vertebral compression fractures. Risk factors for osteoporosis include family history; lack of exercise; thin, small frame; never been pregnant; early menopause; tendency to fractures; loss of height in the past few years; avoidance of dairy products as a child; smoking; drinking alcoholic beverages; diet high in salt, caffeine, or fat; and insufficient intake of vitamin D.

## CHART NOTE QUESTIONS
*Place the correct answer in the space provided.*

1. Signs and symptoms of osteoporosis include loss of height, _____, and pain in the back.

2. What is the prescribed dosage of Actonel (risedronate sodium)? _____

3. Dairy products, fish liver oils, animal liver, and green and yellow vegetables are all good sources of _____.

4. Citrus fruits, tomatoes, melons, fresh berries, raw vegetables, and sweet potatoes are all good sources of _____.

5. Milk, yogurt, cheese, tofu, turnip greens, canned salmon, sardines, beans, egg yolk, molasses, and broccoli are examples of good sources of _____.

6. Give four purposes for using the DEXA scan.

   a. _____    b. _____

   c. _____    d. _____

7. In normal aging, most individuals can lose approximately _____ to _____ in height.

8. Loss of more than 1.5 inches in height can be related to vertebral _____ fractures in asymptomatic women.

9. Name six risk factors for developing osteoporosis.

   a. _____    b. _____    c. _____

   d. _____    e. _____    f. _____

10. Why is a DEXA scan recommended every two years after osteoporosis is diagnosed?

   _____

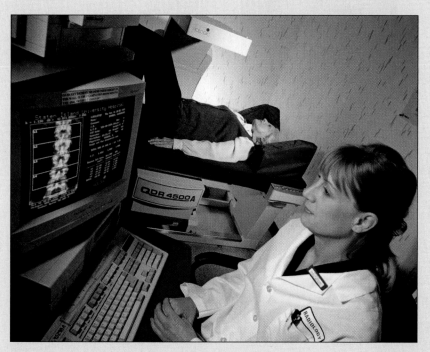

**FIGURE 6–26**  Radiologist monitors a computer screen as a woman undergoes a DEXA scan to measure bone density. (Courtesy of Phototake NYC)

# MULTIMEDIA PREVIEW

*Additional interactive resources and activities for this chapter can be found on the Companion Website. For videos, audio glossary, and review, access the accompanying CD-ROM in this book.*

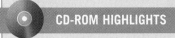
## CD-ROM HIGHLIGHTS

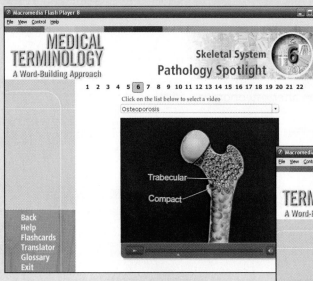

## PATHOLOGY SPOTLIGHT— OSTEOPOROSIS

By viewing concepts in moving, living color, you'll get a fuller picture of the pathologies presented in this chapter. Earlier we discussed osteoporosis. Now click on this feature to watch a video that describes this condition in more detail.

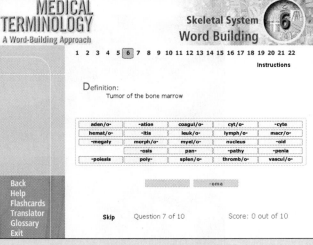

## WORD BUILDING

Are you ready to master the technique of constructing terms using word parts? Put it all together by clicking and dragging the right prefixes, suffixes, roots, and combining forms together to match the definitions provided.

## WEBSITE HIGHLIGHTS—www.prenhall.com/rice

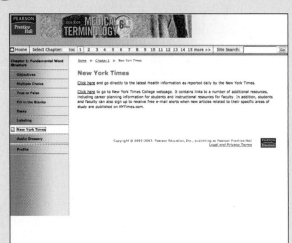

## MEDICINE IN THE NEWS

Click here and take advantage of the free-access on-line study guide that accompanies your textbook. You'll be able to stay current with a link to medical news articles updated daily by the *New York Times*. By clicking on this URL you'll also access a variety of quizzes with instant feedback, links to download mp3 audio reviews, and an audio glossary.

# Muscular System

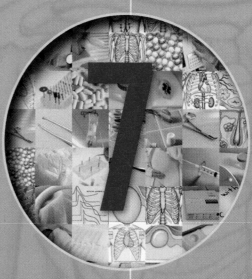

## ■ OUTLINE

## ■ OBJECTIVES

*On completion of this chapter, you will be able to:*

- Describe the muscular system.
- Describe types of muscle tissue.
- Provide the functions of muscles.
- Describe muscular differences of the child and the older adult.
- Analyze, build, spell, and pronounce medical words.
- Comprehend the drugs highlighted in this chapter.
- Describe diagnostic and laboratory tests related to the muscular system.
- Identify and define selected abbreviations.
- Describe each of the conditions presented in the Pathology Spotlights.
- Review the Pathology Checkpoint.
- Complete the Study and Review section and the Chart Note Analysis.

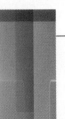

# Anatomy and Physiology Overview

The muscular system is composed of all the **muscles** in the body. This overview describes the three basic types of muscles and some of their functions. The muscles are the primary tissues of the system. They make up approximately 42% of a person's body weight and are composed of long, slender cells known as **fibers.** Muscle fibers are of different lengths and shapes and vary in color from white to deep red. Each muscle consists of a group of fibers held together by connective tissue and enclosed in a fibrous sheath or **fascia.** See Figure 7–1 ▼.

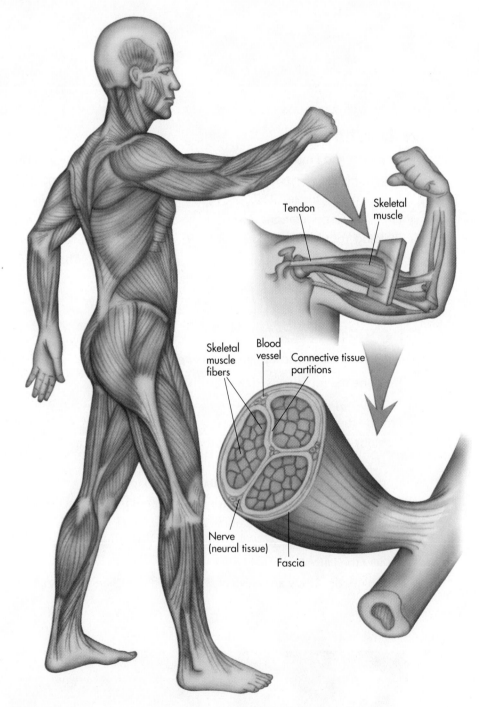

Tendon

Skeletal muscle

Skeletal muscle fibers

Blood vessel

Connective tissue partitions

Nerve (neural tissue)

Fascia

▶ **FIGURE 7–1** Skeletal muscle consists of a group of fibers held together by connective tissue. It is enclosed in a fibrous sheath (fascia).

Each fiber within a muscle receives its own nerve impulses and has its own stored supply of glycogen, which it uses as fuel for energy. Muscle must be supplied with proper nutrition and oxygen to perform properly; therefore, blood and lymphatic vessels permeate its tissues.

# TYPES OF MUSCLE TISSUE

Skeletal muscle, smooth muscle, and cardiac muscle are the three basic types of muscle tissue classed according to their functions and appearance (Figure 7–2 ▼).

## Muscular System

| Organ/Structure | Primary Functions |
|---|---|
| Muscles | Cause movement, help to maintain posture, and produce heat |
| Skeletal | Produces various types of body movement through contractility, extensibility, and elasticity. |
| Smooth | Produce relatively slow contraction with greater degree of extensibility in the internal organs, especially organs of the digestive, respiratory, and urinary tract, plus certain muscles of the eye and skin, and walls of blood vessels |
| Cardiac | Contraction of the myocardium, which is controlled by the autonomic nervous system and specialized neuromuscular tissue located within the right atrium |
| Tendons | Bands of connective tissue that attach muscles to bones |

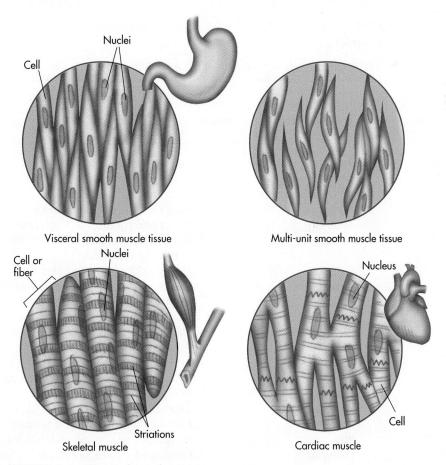

▶ FIGURE 7–2  Types of muscle tissue.

## Skeletal Muscle

Also known as **voluntary** or **striated** muscles, **skeletal muscles** are controlled by the conscious part of the brain and attach to the bones. These muscles have a cross-striped appearance and vary in size, shape, arrangement of fibers, and means of attachment to bones. Selected skeletal muscles are listed with their functions in Table 7–1 and shown in Figures 7–3 ▶ and 7–4 ▶.

There are 600 skeletal muscles that, through contractility, extensibility, excitability, and elasticity, are responsible for the movement of the body. **Contractility** allows muscles to change shape to become shorter and thicker. With **extensibility,** living muscle cells can be stretched and extended. They become longer and thinner. In **excitability,** muscles receive and respond to stimulation. With **elasticity,** once the stretching force is removed, a living muscle cell returns to its original shape.

Muscles have three distinguishable parts: the **body** or main portion, an **origin,** and an **insertion.** The origin is the more fixed attachment and the insertion is the point of attachment of a muscle to the part that it moves. The means of attachment is called a **tendon,** which can vary in length from less than 1 inch to more than 1 foot. A wide, thin, sheetlike tendon is know as an **aponeurois.**

Skeletal muscles move body parts by pulling from one bone across its joint to another bone with movement occurring at the diarthrotic joint. The types of body movement occurring at the diarthrotic joints are described in Chapter 6, Skeletal System, on page 114.

Muscles and nerves function together as a motor unit. For skeletal muscles to contract, it is necessary to have stimulation by impulses from motor nerves. Muscles perform in groups and are classified as follows:

- **Antagonist.** Muscle that counteracts the action of another muscle

- **Prime mover or agonist.** Muscle that is primary in a given movement produced by its contraction

- **Synergist.** Muscle that acts with another muscle to produce movement

## TABLE 7–1  Selected Skeletal Muscles

| Muscle | Direction | Action |
|---|---|---|
| Sternocleidomastoid | Anterior | Rotates and laterally flexes neck |
| Trapezius | Anterior/posterior | Draws head back and to the side; rotates scapula |
| Deltoid | Anterior/posterior | Raises and rotates arm |
| Rectus femoris | Anterior | Extends leg and assists flexion of thigh |
| Sartorius | Anterior | Flexes and rotates the thigh and leg |
| Tibialis anterior | Anterior | Dorsiflexes foot and increases the arch in the beginning process of walking |
| Pectoralis major | Anterior | Flexes, adducts, and rotates arm |
| Biceps brachii | Anterior | Flexes arm and forearm and supinates forearm |
| External oblique | Anterior | Contracts abdomen and viscera (internal organs) |
| Rectus abdominis | Anterior | Compresses or flattens abdomen |
| Gastrocnemius | Anterior/posterior | Plantar flexes foot and flexes knee |
| Soleus | Anterior | Plantar flexes foot |
| Triceps | Posterior | Extends forearm |
| Latissimus dorsi | Posterior | Adducts, extends, and rotates arm; used during swimming |
| Gluteus medius | Posterior | Abducts and rotates thigh |
| Gluteus maximus | Posterior | Extends and rotates thigh |
| Biceps femoris | Posterior | Flexes knee and rotates it outward |
| Semitendinosus | Posterior | Flexes and rotates leg; extends thigh |
| Semimembranosus | Posterior | Flexes and rotates leg; extends thigh |
| Achilles tendon | Posterior | Plantar (sole of the foot) flexion and extension of ankle |

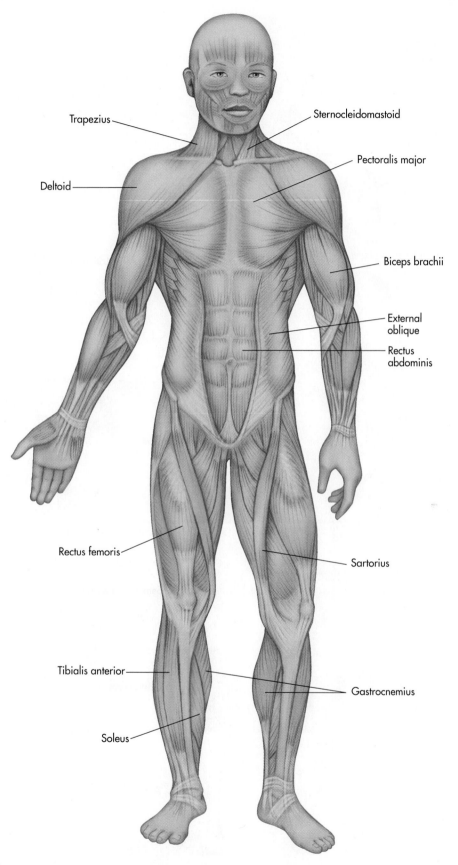

► **FIGURE 7–3** Selected skeletal muscles (anterior view).

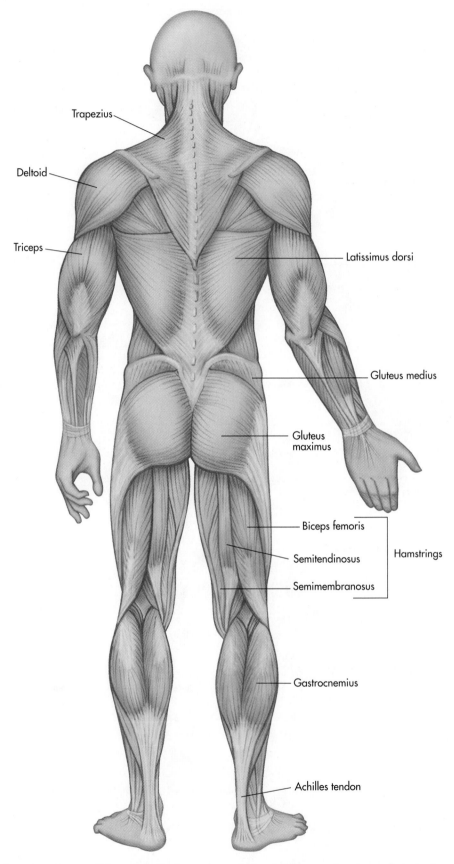

Trapezius

Deltoid

Triceps

Latissimus dorsi

Gluteus medius

Gluteus maximus

Biceps femoris

Semitendinosus

Semimembranosus

Hamstrings

Gastrocnemius

Achilles tendon

▶ **FIGURE 7–4**   Selected skeletal muscles and the Achilles tendon (posterior view).

## Smooth Muscle

Also called *involuntary*, *visceral*, or *unstriated*, **smooth muscles** are not controlled by the conscious part of the brain. They are under the control of the autonomic nervous system and, in most cases, produce relatively slow contraction with greater degree of extensibility. These muscles lack the cross-striped appearance of skeletal muscle and are smooth. Included in this type are the muscles of internal organs of the digestive, respiratory, and urinary tract plus certain muscles of the eye and skin.

## Cardiac Muscle

The muscle of the heart (**myocardium**), the **cardiac muscle,** is *involuntary* but *striated* in appearance. It is controlled by the autonomic nervous system and specialized neuromuscular tissue located within the right atrium.

# FUNCTIONS OF MUSCLES

The following is a list of the primary functions of muscles:

1. Muscles are responsible for movement. The types of movement are locomotion, propulsion of substances through tubes as in circulation and digestion, and changes in the size of openings as in the contraction and relaxation of the iris of the eye.
2. Muscles help to maintain posture through a continual partial contraction of skeletal muscles. This process is known as **tonicity.**
3. Muscles help to produce heat through the chemical changes involved in muscular action.

# LIFE SPAN CONSIDERATIONS

## ■ THE CHILD

At about 6 weeks, the size of the embryo is 12 mm (0.5 inch). The limb buds are extending and the skeletal and muscular systems are developing. At about 7 weeks, the **diaphragm,** a partition of muscles and membranes that separates the chest cavity and the abdominal cavity, is completely developed. At the end of 8 weeks, the embryo is now known as the **fetus.** Fetal growth proceeds from head to tail (**cephalo** to **caudal**), with the head being larger in comparison to the rest of the body.

During fetal development, the bones and muscles continue growing and developing. At about 32 weeks, the developed skeletal system is soft and flexible. Muscle and fat accumulate, and the fetus weighs approximately 2000 g (4 lb, 7 oz). At about 40 weeks, the fetus is ready for birth and extrauterine life.

The movements of the newborn are uncoordinated and random. Muscular development proceeds from head to foot and from the center of the body to the periphery. Head and neck muscles are the first ones that the baby can control. A baby can hold his head up before he can sit erect.

## ■ THE OLDER ADULT

With aging, changes related to mobility are most significant. There is a decrease in muscle strength, endurance, range of motion (ROM), coordination and elasticity, and flexibility of connective tissue. Also, as a person grows older, the number and size of muscle fibers decrease, and the water content of tendons is reduced. Decrease in handgrip strength makes performing routine activities such as opening a jar or turning a key more difficult. The heart muscle becomes less able to propel large quantities of blood quickly to the body. This makes a person tire more quickly and take longer to recover.

To prevent loss of strength, muscles need to be exercised. Regular exercise strengthens muscles and keeps joints, tendons, and ligaments more flexible, allowing active people to move freely and carry out routine activities easily. Exercises such as aerobic dance, brisk walking, and bicycling improve muscle tone and heart and lung function. To maintain aerobic fitness, a person needs to participate in such activities for 20 minutes or more at least three times a week and work at one's target heart rate.

# BUILDING YOUR MEDICAL VOCABULARY

This section provides the foundation for learning medical terminology. Review the following alphabetized word list. Note how common prefixes and suffixes are repeatedly applied to word roots and combining forms to create different meanings.

| P | Prefix |
|---|--------|
| R | Root |
| CF | Combining form |
| S | Suffix |

| Pink words | Terms not built from word parts |
|---|---|
| * | Indicates words covered in the Pathology Spotlights section. |
| ◎ | Check the CD-ROM for more information. |

| MEDICAL WORD | WORD PARTS (WHEN APPLICABLE) | | | DEFINITION |
|---|---|---|---|---|
| | Part | Type | Meaning | |
| **abductor** (ăb-dŭk′tōr) | ab- | P | away from | Muscle that on contraction draws away from the middle |
| | duct | R | to lead | |
| | -or | S | a doer | |
| **adductor** (ă-dŭk′tōr) | ad- | P | toward | Muscle that draws a part toward the middle |
| | duct | R | to lead | |
| | -or | S | a doer | |
| **amputation** (ăm″ pū-tā′shŭn) | amputat | R | to cut through | Removal of a limb, part, or other appendage. See Figure 7–5 ▶. |
| | -ion | S | process | |
| **antagonist** (ăn-tăg′ō-nĭst) | ant- | P | against | Muscle that counteracts the action of another muscle. See Figure 7–6 ▶. |
| | agon | R | agony, a contest | |
| | -ist | S | agent | |

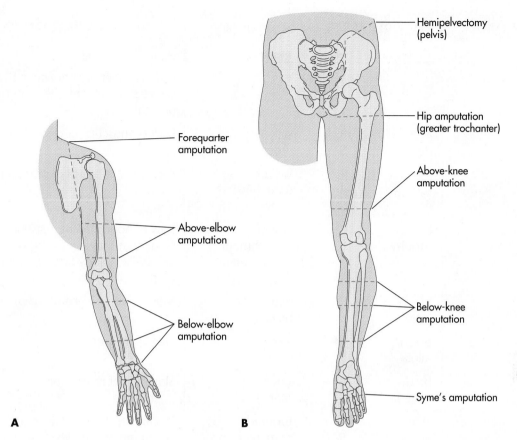

▶ **FIGURE 7–5** Common sites of amputation. (A) Upper extremities. (B) Lower extremities. The surgeon determines the level of amputation based on blood supply and tissue condition.

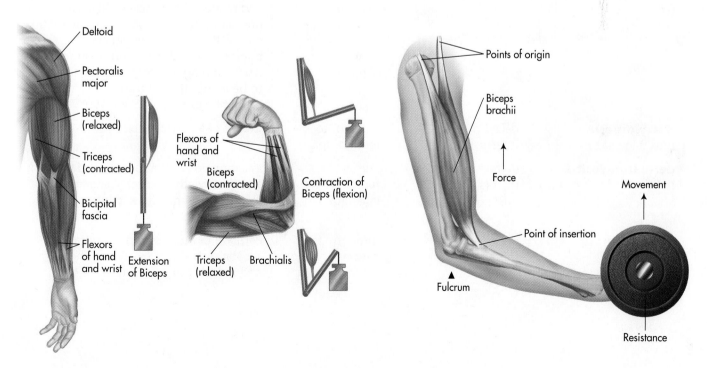

▶ **FIGURE 7–6** Coordination of antagonist muscles to perform movement.

| MEDICAL WORD | WORD PARTS (WHEN APPLICABLE) | | | DEFINITION |
|---|---|---|---|---|
| | Part | Type | Meaning | |
| **aponeurosis** (ăp″ ō-nū-rō′sĭs) | | | | Fibrous sheet of connective tissue that serves to attach muscle to bone or to other tissues |
| **ataxia** (ă-tăks′ĭ-ă) | a- -taxia | P S | lack of order | Lack of muscular coordination |
| **atonic** (ă-tŏn′ĭk) | a- ton -ic | P R S | lack of tone, tension pertaining to | Pertaining to a lack of normal tone or tension |
| **atrophy** (ăt′rō-fē) | a- -trophy | P S | lack of nourishment, development | Lack of nourishment; wasting of muscular tissue that may be caused by lack of use. ✱ See Pathology Spotlight: Atrophy on page 171 and Figure 7–13. |
| **biceps** (bī′sps) | bi- -ceps | P S | two head | Muscle with two heads or points of origin |
| **brachialgia** (brā″ ki-ăl′jĭ-ă) | brach/i -algia | CF S | arm pain | Pain in the arm |
| **bradykinesia** (brăd″ ĭ-kĭ-nē′sĭ-ă) | brady- -kinesia | P S | slow motion | Slowness of motion or movement |
| **clonic** (klŏn′ĭk) | clon -ic | R S | turmoil pertaining to | Pertaining to alternate contraction and relaxation of muscles |
| **contraction** (kŏn-trăk′shŭn) | con- tract -ion | P R S | with, together to draw process | Process of drawing up and thickening of a muscle fiber |
| **contracture** (kŏn-trăk′chūr) | con- tract -ure | P R S | with, together to draw process | Condition in which a muscle shortens and renders the muscle resistant to the normal stretching process. Dupuytren's contracture is a thickening and tightening of subcutaneous tissue of the palm, causing the ring and little fingers to bend into the palm so that they cannot be extended. See Figure 7–7 ▶. |
| **dactylospasm** (dăk′tĭ-lō-spăzm) | dactyl/o -spasm | CF S | finger or toe tension, spasm | Cramp of a finger or toe |
| **dermatomyositis** (dĕr″ mă-tō-mī″ ō-sī′tĭs) | dermat/o my/o(s) -itis | CF CF S | skin muscle inflammation | Inflammation of the muscles and the skin; a connective tissue disease characterized by edema, dermatitis, and inflammation of the muscles. See Figure 7–8 ▶. |
| **diaphragm** (dī′ă-frăm) | dia- -phragm | P S | through a fence, partition | Partition of muscles and membranes that separates the chest cavity and the abdominal cavity. See Figure 7–9 ▶. |

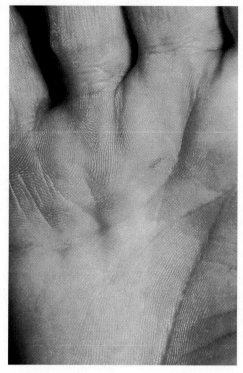

▶ **FIGURE 7–7** Dupuytren's contracture. (Courtesy of Jason L. Smith, MD.)

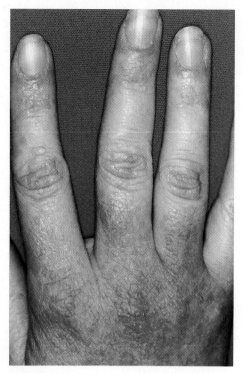

▶ **FIGURE 7–8** Dermatomyositis. (Courtesy of Jason L. Smith, MD.)

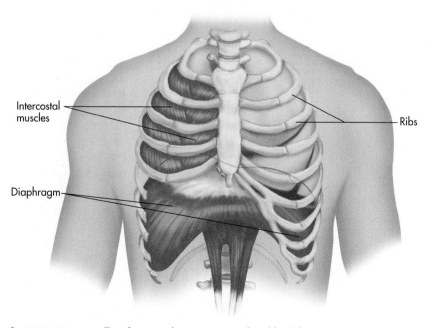

Intercostal muscles

Ribs

Diaphragm

▶ **FIGURE 7–9** Diaphragm, the major muscle of breathing.

| MEDICAL WORD | WORD PARTS (WHEN APPLICABLE) | | | DEFINITION |
|---|---|---|---|---|
| | Part | Type | Meaning | |
| **diathermy** (dĭ′ă-thĕr″ mē) | dia- therm -y | P R S | through hot, heat pertaining to | Treatment using high-frequency current to produce heat within a part of the body; used to increase blood flow but should not be used in acute stage of recovery from trauma. Types: **Microwave.** Electromagnetic radiation directed to specified tissues **Short wave.** High-frequency electric current (wavelength of 3–30 m) directed to specified tissues **Ultrasound.** High-frequency sound waves (20,000–10 billion cycles/sec) directed to specified tissues |
| **dystonia** (dĭs′tō′nĭ-ă) | dys- ton -ia | P R S | difficult tone, tension condition | Condition of impaired muscle tone |
| **dystrophin** (dĭs-trŏf′ĭn) | dys- troph -in | P R S | difficult a turning chemical | Protein found in muscle cells. When the gene that is responsible for this protein is defective and sufficient dystrophin is not produced, muscle wasting occurs. |
| **dystrophy** (dĭs′trō-fē) | dys- -trophy | P S | difficult nourishment, development | Faulty muscular development caused by lack of nourishment |
| **exercise** | | | | Performed activity of the muscles for improvement of health or correction of deformity. Types: **Active.** Muscular contraction and relaxation by patient **Assistive.** Muscular contraction and relaxation with the assistance of a therapist **Isometric.** Active muscular contraction performed against stable resistance, thereby not shortening muscle length **Passive.** Exercise performed by another individual without patient assistance **Range of motion (ROM).** Movement of each joint through its full range of motion; used to prevent loss of mobility or to regain usage after an injury or fracture **Relief of tension.** Technique used to promote relaxation of the muscles and provide relief from tension |
| **fascia** (făsh′ĭ-ă) | fasc -ia | R S | a band condition | Thin layer of connective tissue covering, supporting, or connecting the muscles or inner organs of the body |

| MEDICAL WORD | WORD PARTS (WHEN APPLICABLE) | | | DEFINITION |
|---|---|---|---|---|
| | Part | Type | Meaning | |
| **fascitis** (fă-sī'tĭs) | fasc -itis | R S | a band inflammation | Inflammation of a fascia |
| **fatigue** (fă-tēg') | | | | State of tiredness occurring in a muscle as a result of repeated contractions |
| **fibromyalgia syndrome (FMS)** (fī" brō-mī-ăl'jē-ă sĭn' drōm) | fibr/o my -algia | CF R S | fiber muscle pain | Chronic syndrome with widespread muscular pain and debilitating fatigue. ★ See Figure 7–14 in Pathology Spotlight: Fibromyalgia on page 173. |
| **fibromyitis** (fī" brō-mī-ī'tĭs) | fibr/o my -itis | CF R S | fiber muscle inflammation | Inflammation of muscle and fibrous tissue |
| **First Aid Treatment— (RICE)** **Rest** **Ice** **Compression** **Elevation** | | | | **Cryotherapy** (use of cold) is the treatment of choice for soft tissue and muscle injuries. It causes vasoconstriction of blood vessels and is effective in diminishing bleeding and edema. Ice should not be placed directly onto the skin. **Compression** by an elastic bandage is generally determined by the type of injury and physician preference. Some experts disagree on the use of elastic bandages. When used, the bandage should be 3 to 4 inches wide and applied firmly. Toes or fingers should be periodically checked for blue or white discoloration, indicating that the bandage is too tight. **Elevation** is used to reduce swelling. The injured part should be elevated on two or three pillows. |
| **flaccid** (flăk'sĭd) | | | | Lacking muscle tone; *weak, soft,* and *flabby* |
| **heat** | | | | Thermotherapy; treatment using scientific application of heat can be used 48 to 72 hours after the injury. Types: heating pad, hot water bottle, hot packs, infrared light, and immersion of body part in warm water. Extreme care should be taken when using or applying heat. |
| **hydrotherapy** (hī-drō-thĕr'ă-pē) | hydro- -therapy | P S | water treatment | Treatment using scientific application of water; types: hot tub, cold bath, whirlpool, and vapor bath |

| MEDICAL WORD | WORD PARTS (WHEN APPLICABLE) | | | DEFINITION |
|---|---|---|---|---|
| | **Part** | **Type** | **Meaning** | |
| **insertion**<br>(ĭn″sûr′shŭn) | in-<br>sert<br>-ion | P<br>R<br>S | into<br>to gain<br>process | Point of attachment of a muscle to the part that it moves |
| **intramuscular (IM)**<br>(ĭn″ tră-mŭs′kū-lər) | intra-<br>muscul<br>-ar | P<br>R<br>S | within<br>muscle<br>pertaining to | Pertaining to within a muscle |
| **isometric**<br>(ī″ sō-mĕt′rĭk) | is/o<br>metr<br>-ic | CF<br>R<br>S | equal<br>to measure<br>pertaining to | Pertaining to having equal measure |
| **isotonic**<br>(ī″ sō-tŏn′ĭk) | is/o<br>ton<br>-ic | CF<br>R<br>S | equal<br>tone, tension<br>pertaining to | Pertaining to having the same tone or tension |
| **levator**<br>(lē-vā′ tər) | levat<br>-or | R<br>S | lifter<br>a doer | Muscle that raises or elevates a part |
| **massage**<br>(măh-săhzh) | | | | Kneading that applies pressure and friction to external body tissues |
| **muscular dystrophy (MD)**<br>(mŭs′kū-lār dĭs′trō-fē) | | | | Chronic, progressive wasting and weakening of muscles. Because the leg muscles of children with MD are weak, they must perform the Gowers' maneuver to raise to a standing position. See Figure 7–10 ▶. ✹ See Pathology Spotlight: Muscular Dystrophy on page 173 and Figure 7–15. |
| **myalgia**<br>(mī-ăl′jĭ-ă) | my<br>-algia | R<br>S | muscle<br>pain | Pain in the muscle |
| **myasthenia gravis (MG)**<br>(mī-ăs-thē′nĭ-ă gră vĭs) | my<br>-asthenia<br>gravis | R<br>S<br>R | muscle<br>weakness<br>grave | Chronic disease characterized by progressive muscular weakness. ✹ See Pathology Spotlight: Myasthenia Gravis on page 172. |
| **myoblast**<br>(mī′ō blăst) | my/o<br>-blast | CF<br>S | muscle<br>immature cell, germ cell | Embryonic cell that develops into a cell of muscle fiber |
| **myofibroma**<br>(mī″ ō fī-brō′mă) | my/o<br>fibr<br>-oma | CF<br>R<br>S | muscle<br>fiber<br>tumor | Tumor that contains muscle and fiber |
| **myograph**<br>(mī′ō-grăf) | my/o<br>-graph | CF<br>S | muscle<br>instrument for recording | Instrument used to record muscular contractions |
| **myokinesis**<br>(mī″ ō-kĭn-ē′sĭs) | my/o<br>-kinesis | CF<br>S | muscle<br>motion | Muscular motion or activity |
| **myology**<br>(mĭ-ōl ō-jē) | my/o<br>-logy | CF<br>S | muscle<br>study of | Study of muscles |
| **myoma**<br>(mī-ō′ mă) | my<br>-oma | R<br>S | muscle<br>tumor | Tumor containing muscle tissue |

| MEDICAL WORD | WORD PARTS (WHEN APPLICABLE) | | | DEFINITION |
|---|---|---|---|---|
| | Part | Type | Meaning | |
| **myomalacia**<br>(mī″ ō-mă-lā′sǐ-ă) | my/o<br>-malacia | CF<br>S | muscle<br>softening | Softening of muscle tissue |
| **myoparesis**<br>(mī″ ō-păr′ ĕ-sǐs) | my/o<br>-paresis | CF<br>S | muscle<br>weakness | Weakness or slight paralysis of a muscle |
| **myopathy**<br>(mī-ŏp′ ă-thē) | my/o<br>-pathy | CF<br>S | muscle<br>disease | Muscle disease |
| **myoplasty**<br>(mī′ ŏ-plăs″ tē) | my/o<br>-plasty | CF<br>S | muscle<br>surgical repair | Surgical repair of a muscle |
| **myorrhaphy**<br>(mī-or′ ă-fē) | my/o<br>-rrhaphy | CF<br>S | muscle<br>suture | Suture of a muscle wound |

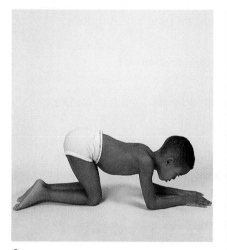

**A**

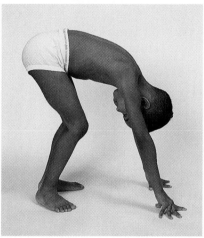

**B**

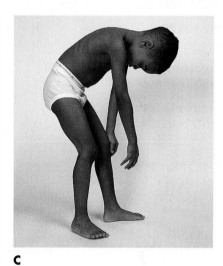

**C**

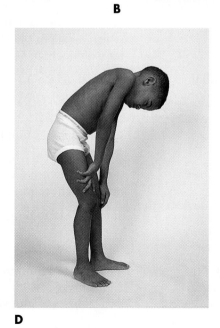

**D**

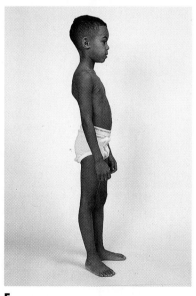

**E**

▶ **FIGURE 7–10**  Because the leg muscles of children with muscular dystrophy are weak, they must perform the Gowers' maneuver to rise to a standing position. (A) and (B) The child first maneuvers to a position supported by arms and legs. (C) The child next pushes off the floor and rests one hand on the knee. (D) and (E) The child then pushes himself upright.

| MEDICAL WORD | WORD PARTS (WHEN APPLICABLE) | | | DEFINITION |
|---|---|---|---|---|
| | **Part** | **Type** | **Meaning** | |
| **myosarcoma**<br>(mĭ″ ō-sar-kō′ mă) | my/o<br>sarc<br>-oma | CF<br>R<br>S | muscle<br>flesh<br>tumor | Malignant tumor derived from muscle tissue |
| **myosclerosis**<br>(mī″ ō-sklĕr-ō′ sĭs) | my/o<br>scler<br>-osis | CF<br>R<br>S | muscle<br>hardening<br>condition (usually abnormal) | Condition of hardening of muscle |
| **myositis**<br>(mī″ ō-s ī ′tĭs) | my/o (s)<br>-itis | CF<br>S | muscle<br>inflammation | Inflammation of muscle tissue, especially skeletal muscles; may be caused by infection, trauma, or parasitic infestation |
| **myospasm**<br>(mī″ ō-spăzm) | my/o<br>-spasm | CF<br>S | muscle<br>tension, spasm | Spasmodic contraction of a muscle |
| **myotome**<br>(mī′ ō-tōm) | my/o<br>-tome | CF<br>S | muscle<br>instrument to cut | Instrument used to cut muscle |
| **myotomy**<br>(mī′ ŏt′ ō-mē) | my/o<br>-tomy | CF<br>S | muscle<br>incision | Incision into a muscle |
| **neuromuscular**<br>(nū″ rō-mŭs′ kū-lăr) | neur/o<br>muscul<br>-ar | CF<br>R<br>S | nerve<br>muscle<br>pertaining to | Pertaining to both nerves and muscles |
| **neuromyopathic**<br>(nū″ rō-m ī″ ō-păth′ ĭk) | neur/o<br>my/o<br>path<br>-ic | CF<br>CF<br>R<br>S | nerve<br>muscle<br>disease<br>pertaining to | Pertaining to a disease condition involving both nerves and muscles |
| **polyplegia**<br>(pŏl″ ē-plē′ jĭ-ă) | poly-<br>-plegia | P<br>S | many<br>stroke, paralysis | Paralysis affecting many muscles |
| **position**<br>(pō-zĭsh′ ŭn) | | | | Bodily posture or attitude; the manner in which a patient's body may be arranged for examination. See Table 7–2. |
| **prosthesis**<br>(prŏs′ thē-sĭs) | prosth/e<br>-sis | CF<br>S | an addition<br>condition | Artificial device used to replace an organ or part, such as a hand, arm, leg, or hip. See Figure 7–11 ▶. |
| **quadriceps**<br>(kwŏd′ rĭ-s ĕps) | quadri-<br>-ceps | P<br>S | four<br>head | Muscle that has four heads or points of origin |
| **relaxation**<br>(rē-lăk-sā′ shŭn) | relaxat<br>-ion | R<br>S | to loosen<br>process | Process in which a muscle loosens and returns to a resting stage |
| **rhabdomyoma**<br>(răb″ dō-m ī-ō′ mă) | rhabd/o<br>my<br>-oma | CF<br>R<br>S | rod<br>muscle<br>tumor | Tumor of striated muscle tissue |
| **rheumatism**<br>(roo′mă-tĭzm) | rheumat<br>-ism | R<br>S | discharge<br>condition | General term used to describe conditions characterized by inflammation, soreness, and stiffness of muscles and pain in joints |
| **rigor mortis**<br>(rĭg′ ur mōr tĭs) | | | | Stiffness of skeletal muscles seen in death |

## TABLE 7–2  Types of Patient Positions

| Position | Description |
| --- | --- |
| **Anatomic** | Body erect, head facing forward, arms by the sides with palms to the front; used as the position of reference in designating the site or direction of a body structure |
| **Dorsal recumbent** | On back with lower extremities flexed and rotated outward; used in application of obstetric forceps, vaginal and rectal examination, and bimanual palpation |
| **Fowler's** | Head of the bed or examining table is raised about 18 inches or 46 cm; patient sitting up with knees also elevated |
| **Knee-chest** | On knees, thighs upright, head and upper part of chest resting on bed or examining table, arms crossed and above head; used in sigmoidoscopy, displacement of prolapsed uterus, rectal exams, and flushing of intestinal canal |
| **Lithotomy** | On back with lower extremities flexed and feet placed in stirrups; used in vaginal examination, Pap smear, vaginal operations, and diagnosis and treatment of diseases of the urethra and bladder |
| **Orthopneic** | Sitting upright or erect; used for patients with dyspnea, shortness of breath (SOB) |
| **Prone** | Lying face downward; used in examination of the back, injections, and massage |
| **Sims'** | Lying on left side, right knee and thigh flexed well up above left leg that is slightly flexed, left arm behind the body, and right arm forward, flexed at elbow; used in examination of rectum, sigmoidoscopy, enema, and intrauterine irrigation after labor |
| **Supine** | Lying flat on back with face upward and arms at the sides; used in examining the head, neck, chest, abdomen, and extremities and in assessing vital signs |
| **Trendelenburg** | Body supine on a bed or examining table that is tilted at about 45° angle with the head lower than the feet; used to displace abdominal organs during surgery and in treating cardiovascular shock; also called the *shock position* |

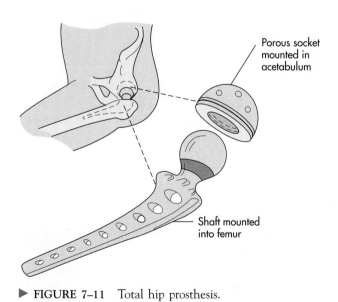

Porous socket
mounted in
acetabulum

Shaft mounted
into femur

▶ FIGURE 7–11  Total hip prosthesis.

| MEDICAL WORD | WORD PARTS (WHEN APPLICABLE) | | | DEFINITION |
|---|---|---|---|---|
| | Part | Type | Meaning | |
| **rotation**<br>(rō-tā′ shŭn) | rotat<br>-ion | R<br>S | to turn<br>process | Process of moving a body part around a central axis |
| **rotator cuff**<br>(rō-tā′ tor kŭf) | | | | Term used to describe the muscles immediately surrounding the shoulder joint that stabilize the shoulder joint while the entire arm is moved |
| **sarcolemma**<br>(sar″ kō-lĕm′ ă) | sarc/o<br>lemma | CF<br>R | flesh<br>a rind | Plasma membrane surrounding each striated muscle fiber |
| **spasticity**<br>(spăs-tĭs′ ĭ-tē) | spastic<br>-ity | R<br>S | convulsive<br>condition | Condition of increased muscular tone causing stiff and awkward movements |
| **sternocleido-mastoid**<br>(stur″ nō-klī″ dō-măs′ toyd) | stern/o<br>cleid/o<br>mast<br>-oid | CF<br>CF<br>R<br>S | sternum<br>clavicle<br>breast<br>resemble | Muscle arising from the sternum and clavicle with its insertion in the mastoid process |
| **strain** | | | | Excessive, forcible stretching of a muscle or the musculotendinous unit |
| **synergetic**<br>(sin″ ĕr-jĕt′ ĭk) | syn-<br>erget<br>-ic | P<br>R<br>S | with, together<br>work<br>pertaining to | Pertaining to certain muscles that work together |
| **synovitis**<br>(sĭn″ o-vī′ tĭs) | synov<br><br>-itis | R<br><br>S | synovial membrane<br>inflammation | Inflammation of a synovial membrane |
| **tendon**<br>(tĕn′ dŭn) | | | | Band of fibrous connective tissue serving for the attachment of muscles to bones; a giant cell tumor of a tendon sheath is a benign, small, yellow, tumorlike nodule. See Figure 7–12 ▼. |
| **tenodesis**<br>(tĕn-ōd′ ĕ-sĭs) | ten/o<br>-desis | CF<br>S | tendon<br>binding | Surgical binding of a tendon |

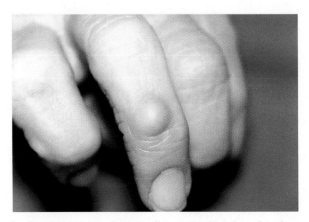

► **FIGURE 7–12** Giant cell tumor of tendon sheath.
(Courtesy of Jason L. Smith, MD.)

| MEDICAL WORD | WORD PARTS (WHEN APPLICABLE) | | | DEFINITION |
|---|---|---|---|---|
| | Part | Type | Meaning | |
| **tenodynia**<br>(tĕn″ ō-dĭn-ĭ-ă) | ten/o<br>-dynia | CF<br>S | tendon<br>pain | Pain in a tendon |
| **tetany**<br>(tĕt′ă-nē) | | | | Condition characterized by cramps, convulsions, twitching of the muscles, and sharp flexion of the wrist and ankle joints; generally caused by an abnormality in calcium (Ca) metabolism |
| **tonic**<br>(tŏn′ ĭk) | ton<br>-ic | R<br>S | tone, tension<br>pertaining to | Pertaining to tone, especially muscular tension |
| **torsion**<br>(tor′ shŭn) | tors<br>-ion | R<br>S | twisted<br>process | Process of being twisted |
| **torticollis**<br>(tor″ tĭ-kŏl′ ĭs) | tort/i<br>-collis | CF<br>R | twisted<br>neck | Stiff neck caused by spasmodic contraction of the muscles of the neck; *wryneck* |
| **triceps**<br>(trī′ sĕps) | tri-<br>-ceps | P<br>S | three<br>head | Muscle having three heads with a single insertion |
| **voluntary**<br>(vŏl′ ŭn-tĕr″ ē) | volunt<br>-ary | R<br>S | will<br>pertaining to | Under the control of one's will |

# DRUG HIGHLIGHTS

**Skeletal muscle relaxants**

Used to treat painful muscle spasms that can result from strains, sprains, and musculoskeletal trauma or disease. Centrally acting muscle relaxants depress the central nervous system (CNS) and can be administered orally or by injection. The patient must be informed of the sedative effect produced by these drugs. Drowsiness, dizziness, and blurred vision can diminish the patient's ability to drive a vehicle, operate equipment, or climb stairs.

*Examples: Lioresal (baclofen), Flexeril (cyclobenzaprine HCl), and Robaxin (methocarbamol)*

**Skeletal muscle stimulants**

Used in the treatment of myasthenia gravis, a disease characterized by progressive weakness of skeletal muscles and their rapid fatiguing. Skeletal muscle stimulants inhibit the action of acetylcholinesterase, the enzyme that halts the action of acetylcholine at the neuromuscular junction. By slowing the destruction of acetylcholine, these drugs foster accumulation of higher concentrations of this neurotransmitter and increase the number of interactions between acetylcholine and the available receptors on muscle fibers.

*Examples: Tensilon (edrophonium chloride), Prostigmin Bromide (neostigmine bromide), and Mestinon (pyridostigmine bromide)*

**Neuromuscular blocking agents**

Used to provide muscle relaxation in patients undergoing surgery and/or electroconvulsive therapy, endotracheal intubation, and to relieve laryngospasm.

*Examples: Tracrium (atracurium besylate), Flaxedil (gallamine triethiodide), and Norcuron (vecuronium)*

**Anti-inflammatory agents and analgesics**

(See Chapter 6, Skeletal System, Drug Highlights on page 130 for a description of anti-inflammatory agents and analgesics.)

# DIAGNOSTIC AND LAB TESTS

| TEST | DESCRIPTION |
|------|-------------|
| **Aldolase (ALD) blood test** (ăl′ dō-lāz) | Test performed on serum that measures ALD enzyme present in skeletal and heart muscle; helpful in the diagnosis of Duchenne's muscular dystrophy before symptoms appear. |
| **Calcium blood test** (kăl′ sē-ŭm) | Test performed on serum to determine levels of calcium, which is essential for muscular contraction, nerve transmission, and blood clotting. |
| **Creatine kinase (CK)** (krē′ ă-tĭn kĭn′ āz) | Blood test to determine the level of CK, which is increased in necrosis or atrophy of skeletal muscle, traumatic muscle injury, strenuous exercise, and progressive muscular dystrophy. |
| **Electromyography (EMG)** (ē-lĕk″ trō-mī-ŏg′ ră-fē) | Test to measure electrical activity across muscle membranes by means of electrodes attached to a needle that is inserted into the muscle. Electrical activity can be heard over a loudspeaker, viewed on an oscilloscope, or printed on a graph (electromyogram). Abnormal results can indicate myasthenia gravis, amyotrophic lateral sclerosis, muscular dystrophy, peripheral neuropathy, and anterior poliomyelitis. |
| **Lactic dehydrogenase (LDH)** (lăk′ tĭk dē-hī-drŏj′ ĕ-nāz) | Blood test to determine the level of LDH enzyme, which is increased in muscular dystrophy, damage to skeletal muscles, after a pulmonary embolism, and during skeletal muscle malignancy. |
| **Muscle biopsy** (mŭs′ ĕl bī′ ŏp-sē) | Operative procedure in which a small piece of muscle tissue is excised and then stained for microscopic examination. Lower motor neuron disease, degeneration, inflammatory reactions, and involvement of specific muscle fibers can indicate myopathic disease. |
| **Serum glutamic oxaloacetic transaminase (SGOT)** (sē′ rŭm gloo-tăm′ ĭk ŏks″ ăl-ō-ă-sē′ tĭk trăns ăm′ ĭn-āz) | Blood test to determine the level of SGOT enzyme, which is increased in skeletal muscle damage and muscular dystrophy; test also called *aspartate aminotransferase* (AST). |
| **Serum glutamic pyruvic transaminase (SGPT)** (sē′ rŭm gloo-tăm′ ĭk pī-roo′ vĭk trăns-ăm′ ĭn-āz) | Blood test to determine the level of SGPT enzyme, which is increased in skeletal muscle damage; test also called *alanine aminotransferase* (ALT). |

# ABBREVIATIONS

| ABBREVIATION | MEANING | ABBREVIATION | MEANING |
|---|---|---|---|
| ACR | American College of Rheumatology | MD | muscular dystrophy |
| AE | above elbow | MG | myasthenia gravis |
| AK | above knee | MS | musculoskeletal |
| ALD | aldolase | NSAIDs | nonsteroidal anti-inflammatory drugs |
| ALT | alanine aminotransferase | PM | physical medicine |
| AST | aspartate aminotransferase | PMR | physical medicine and rehabilitation |
| BE | below elbow | | |
| BK | below knee | ROM | range of motion |
| Ca | calcium | SGOT | serum glutamic oxaloacetic transaminase |
| CPM | continuous passive motion | | |
| DTRs | deep tendon reflexes | SGPT | serum glutamic pyruvic transaminase |
| EMG | electromyography | | |
| FMS | fibromyalgia syndrome | sh | shoulder |
| FROM | full range of motion | SOB | shortness of breath |
| IM | intramuscular | TBW | total body weight |
| LDH | lactic dehydrogenase | TJ | triceps jerk |
| LOM | limitation or loss of motion | | |

# PATHOLOGY SPOTLIGHTS

 ✷ **Atrophy**

**Atrophy** occurs with the disuse of muscles over a long period of time. Bedrest and immobility can cause loss of muscle mass and strength. When immobility is due to a treatment mode, such as casting or traction, isometric exercise of the muscles of the immobilized part can decrease the effects of immobility. Isometric exercise involves active muscular contraction performed against stable resistance, such as tightening the muscles of the thigh and/or tightening the muscles of the buttocks. Active exercise of uninjured parts of the body helps prevent muscle atrophy.

Other benefits of exercise follow:

- Can slow down the progression of osteoporosis.
- Reduces the levels of triglycerides and raises the "good" cholesterol (high-density lipoproteins).
- Can lower systolic and diastolic blood pressure.
- Can improve blood glucose levels in the diabetic person.
- Combined with a low-fat, low-calorie diet, is effective in preventing obesity and helping individuals maintain a proper body weight.
- Can elevate mood and reduce anxiety and tension.

*Lipoatrophy* is atrophy of fat tissue. This condition can occur at the site of an insulin and/or corticosteroid injection. It is also known as *lipodystrophy*. See Figure 7–13 ▶.

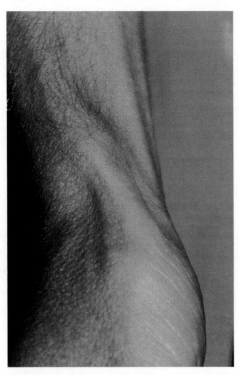

▶ **FIGURE 7–13** Lipoatrophy, wrist.
(Courtesy of Jason L. Smith, MD.)

## ✴ Fibromyalgia

**Fibromyalgia,** or **fibromyalgia syndrome** (FMS), is a widespread musculoskeletal pain and fatigue disorder. An estimated 3 million people are affected in the United States. It affects women more than men but occurs in people of all ages.

Symptoms include mild to severe muscle pain and fatigue, sleep disorders, irritable bowel syndrome, depression, and chronic headaches. Although the exact cause is still unknown, fibromyalgia is often traced to an injury or physical or emotional trauma.

The American College of Rheumatology (ACR) has identified specific criteria for fibromyalgia. The ACR classifies a patient with fibromyalgia if at least 11 of 18 specific areas of the body are painful under pressure. These specific areas are often called *trigger points*. See Figure 7–14 ▶. The location of some of these trigger points includes the inside of the elbow joint, the front of the collarbone, and the base of the skull.

Treatments are geared toward improving the quality of sleep and reducing pain. Because deep sleep is so crucial for many body functions, such as tissue repair and antibody production, the sleep disorders that frequently occur in fibromyalgia are thought to be a major contributing factor to the symptoms. Medications that boost the body's level of serotonin and norepinephrine—neurotransmitters that modulate sleep, pain, and immune system function—are commonly prescribed. In addition, nonsteroidal, anti-inflammatory drugs (NSAIDs) such as ibuprofen may also be beneficial.

## ✴ Myasthenia Gravis

**Myasthenia gravis** (MG) is a chronic autoimmune neuromuscular disease characterized by varying degrees of weakness of the skeletal (voluntary) muscles of the body. The name *myasthenia gravis*, which is Latin and Greek in origin, literally means *grave muscle weakness*. With current therapies, however, most cases of myasthenia gravis are not as "grave" as the

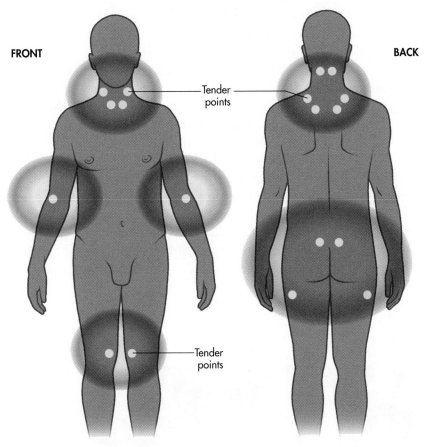

FRONT

BACK

Tender points

Tender points

▶ **FIGURE 7–14** The 18 tender points of fibromyalgia.

name implies. For the majority of individuals with myasthenia gravis, life expectancy is not lessened by the disorder.

The primary symptom of myasthenia gravis is muscle weakness that increases during periods of activity and improves after periods of rest. Certain muscles such as those that control eye and eyelid movement, facial expression, chewing, talking, and swallowing are often, but not always, involved in the disorder. The muscles that control breathing and neck and limb movements can also be affected.

Myasthenia gravis is caused by a defect in the transmission of nerve impulses to muscles. It occurs when normal communication between the nerve and muscle is interrupted at the neuromuscular junction—the place where nerve cells connect with the muscles they control.

Myasthenia gravis occurs in all ethnic groups and both genders. It most commonly affects young adult women (under 40) and older men (over 60), but it can occur at any age. Treatment includes lifestyle adjustments that can enable continuation of many activities, including planning activity to allow for scheduled rest periods and avoiding stress and excessive heat exposure.

## ✷ Muscular Dystrophy

**Muscular dystrophy** (MD) refers to a group of genetic diseases characterized by progressive weakness and degeneration of the skeletal or voluntary muscles that control movement. The muscles of the heart and some other involuntary muscles are also affected in some forms of MD, and a few forms involve other organs as well.

The major forms of MD include myotonic, Duchenne, Becker, limb-girdle, facioscapulohumeral, congenital, oculopharyngeal, distal, and Emery-Dreifuss. Duchenne is the most common form of MD affecting children, and myotonic MD is the most common form affecting adults. MD can affect people of all ages. Although some forms first become apparent in infancy or childhood, others do not appear until middle age or later.

The prognosis of MD varies according to the type of MD and the progression of the disorder. Some cases are mild and very slowly progressive, allowing a normal life span, while other cases have more marked progression of muscle weakness, functional disability, and loss of ambulation. See Figure 7–15 ▼.

Life expectancy depends on the degree of progression and late respiratory deficit. In Duchenne MD, death usually occurs in the late teens to early twenties.

There is no specific treatment for any of the forms of MD. Physical therapy to prevent contractures (a condition in which shortened muscles around joints cause abnormal and sometimes painful positioning of the joints), orthoses (orthopedic appliances used for support), and corrective orthopedic surgery could be needed to improve the quality of life in some cases.

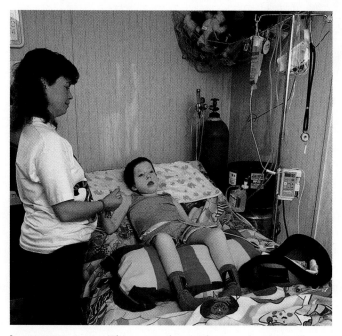

▶ FIGURE 7–15   This young boy with muscular dystrophy needs to receive tube feedings and home nursing care. He attends school when possible and is able to use an adapted computer.

# ✔PATHOLOGY CHECKPOINT

*Following is a concise list of the pathology-related terms that you have seen in the chapter. Review this checklist to make sure that you are familiar with the meaning of each term before moving to the next section.*

## Conditions and Symptoms

- ❑ amputation
- ❑ ataxia
- ❑ atonic
- ❑ atrophy
- ❑ brachialgia
- ❑ bradykinesia
- ❑ contracture
- ❑ dactylospasm
- ❑ dermatomyositis
- ❑ dystonia
- ❑ Duchenne muscular dystrophy
- ❑ dystrophy
- ❑ fascitis
- ❑ fatigue
- ❑ fibromyalgia
- ❑ fibromyitis
- ❑ flaccid
- ❑ muscular dystrophy

- ❑ myalgia
- ❑ myasthenia
- ❑ myasthenia gravis
- ❑ myofibroma
- ❑ myokinesis
- ❑ myoma
- ❑ myomalacia
- ❑ myoparesis
- ❑ myopathy
- ❑ myosarcoma
- ❑ myosclerosis
- ❑ myositis
- ❑ myospasm
- ❑ neuromyopathic
- ❑ polyplegia
- ❑ rhabdomyoma
- ❑ rheumatism
- ❑ rigor mortis
- ❑ spasticity
- ❑ strain

- ❑ synovitis
- ❑ tenodynia
- ❑ torsion
- ❑ torticollis

## Diagnosis and Treatment

- ❑ diathermy
- ❑ exercise
- ❑ first aid—RICE
- ❑ heat
- ❑ hydrotherapy
- ❑ massage
- ❑ myograph
- ❑ myoplasty
- ❑ myorrhaphy
- ❑ myotome
- ❑ myotomy
- ❑ position
- ❑ prosthesis
- ❑ tenodesis

# STUDY AND REVIEW

## Anatomy and Physiology

*Write your answers to the following questions. Do not refer to the text.*

1. The muscular system is made up of three types of muscle tissue. Name the three types.

    a. _____    b. _____

    c. _____

2. Muscles make up approximately _____ percent of a person's body weight.

3. Name the two essential ingredients that are needed for a muscle to perform properly.

    a. _____    b. _____

4. Name the two points of attachment for a skeletal muscle.

    a. _____    b. _____

5. Skeletal muscle is also known as _____ or _____.

6. A wide, thin, sheetlike tendon is known as an _____.

7. Name the three distinguishable parts of a muscle.

    a. _____    b. _____

    c. _____

8. Define the following:

    a. Antagonist _____

    b. Prime mover _____

    c. Synergist _____

9. Smooth muscle is also called _____, _____, or

    _____.

10. Smooth muscles are found in the internal organs. Name five examples of these locations.

    a. _____    b. _____

    c. _____    d. _____

    e. _____

11. _____ is the muscle of the heart.

12. Name the three primary functions of the muscular system.

a. _____     b. _____

c. _____

## Word Parts

1. In the spaces provided, write the definition of these prefixes, roots, combining forms, and suffixes. Do not refer to the listings of medical words. Leave blank those words you cannot define.

2. After completing as many as you can, refer to the medical word listings to check your work. For each word missed or left blank, write the word and its definition several times on the margins of these pages or on a separate sheet of paper.

3. To maximize the learning process, it is to your advantage to do the following exercises as directed. To refer to the word-building section before completing these exercises invalidates the learning process.

## PREFIXES

*Give the definitions of the following prefixes.*

1. a- _____     2. ab- _____

3. ad- _____     4. ant- _____

5. bi- _____     6. brady- _____

7. con- _____     8. dia- _____

9. dys- _____     10. in- _____

11. intra- _____   12. hydro- _____

13. quadri- _____  14. syn- _____

15. tri- _____

## ROOTS AND COMBINING FORMS

*Give the definitions of the following roots and combining forms.*

1. agon _____     2. brach/i _____

3. cleid/o _____   4. amputat _____

5. collis _____    6. dactyl/o _____

7. duct _____      8. erget _____

9. fasc _____      10. dermat/o _____

11. rheumat _____

12. fibr _____

13. fibr/o _____

14. is/o _____

15. lemma _____

16. levat _____

17. prosth/e _____

18. mast _____

19. therm _____

20. metr _____

21. muscul _____

22. my _____

23. my/o _____

24. my/o(s) _____

25. neur/o _____

26. path _____

27. relaxat _____

28. rhabd/o _____

29. rotat _____

30. troph _____

31. sarc/o _____

32. scler _____

33. sert _____

34. spastic _____

35. stern/o _____

36. teno _____

37. ton _____

38. torti _____

39. tract _____

40. volunt _____

41. synov _____

42. tors _____

## SUFFIXES

*Give the definitions of the following suffixes.*

1. -algia _____

2. -ar _____

3. -ary _____

4. -asthenia _____

5. -blast _____

6. -ceps _____

7. -desis _____

8. -dynia _____

9. -in _____

10. -therapy _____

11. -graph _____

12. -ia _____

13. -ic _____

14. -ion _____

15. -ist _____

16. -itis _____

17. -ity _____

18. -kinesia _____

19. -kinesis _____

20. -logy _____

21. -ure _____

22. -malacia _____

23. -oid _____

24. -oma _____

25. -or _____

26. -osis _____

27. -paresis _____

28. -pathy _____

29. -phragm _____

30. -plasty _____

31. -plegia _____

32. -rrhaphy _____

33. -y _____

34. -spasm _____

35. -taxia _____

36. -tome _____

37. -tomy _____

38. -trophy _____

39. -sis _____

40. -ism _____

## Identifying Medical Terms

*In the spaces provided, write the medical terms for the following meanings.*

1. _____ Pertaining to a lack of normal tone or tension

2. _____ Slowness of motion or movement

3. _____ Cramp of a finger or toe

4. _____ Faulty muscular development caused by lack of nourishment

5. _____ Pertaining to within a muscle

6. _____ Muscle that raises or elevates a part

7. _____ Muscle weakness

8. _____ Study of muscles

9. _____ Weakness or slight paralysis of a muscle

10. _____ Surgical repair of a muscle

11. _____ Malignant tumor derived from muscle tissue

12. _____ Incision into a muscle

13. _____ Paralysis affecting many muscles

14. _____ Surgical binding of a tendon

15. _____ Pertaining to certain muscles that work together

16. _____ Muscle having three heads with a single insertion

## Spelling

*In the spaces provided, write the correct spelling of these misspelled terms.*

1. facia _____

2. mykinesis _____

3. dermatomyoitis _____

4. rhadomyoma _____

5. sarclemma _____

6. sterncleidomastoid _____

7. dystropin _____

8. torticolis _____

## Matching

*Select the appropriate lettered meaning for each of the following words.*

_____ 1. dermatomyositis

_____ 2. fibromyalgia

_____ 3. muscular dystrophy

_____ 4. flaccid

_____ 5. prosthesis

_____ 6. rotator cuff

_____ 7. strain

_____ 8. tenodynia

_____ 9. torsion

_____ 10. voluntary

a. Term used to describe the muscles immediately surrounding the shoulder joint
b. Process of being twisted
c. Pain in a tendon
d. Inflammation of the muscles and the skin
e. Lacking muscle tone
f. Under the control of one's will
g. Chronic, progressive wasting and weakening of muscles
h. Excessive, forcible stretching of a muscle or the musculotendinous unit
i. Condition with widespread muscular pain and debilitating fatigue
j. Artificial device, organ, or part
k. Pain in a joint

## Abbreviations

*Place the correct word, phrase, or abbreviation in the space provided.*

1. AE _____

2. AST _____

3. calcium _____

4. electromyography _____

5. FROM _____

6. MS _____

7. range of motion _____

8. shoulder _____

9. TBW _____

10. TJ _____

## Diagnostic and Laboratory Tests

*Select the best answer to each multiple choice question. Circle the letter of your choice.*

1. Diagnostic test to help diagnose Duchenne muscular dystrophy before symptoms appear.
   a. creatine kinase
   b. aldolase blood test
   c. calcium blood test
   d. muscle biopsy

2. Test to measure electrical activity across muscle membranes by means of electrodes that are attached to a needle that is inserted into the muscle.
   a. muscle biopsy
   b. lactic dehydrogenase
   c. creatine kinase
   d. electromyography

3. Test that is also called *aspartate aminotransferase.*
   a. lactic dehydrogenase
   b. serum glutamic oxaloacetic transaminase
   c. serum glutamic pyruvic transaminase
   d. creatine kinase

4. Test that is also called *alanine aminotransferase.*
   a. lactic dehydrogenase
   b. serum glutamic oxaloacetic transaminase
   c. serum glutamic pyruvic transaminase
   d. creatine kinase

5. For a/an _____, a small piece of muscle tissue is excised and then stained for microscopic examination.
   a. muscle biopsy
   b. electromyography
   c. bone biopsy
   d. electrocardiography

# PRACTICAL APPLICATION

## S O A P : Chart Note Analysis

*This exercise will make you aware of information, abbreviations, and medical terminology typically found in a pediatric patient's chart.*

### Abbreviations Key

| | | | | |
|---|---|---|---|---|
| Abd | abdomen | | MS | musculoskeletal |
| BP | blood pressure | | Neuro | neurology |
| CK | creatine kinase | | P | pulse |
| CTA | clear to auscultation | | R | respiration |
| DMD | Duchenne muscular dystrophy | | SOAP | subjective, objective, assessment, plan |
| EMG | electromyography | | | |
| F | Fahrenheit | | T | temperature |
| Ht | height | | Wt | weight |
| lb | pound | | y/o | year(s) old |

*Read the following chart note and then answer the questions that follow.*

**PATIENT:** Davis, Christopher  **DATE:** 01/15/2007
**DOB:** 11/24/2003  **AGE:** 3  **SEX:** Male
**INSURANCE:** Best Care Insurance

**Vital Signs:**
T: 98.4 F
P: 90
R: 20
BP: 85/60
Ht: 3' 2"
Wt: 36 lb
**Allergies:** penicillin
**Chief Complaint:** Waddling gait with increasing episodes of falling and apparent clumsiness. Activities of running and climbing very slow in comparison to peers.

**S** | **Subjective:** Mother of 3 y/o white male states that she has noticed her son is beginning to appear "clumsy" with increasing episodes of falling. She has noticed that he looks like he is "waddling" when he walks. "He runs very slow, has trouble climbing playground equipment and trouble getting up off the floor. He isn't able to jump from a standing position, like his feet are glued to the floor. At times, he appears to be walking on his toes." She expresses concern that he did not learn to walk until after he was 18 months old and that she is at risk for carrying the gene that causes muscular dystrophy.

**O    Objective:**

**General Appearance:** Pleasant child who exhibits no distress while sitting and playing on the floor. Noted difficulty rising from floor to standing position. Child used Gowers' maneuver to push himself upright.

**Lungs:** CTA

**Heart:** No murmurs, gallops or rubs. Normal rate and rhythm.

**Abd:** Bowel sounds all 4 quadrants. Soft, no masses or tenderness.

**MS:** Abduction of arms to full 180° above head impaired, due to muscle weakness. Noted muscle weakness of bilateral lower extremities. No contractures with joint involvement. Calf muscles appear enlarged by connective tissue and fat. Upon palpation, felt "rubbery."

**Neuro:** Oriented to person and place. Reflexes intact.

**Skin:** Cool and moist, soft to touch. Noted generalized bruising at various stages on legs and arms.

**A    Assessment:** Duchenne Muscular Dystrophy

**P    Plan:**

1. Schedule physical therapy to help delay permanent muscular contracture.
2. Recommend supportive measures such as splints and braces to minimize deformities and preserve mobility.
3. Recommend deep breathing exercises to help delay weakening of the muscles of respiration.
4. Suggest counseling and referral services as supportive measures for parent and child.
5. Provide the family with information on the Muscular Dystrophy Association which is located 3561 E. Sunrise Drive, Tucson, AZ 85718. Telephone: 1-602-529-2000 or 1-800-572-1717. E-mail: mda@mdausa.org.

**FYI:** Duchenne muscular dystrophy is an X-linked disorder seen only in males. The body needs a chemical substance, **dystrophin,** as a muscle membrane stabilizer, but it is absent in DMD. This leads to necrosis in muscle fibers and their replacement with connective tissue and fat.

The Gowers' maneuver is the use of the upper extremity muscles to raise oneself to a standing position. It is a "butt-first" maneuver by which the child sticks his posterior up in the air and then "walks" up the legs with his hands, leaning on his arms for support. This is a good indicator of muscle weakness of the legs. Early in the diagnostic process, a serum creatine kinase (CK) test, an electromyography (EMG), and a muscle biopsy is ordered. Creatine kinase is an enzyme that leaks out of damaged muscles. When elevated CK levels are found in blood samples, a high CK level suggests muscular dystrophy or inflammation.

## Chart Note Questions
*Place the correct answer in the space provided.*

1. Signs and symptoms of Duchenne muscular dystrophy include a _____ gait, frequent falls, clumsiness, slowness in running and climbing, and walking on toes.

2. The diagnosis can be determined by the characteristic symptoms, family history, a muscle biopsy, an _____, and an elevated creatine kinase level.

3. As part of the treatment for Duchenne muscular dystrophy, the use of splints and braces help to _____ and _____.

4. Use of Gowers' maneuver is a good indicator of _____.

5. What chemical is important to muscle fibers and, when present in abnormally high amounts in the blood serum, can be an indicator of DMD? _____

6. What is the name of the test used to evaluate the electrical activity generated by a contracted muscle? _____

7. State the purpose of physical therapy for this patient. _____

8. In the chart note, it indicated that the patient was allergic to _____.

9. Is the pulse rate within normal range for a child of this age? _____

10. Were the activities of running and climbing within normal range for a child of this age? _____

# MULTIMEDIA PREVIEW

*Additional interactive resources and activities for this chapter can be found on the Companion Website. For videos, audio glossary, and review, access the accompanying CD-ROM in this book.*

 **CD-ROM HIGHLIGHTS**

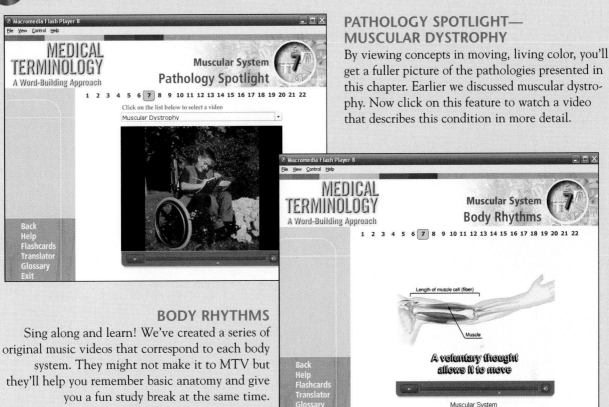

## PATHOLOGY SPOTLIGHT— MUSCULAR DYSTROPHY

By viewing concepts in moving, living color, you'll get a fuller picture of the pathologies presented in this chapter. Earlier we discussed muscular dystrophy. Now click on this feature to watch a video that describes this condition in more detail.

## BODY RHYTHMS

Sing along and learn! We've created a series of original music videos that correspond to each body system. They might not make it to MTV but they'll help you remember basic anatomy and give you a fun study break at the same time.

 **WEBSITE HIGHLIGHTS—www.prenhall.com/rice**

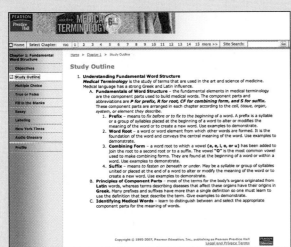

## STUDY OUTLINES

Click here and take advantage of the free-access online study guide that accompanies your textbook. You'll find outline summaries of each chapter to give you a snapshot of the important concepts. By clicking on this URL you'll also access a variety of quizzes with instant feedback, links to download mp3 audio reviews, news updates, and an audio glossary.

# Digestive System

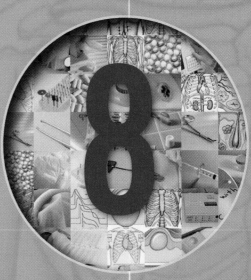

**8**

## ■ OUTLINE

## ■ OBJECTIVES

*On completion of this chapter, you will be able to:*

- Describe the digestive system.
- Describe the primary organs of the digestive system and state their functions.
- Describe the two sets of teeth with which humans are provided.
- Describe the three main portions of a tooth.
- Describe the accessory organs of the digestive system and state their functions.
- Describe digestive differences of the child and the older adult.
- Analyze, build, spell, and pronounce medical words.
- Comprehend the drugs highlighted in this chapter.
- Describe diagnostic and laboratory tests related to the digestive system.
- Identify and define selected abbreviations.
- Describe each of the conditions presented in the Pathology Spotlights.
- Review the Pathology Checkpoint.
- Complete the Study and Review section and the Chart Note Analysis.

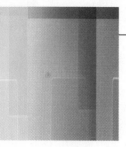

# Anatomy and Physiology Overview

A general description of the digestive system is that of a continuous tube beginning with the mouth and ending at the anus. This tube is known as the **alimentary canal** and/or **gastrointestinal tract.** It measures about 30 feet in adults and contains both primary and accessory organs for the conversion of food and fluids into a semiliquid that can be absorbed for the body to use. The three main functions of the digestive system are digestion, absorption, and elimination. **Digestion** is the process by which food is changed in the mouth, stomach, and intestines by chemical, mechanical, and physical action, so that the body can absorb it. Digestive enzymes increase chemical reactions and, in so doing, break down complex nutrients. Complex proteins are broken down into simple amino acids, complicated sugars are reduced to simple sugars (glucose), and large fat molecules (triglycerides) are broken down to fatty acids and glycerol. **Absorption** is the process by which nutrient material is taken into the bloodstream or lymph and travels to all cells of the body. Valuable nutrients such as amino acids, glucose, fatty acids, and glycerol can then be utilized for energy, growth, and development of the body. **Elimination** is the process whereby the solid waste (end) products of digestion are excreted. Each of the various organs commonly associated with digestion is described in this chapter. The organs of digestion are shown in Figure 8–1 ▶.

## Digestive System

| Organ | Functions |
|---|---|
| Mouth | Breaks food apart by the action of the teeth, moistens and lubricates food with saliva; food formed into a bolus |
| Teeth | Serve as organs of mastication |
| Pharynx | Is common passageway for both respiration and digestion; muscular constrictions move the bolus into the esophagus |
| Esophagus | Moves the food by peristalsis down the esophagus into the stomach |
| Stomach | Reduces food to a digestible state, converts the food to a semiliquid form |
| Small Intestine | Digests and absorbs food, nutrients absorbed into tiny capillaries and lymph vessels in the walls of the small intestine and transmitted to body cells by the circulatory system |
| Large Intestine | Removes water from the fecal material, stores, and then eliminates waste from the body via the rectum and anus |
| Salivary glands | Secrete saliva to moisten and lubricate food |
| Liver | Changes glucose to glycogen and stores it until needed; changes glycogen back to glucose; desaturates fats; assists in protein catabolism; manufactures bile, fibrinogen, prothrombin, heparin, and blood proteins; stores vitamins; produces heat; and detoxifies substances |
| Gallbladder | Stores and concentrates bile |
| Pancreas | Secretes pancreatic juice into the small intestine, contains cells that produce digestive enzymes, secretes insulin and glucagon |

# MOUTH

The **mouth** is the cavity formed by the palate or roof, the lips and cheeks on the sides, and the tongue at its floor. Contained within are the teeth and salivary glands. The cheeks form the lateral walls and are continuous with the lips. The vestibule includes the space between the cheeks and the teeth. The **gingivae** (gums) surround the necks of the teeth. See Figure 8–2A ▶. The hard and soft palates provide a roof for the oral cavity with the tongue at its floor. The free portion of the tongue is connected to the underlying epithelium by a thin

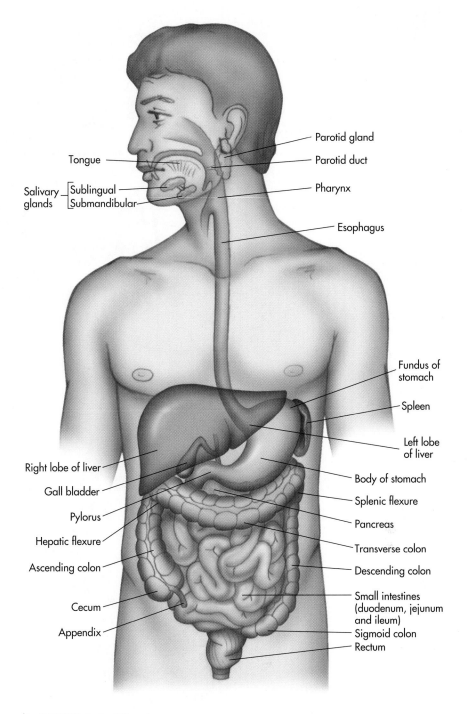

Tongue

Salivary glands
Sublingual
Submandibular

Parotid gland

Parotid duct

Pharynx

Esophagus

Fundus of stomach

Spleen

Left lobe of liver

Body of stomach

Splenic flexure

Pancreas

Transverse colon

Descending colon

Small intestines (duodenum, jejunum and ileum)

Sigmoid colon

Rectum

Right lobe of liver

Gall bladder

Pylorus

Hepatic flexure

Ascending colon

Cecum

Appendix

▶ **FIGURE 8–1**  Digestive system.

fold of mucous membrane, the **lingual frenulum,** which prevents extreme movement of the tongue. See Figure 8–2B.

The **tongue** is made of skeletal muscle and is covered with mucous membrane. The tongue can be divided into a blunt rear portion called the **root,** a pointed **tip,** and a central **body.** Located on the surface of the tongue are **papillae** (elevations) and **taste buds** (sweet, salt, sour, and bitter). Three pairs of salivary glands secrete fluids into the oral cavity. These glands are the **parotid, sublingual,** and **submandibular.** The posterior margin of the soft palate supports the dangling uvula and two pairs of muscular pharyngeal arches. On either side, a palatine tonsil lies between an anterior

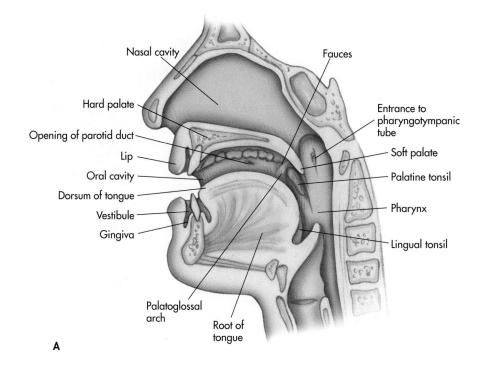

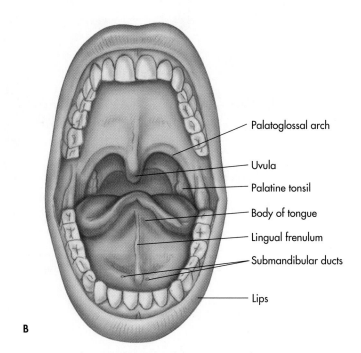

▶ **FIGURE 8–2** Oral cavity: (A) sagittal section; (B) anterior view as seen through the open mouth.

palatoglossal arch and a posterior palatopharyngeal arch. A curving line that connects the palatoglossal arches and uvula forms the boundaries of the fauces, the passageway between the oral cavity and the pharynx. See Figure 8–2A. Digestion begins as food is broken apart by the action of the teeth, moistened and lubricated by saliva, and formed into a **bolus** (see Figure 8–3 ▶). A bolus is a small mass of masticated food ready to be swallowed.

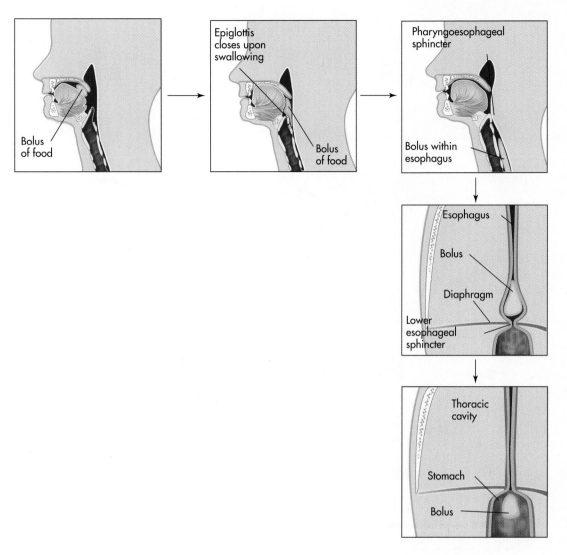

▶ FIGURE 8–3  Movement of a bolus of food from the mouth to the stomach via the esophagus.

## TEETH

Human beings are provided two sets of teeth. The 20 **deciduous** teeth, the temporary teeth of the primary dentition, include 8 incisors, 4 canines (cuspids), and 8 molars. Deciduous teeth are also referred to as *milk teeth* or *baby teeth*. There are 32 **permanent** or secondary dentition teeth: 8 incisors, 4 canines, 8 premolars, and 12 molars. See Figure 8–4 ▶.

The **incisors** are so named because they present a sharp cutting edge, adapted for biting into food. They form the four front teeth in each dental arch. The **canine** or **cuspid** teeth are larger and stronger than the incisors. Their roots sink deeply into the bones and cause well-marked prominences upon the surface. The **premolars** or **bicuspid** teeth are situated lateral to and behind the canine teeth. The **molar** teeth are the largest of the permanent set, and their broad crowns are adapted for grinding and pounding the food. The deciduous teeth are smaller than, but generally resemble in form, the teeth that bear the same names in the permanent set.

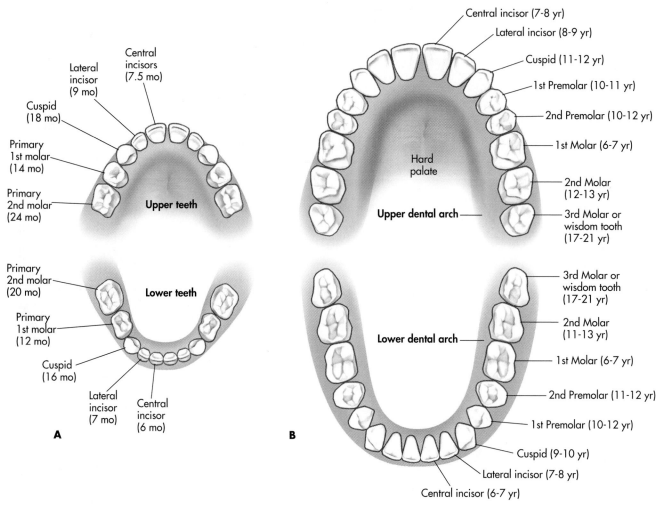

**FIGURE 8–4**  Deciduous and permanent teeth. (A) The deciduous teeth, with the age of eruption given in months; (B) the permanent teeth, with the age at eruption given in years.

Each tooth consists of three main portions: the **crown,** projecting above the gum; the **root,** embedded in the alveolus; and the **neck,** the constricted portion between the crown and root. On making a vertical section of a tooth, a cavity will be found in the interior of the crown and the center of each root; it opens by a minute orifice at the extremity of the latter. See Figure 8–5 ▶. This cavity is called the **pulp cavity,** which contains the dental pulp, a loose connective tissue richly supplied with vessels and nerves that enter the cavity through the small aperture at the point of each root. The pulp cavity receives blood vessels and nerves from the **root canal,** a narrow tunnel located at the root, or base, of the tooth. Blood vessels and nerves enter the root canal through an opening called the **apical foramen** to supply the pulp cavity.

The root of each tooth sits in a bony socket called an *alveolus*. Collagen fibers of the **periodontal ligament** extend from the dentin of the root to the bone of the alveolus, creating a strong articulation known as a *gomphosis*, which binds the teeth to bony sockets in the maxillary bone and mandible. A layer of **cementum** (a thin layer of bone) covers the dentin of the root, providing protection and firmly anchoring the periodontal ligament.

The solid portion of the tooth consists of the **dentin,** which forms the bulk of the tooth; the **enamel,** which covers the exposed part of the crown and is the hardest and most compact part of a tooth; and the cementum, which is disposed on the surface of the root.

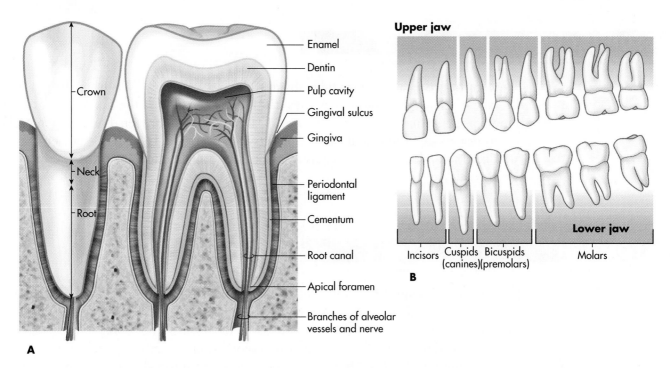

**▶ FIGURE 8–5**    Teeth. (A) Diagrammatic section through a typical adult tooth; (B) the adult teeth.

The neck of the tooth marks the boundary between the root and the crown, the exposed portion of the tooth that projects above the soft tissue of the **gingiva.** A shallow groove called the **gingival sulcus** surrounds the neck of each tooth.

When the calcification of the different tissues of the tooth is sufficiently advanced to enable it to bear the pressure to which it will be afterward subjected, eruption takes place, and the tooth makes its way through the gums. The eruption of the deciduous teeth commences about the seventh month after birth and is completed about the end of the second year, the teeth of the lower jaw preceding those of the upper. At the age of 2½ years, a child should have 20 teeth.

# PHARYNX

Just beyond the mouth, at the beginning of the tube leading to the stomach, is the **pharynx,** a musculomembranous tube extending from the base of the skull to the level of the sixth cervical vertebra where it becomes continuous with the esophagus. The upper portion, the **nasopharynx,** is above the soft palate. The middle portion, the **oropharynx,** lies between the palate and the hyoid bone and has an opening to the oral cavity. The lowest portion, the **laryngopharynx,** is below the hyoid bone and opens inferiorly to the larynx anteriorly and the esophagus posteriorly.

Simply put, the pharynx is a common passageway for both respiration and digestion. Both the **larynx,** or voice box, and the esophagus begin in the pharynx. Food that is swallowed passes through the pharynx into the esophagus reflexively. Muscular constrictions move the bolus into the esophagus while blocking the opening to the larynx and preventing the food from entering the airway leading to the trachea or windpipe.

# ESOPHAGUS

The **esophagus** is a muscular tube about 10 inches long that leads from the pharynx to the stomach. Food and liquids pass down the esophagus and into the stomach. At the junction with the stomach is the lower esophageal or cardiac sphincter. This sphincter relaxes to permit passage of food and then contracts to prevent the backup of stomach contents. Food is carried along the esophagus by a series of wavelike muscular contractions called **peristalsis.**

# STOMACH

The **stomach** is a muscular, distensible saclike portion of the alimentary canal between the esophagus and duodenum (see Figure 8–6 ▶). Food and liquids pass from the esophagus into the stomach where some of the early processes of digestion takes place. In the stomach, food is reduced to a digestible state as hydrochloric acid and gastric juices convert the food to a semiliquid state called **chyme.** Chyme is passed at intervals into the small intestine.

# SMALL INTESTINE

The **small intestine** is about 21 feet long and 1 inch in diameter. It extends from the pyloric sphincter at the base of the stomach to the entrance of the large intestine. The small intestine is considered to have three parts: the **duodenum,** the **jejunum,** and the **ileum.** The duodenum is the first 12 inches just beyond the stomach. The jejunum is the next 8 feet or so, and the ileum is the remaining 12 feet of the tube (see Figure 8–7 ▶).

Chyme is received from the stomach through the pylorus and is mixed with bile from the liver and gallbladder along with pancreatic juice from the pancreas. Digestion and absorption take place chiefly in the small intestine. Nutrients are absorbed into tiny capillaries and lymph vessels in the walls of the small intestine and transmitted to body cells by the circulatory system.

# LARGE INTESTINE

The **large intestine** is about 5 feet long and 2.5 inches in diameter. It extends from the ileocecal valve at the small intestine to the anus. The large intestine may be divided into the **cecum,** the **colon,** the **rectum,** and the **anal canal.** The cecum is a pouchlike structure forming the beginning of the large intestine. It is about 3 inches long and has the **appendix** attached to it. The colon makes up the bulk of the large intestine and is divided into several parts: the ascending colon, the transverse colon, the descending colon, and, at its end, the sigmoid colon (see Figure 8–8 ▶). Digestion and absorption continue in the large intestine on a reduced scale. The waste products of digestion are eliminated from the body via the rectum and the anus.

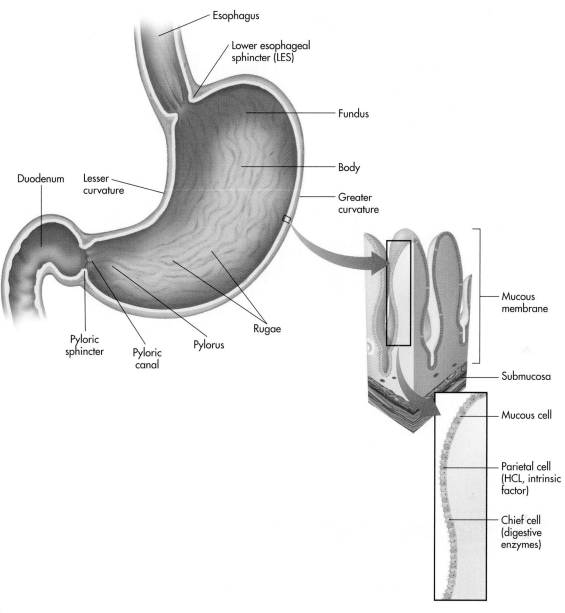

▶ FIGURE 8–6   Stomach.

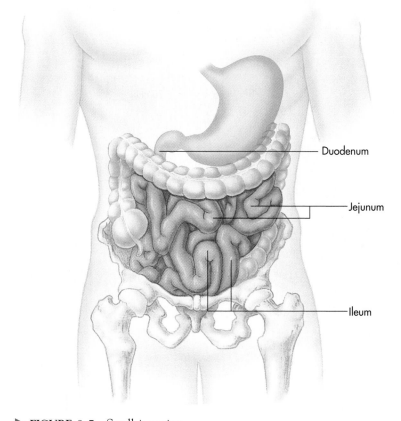

▶ **FIGURE 8–7**   Small intestine.

## ACCESSORY ORGANS

The salivary glands, the liver, the gallbladder, and the pancreas are not actually part of the digestive tube; however, they are closely related to it in their functions.

### Salivary Glands

Located in or near the mouth, the **salivary glands** secrete **saliva** in response to the sight, smell, taste, or mental image of food. The various salivary glands are the **parotid,** located on either side of the face slightly below the ear; the **submandibular,** located in the floor of the mouth; and the **sublingual,** located below the tongue. All salivary glands secrete through openings into the mouth to moisten and lubricate food.

### Liver

The largest glandular organ in the body, the **liver,** weighs about 3½ lb and is located in the upper right part of the abdomen (see Figure 8–9 ▶). The liver plays an essential role in the normal metabolism of carbohydrates, fats, and proteins. In carbohydrate metabolism, it changes glucose to glycogen and stores it until needed by body cells. It also changes glycogen back to glucose. In fat metabolism, the liver serves as a storage place and acts to desaturate fats before releasing them into the bloodstream. In protein metabolism, the liver acts as a storage place and assists in protein **catabolism.**

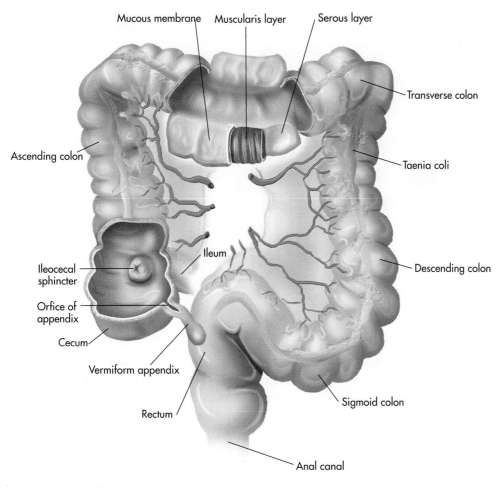

Mucous membrane  Muscularis layer  Serous layer

Transverse colon

Ascending colon

Taenia coli

Ileum

Descending colon

Ileocecal
sphincter

Orfice of
appendix

Cecum

Vermiform appendix

Sigmoid colon

Rectum

Anal canal

▶ **FIGURE 8–8**  Large intestine.

The liver manufactures the following important substances:

- **Bile.** Digestive juice
- **Fibrinogen and prothrombin.** Coagulants essential for blood clotting
- **Heparin.** Anticoagulant that helps to prevent the clotting of blood
- **Blood proteins.** Albumin, gamma globulin

Additionally, the liver stores iron and vitamins $B_{12}$, A, D, E, and K. It also produces body heat and detoxifies many harmful substances such as drugs and alcohol.

## Gallbladder

The **gallbladder** is a membranous sac attached to the liver in which excess bile is stored and concentrated. Bile leaving the gallbladder is 6 to 10 times as concentrated as that which comes to it from the liver. Concentration is accomplished by absorption of water from the bile into the mucosa of the gallbladder.

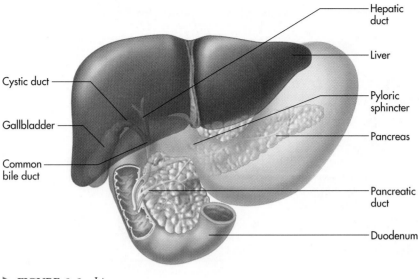

▶ **FIGURE 8–9**    Liver.

## Pancreas

The **pancreas** is a large, elongated gland situated behind the stomach and secreting pancreatic juice into the small intestine (see Figure 8–10 ▼). The pancreas is 6 to 9 inches long and contains cells that produce digestive **enzymes.** Other cells in the pancreas secrete the hormones insulin and glucagon directly into the bloodstream.

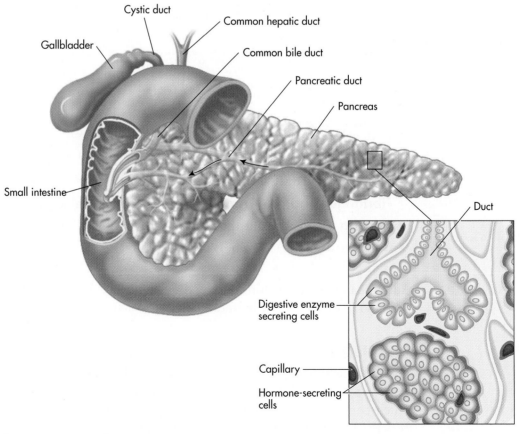

▶ **FIGURE 8–10**    Pancreas.

# LIFE SPAN CONSIDERATIONS

## ■ THE CHILD

The primitive digestive tract is formed by the embryonic membrane (yolk sac) and is divided into three sections. The **foregut** evolves into the pharynx, lower respiratory tract, esophagus, stomach, duodenum, and beginning of the common bile duct. The **midgut** elongates in the fifth week to form the primary intestinal loop. The remainder of the large colon is derived from the primitive **hindgut.** The liver, pancreas, and biliary tract evolve from the foregut. At 8 weeks, the anal membrane ruptures, forming the anal canal and opening.

The functioning of the gastrointestinal tract normally begins after birth. Food is prepared for absorption and absorbed, and waste products are eliminated. **Meconium,** the first stool, is a mixture of amniotic fluid and secretions of the intestinal glands. It is thick and sticky, and dark green in color. It is usually passed 8 to 24 hours following birth. The stools change during the first week and become loose and greenish-yellow. The stools of a breast-fed baby are bright yellow, soft, and pasty. The stools of a bottle-fed baby are more solid than those of a breast-fed baby, and they vary from yellow to brown in color.

The infant's stomach is small and empties rapidly. Newborns produce very little saliva until they are 3 months of age. Swallowing is a reflex action for the first 3 months. The hepatic efficiency of the newborn is often immature, thereby causing **jaundice.** Fat absorption is poor because of a decreased level of bile production.

## ■ THE OLDER ADULT

With aging, the digestive system becomes less motile as muscle contractions become weaker. Glandular secretions decrease, thus causing a drier mouth and a lower volume of gastric juices. Nutrient absorption is mildly reduced due to **atrophy** of the mucosal lining. The teeth are mechanically worn down with age, and the gums begin to recede from the teeth. There is a loss of tastebuds, and food preferences change. Gastric motor activity slows; as a result, gastric emptying is delayed and hunger contractions diminish. There are no significant changes in the small intestine, but in the large intestine, the muscle layer and mucosa atrophy. Smooth muscle tone and blood flow decrease, and connective tissue increases.

**Constipation** is a frequent problem among older adults. It is believed that constipation is not a normal age-related change but is caused by low fluid intake, lack of dietary fiber, inactivity, medicines, depression, and other health-related conditions.

# BUILDING YOUR MEDICAL VOCABULARY

This section provides the foundation for learning medical terminology. Review the following alphabetized word list. Note how common prefixes and suffixes are repeatedly applied to word roots and combining forms to create different meanings.

| | |
|---|---|
| **P** | Prefix |
| **R** | Root |
| **CF** | Combining form |
| **S** | Suffix |

| | |
|---|---|
| Pink words | Terms not built from word parts. |
| * | Indicates words covered in the Pathology Spotlights section. |
| 💿 | Check the CD-ROM for more information. |

| MEDICAL WORD | WORD PARTS (WHEN APPLICABLE) | | | DEFINITION |
|---|---|---|---|---|
| | **Part** | **Type** | **Meaning** | |
| **absorption**<br>(ăb-sōrp′ shŭn) | absorpt<br>-ion | R<br>S | to suck in<br>process | Process by which nutrient material is taken into the bloodstream or lymph |
| **amylase**<br>(ăm′ ĭ-lās) | amyl<br>-ase | R<br>S | starch<br>enzyme | Enzyme that breaks down starch. Ptyalin is a salivary amylase and amylopsin is a pancreatic amylase. |
| **anabolism**<br>(ă-năb′ ō-lĭzm) | anabol<br>-ism | R<br>S | a building up<br>condition | Building up of the body substance in the constructive phase of metabolism |
| **anorexia**<br>(ăn″ ō-rĕks′ ĭ-ă) | an-<br>-orexia | P<br>S | lack of<br>appetite | Lack of appetite |
| **appendectomy**<br>(ăp″ ĕn-dĕk′ tō-mē) | append<br>-ectomy | R<br>S | appendix<br>surgical excision | Surgical excision of the appendix. See Figure 8–11 ▼. |

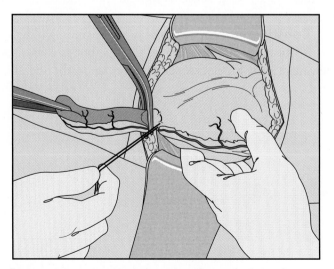

▶ **FIGURE 8–11** Appendectomy. The appendix and cecum are brought through the incision to the surface of the abdomen. The base of the appendix is clamped and ligated, and the appendix is then removed.

| MEDICAL WORD | WORD PARTS (WHEN APPLICABLE) | | | DEFINITION |
|---|---|---|---|---|
| | Part | Type | Meaning | |
| **appendicitis**<br>(ă-pĕn″ dĭ-sī′ tĭs) | appendic<br>-itis | R<br>S | appendix<br>inflammation | Inflammation of the appendix. A point of tenderness in acute appendicitis is known as *McBurney's point,* located 1 to 2 inches above the anterosuperior spine of the ilium on a line between the ilium and the umbilicus. See Figure 8–12 ▼. |
| **ascites**<br>(ă-sī′ tēz) | | | | Accumulation of serous fluid in the peritoneal cavity |
| **biliary**<br>(bĭl′ ĭ-ār″ ē) | bil/i<br>-ary | CF<br>S | gall, bile<br>pertaining to | Pertaining to or conveying bile |
| **bilirubin**<br>(bĭl″ ĭ-rōō′ bĭn) | | | | Orange-colored bile pigment produced by the separation of hemoglobin into parts that are excreted by the liver cells |
| **black hairy tongue** | | | | Condition in which the tongue is covered by hairlike papillae entangled with threads produced by *Aspergillus niger* or *Candida albicans* fungi. This unusual condition could be caused by poor oral hygiene and/or overgrowth of fungi due to antibiotic therapy. See Figure 8–13 ▼. |

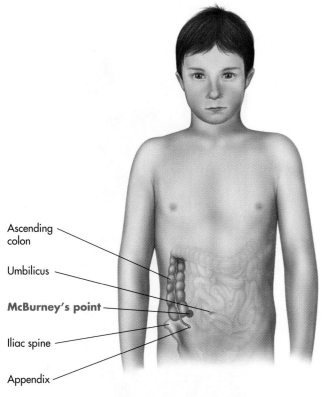

Ascending colon

Umbilicus

**McBurney's point**

Iliac spine

Appendix

▶ **FIGURE 8–12**  McBurney's point is the common location of pain in children and adolescents with appendicitis.

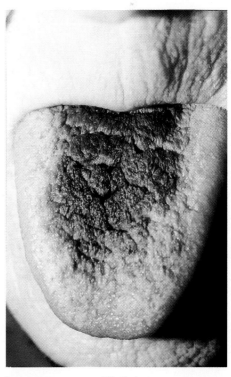

▶ **FIGURE 8–13**  Black hairy tongue.
(Courtesy of Jason L. Smith, MD)

| MEDICAL WORD | WORD PARTS (WHEN APPLICABLE) | | | DEFINITION |
|---|---|---|---|---|
| | **Part** | **Type** | **Meaning** | |
| **bowel**<br>(bou′əl) | | | | Intestine |
| **buccal**<br>(bək′ əl) | bucc<br>-al | R<br>S | cheek<br>pertaining to | Pertaining to the cheek |
| **catabolism**<br>(kă-tăb′ ō-lĭzm) | catabol<br>-ism | R<br>S | a casting down<br>condition | Literally *a casting down;* a breaking of complex substances into more basic elements |
| **celiac**<br>(sē′ lĭ-ăk) | celi<br>-ac | R<br>S | abdomen, belly<br>pertaining to | Pertaining to the abdomen |
| **cheilosis**<br>(kī-lō′ sĭs) | cheil<br>-osis | R<br>S | lip<br>condition (usu-<br>(ally abnormal) | Abnormal condition of the lip as seen in riboflavin and other B-complex deficiencies |
| **cholecystectomy**<br>(kō″ lē-sĭs-těk′ tō-mē) | chol/e<br>cyst<br>-ectomy | CF<br>R<br>S | gall, bile<br>bladder<br>surgical excision | Surgical excision of the gallbladder. With laparoscopic cholecystectomy, the gallbladder is removed through a small incision near the navel. *Cholelithiasis* (gallstones) are usually present in the removed gallbladder. See Figure 8–14 ▼. |
| **cholecystitis**<br>(kō″ lē-sĭs-tī′ tĭs) | chol/e<br>cyst<br>-itis | CF<br>R<br>S | gall, bile<br>bladder<br>inflammation | Inflammation of the gallbladder |

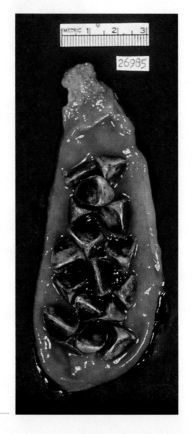

▶ **FIGURE 8–14**   Gallbladder with gallstones.
(MartinRotker/Phototake, New York City)

| MEDICAL WORD | WORD PARTS (WHEN APPLICABLE) | | | DEFINITION |
|---|---|---|---|---|
| | **Part** | **Type** | **Meaning** | |
| **choledochotomy** (kō-lĕd" ō-kŏt' ō-mē) | choledoch/o | CF | common bile duct | Surgical incision of the common bile duct |
| | -tomy | S | incision | |
| **chyle** (kīl) | | | | Milky fluid of intestinal digestion composed of lymph and emulsified fats |
| **cirrhosis** (sĭ-rō' sĭs) | cirrh | R | orange-yellow | Chronic degenerative liver disease characterized by changes in the lobes; parenchymal cells and the lobules are infiltrated with fat |
| | -osis | S | condition (usually abnormal) | |
| **colectomy** (kō-lĕk' tō-mē) | col | R | colon | Surgical excision of part of the colon |
| | -ectomy | S | surgical excision | |
| **colon cancer** (kō-lŏn kăn' ser) | | | | Malignancy of the colon; sometimes called *colorectal cancer* |
| **colonic** (kō-lŏn' ĭk) | colon | R | colon | Pertaining to the colon |
| | -ic | S | pertaining to | |
| **colonoscope** (kō-lŏn' ŏ-skōp) | colon | R | colon | Thin, lighted flexible instrument that is moved through the colon during a colonoscopy |
| | -scope | S | instrument for examining | |
| **colonoscopy** (kō-lŏn-ŏs' kō-pē) | colon/o | CF | colon | Visual examination of the colon via a colonoscope |
| | -scopy | S | visual examination, to view, examine | |
| **colostomy** (kō-lŏs' tō-mē) | col/o | CF | colon | Literally means *the creation of a new opening into the colon,* performed for the purpose of evacuating the bowel and can be required because of colon cancer, intestinal obstruction, perforation, birth defects, and Crohn's disease. A colostomy can be permanent or temporary. The most common types are transverse, descending, and sigmoid, so named due to the site of the disorder and the location of the stoma. See Figure 8–15 ▶. |
| | -stomy | S | new opening | |
| **constipation** (kon" stĭ-pā' shŭn) | constipat | R | to press together | Infrequent passage of unduly hard and dry feces; *difficult defecation* |
| | -ion | S | process | |
| **Crohn's disease** (krōnz dĭ-zez') | | | | Chronic autoimmune disease that can affect any part of the gastrointestinal tract but most commonly occurs in the ileum |
| **defecation** (dĕf-ĕ-kā' shŭn) | defecat | R | to remove dregs | Evacuation of the bowel |
| | -ion | S | process | |
| **deglutition** (dē" glōō-tĭsh' ūn) | | | | Act or process of swallowing |

| MEDICAL WORD | WORD PARTS (WHEN APPLICABLE) | | | DEFINITION |
|---|---|---|---|---|
| | Part | Type | Meaning | |
| **dentalgia**<br>(děn-tǎl' jǐ-ǎ) | dent<br>-algia | R<br>S | tooth<br>pain, ache | Pain in a tooth; *toothache* |
| **dentist** | dent<br>-ist | R<br>S | tooth<br>one who specializes | One who specializes in dentistry |
| **dentition**<br>(děn-tǐ'shǔn) | | | | Type, number, and arrangement of teeth in the dental arch |
| **diarrhea**<br>(dǐ' ǎ-rē' ǎ) | dia-<br>-rrhea | P<br>S | through<br>flow | Frequent passage of unformed watery stools |
| **digestion**<br>(dī-jěst' chǔn) | | | | Process by which food is changed in the mouth, stomach, and intestines by chemical, mechanical, and physical action so that it can be absorbed by the body |
| **diverticulitis**<br>(dī" věr-tǐk" ū-lǐ' tǐs) | diverticul<br>-itis | R<br>S | diverticula<br>inflammation | Inflammation of the diverticula in the colon. ✳ See Pathology Spotlight: Diverticulitis on page 216 and Figure 8–23. |
| **duodenal**<br>(dū" ō-dē' nǎl) | duoden<br>-al | R<br>S | duodenum<br>pertaining to | Pertaining to the duodenum; the first part of the small intestine |
| **dysentery**<br>(dǐs' ěn-těr" ē) | dys-<br>enter<br>-y | P<br>R<br>S | difficult<br>intestine<br>pertaining to | An intestinal disease characterized by inflammation of the mucous membrane |
| **dyspepsia**<br>(dǐs-pěp' sǐ-ǎ) | dys-<br>-pepsia | P<br>S | difficult<br>to digest | Difficulty in digestion; *indigestion* |
| **dysphagia**<br>(dǐs-fā' jǐ-ǎ) | dys-<br>-phagia | P<br>S | difficult<br>to eat, to swallow | Difficulty in swallowing |

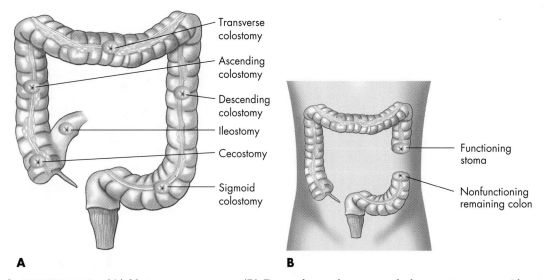

**A**            **B**

▶ **FIGURE 8–15** (A) Various -ostomy sites. (B) Descending colostomy with functioning stoma. Also illustrates nonfunctioning sigmoid colon, rectum, and anus.

| MEDICAL WORD | WORD PARTS (WHEN APPLICABLE) | | | DEFINITION |
|---|---|---|---|---|
| | **Part** | **Type** | **Meaning** | |
| **emesis**<br>(ĕm′ ĕ-sĭs) | eme<br>-sis | R<br>S | to vomit<br>condition | Vomiting |
| **enteric**<br>(ĕn-tĕr′ ĭk) | enter<br>-ic | R<br>S | small intestine<br>pertaining to | Pertaining to the small intestine |
| **enteritis**<br>(ĕn″ tĕr-ī′ tĭs) | enter<br>-itis | R<br>S | small intestine<br>inflammation | Inflammation of the small intestine |
| **enzyme**<br>(ĕn′ zīm) | | | | Protein substance capable of causing chemical changes in other substances without being changed itself |
| **epigastric**<br>(ĕp′ ĭ-găs′ trĭc) | epi-<br>gastr<br>-ic | P<br>R<br>S | above<br>stomach<br>pertaining to | Pertaining to the region above the stomach |
| **eructation**<br>(ē-rk-tā′ shŭn) | eructat<br>-ion | R<br>S | a breaking out<br>process | Belching |
| **esophageal**<br>(ē-sŏf″ ă-jē′ ăl) | esophage/(o)<br>-al | CF<br>S | esophagus<br>pertaining to | Pertaining to the esophagus. *Note that the suffix begins with a vowel; drop the (o) from the combining form and add -al to form esophageal.* |
| **feces**<br>(fē′ sēz) | | | | Body waste expelled from the bowels; *stools, excreta* |
| **fibroma**<br>(fĭ-brō′ mă) | fibr<br>-oma | R<br>S | fibrous tissue<br>tumor | Fibrous, encapsulated connective tissue tumor |
| **flatus**<br>(flā′ tŭs) | | | | Gas in the digestive tract. Also, the expelling of gas from a body orifice, especially the anus. The average person passes 400 to 1200 mL of gas each day. |
| **gastrectomy**<br>(găs-trĕk′ tō-mē) | gastr<br>-ectomy | R<br>S | stomach<br>surgical excision | Surgical excision of a part or the whole stomach. See Figure 8–16 ▼. |

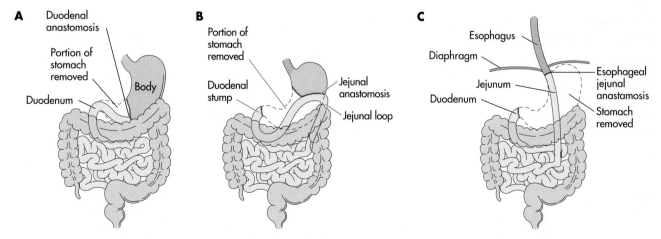

▶ **FIGURE 8–16** Partial and total gastrectomy procedures. (A) Partial gastrectomy with anastomosis to the duodenum. (B) Partial gastrectomy with anastomosis to the jejunum. (C) Total gastrectomy with anastomosis of the esophagus to the jejunum.

| MEDICAL WORD | WORD PARTS (WHEN APPLICABLE) | | | DEFINITION |
|---|---|---|---|---|
| | **Part** | **Type** | **Meaning** | |
| **gastric**<br>(găs′ trĭk) | gastr<br>-ic | R<br>S | stomach<br>pertaining to | Pertaining to the stomach |
| **gastroenterology**<br>(găs″ trō-ĕn″ tĕr-ŏl′ ō-jē) | gastr/o<br>enter/o<br>-logy | CF<br>CF<br>S | stomach<br>intestine<br>study of | Study of the stomach and the intestines |
| **gastroesophageal**<br>(găs′ trō ē-sŏf″ ă-jē-ăl) | gastr/o<br>esophage/(o)<br>-al | CF<br>CF<br>S | stomach<br>esophagus<br>pertaining to | Pertaining to the stomach and esophagus |
| **gastroesophageal reflux**<br>(găs′ trō ē-sŏf″ ă-jē-ăl rē′ flŭcks) | | | | Condition that occurs when the muscle between the esophagus and the stomach, the lower esophageal sphincter, is weak or relaxes inappropriately, allowing the stomach's contents to back up (*reflux*) into the esophagus. ✱ See Pathology Spotlight: Gastroesophageal Reflux Disease on page 216. |
| **gavage**<br>(gă-văzh′) | | | | To feed liquid or semiliquid food via a tube (stomach or nasogastric) |
| **gingivitis**<br>(jĭn″ jĭ-vī′ tĭs) | gingiv<br>-itis | R<br>S | gums<br>inflammation | Inflammation of the gums |
| **glossotomy**<br>(glŏ-sŏt′ ō-mē) | gloss/o<br>-tomy | CF<br>S | tongue<br>incision | Surgical incision into the tongue |
| **glycogenesis**<br>(glī″ kŏ-jĕn′ ĕ-sĭs) | glyc/o<br>-genesis | CF<br>S | sweet, sugar<br>formation, produce | Formation of glycogen from glucose |
| **halitosis**<br>(hăl″ ĭ-tō′ sĭs) | halit<br>-osis | R<br>S | breath<br>condition (usually abnormal) | Bad breath |
| **hematemesis**<br>(hĕm″ ăt-ĕm′ ĕ-sĭs) | hemat<br>-emesis | R<br>S | blood<br>vomiting | Vomiting of blood |
| **hematochezia**<br>(hĕm″ă-tō-kē′zē-ă) | | | | Passage of stools that contain red blood rather than tarry stools |
| **hemorrhoid**<br>(hĕm′ ō-royd) | hemorrh<br><br>-oid | R<br><br>S | vein liable to bleed<br>resemble | Mass of dilated, tortuous veins in the anorectum; can be internal or external. See Figure 8–17 ▶. |
| **hepatitis**<br>(hĕp″ ă-tī′ tĭs) | hepat<br>-itis | R<br>S | liver<br>inflammation | Inflammation of the liver |
| **hepatoma**<br>(hĕp″ ă-tō′ mă) | hepat<br>-oma | R<br>S | liver<br>tumor | Tumor of the liver |
| **hernia**<br>(hĕr′ nē-ă) | | | | Abnormal protrusion of an organ or a part of an organ through the wall of the body cavity that normally contains it. ✱See Pathology Spotlight: Hernia on page 218 and Figure 8–25. |

| MEDICAL WORD | WORD PARTS (WHEN APPLICABLE) | | | DEFINITION |
|---|---|---|---|---|
| | **Part** | **Type** | **Meaning** | |
| **herniorrhaphy**<br>(hĕr″ nĕ-or′ ă-fē) | herni/o<br>-rrhaphy | CF<br>S | hernia<br>suture | Surgical repair of a hernia |
| **hyperalimen-<br>tation**<br>(hī″ pĕr-ăl″ ĭ mĕn-<br>tā′ shŭn) | hyper-<br>alimentat<br>-ion | P<br>R<br>S | excessive<br>nourishment<br>process | Intravenous infusion of a hypertonic solution to sustain life; used in patients whose gastrointestinal tracts are not functioning properly |
| **hyperemesis**<br>(hī″ pĕr-ĕm′ ĕ-sĭs) | hyper-<br>-emesis | P<br>S | excessive, above<br>vomiting | Excessive vomiting |
| **hypogastric**<br>(hī″ pō-găs′ trĭk) | hypo-<br>gastr<br>-ic | P<br>R<br>S | deficient, below<br>stomach<br>pertaining to | Pertaining to below the stomach |
| **ileitis**<br>(ĭl″ ē-ī′ tis) | ile<br>-itis | R<br>S | ileum<br>inflammation | Inflammation of the ileum |
| **ileostomy**<br>(ĭl″ ē-ŏs′ tō-mē) | ile/o<br>-stomy | CF<br>S | ileum<br>new opening | Creation of a new opening through the abdominal wall into the ileum |
| **irritable bowel<br>syndrome (IBS)**<br>(ĭr′ ă-tă-bl bŏu′ ĕl<br>sĭn′ drōm) | | | | Disorder that interferes with the normal functions of the large intestine (colon); characterized by a group of symptoms, including crampy abdominal pain, bloating, constipation, and diarrhea.<br>＊See Pathology Spotlight: Irritable Bowel Syndrome on page 218. |

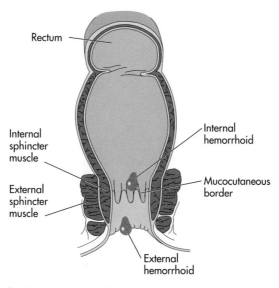

▶ FIGURE 8–17  Location of internal and external hemorrhoids.

| MEDICAL WORD | WORD PARTS (WHEN APPLICABLE) | | | DEFINITION |
|---|---|---|---|---|
| | **Part** | **Type** | **Meaning** | |
| **labial** (lā′ bĭ-ăl) | labi -al | R S | lip pertaining to | Pertaining to the lip |
| **laparotomy** (lăp″ ăr-ŏt′ ō-mē) | lapar/o -tomy | CF S | abdomen incision | Surgical incision into the abdomen |
| **lavage** (lă-văzh′) | | | | To wash out a cavity. Gastric lavage is used to remove or dilute gastric contents in cases of acute poisoning or ingestion of a caustic substance. *Vomiting should not be induced.* A closed system irrigation uses an ordered amount of solution until the desired results are obtained. See Figure 8–18 ▼. |
| **laxative** (lăk′ să-tĭv) | laxat -ive | R S | to loosen nature of, quality of | Substance that acts to loosen the bowels |
| **lingual** (lĭng′ gwal) | lingu -al | R S | tongue pertaining to | Pertaining to the tongue |
| **lipolysis** (lĭp-ŏl′ ĭ-sĭs) | lip/o -lysis | CF S | fat destruction, to separate | Destruction of fat |
| **liver transplant** | | | | Surgical process of transferring the liver from a donor to a patient |
| **malabsorption** (măl″ ăb-sōrp′ shŭn) | mal- absorpt -ion | P R S | bad to suck in process | Process of bad or inadequate absorption of nutrients from the intestinal tract |

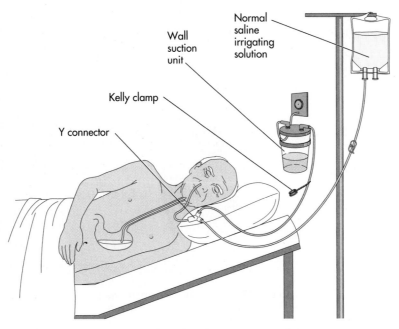

▶ **FIGURE 8–18** Patient with a closed system gastric lavage.

| MEDICAL WORD | WORD PARTS (WHEN APPLICABLE) | | | DEFINITION |
|---|---|---|---|---|
| | Part | Type | Meaning | |
| **mastication**<br>(măs″ tĭ-kā′ shŭn) | masticat<br>-ion | R<br>S | to chew<br>process | Chewing |
| **melena**<br>(měl′ ĕ-nă) | | | | Black, tarry feces (stools) caused by the action of intestinal juices on blood |
| **mesentery**<br>(měs′ ĕn-tĕr″ ē) | mes<br>enter<br>-y | R<br>R<br>S | middle<br>small intestine<br>pertaining to | Pertaining to the peritoneal fold encircling the small intestines and connecting the intestines to the posterior abdominal wall |
| **nausea**<br>(naw′ sē-ă) | | | | Feeling of the inclination to vomit |
| **pancreas transplant**<br>(păn′ krē-ăs trăns plănt) | | | | Surgical process of transferring the pancreas from a donor to a patient |
| **pancreatitis**<br>(păn″ krē-ă-tī′ tĭs) | pancreat<br>-itis | R<br>S | pancreas<br>inflammation | Inflammation of the pancreas |
| **paralytic ileus**<br>(păr″ ă-lĭt′ ĭk ĭl′ ē-ŭs) | paralyt<br>-ic<br>ile<br>-us | R<br>S<br>R<br>S | to disable; paralysis<br>pertaining to<br>a twisting<br>pertaining to | Paralysis of the intestines that causes distention and symptoms of acute obstruction and prostration |
| **peptic**<br>(pĕp′ tĭk) | pept<br>-ic | R<br>S | to digest<br>pertaining to | Pertaining to gastric digestion |
| **periodontal**<br>(pĕr″ ē-ō-dŏn′ tăl) | peri-<br>odont<br>-al | P<br>R<br>S | around<br>tooth<br>pertaining to | Pertaining to the area around the tooth |
| **periodontal disease**<br>(pĕr″ ē-ō-dŏn′ tăl) | | | | Inflammation and degeneration of the gums and surrounding bone, which frequently causes loss of the teeth |
| **peristalsis**<br>(pĕr″ ĭ-stăl′ sĭs) | peri-<br>-stalsis | P<br>S | around<br>contraction | Wavelike contraction that occurs involuntarily in hollow tubes of the body, especially the alimentary canal |
| **pharyngeal**<br>(făr-ĭn′ jē-ăl) | pharyng/e<br>-al | CF<br>S | pharynx<br>pertaining to | Pertaining to the pharynx |
| **pilonidal cyst**<br>(pī″ lō-nī′ dăl sĭst) | pil/o<br>nid<br>-al<br>cyst | CF<br>R<br>S<br>R | hair<br>nest<br>pertaining to<br>sac | Closed sac in the crease of the sacrococcygeal region caused by a developmental defect that permits epithelial tissue and hair to be trapped below the skin |
| **postprandial (PP)**<br>(pōst-prăn′ dĭ-ăl) | post-<br>prand/i<br>-al | P<br>CF<br>S | after<br>meal<br>pertaining to | After a meal |
| **proctologist**<br>(prŏk-tŏl′ ō-jĭst) | proct/o<br>log<br>-ist | CF<br>R<br>S | anus and rectum<br>study of<br>one who specializes | Physician who specializes in the study of the anus and the rectum |
| **proctoscope**<br>(prŏk′ tō-scōp) | proct/o<br>-scope | CF<br>S | anus and rectum<br>instrument for examining | Instrument used to view the anus and rectum |

| MEDICAL WORD | WORD PARTS (WHEN APPLICABLE) | | | DEFINITION |
|---|---|---|---|---|
| | **Part** | **Type** | **Meaning** | |
| **pyloric**<br>(pī-lōr′ ĭk) | pylor<br><br>-ic | R<br><br>S | pylorus,<br>gatekeeper<br>pertaining to | Pertaining to the gatekeeper, the opening between the stomach and the duodenum. In *pyloric stenosis* seen in an infant, the hypertrophied pyloric muscle causes symptoms of projectile vomiting and visible peristalsis. |
| **rectocele**<br>(rĕk′ tō-sēl) | rect/o<br>-cele | CF<br>S | rectum<br>hernia | Hernia of part of the rectum into the vagina |
| **sialadenitis**<br>(sī″ ăl-ăd″ ĕ-nī′ tĭs) | sial<br>aden<br>-itis | R<br>R<br>S | saliva<br>gland<br>inflammation | Inflammation of the salivary gland |
| **sigmoidoscope**<br>(sĭg-moy′ dō-skōp) | sigmoid/o<br>-scope | CF<br>S | sigmoid<br>instrument for<br>examining | Instrument used to view the sigmoid |
| **splenomegaly**<br>(splē″ nō-mĕg′ ă-lē) | splen/o<br>-megaly | CF<br>S | spleen<br>enlargement,<br>large | Enlargement of the spleen |
| **stomatitis**<br>(stō″ mă-tī′ tĭs) | stomat<br>-itis | R<br>S | mouth<br>inflammation | Inflammation of the mouth |
| **sublingual**<br>(sŭb-lĭng′ gwăl) | sub-<br>lingu<br>-al | P<br>R<br>S | below<br>tongue<br>pertaining to | Pertaining to below the tongue. See Figure 8–19 ▼. |

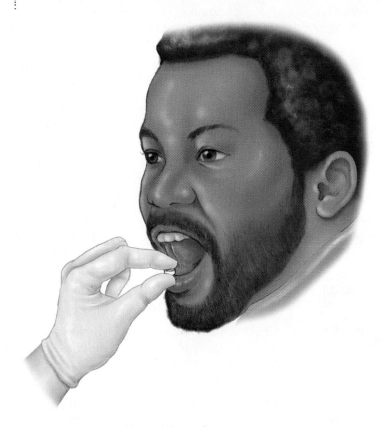

► FIGURE 8–19   Sublingual drug administration.

| MEDICAL WORD | WORD PARTS (WHEN APPLICABLE) | | | DEFINITION |
|---|---|---|---|---|
| | Part | Type | Meaning | |
| **ulcer** | | | | Open lesion or sore of the epidermis or mucous membrane. A *peptic ulcer* forms in the mucosal wall of the stomach, the pylorus, the duodenum, or the esophagus. It is referred to as a *gastric, duodenal,* or *esophageal ulcer,* depending on the location. ✱ See Pathology Spotlight: Peptic Ulcer Disease on page 219 and Figure 8–26. |
| **ulcerative colitis**<br>(ŭl′ sĕr-ă-tĭv kō-lī′ tĭs) | | | | Disease that causes inflammation and ulcers in the lining of the large intestine. The inflammation usually occurs in the rectum and lower part of the colon but can affect the entire colon; also called *colitis* or *proctitis.* |
| **vermiform**<br>(vĕr′ mĭ-form) | verm/i<br>-form | CF<br>S | worm<br>shape | Shaped like a worm; *vermiform appendix* |
| **volvulus**<br>(vŏl′ vū-lŭs) | volvul<br>-us | R<br>S | to roll<br>pertaining to | Twisting of the bowel on itself that causes an obstruction. See Figure 8–20 ▼. |
| **vomit** | | | | To eject stomach contents through the mouth |

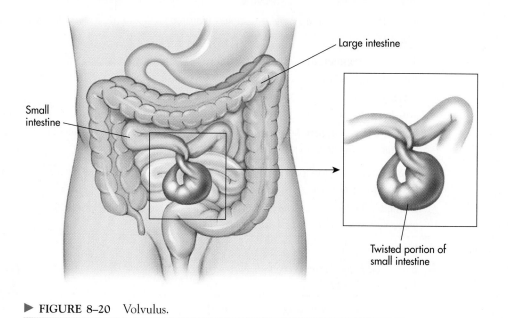

Large intestine

Small intestine

Twisted portion of small intestine

▶ **FIGURE 8–20**  Volvulus.

# DRUG HIGHLIGHTS

| | |
|---|---|
| **Antacids** | Neutralize hydrochloric acid in the stomach; classified as nonsystemic and systemic. |
| Nonsystemic | *Examples: Amphojel (aluminum hydroxide), Tums (calcium carbonate), Riopan (magaldrate), and Milk of Magnesia (magnesium hydroxide)* |
| Systemic | *Example: sodium bicarbonate* |
| **Antacid mixtures** | Products that combine aluminum (can cause constipation) and/or calcium compounds with magnesium salts (can cause diarrhea). By combining the antacid properties of two single-entity agents, these products provide the antacid action of both yet tend to counter the adverse effects of each other. |
| | *Examples: Gaviscon, Gelusil, Maalox Plus, and Mylanta* |
| **Histamine H$_2$-receptor antagonists** | Inhibit both daytime and nocturnal basal gastric acid secretion and inhibit gastric acid stimulated by food, histamines, caffeine, insulin, and pentagastrin; used in the treatment of active duodenal ulcer. |
| | *Examples: Tagamet (cimetidine), Pepcid (famotidine), Axid (nizatidine), and Zantac (ranitidine)* |
| **Mucosal protective medications** | Medicines that protect the stomach's mucosal lining from acids but do not inhibit the release of acid. |
| | *Examples: Carafate (sucralfate) and Cytotec (misoprostol)* |
| **Gastric acid pump inhibitors (proton-pump inhibitor—PPI)** | Antiulcer agents that suppress gastric acid secretion by specific inhibition of the H + /K + ATPase enzyme at the secretory surface of the gastric parietal cell. Because this enzyme system is regarded as the acid (proton) pump within the gastric mucosa, gastric acid pump inhibitors are so classified, because they block the final step of acid production. |
| | *Examples: Prilosec (omeprazole), Aciphex (rabeprazole sodium), Prevacid (lansoprazole), and Protonix (pantoprazole)* |
| **Other ulcer medications** | Treatment regimen for active duodenal ulcers associated with *H. pylori* can involve a two- or three-drug program. |
| | *Examples: a two-drug program—Biaxin (clarithromycin) and Prilosec (omeprazole); and a three-drug program—Flagyl (metronidazole) and either tetracycline or amoxicillin and Pepto Bismol* |
| | *Note: For the treatment program to be effective, the patient must complete the full treatment program that involves taking 15 pills a day for a total of at least 2 weeks.* |
| **Laxatives** | Used to relieve constipation and to facilitate the passage of feces through the lower gastrointestinal tract. |
| | *Examples: Dulcolax (bisacodyl), Milk of Magnesia (magnesium hydroxide), Metamucil (psyllium hydrophilic muciloid), and Ex-Lax (phenolphthalein)* |
| **Antidiarrheal agents** | Used to treat diarrhea. |
| | *Examples: Pepto-Bismol (bismuth subsalicylate), Kaopectate (kaolin mixture with pectin), and Imodium (loperamide HCl)* |
| **Antiemetics** | Prevent or arrest vomiting; also used in the treatment of vertigo, motion sickness, and nausea. |
| | *Examples: Dramamine (dimenhydrinate), Phenergan (promethazine HCl), Tigan (trimethobenzamide HCl), and Transderm Scop (scopolamine)* |
| **Emetics** | Used to induce vomiting in people who have taken an overdose of oral drugs or who have ingested certain poisons. An emetic agent should not be given to a person who is unconscious, in shock, or in a semicomatose state. Emetics are also contraindicated in individuals who have ingested strongly caustic substances, such as lye or acid, because their use could result in additional injury to the person's esophagus. |
| | *Example: Ipecac syrup* |

# DIAGNOSTIC AND LAB TESTS

| TEST | DESCRIPTION |
| --- | --- |
| **Alcohol toxicology (ethanol and ethyl)** (ăl′ kō-hōl tŏks″ ĭ-kŏl′ ō-jē) | Test performed on blood serum or plasma to determine levels of alcohol. All 50 states and the District of Columbia have laws defining it as a crime to drive with a blood alcohol concentration (BAC) at or above 0.08%. Increased values indicate alcohol consumption that could lead to cirrhosis of the liver, gastritis, malnutrition, vitamin deficiencies, and other gastrointestinal disorders. |
| **Ammonia (NH 4)** (ă-mō′ nē-ă) | Test performed on blood plasma to determine the level of ammonia (end product of protein breakdown). Increased values can indicate hepatic failure, hepatic encephalopathy, and high protein diet in hepatic failure. |
| **Barium enema (BE)** (bă′ rē-ūm ĕn′ ĕ-mă) | Test performed by administering barium (Ba) via the rectum to determine the condition of the colon. X-rays are taken to ascertain the structure and to check the filling of the colon. Abnormal results can indicate cancer of the colon, polyps, fistulas, ulcerative colitis, diverticulitis, hernias, and intussusception. |
| **Bilirubin blood test (total)** (bĭl-ĭ-roo′ bĭn blod test) | Test done on blood serum to determine whether bilirubin is conjugated and excreted in the bile. Abnormal results can indicate obstructive jaundice, hepatitis, and cirrhosis. |
| **Carcinoembryonic antigen (CEA)** (kăr″ sĭn-ō-ĕm″ brē-ŏn′ ĭk ăn′ tĭ-jĕn) | Test performed on whole blood or plasma to determine the presence of CEA (antigens originally isolated from colon tumors). Increased values can indicate stomach, intestinal, rectal, and various other cancers and conditions. This test is nonspecific and must be combined with other tests for a final diagnosis. It is being used to monitor the course of cancer therapy. |
| **Cholangiography** (kō-lăn″ jē-ŏg′ ră-fē) | X-ray examination of the common bile duct, cystic duct, and hepatic ducts in which radiopaque dye is injected, and then films are taken. Abnormal results can indicate obstruction, stones, and tumors. |
| **Cholecystography** (kō″ lē-sĭs-tŏg′ ră-fē) | X-ray examination of the gallbladder in which radiopaque dye is injected, and then films are taken. Abnormal results can indicate cholecystitis, cholelithiasis, and tumors. |
| **Colonofiberoscopy** (kŏ′ lō-nŏ-fī″ bĕr-ŏs′ kō-pē) | Fiberoptic colonoscopy, a direct visual examination of the colon via a flexible colonoscope; used as a diagnostic aid, for removal of foreign bodies, polyps, and tissue. The patient is lightly sedated during the procedure. |
| **Colonoscopy** (kŏ′ lŏn-ŏs′ kō-pē) | Direct visual examination of the colon via a colonoscope; used to diagnose growths and to confirm findings of other tests. It can also be used to remove small polyps and to collect tissue samples for analysis. The patient is lightly sedated during the procedure. |
| **Endoscopic retrograde cholangiopancreatography (ERCP)** (ĕn′ dō-skōp-ĭk rĕt′ rō-grād kō-lăn″ jē-ō-păn″ krē-ă-tŏg′ ră-fē) | X-ray examination of the biliary and pancreatic ducts by injecting a contrast medium, and then films are taken. Abnormal results can indicate fibrosis, biliary or pancreatic cysts, strictures, stones, and chronic pancreatitis. |
| **Esophagogastroduodenalendoscopy** (ĕ-sŏf″ ă-gō′ găs″ trō-dū″ ō-dē′ năl ĕn-dŏs′kō-pē) | Endoscopic examination of the esophagus, stomach, and small intestine. During the procedure, photographs, biopsy, or brushings may be done. |

| | |
|---|---|
| **Gamma-glutamyl transferase (GGT)** (găm′ ă glōō-tăm′ ĭl trăns′ fĕr-ās) | Test performed on blood serum to determine the level of GGT (enzyme found in the liver, kidney, prostate, heart, and spleen). Increased values can indicate cirrhosis, liver necrosis, hepatitis, alcoholism, neoplasms, acute pancreatitis, acute myocardial infarction, nephrosis, and acute cholecystitis. |
| **Gastric analysis** (găs′ trĭk ă-năl′ ĭ sĭs) | Test performed to determine quality of secretion, amount of free and combined HCl, and absence or presence of blood, bacteria, bile, and fatty acids. Increased level of HCl can indicate peptic ulcer disease, Zollinger-Ellison syndrome (a condition caused by non insulin-secreting pancreatic tumors, which secrete excess amounts of gastrin), and hypergastremia. Decreased level of HCl can indicate stomach cancer, pernicious anemia, and atrophic gastritis. |
| **Gastrointestinal (GI) series** (găs″ trō-ĭn-tes′ tĭn″ ăl sēr′ ēz) | Fluoroscopic examination of the esophagus, stomach, and small intestine in which barium is given orally and is observed as it flows through the GI system. See Figure 8–21 ▶. Abnormal results can indicate esophageal varices, ulcers, gastric polyps, malabsorption syndrome, hiatal hernias, diverticuli, pyloric stenosis, and foreign bodies. |
| **Hepatitis-associated antigen (HAA)** (hĕp″ ă-tī-tĭs ă-sō′ shē-āt′ ĕd ăn′ tĭ-jĕn) | Test performed to determine the presence of the hepatitis B virus. |
| **Liver biopsy** | Microscopic examination of liver tissue. Abnormal results can indicate cirrhosis, hepatitis, and tumors. |
| **Occult blood** (ŭ-kŭlt) | Test performed on feces to determine gastrointestinal bleeding that is invisible (hidden). Positive results can indicate gastritis, stomach cancer, peptic ulcer, ulcerative colitis, bowel cancer, bleeding esophageal varices, portal hypertension, pancreatitis, and diverticulitis. |
| **Ova and parasites (O&P)** (o′ vă păr′ ă-sīts) | Test performed on stool to identify ova and parasites. Positive results indicate protozoa infestation. |
| **Stool culture** | Test performed on stool to identify the presence of organisms. |
| **Ultrasonography, gallbladder** (ŭl-tră-sŏn-ŏg′ ră-fē găl″ blăd′ dĕr) | Test to visualize the gallbladder by using high-frequency sound waves. The echoes are recorded on an oscilloscope and film. See Figure 8–22 ▶. Abnormal results can indicate biliary obstruction, cholelithiasis, and acute cholecystitis. |
| **Ultrasonography, liver** (ŭl-tră-sŏn-ŏg′ ră-fē lĭv′ ĕr) | Test to visualize the liver by using high-frequency sound waves. The echoes are recorded on an oscilloscope and film. Abnormal results can indicate hepatic tumors, cysts, abscess, and cirrhosis. |
| **Upper gastrointestinal fiberoscopy** (ŭp′ ir găs′ trō-ĭn-tĕs′ tĭn″ ăl fī′ bĕr-ŏs′ kō-pē) | Direct visual examination of the gastric mucosa via a flexible fiberscope when gastric neoplasm is suspected. Colored photographs or motion pictures can be taken during the procedure. |

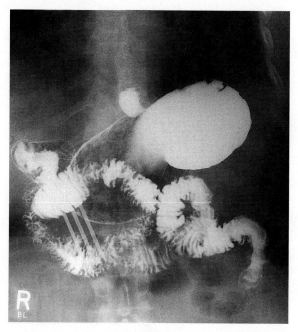

► **FIGURE 8–21** Upper GI series. (Courtesy of Teresa Resch)

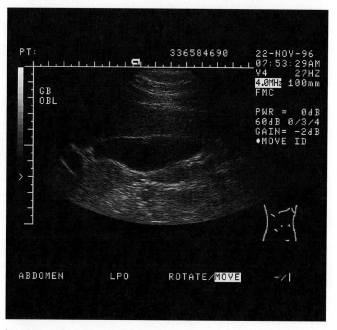

► **FIGURE 8–22** Gallbladder ultrasound. (Courtesy of Teresa Resch)

# ABBREVIATIONS

| ABBREVIATION | MEANING | ABBREVIATION | MEANING |
|---|---|---|---|
| ac | before meals (ante cibum) | HBIG | hepatitis B immune globulin |
| A/G | albumin/globulin (ratio) | HBV | hepatitis B virus |
| Ba | barium | HCl | hydrochloric acid |
| BAC | blood alcohol concentration | IBS | irritable bowel syndrome |
| BE | barium enema | LES | lower esophageal sphincter |
| BM | bowel movement | MALT | mucosal-associated-lymphoid |
| BRP | bathroom privileges | | type (lymphoma) |
| BS | bowel sounds | NANBH | non-A, non-B hepatitis virus |
| CEA | carcinoembryonic antigen | NG | nasogastric (tube) |
| CHO | carbohydrate | NH$_4$ | ammonia |
| chol | cholesterol | NPO, npo | nothing by mouth |
| CUC | chronic ulcerative colitis | N&V | nausea and vomiting |
| E. coli | Escherichia coli | O&P | ova and parasites |
| ERCP | endoscopic retrograde | pc | after meals (post cibum) |
| | cholangiopancreatography | PEG | percutaneous endoscopic |
| GB | gallbladder | | gastrostomy |
| GERD | gastroesophageal reflux disease | PP | postprandial (after meals) |
| GGT | gamma-glutamyl transferase | PUD | peptic ulcer disease |
| GI | gastrointestinal | RDA | recommended dietary or |
| GTT | glucose tolerance test | | daily allowance |
| HAA | hepatitis-associated antigen | TPN | total parenteral nutrition |
| HAV | hepatitis A virus | UGI | upper gastrointestinal |

# PATHOLOGY SPOTLIGHTS

## \* Diverticulitis

**Diverticulitis** is an inflammation of the diverticula in the colon. Pain is a common symptom of diverticulitis. Diverticulitis occurs when a **diverticulum** (a pouch or sac in the walls of an organ or canal) becomes inflamed or infected. See Figure 8–23 ▼. The exact cause of this condition is unknown, but it generally begins when stool lodges in the diverticula. Infection can lead to complications such as swelling or rupturing of the diverticula. Symptoms include pain, fever, chills, cramping, bloating, constipation, and diarrhea. Treatment depends on the severity of the condition. A liquid diet and oral antibiotics are used for mild conditions, generally followed by a high-fiber diet. If the condition is severe, hospitalization, bedrest, IV antibiotics and fluids, and/or surgery is recommended.

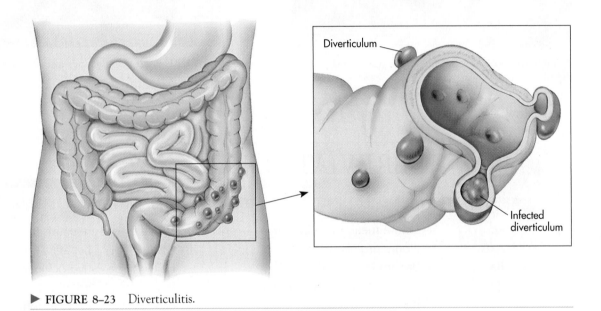

Diverticulum

Infected
diverticulum

▶ **FIGURE 8–23**   Diverticulitis.

 ## \* Gastroesophageal Reflux Disease

**Gastroesophageal reflux disease** (GERD) occurs when the muscle between the esophagus and the stomach, the lower esophageal sphincter, is weak or relaxes inappropriately. This allows the stomach's contents to back up (*reflux*) into the esophagus (see Figure 8–24 ▶). It is also called *esophageal reflux* or *reflux esophagitis*. Symptoms include heartburn, belching, and regurgitation of food.

Most GERD sufferers have frequent, severe heartburn. This tears down and damages the cell wall lining of the esophagus. Without treatment, GERD can lead to the following conditions: **Barrett's esophagus,** a precancerous change in the cells lining the esophagus; esophageal cancer; esophageal perforation, or a hole in the esophagus; esophageal ulcers, which damage the lining further; **esophagitis,** inflammation of the esophagus or **esophageal stricture,** narrowing of the esophagus that can interfere with eating. When deemed necessary, a surgical procedure known as **dilation** is done to treat esophageal stricture. The surgeon passes a series of dilators down the esophagus, stretching the narrowed opening.

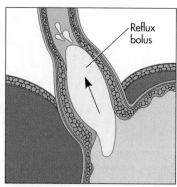 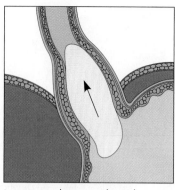 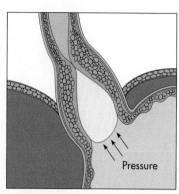

Transient lower esophageal sphincter relaxation

Incompetent lower esophageal sphincter

Increased intragastric pressure

▶ **FIGURE 8–24** Mechanisms of gastroesophageal reflux.

Dietary and lifestyle choices can contribute to GERD. Studies show that cigarette smoking relaxes the lower esophageal sphincter. Obesity and pregnancy can also cause GERD. Some doctors believe a hiatal hernia weakens the lower esophageal sphincter (LES) and causes reflux.

Some medical and surgical treatments for GERD include use of medications such as $H_2$ blockers and proton-pump inhibitors and **fundoplication,** a surgical reduction of the opening into the fundus of the stomach and suturing of the previously removed end of the esophagus to the opening.

## ✳ Hernia

A **hernia** is the abnormal protrusion of an organ or a part of an organ through the wall of the body cavity that normally contains it. Most often, *hernia* refers to an abdominal hernia. The two most common types of abdominal hernia are hiatal and inguinal.

**Hiatal hernia** occurs when the upper part of the stomach moves up into the chest through a small opening in the diaphragm. See Figure 8–25A ▶.

Coughing, vomiting, straining, or sudden physical exertion can cause increased pressure in the abdomen that results in hiatal hernia. Obesity and pregnancy also contribute to this condition.

Hiatal hernias usually do not require treatment. However, treatment can be necessary if the hernia is in danger of becoming strangulated (twisted in a way that cuts off blood supply) or is complicated by severe GERD or esophagitis. The physician can perform surgery to reduce the size of the hernia or to prevent strangulation.

An **inguinal hernia** occurs when a loop of intestine enters the inguinal canal, a tubular passage through the lower layers of the abdominal wall. See Figure 8–25B. Symptoms include groin discomfort or pain, and in the male, a scrotum lump.

Infants and children can also develop inguinal hernias. In these populations, hernias can occur when a portion of the peritoneum (the lining around all of the organs in the abdomen) does not close properly before birth. This causes a small portion of the intestine to push out into the opening (a bulge might be seen in the groin or scrotum). Diagnosis is typically made through a physical examination in which the hernia mass is palpated and increases in size when coughing, bending, lifting, or straining. The hernia (bulge) is not necessarily obvious in infants and children except when the child is crying or coughing. Treatment is usually a **herniorrhaphy,** a hernia repair surgery, in which the hernia is pushed back into the abdominal cavity.

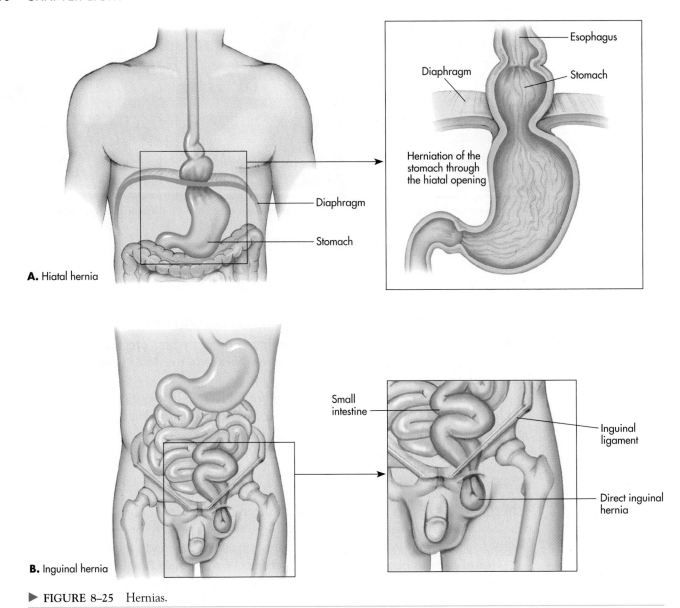

Esophagus

Diaphragm

Stomach

Herniation of the stomach through the hiatal opening

Diaphragm

Stomach

**A.** Hiatal hernia

Small intestine

Inguinal ligament

Direct inguinal hernia

**B.** Inguinal hernia

▶ **FIGURE 8–25**   Hernias.

## ✳ Irritable Bowel Syndrome

**Irritable bowel syndrome** (IBS) is a disorder that interferes with the normal functions of the large intestine (colon). It is characterized by a group of symptoms, including crampy abdominal pain, bloating, constipation, and diarrhea. The cause is not known, but the symptoms are often worsened by emotional stress.

Symptoms of irritable bowel syndrome include abdominal distress that is often relieved with a bowel movement; bloating, or feeling that the stomach is inflated; excess gas; and changes in stool. Some people with IBS have painful, loose stools, or diarrhea; others have painful hard stools, or constipation. Some people alternate between diarrhea and constipation.

One in five Americans has IBS, making it one of the most common disorders diagnosed by doctors. It occurs more often in women than in men, and it usually begins between the ages of 20 and 30. Predisposing factors include a low-fiber diet, emotional stress, and use of laxatives.

Treatment of irritable bowel syndrome often focuses on treating the symptoms and preventing flareups. Most people can control their symptoms with diet, stress management, and medications prescribed by their physician.

## ✳ Peptic Ulcer Disease

**Peptic ulcer disease** (PUD) occurs when the lining of the esophagus, stomach, or duodenum is worn away. See Figure 8–26 ▼. Peptic ulcer disease most commonly occurs in the upper part of the small intestine called the *duodenum*.

The most common ulcer symptom is gnawing or burning pain in the epigastrium. This pain typically occurs when the stomach is empty, between meals, and in the early morning hours, but it can also occur at other times. It can last from minutes to hours and can be relieved by eating or by taking antacids. Less common ulcer symptoms include nausea, vomiting, and loss of appetite. Bleeding can also occur; prolonged bleeding can cause anemia, leading to weakness and fatigue. If bleeding is heavy, **hematemesis, hematochezia,** or **melena** can occur.

In peptic ulcer disease there is an imbalance between acid and pepsin (an enzyme) secretion and the defenses of the mucosal lining. This leads to inflammation, which can be caused by aspirin and nonsteroidal anti-inflammatory medications (NSAIDs). Contrary to

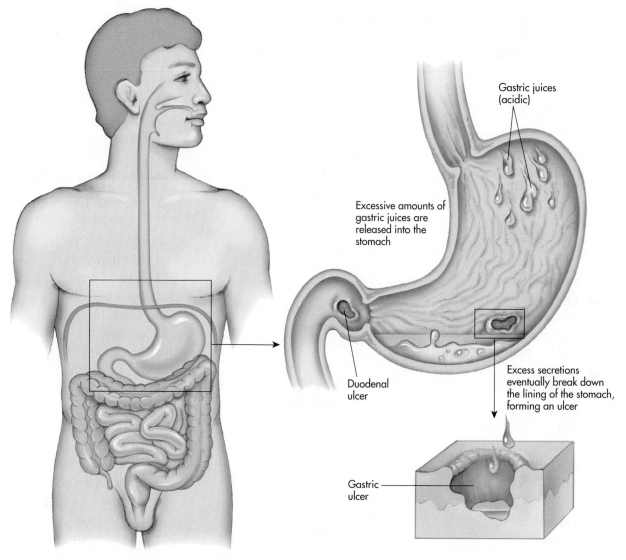

▶ **FIGURE 8–26**   Peptic ulcer disease (PUD).

popular belief, ulcers are *not* caused by spicy foods or stress but are aggravated by them. The erosion of the mucosa that characterizes peptic ulcers is often caused by infection with a bacterium called *Helicobacter pylori* (*H. pylori*). Approximately 90% of duodenal ulcers and 80% of peptic ulcers are associated with *Helicobacter pylori*. By killing the bacteria with antibiotics, it is estimated that 90% of the ulcers caused by *H. pylori* can be cured. Infected persons who are not treated have a two- to sixfold increased risk of developing gastric cancer and mucosal-associated-lymphoid-type (MALT) lymphoma compared with those who are not infected.

Treatment of peptic ulcer disease depends on the cause. If aspirin or other medications are the cause, these medications must be stopped. Smoking and drinking alcohol should be stopped as well because they can delay healing. Medications are given to help protect the stomach lining and allow faster healing. Most of these medications work by neutralizing stomach acid or preventing its production. If an infection with *H. pylori* is present, antibiotics are given. Surgery can be needed for severe ulcers that bleed, are unresponsive to medication, or cause a hole in the stomach.

# ✔ PATHOLOGY CHECKPOINT

*Following is a concise list of the pathology-related terms that you have seen in the chapter. Review this checklist to make sure that you are familiar with the meaning of each term before moving to the next section.*

## Conditions and Symptoms

- ❏ anorexia
- ❏ appendicitis
- ❏ ascites
- ❏ Barrett's esophagus
- ❏ cheilosis
- ❏ cholecystitis
- ❏ cirrhosis
- ❏ colon cancer
- ❏ constipation
- ❏ Crohn's disease
- ❏ dentalgia
- ❏ diarrhea
- ❏ diverticulitis
- ❏ dysentery
- ❏ dyspepsia
- ❏ dysphagia
- ❏ emesis
- ❏ enteritis
- ❏ eructation
- ❏ flatus
- ❏ gastroesophageal reflux
- ❏ gastroesophageal reflux disease
- ❏ gingivitis

- ❏ halitosis
- ❏ hematemesis
- ❏ hematochezia
- ❏ hemorrhoid
- ❏ hepatitis
- ❏ hepatoma
- ❏ hernia
- ❏ hiatal hernia
- ❏ hyperemesis
- ❏ ileitis
- ❏ inguinal hernia
- ❏ irritable bowel syndrome
- ❏ malabsorption
- ❏ melena
- ❏ nausea
- ❏ pancreatitis
- ❏ paralytic ileus
- ❏ peptic ulcer disease
- ❏ periodontal disease
- ❏ pilonidal cyst
- ❏ rectocele
- ❏ sialadentitis
- ❏ splenomegaly
- ❏ stomatitis
- ❏ ulcer

- ❏ ulcerative colitis
- ❏ volvulus
- ❏ vomit

## Diagnosis and Treatment

- ❏ appendectomy
- ❏ cholecystectomy
- ❏ choledochotomy
- ❏ colectomy
- ❏ colonoscopy
- ❏ colostomy
- ❏ gastrectomy
- ❏ gavage
- ❏ glossotomy
- ❏ herniorrhaphy
- ❏ hyperalimentation
- ❏ ileostomy
- ❏ laparotomy
- ❏ lavage
- ❏ laxative
- ❏ liver transplant
- ❏ pancreas transplant
- ❏ proctoscope
- ❏ sigmoidscope

# STUDY AND REVIEW

## Anatomy and Physiology

*Write your answers to the following questions. Do not refer to the text.*

1. Name the primary organs commonly associated with digestion.

   a. _____    b. _____

   c. _____    d. _____

   e. _____    f. _____

2. Name four accessory organs of digestion.

   a. _____    b. _____

   c. _____    d. _____

3. State the three main functions of the digestive system.

   a. _____

   b. _____

   c. _____

4. Define *bolus*. _____

   _____

5. Define *peristalsis*. _____

   _____

6. _____ _____ and _____ _____ convert the food into a semiliquid state.

7. The _____ is the first portion of the small intestine.

8. Semiliquid food is called _____.

9. The _____ _____ transports nutrients to body cells.

10. The large intestine can be divided into four distinct sections called the _____, the _____, the _____, and the _____.

11. The _____ is the largest glandular organ in the body.

12. State the function of the gallbladder. _____

13. Name an important function of the pancreas. _____

14. State three functions of the liver.

    a. _____            b. _____

    c. _____

15. Where does digestion and absorption chiefly take place? _____

16. The salivary glands located in and about the mouth are called the _____,

    the _____, and the _____.

17. Name the two hormones secreted into the bloodstream by the pancreas.

    a. _____            b. _____

## Word Parts

1. In the spaces provided, write the definition of these prefixes, roots, combining forms, and suffixes. Do not refer to the listings of medical words. Leave blank those words you cannot define.

2. After completing as many as you can, refer to the medical word listings to check your work. For each word missed or left blank, write the word and its definition several times on the margins of these pages or on a separate sheet of paper.

3. To maximize the learning process, it is to your advantage to do the following exercises as directed. To refer to the word-building section before completing these exercises invalidates the learning process.

## PREFIXES

*Give the definitions of the following prefixes.*

1. an- _____        2. dys- _____

3. epi- _____       4. hyper- _____

5. hypo- _____       6. mal- _____

7. peri- _____       8. post- _____

9. dia- _____      10. sub- _____

## ROOTS AND COMBINING FORMS

*Give the definitions of the following roots and combining forms.*

1. absorpt _____      2. aden _____

3. amyl _____       4. anabol _____

5. catabol _____      6. cirrh _____

7. append _____       8. appendic _____

9. bil/i _____

10. bucc _____

11. celi _____

12. cheil _____

13. chol/e _____

14. choledoch/o _____

15. col _____

16. col/o _____

17. colon _____

18. colon/o _____

19. cyst _____

20. dent _____

21. constipat _____

22. diverticul _____

23. duoden _____

24. enter _____

25. defecat _____

26. esophage/(o) _____

27. gastr _____

28. gastr/o _____

29. gingiv _____

30. gloss/o _____

31. glyc/o _____

32. hemat _____

33. hepat _____

34. hepat/o _____

35. herni/o _____

36. ile _____

37. ile/o _____

38. labi _____

39. lapar/o _____

40. laxat _____

41. lingu _____

42. lip/o _____

43. log _____

44. mes _____

45. pancreat _____

46. pept _____

47. pharyng/e _____

48. prand/i _____

49. eme _____

50. proct/o _____

51. pylor _____

52. rect/o _____

53. sial _____

54. sigmoid/o _____

55. splen/o _____

56. stomat _____

57. tox _____

58. eructat _____

59. verm/i _____

60. halit _____

61. hemorrh _____

62. alimentat _____

63. masticat _____

64. paralyt _____

65. pil/o _____

66. nid _____

67. volvul _____

68. odont _____

## SUFFIXES

*Give the definitions of the following suffixes.*

1. -ac _____
2. -al _____
3. -algia _____
4. -ary _____
5. -ase _____
6. -cele _____
7. -oid _____
8. -sis _____
9. -ectomy _____
10. -emesis _____
11. -form _____
12. -genesis _____
13. -ic _____
14. -in _____
15. -ion _____
16. -ism _____
17. -ist _____
18. -itis _____
19. -ive _____
20. -logy _____
21. -lysis _____
22. -megaly _____
23. -oma _____
24. -orexia _____
25. -osis _____
26. -rrhea _____
27. -pepsia _____
28. -us _____
29. -phagia _____
30. -scope _____
31. -scopy _____
32. -stalsis _____
33. -stomy _____
34. -tomy _____
35. -y _____
36. -rrhaphy _____

## Identifying Medical Terms

*In the spaces provided, write the medical terms for the following meanings.*

1. _____ Enzyme that breaks down starch

2. _____ Building up of the body substance in the constructive phase of metabolism

3. _____ Lack of appetite

4. _____ Surgical excision of the appendix

5. _____ Inflammation of the appendix

6. _____ Pertaining to or conveying bile

7. _____ Pertaining to the abdomen

8. _____ Difficulty in swallowing

9. _____ Inflammation of the liver

10. _____ Surgical repair of a hernia

11. _____ Pertaining to after meals

12. _____ Enlargement of the spleen

13. _____ Instrument used to view the sigmoid

## Spelling

*In the spaces provided, write the correct spelling of these misspelled terms.*

1. bilery _____

2. colonscopy _____

3. degultition _____

4. gastorentreology _____

5. haltosis _____

6. laxtive _____

7. persitalsis _____

8. salademitis _____

9. peridontal _____

10. verimform _____

## Matching

*Select the appropriate lettered meaning for each of the following words.*

_____ 1. cirrhosis

_____ 2. constipation

_____ 3. diarrhea

_____ 4. gavage

_____ 5. hemorrhoid

_____ 6. hernia

_____ 7. hyperalimentation

_____ 8. lavage

_____ 9. pilonidal cyst

_____ 10. volvulus

a. To wash out a cavity
b. To feed liquid or semiliquid food via a tube
c. Twisting of the bowel on itself
d. Frequent passage of unformed watery stools
e. Chronic degenerative liver disease
f. Infrequent passage of unduly hard and dry feces
g. Closed sac in the crease of the sacrococcygeal region
h. Abnormal protrusion of an organ or a part of an organ through the wall of the body cavity that normally contains it
i. Mass of dilated, tortuous veins in the anorectum
j. Intravenous infusion of a hypertonic solution to sustain life
k. Evacuation of the bowel

## Abbreviations

*Place the correct word, phrase, or abbreviation in the space provided.*

1. before meals _____

2. BM _____

3. BS _____

4. chol _____

5. gallbladder _____

6. hepatitis A virus _____

7. NG _____

8. NPO, npo _____

9. after meals _____

10. total parenteral nutrition _____

## Diagnostic and Laboratory Tests

*Select the best answer to each multiple choice question. Circle the letter of your choice.*

1. X-ray examination of the common bile duct, cystic duct, and hepatic ducts.
   a. cholangiography
   b. cholecystography
   c. cholangiopancreatography
   d. ultrasonography

2. Direct visual examination of the colon via a flexible colonoscope.
   a. cholangiography
   b. ultrasonography
   c. colonofiberoscopy
   d. cholecystography

3. Fluoroscopic examination of the esophagus, stomach, and small intestine.
   a. barium enema
   b. ultrasonography
   c. cholangiography
   d. gastrointestinal series

4. Endoscopic examination of the esophagus, stomach, and small intestine.
   a. cholangiography
   b. gastroduodenoesophagoscopy
   c. esophagogastroduodenoscopy
   d. gastric analysis

5. Test performed to determine the presence of the hepatitis B virus.
   a. occult blood test
   b. stool culture
   c. hepatic antigen
   d. ova and parasites test

# PRACTICAL APPLICATION

## S O A P : Chart Note Analysis

*This exercise will make you aware of information, abbreviations, and medical terminology typically found in a gastroenterology patient's chart.*

### Abbreviations Key

| | | | | |
|---|---|---|---|---|
| Abd | abdomen | | Neuro | neurology |
| ACE | angiotensin converting enzyme (inhibitor) | | NSAIDs | nonsteroidal anti-inflammatory drugs |
| bid | twice a day | | P | pulse |
| BP | blood pressure | | PO | orally, by mouth |
| c/o | complains of | | PPD | pack(s) per day |
| CTA | clear to auscultation | | PPI | proton-pump inhibitor |
| F | Fahrenheit | | PUD | peptic ulcer disease |
| g | gram | | R | respiration |
| *H. pylori* | *Helicobacter pylori* | | SOAP | subjective, objective, assessment, plan |
| Ht | height | | | |
| HTN | hypertension | | T | temperature |
| lb | pound | | Wt | weight |
| mg | milligram | | y/o | year(s) old |
| MS | musculoskeletal | | | |

*Read the following chart note and then answer the questions that follow.*

**PATIENT:** Schmidt, Thomas C.      **DATE:** 06/10/2007
**DOB:** 05/29/72    **AGE:** 35    **SEX:** Male
**INSURANCE:** Physicare Health Insurance

    **Vital Signs:**
       T: 98.8F
       P: 88
       R: 18
       BP: 132/86
       Ht: 6' 2"
       Wt: 226 lb

**Allergies:** Zestril (lisinopril)—angiotensin converting enzyme (ACE inhibitor) that he took for hypertension
**Chief Complaint:** Dull, aching pain and burning sensation in the epigastruim. Pyrosis (heartburn) and sour eructation (belching).

**S**   **Subjective:** 35 y/o white male c/o dull, aching pain in stomach and back. He states that he is experiencing increased episodes of "heartburn and belching" which occur "two to three hours after meals and during the night." He describes a four-month history of "heartburn," which lasts for several days but is relieved by eating. "It stops for a couple of weeks, but it always returns." Patient was diagnosed with HTN six years ago.

He is taking Catapres (clonidine) 0.4 mg per day with apparent good control. Patient is a smoker with a history of 1 PPD for 18 years. Denies use of NSAIDs or regular alcohol consumption but drinks two to four cups of coffee and two colas daily. He denies recent history of back injury.

**O    Objective:**

**General Appearance:** Appears uneasy and tense; in apparent discomfort as indicated by facial expression (grimace)

**Lungs:** CTA

**Heart:** Regular rate and rhythm, no murmurs, gallops, or rubs

**Abd:** Tenderness in the epigastric area, rigidity, bowel sounds in all 4 quadrants, no masses or liver/spleen enlargement

**MS:** Well-developed musculature of upper body

**Neuro:** No recent history of back injury; no irregularities of the spine

**Skin:** Slight flushing of cheeks and redness of the nose, overall suntan of body

**A    Assessment:** Peptic ulcer disease (PUD)

**P    Plan:**

1. Patient is treated for *H. pylori* due to positive results of culture. Treatment regimen includes two antibiotics and a proton-pump inhibitor (PPI). Instruct the patient to take the following medications PO: Biaxin (clarithromycin) 500 mg bid + amoxicillin 1 g bid + Prilosec (omeprazole) 20 mg bid for 10 days. Inform patient that the cure rate ranges from 70% to 90%, not 100 %, because of patients' failure to adhere to regimen. Encourage patient to take the medication as ordered for the total of 10 days.

2. Inform patient of the three complications of an ulcer—bleeding, obstruction, and perforation. **Bleeding** occurs when the acid or ulcer breaks a blood vessel. **Obstruction** occurs when the ulcer blocks the path of food trying to leave the stomach. A **perforation** occurs when ulcer burrows through stomach lining. Instruct patient to immediately report any signs of bleeding, such as black, tarry stools or the passing of or vomiting of blood to his physician Also to report sudden weight loss or severe pain in the epigastric area of the abdomen.

3. Stress importance of smoking cessation and consequences if the patient continues. Provide patient with information to contact the local smoking cessation program through American Heart Association.

4. Educate the patient that ulcers are the end result of an imbalance between digestive enzymes, acid, and pepsin in the stomach and the mucosal lining of the duodenum caused by several factors: a bacterial infection by *H. pylori;* overuse of NSAIDs, overuse of caffeine or alcohol; smoking; or the formation of **gastrinomas,** tumors of the acid-producing cells of the stomach that increase acid output.

5. Discuss with the patient that ulcers are *not* caused by spicy foods or stress but are aggravated by them. Also, milk cannot cure an ulcer. Milk provides brief relief of ulcer pain by coating the stomach lining. Milk can also stimulate the stomach to produce more acid and digestive juices, which may aggravate ulcers.

**FYI:** Upper esophagogastroduodenal endoscopy is considered the reference method of diagnosis. Endoscopy obtains biopsy specimens of the stomach and duodenum. The diagnosis of *H. pylori* can be made by several methods: The biopsy urease test is a colorimetric test based on the ability of *H. pylori* to produce urease; it provides rapid testing at the time of biopsy. Histologic identification of organisms is considered the gold standard of diagnostic tests. Culture of biopsy specimens for *H. pylori,* which requires an experienced laboratory, is necessary when antimicrobial susceptibility testing is desired.

## Chart Note Questions
*Place the correct answer in the space provided.*

1. Signs and symptoms of a peptic ulcer include a dull, aching pain and a burning sensation in the _____ area of the abdomen.

2. The diagnosis of a peptic ulcer caused by *H. plyori* can be determined by a biopsy urease test, histologic identification of organisms, or a _____ of biopsy specimens.

3. Three complications of an ulcer are _____.

4. A triple regimen of medication contains a proton-pump inhibitor and two _____.

5. Prevention activities include avoidance of alcohol, caffeine, _____, and overuse of NSAIDS.

6. What does the abbreviation HTN mean? _____

7. Pyrosis is _____.

8. If milk coats the stomach lining, why is it not beneficial for treatment of ulcers? _____

9. Tumors of the acid-producing cells of the stomach that increase acid output are known as _____.

10. Why is the cure rate for *H. pylori* not 100%? _____

# MULTIMEDIA PREVIEW

*Additional interactive resources and activities for this chapter can be found on the Companion Website. For videos, audio glossary, and review, access the accompanying CD-ROM in this book.*

 **CD-ROM HIGHLIGHTS**

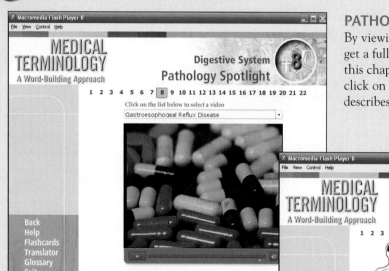

## PATHOLOGY SPOTLIGHT—GERD

By viewing concepts in moving, living color, you'll get a fuller picture of the pathologies presented in this chapter. Earlier we discussed GERD. Now click on this feature to watch a video that describes this condition in more detail.

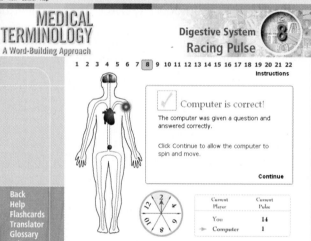

## RACING PULSE

Don't miss a beat! Your challenge is to answer quiz show questions to top the computer. With each correct answer you earn a spin of the dial which tells you how many pulses to advance. First around the body is the winner.

 **WEBSITE HIGHLIGHTS—www.prenhall.com/rice**

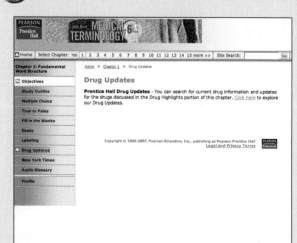

## DRUG UPDATES

Click here and take advantage of the free-access on-line study guide that accompanies your textbook. You'll find a feature that allows you to search for current information on the drugs discussed in this chapter. By clicking on this URL you'll also access links to download mp3 audio reviews, current news articles, review questions, and an audio glossary.

# Cardiovascular System

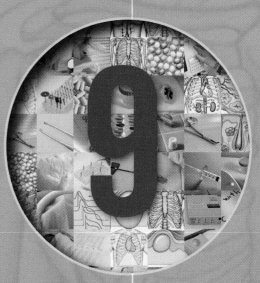

**9**

## ■ OBJECTIVES

*On completion of this chapter, you will be able to:*

- Describe the cardiovascular system.
- Describe and state the functions of arteries, veins, and capillaries.
- Describe cardiovascular differences of the child and the older adult.
- Identify the commonly used pulse checkpoints of the body.
- Describe blood pressure.
- Analyze, build, spell, and pronounce medical words.
- Comprehend the drugs highlighted in this chapter.
- Describe diagnostic and laboratory tests related to the cardiovascular system.
- Identify and define selected abbreviations.
- Describe each of the conditions presented in the Pathology Spotlights.
- Review the Pathology Checkpoint.
- Complete the Study and Review section and the Chart Note Analysis.

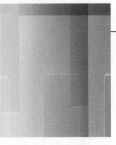

# Anatomy and Physiology Overview

The cardiovascular system circulates blood to all parts of the body by the action of the heart. This process provides the body's cells oxygen and nutritive elements and removes waste materials and carbon dioxide. The heart, a muscular pump, is the central organ of the system, which also includes arteries, veins, and capillaries. The various organs and components of the cardiovascular system are described in this chapter as well as some of their functions.

## Cardiovascular System

| Organ/Structure | Primary Functions |
|---|---|
| Heart | Hollow muscular pump that circulates blood throughout the cardiovascular system |
| Arteries | Branching system of vessels that transports blood from the right and left ventricles of the heart to all body parts |
| Veins | Vessels that transport blood from peripheral tissues to the heart |
| Capillaries | Microscopic blood vessels that connect arterioles with venules; facilitate passage of life-sustaining fluids containing oxygen and nutrients to cell bodies and the removal of accumulated waste and carbon dioxide |

# HEART

The **heart** is a four-chambered, hollow muscular pump that circulates blood throughout the cardiovascular system. The heart is the center of the cardiovascular system from which the various blood vessels originate and later return. It is slightly larger than a man's fist and weighs approximately 300 g in the average adult male. It lies slightly to the left of the midline of the body and is shaped like an inverted cone with its apex downward. The heart has three layers or linings (see Figure 9–1 ▼).

**Endocardium.** The inner lining of the heart.

**Myocardium.** The muscular middle layer of the heart.

**Pericardium.** The outer membranous sac surrounding the heart.

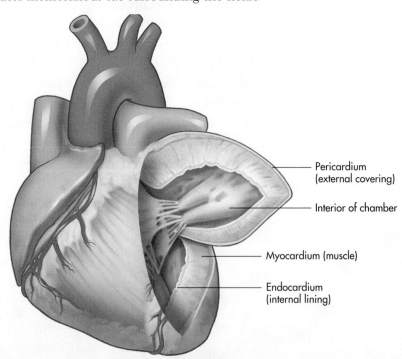

Pericardium (external covering)

Interior of chamber

Myocardium (muscle)

Endocardium (internal lining)

▶ FIGURE 9–1    Tissues of the heart.

## Chambers of the Heart

The human heart acts as a double pump and is divided into the right and left heart by a partition called the **septum.** Each side contains an upper and lower chamber. The **atria,** or upper chambers, are separated by the interatrial septum. The **ventricles,** or lower chambers, are separated by the interventricular septum. The atria receive blood from the various parts of the body whereas the ventricles pump blood to body parts. A description of the heart's four chambers and some of their functions is given in the following paragraphs.

### Right Atrium

The right upper portion of the heart is called the **right atrium** (RA). It is a thin-walled space that receives blood from all body parts except the lungs. Two large veins bring the blood into the right atrium and are known as the superior and inferior vena cavae.

### Right Ventricle

The right lower portion of the heart is called the **right ventricle** (RV). It receives blood from the right atrium through the atrioventricular valve and pumps it through a semilunar valve to the lungs.

### Left Atrium

The left upper portion of the heart is called the **left atrium** (LA). It receives blood rich in oxygen as it returns from the lungs via the left and right pulmonary veins.

### Left Ventricle

The left lower portion of the heart is called the **left ventricle** (LV). It receives blood from the left atrium through an atrioventricular (AV) valve and pumps it through a semilunar valve to a large artery known as the *aorta* and from there to all parts of the body except the lungs.

## Heart Valves

The **valves** of the heart are located at the entrance and exit of each ventricle. See Figure 9–2 ▶. The functions of each of the four heart valves are described in this section.

### Tricuspid Valve

The **tricuspid** or **right atrioventricular valve** guards the opening between the right atrium and the right ventricle. The tricuspid valve allows the flow of blood into the ventricle and prevents its return to the right atrium.

### Pulmonary Semilunar Valve

The exit point for blood leaving the right ventricle is called the **pulmonary semilunar valve.** Located between the right ventricle and the pulmonary artery, it allows blood to flow from the right ventricle through the pulmonary artery to the lungs.

### Bicuspid or Mitral Valve

The left atrioventricular valve between the left atrium and ventricle is called the **bicuspid** or **mitral valve** (MV). It allows blood to flow to the left ventricle and closes to prevent its return to the left atrium.

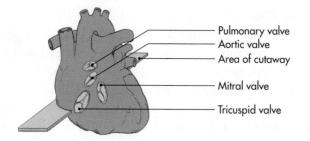

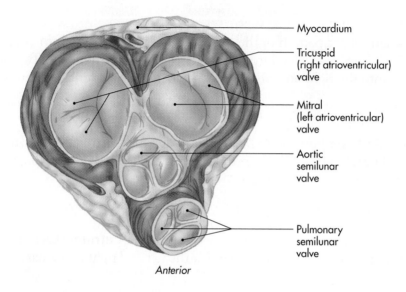

▶ **FIGURE 9–2** Valves of the heart.

### Aortic Semilunar Valve

Blood exits from the left ventricle through the **aortic semilunar valve.** Located between the left ventricle and the aorta, it allows blood to flow into the aorta and prevents its return to the ventricle.

### Vascular System of the Heart

Due to the membranous lining of the heart (endocardium) and the thickness of the myocardium, it is essential that the heart have its own vascular system. The coronary arteries supply the heart with blood, and the cardiac veins, draining into the coronary sinus, collect the blood and return it to the right atrium (see Figure 9–3 ▶).

## FLOW OF BLOOD

Blood flows through the heart, to the lungs, back to the heart, and on to the various body parts as indicated in Figure 9–4 ▶.

Blood from the superior and inferior vena cavae enters the right atrium and subsequently passes through the tricuspid valve and into the right ventricle, which pumps it through the pulmonary semilunar valve into the left and right pulmonary arteries, which carry it to the lungs. In the lungs, the blood gives up wastes and takes on oxygen as it passes through capillaries into veins. Blood leaves the lungs through the left and right pulmonary veins, which carry it to the heart's left atrium. The oxygenated blood then passes through the bicuspid or mitral valve into the left ventricle, which pumps it out through the aortic

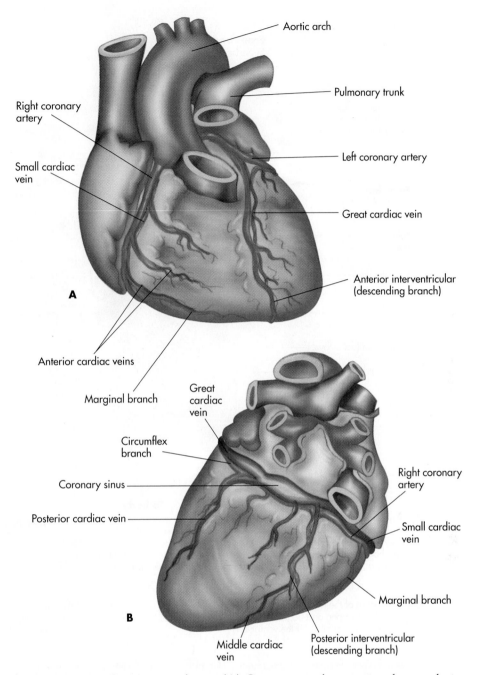

▶ **FIGURE 9–3** Coronary circulation. (A) Coronary vessels portraying the complexity and extent of the coronary circulation. (B) Coronary vessels that supply the anterior surface of the heart.

valve and into the **aorta.** This large artery supplies a branching system of smaller arteries that connect to tiny capillaries throughout the body.

**Capillaries** are microscopic blood vessels with thin walls that allow the passage of oxygen and nutrients to the body and let the blood pick up waste and carbon dioxide. Veins lead away from the capillaries as tiny vessels and increase in size until they join the superior and inferior vena cavae as they return to the heart.

## Heartbeat

The autonomic nervous system controls the **heartbeat**. It normally is generated by specialized neuromuscular tissue of the heart that is capable of causing cardiac muscle to contract rhythmically. This tissue of the heart comprises the

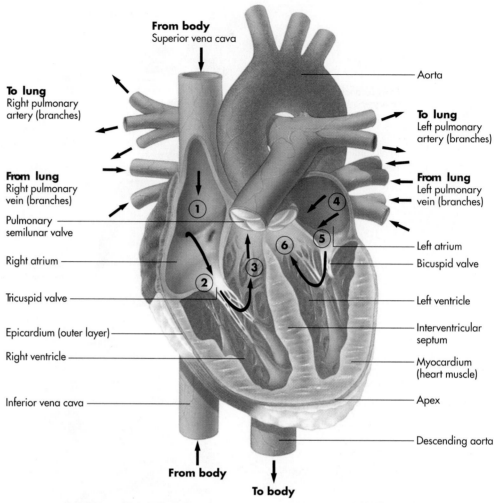

**From body**
Superior vena cava

Aorta

**To lung**
Right pulmonary
artery (branches)

**To lung**
Left pulmonary
artery (branches)

**From lung**
Right pulmonary
vein (branches)

**From lung**
Left pulmonary
vein (branches)

Pulmonary
semilunar valve

Left atrium

Right atrium

Bicuspid valve

Tricuspid valve

Left ventricle

Epicardium (outer layer)

Interventricular
septum

Right ventricle

Myocardium
(heart muscle)

Inferior vena cava

Apex

Descending aorta

**From body**

**To body**

### RIGHT HEART PUMP

1. Deoxygenated blood returns from the upper and lower body to fill the right atrium of the heart creating a pressure against the tricuspid valve.

2. This pressure of the returning blood forces the tricuspid valve open and begins filling the ventricle. The final filling of the ventricle is achieved by the contracting of the right atrium.

3. The right ventricle contracts increasing the internal pressure. This pressure closes the tricuspid valve and forces open the pulmonary semilunar valve thus sending blood toward the lung via the pulmonary artery. This blood will become oxygenated as it travels through the capillary beds of the lung and then return to the left side of the heart.

### LEFT HEART PUMP

4. Oxygenated blood returns from the lung via the pulmonary vein and fills the left atrium creating a pressure against the bicuspid valve.

5. This pressure of returning blood forces the bicuspid valve open and begins filling the left ventricle. The final filling of the left ventricle is achieved by the contracting of the left atrium.

6. The left ventricle contracts increasing internal pressure. This pressure closes the bicuspid valve and forces open the aortic valve causing oxygenated blood to flow through the aorta to deliver oxygen throughout the body.

▶ **FIGURE 9–4**   The functioning of the heart valves and blood flow.

**sinoatrial node,** the **atrioventricular node,** and the **atrioventricular bundle** (see Figure 9–5 ▶).

### Sinoatrial Node (SA Node)

Often called the **pacemaker of the heart,** the **SA node** is located in the upper wall of the right atrium, just below the opening of the superior vena cava. It consists of a dense

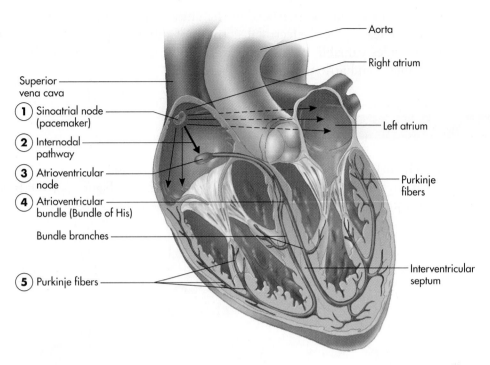

Superior
vena cava

(1) Sinoatrial node
(pacemaker)

(2) Internodal
pathway

(3) Atrioventricular
node

(4) Atrioventricular
bundle (Bundle of His)

Bundle branches

(5) Purkinje fibers

Aorta

Right atrium

Left atrium

Purkinje
fibers

Interventricular
septum

1. The sinoatrial (SA) node fires a stimulus across the walls of both
   left and right atria causing them to contract.

2. The stimulus arrives at the atrioventricular (AV) node.

3. The stimulus is directed to follow the AV bundle (Bundle of His).

4. The stimulus now travels through the apex of the heart through
   the bundle branches.

5. The Purkinje fibers distribute the stimulus across both ventricles
   causing ventricular contraction.

▶ **FIGURE 9–5**   Conduction system of the heart.

network of **Purkinje fibers** *(atypical muscle fibers)* considered to be the source of impulses initiating the heartbeat. Electrical impulses discharged by the SA node are distributed to the right and left atria and cause them to contract.

### Atrioventricular Node (AV Node)

Located beneath the endocardium of the right atrium, the **AV node** transmits electrical impulses to the **bundle of His** *(atrioventricular bundle)*.

### Atrioventricular Bundle (Bundle of His)

The **bundle of His** forms a part of the conducting system of the heart. It extends from the AV node into the intraventricular septum, where it divides into two branches within the two ventricles. The **Purkinje system** includes the bundle of His and the peripheral fibers. These fibers end in the ventricular muscles, where the excitation of muscle is initiated, causing contraction. The average heartbeat *(pulse)* is between 60 and 100 beats per minute for the average adult. The rate of heartbeat can be affected by emotions, smoking, disease, body size, age, stress, the environment, and many other factors.

### Electrocardiogram

An **electrocardiogram** (ECG, EKG) records the heart's electrical activity. A standard electrocardiogram consists of 12 different leads. With electrodes placed on the patient's arms, legs, and six positions on the chest, a 12-lead ECG can be recorded. Six unipolar chest leads record electrical activity of different parts of the heart. An ECG (EKG) provides valuable information in diagnosing cardiac abnormalities, such as myocardial damage and arrhythmias (see Figure 9–6 ▼).

## ARTERIES

The **arteries** constitute a branching system of vessels that transports blood from the right and left ventricles of the heart to all body parts (see Figure 9–7 ▶). In a normal state, arteries are elastic tubes that recoil and carry blood in pulsating waves. All arteries have a pulse,

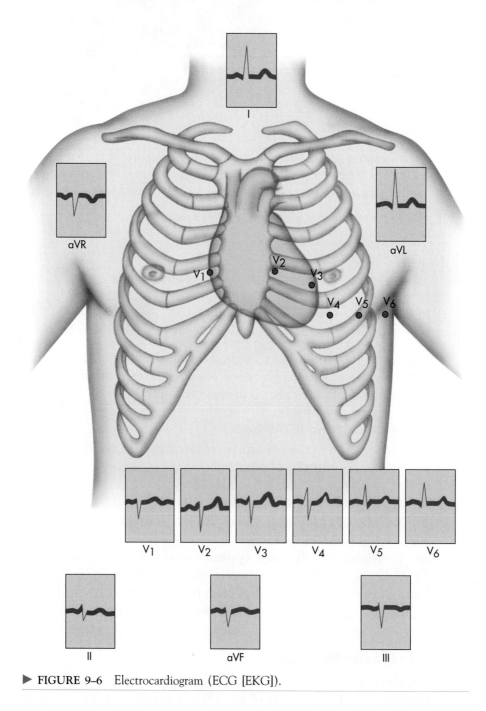

▶ **FIGURE 9–6**   Electrocardiogram (ECG [EKG]).

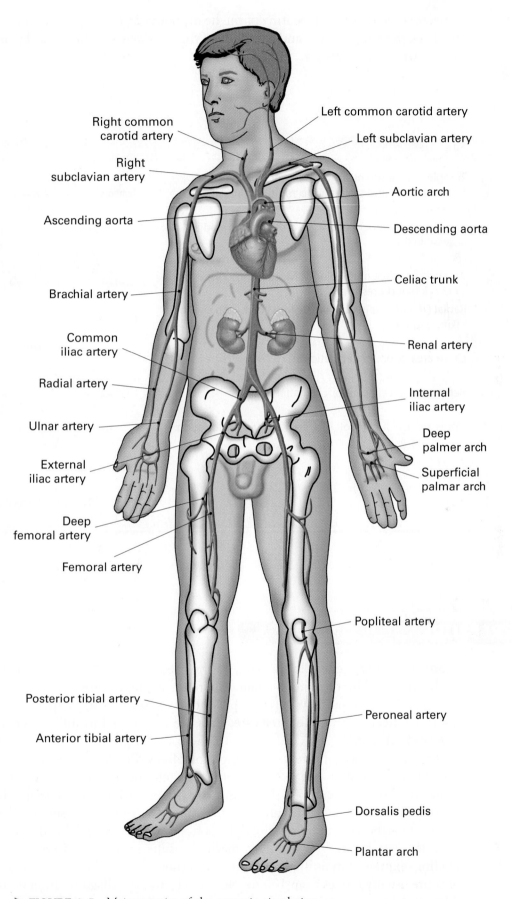

▶ **FIGURE 9–7** Major arteries of the systemic circulation.

reflecting the rhythmical beating of the heart; however, certain points are commonly used to check the rate, rhythm, and condition of the arterial wall. These checkpoints follow and are shown in Figure 9–8 ▼.

| Checkpoint | Site/Use |
| --- | --- |
| Temporal | Temple area of the head. Used to control bleeding from the head and scalp and to monitor circulation. |
| Carotid | Neck. In an emergency (*cardiac arrest*), most readily accessible site. |
| Brachial | Antecubital space of the elbow. Most common site used to check blood pressure. |
| Radial | Radial (*thumb side*) of the wrist. Most common site for taking a pulse. |
| Femoral | Groin area. Monitor circulation. |
| Popliteal | Behind the knee. Monitor circulation. |
| Dorsalis pedis | Upper surface of the foot. Monitor lower limb circulation. |

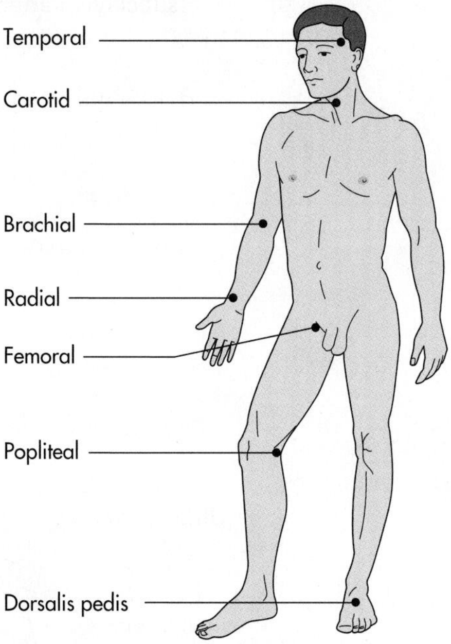

▶ **FIGURE 9–8**   Primary pulse points of the body.

# BLOOD PRESSURE

**Blood pressure,** generally speaking, is the pressure exerted by the blood on the walls of the vessels. The term most commonly refers to the pressure exerted in large arteries at the peak of the pulse wave. This pressure is measured with a **sphygmomanometer** used in concert with a **stethoscope.** Pressure is reported in millimeters of mercury as observed on a graduated column. With the use of a pressure cuff, circulation is interrupted in the brachial artery just above the elbow. Pressure from the cuff is shown on the graduated column of the sphygmomanometer, and as the pressure is released, blood again flows past the cuff. At this point, the person, using a stethoscope, hears a heartbeat and records the systolic pressure. Continued release of pressure results in a change in the heartbeat sound from loud to soft, at which point the diastolic pressure is recorded (see Figure 9–9 ▶). This method results in a ratio of systolic over diastolic readings expressed in millimeters of mercury (mm Hg). In the average adult, the systolic pressure usually ranges from 100 to 140 mm Hg and the diastolic from 60 to 90 mm Hg. A typical blood pressure showing systolic over diastolic readings might be expressed as 120/80.

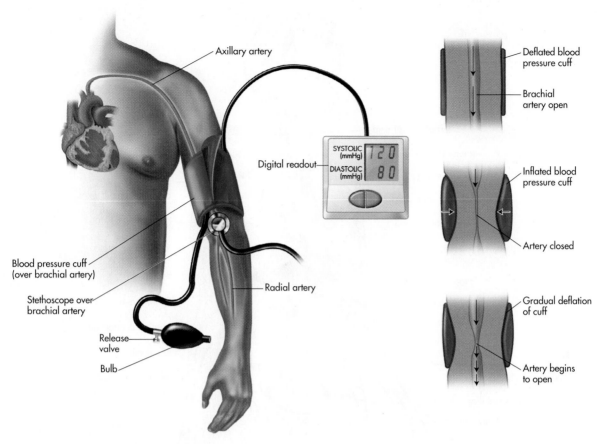

Axillary artery

Digital readout

SYSTOLIC (mmHg)  120
DIASTOLIC (mmHg)  80

Radial artery

Blood pressure cuff (over brachial artery)

Stethoscope over brachial artery

Release valve

Bulb

Deflated blood pressure cuff

Brachial artery open

Inflated blood pressure cuff

Artery closed

Gradual deflation of cuff

Artery begins to open

▶ FIGURE 9–9  Blood pressure measurement.

### Pulse Pressure

The **pulse pressure** is the difference between the systolic and diastolic readings. This reading indicates the tone of the arterial walls. The normal pulse pressure is found when the systolic pressure is about 40 points higher than the diastolic reading. For example, if the blood pressure is 120/80, the pulse pressure would be 40. A pulse pressure over 50 points or under 30 points is considered abnormal.

## VEINS

The vessels that transport blood from peripheral tissues and from the lungs to the heart are the **veins** (see Figure 9–10 ▶). In a normal state, veins have thin walls and valves that prevent the backflow of blood. Veins are the vessels used when blood is removed for analysis. The process of removing blood from a vein is called **venipuncture.**

## CAPILLARIES

The **capillaries** are microscopic blood vessels with single-celled walls that connect **arterioles** (*small arteries*) with **venules** (*small veins*). Blood passing through capillaries gives up the oxygen and nutrients carried to this point by the arteries and picks up waste and carbon dioxide as it enters veins. The extremely thin walls of capillaries facilitate passage of life-sustaining fluids containing oxygen and nutrients to cell bodies and the removal of accumulated waste and carbon dioxide.

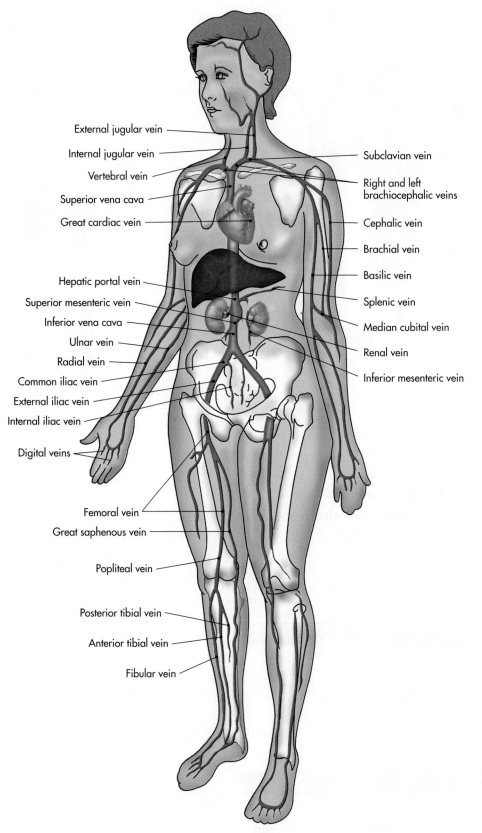

External jugular vein

Internal jugular vein

Vertebral vein

Superior vena cava

Great cardiac vein

Hepatic portal vein

Superior mesenteric vein

Inferior vena cava

Ulnar vein

Radial vein

Common iliac vein

External iliac vein

Internal iliac vein

Digital veins

Femoral vein

Great saphenous vein

Popliteal vein

Posterior tibial vein

Anterior tibial vein

Fibular vein

Subclavian vein

Right and left
brachiocephalic veins

Cephalic vein

Brachial vein

Basilic vein

Splenic vein

Median cubital vein

Renal vein

Inferior mesenteric vein

▶ **FIGURE 9–10**   Major veins of the systemic circulation.

# LIFE SPAN CONSIDERATIONS

## ■ THE CHILD

The development of the fetal heart is usually completed during the first 2 months of intrauterine life. It is completely formed and functioning by 10 weeks. At 16 weeks, fetal heart tones can be heard with a **fetoscope.** Oxygenated blood is transported by the umbilical vein from the placenta to the fetus. Fetal circulation is terminated at birth when the umbilical cord is clamped. The newborn's circulation begins to function shortly after birth and if proper adaptations do not take place, congenital heart disease can occur. Most congenital heart defects develop before the 10th week of pregnancy. Pediatric cardiologists have recognized more than 50 congenital heart defects. If the left side of the heart is not completely separated from the right side, various septal defects develop. If the four chambers of the heart do not occur normally, complex anomalies form, such as tetralogy of Fallot (TOF), a congenital heart condition involving four defects: pulmonary stenosis, ventricular septal defect (VSD), dextroposition of the aorta, and hypertrophy of the right ventricle.

The **pulse** (P), **blood pressure** (BP), and **respiration** (R) vary according to the child's age. A newborn's pulse rate is irregular and rapid, varying from 120 to 140 beats/minute. Blood pressure is low and can vary with the size of the cuff used. The average blood pressure at birth is 80/46. The respirations are approximately 35 to 50 per minute.

## ■ THE OLDER ADULT

Current evidence indicates that cardiac changes that were once attributed to the aging process can be minimized by modifying lifestyle and personal habits, such as following a low-sodium, low-fat diet, not smoking, drinking in moderation, managing stress, and exercising regularly. Studies have shown that the normal aging heart is able to provide an adequate cardiac output. In some older adults, however, the heart must work harder to pump blood because of hardening of the arteries (**arteriosclerosis**) and a buildup of fatty plaques (cholesterol deposits and triglycerides) in the arterial walls (**atherosclerosis**). Arteries can gradually become stiff and lose their elastic recoil. The aorta and arteries supplying the heart and brain are generally affected first. Arteriosclerotic heart disease (AHD) occurs when the arterial vessels are marked by thickening, hardening, and loss of elasticity in the arterial walls. Reduced blood flow, elevated blood lipids, and defective endothelial repair that can be seen in aging accelerate the course of cardiovascular disease.

**Heart failure** (HF) is one of the most common types of cardiovascular disease seen in the older adult. It can be caused by coronary artery disease, diabetes, chronic hypertension, myocardial infarction, infection, and valvular disorders such as mitral stenosis.

Heart failure can involve the heart's left side, right side, or both sides. It usually affects the left side first. Left-sided or left ventricular (LV) heart failure involves the heart's left ventricle. If the left ventricle loses its ability to contract normally (called **systolic failure**), the heart cannot pump with enough force to push sufficent blood into circulation. If the ventricle loses its ability to relax normally (**diastolic failure**) because the muscle has become stiff, the heart can't properly fill with blood during the resting period between each beat. This is an important distinction because the drug treatments for each type of failure are different.

Left-sided failure leads to a buildup of fluid in the lungs, or **pulmonary edema,** which causes **dyspnea** and shortness of breath. Left-sided heart failure is commonly called **congestive heart failure** (CHF).

Right-sided or right ventricular (RV) heart failure usually occurs as a result of left-sided failure. When the left ventricle fails, increased fluid pressure is, in effect, transferred back through the lungs, ultimately damaging the heart's right side. Right-sided failure is a result of a buildup of blood flowing into the right side of the heart, which causes edema of the ankles, distention of the neck veins, and enlargement of the spleen and/or liver. See Figure 9–11 ▼ for some signs and symptoms of a patient with heart failure and Figure 9–12 ▶ for multisystem effects of heart failure.

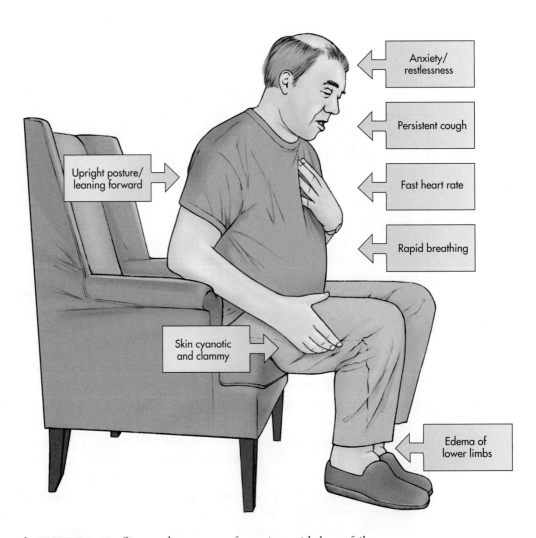

▶ **FIGURE 9–11** Signs and symptoms of a patient with heart failure.

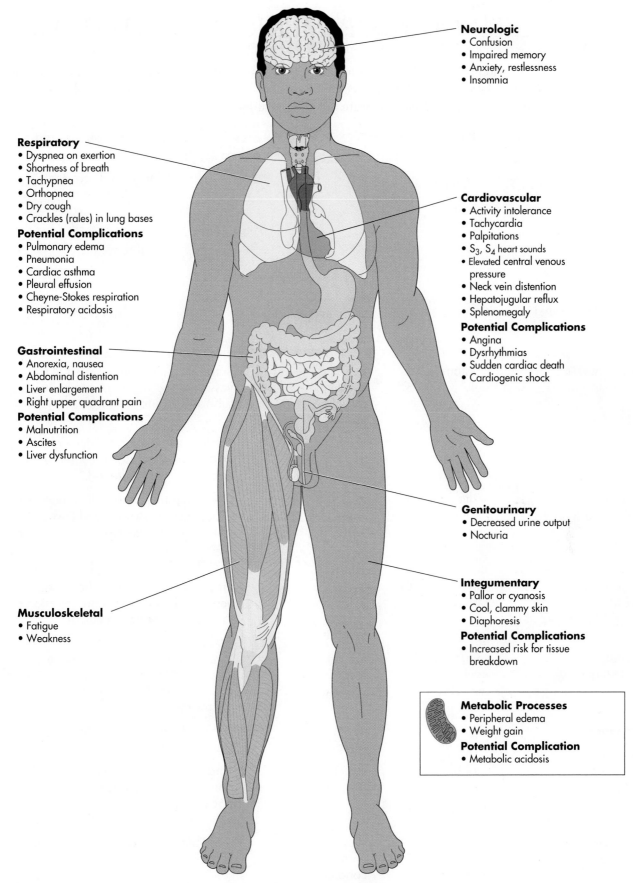

**Neurologic**
• Confusion
• Impaired memory
• Anxiety, restlessness
• Insomnia

**Respiratory**
• Dyspnea on exertion
• Shortness of breath
• Tachypnea
• Orthopnea
• Dry cough
• Crackles (rales) in lung bases
**Potential Complications**
• Pulmonary edema
• Pneumonia
• Cardiac asthma
• Pleural effusion
• Cheyne-Stokes respiration
• Respiratory acidosis

**Cardiovascular**
• Activity intolerance
• Tachycardia
• Palpitations
• $S_3$, $S_4$ heart sounds
• Elevated central venous
  pressure
• Neck vein distention
• Hepatojugular reflux
• Splenomegaly
**Potential Complications**
• Angina
• Dysrhythmias
• Sudden cardiac death
• Cardiogenic shock

**Gastrointestinal**
• Anorexia, nausea
• Abdominal distention
• Liver enlargement
• Right upper quadrant pain
**Potential Complications**
• Malnutrition
• Ascites
• Liver dysfunction

**Genitourinary**
• Decreased urine output
• Nocturia

**Integumentary**
• Pallor or cyanosis
• Cool, clammy skin
• Diaphoresis
**Potential Complications**
• Increased risk for tissue
  breakdown

**Musculoskeletal**
• Fatigue
• Weakness

**Metabolic Processes**
• Peripheral edema
• Weight gain
**Potential Complication**
• Metabolic acidosis

▶ **FIGURE 9–12**  Multisystem effects of heart failure.

# BUILDING YOUR MEDICAL VOCABULARY

This section provides the foundation for learning medical terminology. Review the following alphabetized word list. Note how common prefixes and suffixes are repeatedly applied to word roots and combining forms to create different meanings.

| | |
|---|---|
| **P** | Prefix |
| **R** | Root |
| **CF** | Combining form |
| **S** | Suffix |

| | |
|---|---|
| Pink words | Terms not built from word parts. |
| ∗ | Indicates words covered in the Pathology Spotlights section. |
|  | Check the CD-ROM for more information. |

| MEDICAL WORD | WORD PARTS (WHEN APPLICABLE) | | | DEFINITION |
|---|---|---|---|---|
| | **Part** | **Type** | **Meaning** | |
| **anastomosis** (ă-năs″ tō-mō′sĭs) | anastom -osis | R S | opening condition (usually abnormal) | Surgical connection between blood vessels or the joining of one hollow or tubular organ to another |
| **aneurysm** (ăn′ ū-rĭzm) | | | | Sac formed by a local widening of the wall of an artery usually caused by injury or disease. See Figure 9–13 ▶. |
| **angina pectoris** (ăn′ jĭ-nă pĕk′tŏr″ĭs) | angin (a) pector -is | R R S | to choke chest pertaining to | Chest pain that occurs when diseased blood vessels restrict blood flow to the heart. It is often referred to as angina. ∗ See Pathology Spotlight: Coronary Heart Disease and Heart Attack on pages 267, 270. |
| **angiocardiography (ACG)** (ăn″ jĭ-ō-kăr″ dĭ-ŏg′ ră-fē) | angi/o cardi/o -graphy | CF CF S | vessel heart recording | Process of recording the heart and vessels after an intravenous injection of a radiopaque contrast medium |
| **angiogram** (ăn′jē-ō-grăm) | angi/o -gram | CF S | vessel record | X-ray record of the size, shape, and location of the heart and its blood vessels after the introduction of an radiopaque contrast medium. |
| **angioma** (ăn″ jĭ-ō′ mă) | ang/i -oma | CF S | vessel tumor | Tumor of a blood vessel. See Figure 9–14 ▶. |
| **angioplasty** (ăn′ jĭ-ō-plăs″ tē) | angi/o -plasty | CF S | vessel surgical repair | Surgical repair of a blood vessel(s) or a nonsurgical technique for treating diseased arteries by temporarily inflating a tiny balloon inside an artery |
| **angiostenosis** (ăn″ jĭ-ō-stě-n ō′ sĭs) | angi/o sten -osis | CF R S | vessel narrowing condition (usually abnormal) | Condition of the narrowing of a blood vessel |

| MEDICAL WORD | WORD PARTS (WHEN APPLICABLE) | | | DEFINITION |
|---|---|---|---|---|
| | **Part** | **Type** | **Meaning** | |
| **arrhythmia**<br>(ă-rĭth′ mĭ-ă) | a-<br>rrhythm<br>-ia | P<br>R<br>S | lack of<br>rhythm<br>condition | Condition in which there is a lack of rhythm of the heartbeat; also called *dysrhythmia* |
| **arterial**<br>(ăr-tē′ rĭ-ăl) | arter/i<br>-al | CF<br>S | artery<br>pertaining to | Pertaining to an artery |
| **arteriosclerosis**<br>(ăr-tē″ rĭ-ō-sklĕ-rō′ sĭs) | arteri/o<br>scler<br>-osis | CF<br>R<br>S | artery<br>hardening<br>condition (usually abnormal) | Condition of hardening of arteries |
| **arteritis**<br>(ăr″ tĕ-rĭ′ tĭs) | arter<br>-itis | R<br>S | artery<br>inflammation | Inflammation of an artery. See Figure 9–15 ▶. |
| **artificial pacemaker**<br>(ăr″ tĭ-fĭsh′ al pās′ māk-ĕr) | | | | Electronic device that stimulates impulse initiation within the heart. It is a small battery-operated device that helps the heart beat in a regular rhythm. Some are permanent (internal) and some are temporary (external). They can replace a defective natural pacemaker or blocked pathway. See Figure 9–16 ▶. |
| **atheroma**<br>(ăth″ ĕr-ō mă) | ather<br><br><br>-oma | R<br><br><br>S | fatty substance, porridge<br>tumor | Tumor of an artery containing a fatty substance |

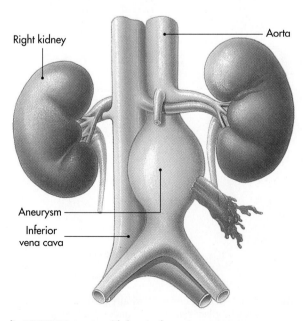

▶ **FIGURE 9–13**   Abdominal aortic aneurysm.

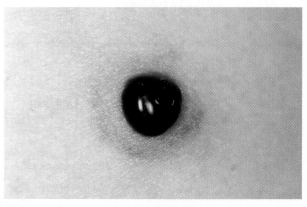

▶ **FIGURE 9–14**   Infarction angioma. (Courtesy of Jason L. Smith, MD)

| MEDICAL WORD | WORD PARTS (WHEN APPLICABLE) | | | DEFINITION |
|---|---|---|---|---|
| | **Part** | **Type** | **Meaning** | |
| **atherosclerosis** (ăth″ ĕr-ō-sklĕ-rō′ sĭs) | ather/o | CF | fatty substance, porridge | Condition of the arteries characterized by the buildup of fatty substances (cholesterol deposits and triglycerides) and hardening of the walls. ✷ See Pathology Spotlight: Coronary Heart Disease on page 267 and Figures 9–34 and 9–35. |
| | scler -osis | R S | hardening condition (usually abnormal) | |
| **atrioventricular (AV)** (ăt″ rĭ-ō-vĕn-trĭk′ ū-lăr) | atri/o ventricul -ar | CF R S | atrium ventricle pertaining to | Pertaining to the atrium and the ventricle |
| **auscultation** (ŏs″ kool-tā′ shŭn) | auscultat -ion | R S | listen to process | Method of physical assessment using a stethoscope to listen to sounds within the chest, abdomen, and other parts of the body |
| **automated external defibrillator (AED)** (aw-tōm′ăt-ĕd ēx′tĕr′năl dē-fĭb″rĭ-lā′tor) | | | | Portable automatic device used to restore normal heart rhythm to patients in cardiac arrest. An AED is applied outside the body. It automatically analyzes the patient's heart rhythm and advises the rescuer whether or not a shock is needed to restore a normal heart beat. If the patient's heart resumes beating normally, the heart has been defibrillated. See Figure 9–17 ▶. |

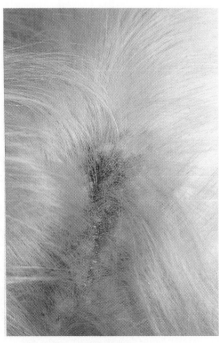

▶ **FIGURE 9–15** Temporal arteritis. (Courtesy of Jason L. Smith, MD)

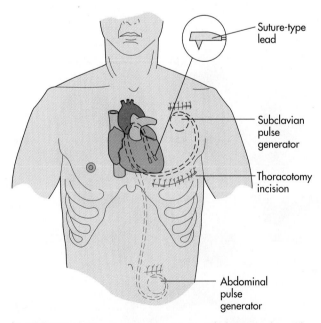

▶ **FIGURE 9–16** A permanent epicardial pacemaker. The pulse generator can be placed in subcutaneous pockets in the subclavian or abdominal regions.

| MEDICAL WORD | WORD PARTS (WHEN APPLICABLE) | | | DEFINITION |
|---|---|---|---|---|
| | Part | Type | Meaning | |
| **bicuspid** (bī-kŭs′ pĭd) | bi- -cuspid | P S | two point | Having two points or cusps; pertaining to the mitral valve |
| **bradycardia** (brăd″ ĭ-kăr′ dĭ-ă) | brady- card -ia | P R S | slow heart condition | Condition of abnormally slow heartbeat that is less than 60 beats per minute |
| **bruit** (brōōt) | | | | Noise; a sound of venous or arterial origin heard on auscultation |
| **cardiac** (kăr′ dĭ-ăk) | card/i -ac | CF S | heart pertaining to | Pertaining to the heart |
| **cardiac arrest** (kăr′ dĭ-ăk ă-rĕst′) | | | | Loss of effective heart function, which results in cessation of functional circulation. Sudden cardiac arrest (SCA) results in sudden death due to cardiac causes rather than to trauma. |
| **cardiologist** (kăr-dē-ŏl′ ō-jĭst) | cardi/o log -ist | CF R S | heart study of one who specializes | Physician who specializes in the study of the heart |
| **cardiology** (kăr″ dĭ-ōl′ ō-jē) | cardi/o -logy | CF S | heart study of | Study of the heart |
| **cardiomegaly** (kăr″ dĭ-ō-mĕg′ ă-lē) | cardi/o -megaly | CF S | heart enlargement, large | Enlargement of the heart |
| **cardiometer** (kăr″ dĭ-ōm′ ĕ-tĕr) | cardi/o -meter | CF S | heart instrument to measure | Instrument used to measure the action of the heart |

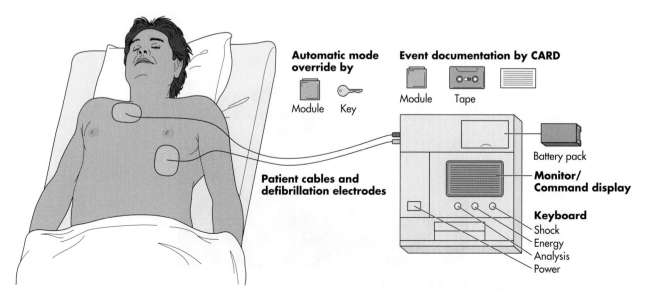

▶ **FIGURE 9–17** Schematic of an automated external defibrillator (AED) attached to a patient.

| MEDICAL WORD | WORD PARTS (WHEN APPLICABLE) | | | DEFINITION |
|---|---|---|---|---|
| | Part | Type | Meaning | |
| **cardiomyopathy (CMP)** (kăr″ dē-ō-mī-ŏp′ ă-thē) | cardi/o my/o -pathy | CF CF S | heart muscle disease | Disease of the heart muscle that leads to generalized deterioration of the muscle and its pumping ability. It can be caused by a viral infection, a parasitic infection, or overconsumption of alcohol. See Figure 9–18 ▼. |
| **cardiopulmonary** (kăr″ dĭ-ō-pŭl′ mō-něr-ē) | cardi/o pulmonar -y | CF R S | heart lung pertaining to | Pertaining to the heart and lungs (H & L) |
| **cardiotonic** (kăr″ dĭ-ō-tŏn′ ĭk) | cardi/o ton -ic | CF R S | heart tone pertaining to | Pertaining to increasing the tone of the heart; a type of medication |
| **cardiovascular (CV)** (kăr″ dĭ-ō-văs′ kū-lar) | cardi/o vascul -ar | CF R S | heart small vessel pertaining to | Pertaining to the heart and small blood vessels |
| **cardioversion** (kăr′ dē-ō-věr″ zhŭn) | cardi/o vers -ion | CF R S | heart turning process | Procedure used to treat different types of disruptions in the normal heart rhythm (cardiac arrhythmias). An electrical shock is delivered to the heart to restore its rhythm to a normal pattern. ✳ See Pathology Spotlight: Dysrythmias on page 269. |
| **cholesterol (chol)** (kō-lěs′ těr-ŏl) | chol/e sterol | CF R | bile solid (fat) | Waxy, fatlike substance in the bloodstream of all animals. It is believed to be dangerous when it builds up on arterial walls and contributes to the risk of coronary heart disease. |
| **circulation** (sər″-kyəlā′ shūn) | circulat -ion | R S | circular process | Process of moving the blood in the veins and arteries throughout the body |

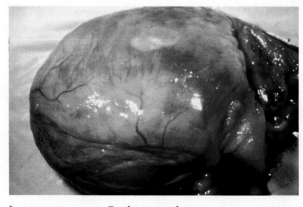

▶ **FIGURE 9–18** Cardiomyopathy.

| MEDICAL WORD | WORD PARTS (WHEN APPLICABLE) | | | DEFINITION |
|---|---|---|---|---|
| | **Part** | **Type** | **Meaning** | |
| **claudication** (klaw-dĭ-kā′ shŭn) | claudicat -ion | R S | to limp process | Process of lameness or limping. It is a dull, cramping pain in the hips, thighs, calves, or buttocks caused by an inadequate supply of oxygen to the muscles, usually due to narrowed arteries. It is one of the major symptoms in peripheral artery disease (PAD). ✳ See Pathology Spotlight: Peripheral Artery Disease on page 269. |
| **constriction** (kən-strĭk′ shŭn) | con- strict -ion | P R S | together, with to draw, to bind process | Process of drawing together, as in the narrowing of a vessel |
| **coronary bypass** (kŏr′ ō-nă-rē bī′ păs) | | | | Surgical procedure performed to increase blood flow to the myocardium by using a section of a saphenous vein or internal mammary artery to bypass the obstructed or occluded coronary artery |
| **coronary heart disease (CHD)** (kŏr′ ō-nă-rē hart dĭ-zēz′) | | | | Also referred to as *coronary artery disease* (CAD), refers to the narrowing of the coronary arteries sufficient to prevent adequate blood supply to the myocardium. ✳ See Pathology Spotlight: Coronary Heart Disease on page 267. |
| **cyanosis** (sī-ă n-ō′ sĭs) | cyan -osis | R S | dark blue condition (usually abnormal) | Abnormal condition of the skin and mucous membranes caused by oxygen deficiency in the blood. The skin, fingernails, and mucous membranes can appear slightly bluish or grayish. |
| **defibrillator** (dē-fĭb″rĭ-lā′tor) | | | | Machine that helps restore a normal heart rhythm by delivering an electric shock; also called a *cardioverter*. See Figure 9–19 ▼. |

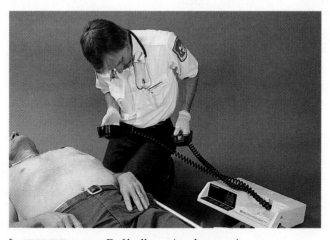

▶ FIGURE 9–19  Defibrillator (cardioverter).

| MEDICAL WORD | WORD PARTS (WHEN APPLICABLE) | | | DEFINITION |
|---|---|---|---|---|
| | **Part** | **Type** | **Meaning** | |
| **diastole**<br>(dī-ăs′ tō-lē) | | | | Relaxation phase of the heart cycle during which the heart muscle relaxes and the heart chambers fill with blood |
| **dysrhythmia**<br>(dĭs-rĭth′ mē-ă) | dys-<br><br>rhythm<br>-ia | P<br><br>R<br>S | difficult, abnormal<br>rhythm<br>condition | Abnormal, difficult, or bad rhythm. Dysrhythmia is also referred to as an *arrhythmia*. ✱ See Pathology Spotlight: Dysrythmias on page 269. |
| **echocardiography (ECHO)**<br>(ĕk″ ō-kăr″ dē-ŏg′ rah-fē) | ech/o<br>cardi/o<br>-graphy | CF<br>CF<br>S | reflected sound<br>heart<br>recording | Noninvasive ultrasound method for evaluating the heart for valvular or structural defects and coronary artery disease |
| **electrocardiograph (ECG, EKG)**<br>(ē-lĕk″ trō-kăr′ dĭ-ō-grăf) | electr/o<br>cardi/o<br>-graph | CF<br>CF<br>S | electricity<br>heart<br>instrument for recording | Device used for recording the electrical impulses of the heart muscle |
| **electrocardio-phonograph**<br>(ē-lĕk″ trō-kăr″ dĭ-ō-fō′ nō-grăf) | electr/o<br>cardi/o<br>phon/o<br>-graph | CF<br>CF<br>CF<br>S | electricity<br>heart<br>sound<br>instrument for recording | Device used to record heart sounds |
| **embolism**<br>(ĕm′ bō-lĭzm) | embol<br>-ism | R<br>S | a throwing in<br>condition | Condition in which there is an obstruction of a blood vessel by foreign substances or a blood clot |
| **endarterectomy**<br>(ĕn″ dăr-tĕr-ĕk′ tō-mē) | end-<br>arter<br>-ectomy | P<br>R<br>S | within<br>artery<br>surgical excision | Surgical excision of the inner portion of an artery |
| **endocarditis**<br>(ĕn″ dō-kăr-dī′ tĭs) | endo-<br>card<br>-itis | P<br>R<br>S | within<br>heart<br>inflammation | Inflammation of the endocardium. See Figure 9–20 ▶. |
| **endocardium**<br>(ĕn″ dō-kăr′ dē-ŭm) | endo-<br>card/i<br>-um | P<br>CF<br>S | within<br>heart<br>tissue | Inner lining of the heart |
| **extracorporeal circulation (ECC)**<br>(ĕks-tră-kor-pōr′ ē-ăl sər″-kyəlā′ shŭn) | extra-<br>corpor/e<br>-al<br>circulat<br>-ion | P<br>CF<br>S<br>R<br>S | outside<br>body<br>pertaining to<br>circular<br>process | Pertaining to the circulation of the blood outside the body via a heart–lung machine or hemodialyzer |
| **fibrillation**<br>(fī″ brĭl-ā′ shŭn) | fibrillat<br>-ion | R<br>S | fibrils (small fibers)<br>process | Quivering or spontaneous contraction of individual muscle fibers, an abnormal bioelectric potential occurring in neuropathies and myopathies |
| **flutter**<br>(flŭt′ ər) | | | | Condition of the heartbeat in which the contractions become extremely rapid. With atrial flutter, the heartbeat is 200 to 400 beats per minute. With ventricular flutter, the heartbeat is 250 beats or more per minute. |

| MEDICAL WORD | WORD PARTS (WHEN APPLICABLE) | | | DEFINITION |
|---|---|---|---|---|
| | Part | Type | Meaning | |
| **heart failure (HF)** | | | | Disorder in which the heart loses its ability to pump blood efficiently. Left-sided heart failure is commonly called *congestive heart failure* (CHF). See Figure 9–11 on page 244. |
| **heart–lung transplant** | | | | Surgical process of transferring the heart and lungs from a donor to a patient |
| **heart transplant** | | | | Surgical process of transferring the heart from a donor to a patient |

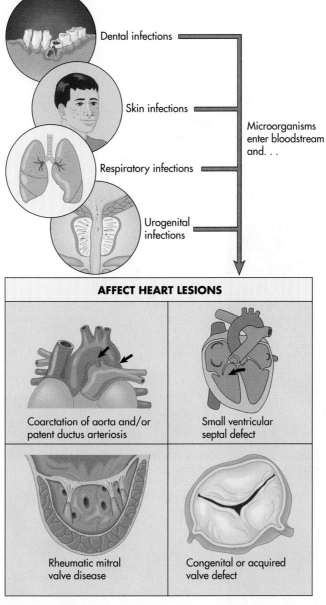

▶ FIGURE 9–20   How microorganisms enter bloodstream and affect heart lesions, which could result in bacterial endocarditis.

| MEDICAL WORD | WORD PARTS (WHEN APPLICABLE) | | | DEFINITION |
|---|---|---|---|---|
| | **Part** | **Type** | **Meaning** | |
| **hemangioma**<br>(hē-măn″ jĭ-ō′ mă) | hem<br>ang/i<br>-oma | R<br>CF<br>S | blood<br>vessel<br>tumor | Benign tumor of a blood vessel. See Figures 9–21 ▼ and 9–22 ▼. |
| **hemodynamic**<br>(hē″ mō-dī-năm′ ĭk) | hem/o<br>dynam<br>-ic | CF<br>R<br>S | blood<br>power<br>pertaining to | Pertaining to the study of the heart's ability to function as a pump; the movement of the blood and its pressure |
| **hyperlipidemia**<br>(hī″pĕr-lĭp′ ĭd- ē′ mĭ-ă) | hyper-<br>lipid<br>-emia | P<br>R<br>S | excessive<br>fat<br>blood condition | Excessive amount of fatty substances (lipids) in the blood. Lipids include sterols (cholesterol and cholesterol esters), free fatty acids (FFA), triglycerides (glycerol esters of FFA), and phospholipids (phosphoric acid esters of lipid substances). |
| **hypertension (HTN)**<br>(hī″pĕr-tĕn′ shŭn) | hyper-<br>tens<br>-ion | P<br>R<br>S | excessive, above<br>pressure<br>process | High blood pressure (HBP); a disease of the arteries caused by such pressure. ✱ See Pathology Spotlight: Hypertension on page 270 and Figure 9–36. |
| **hypotension**<br>(hī″pō-tĕn′ shŭn) | hypo-<br>tens<br>-ion | P<br>R<br>S | deficient, below<br>pressure<br>process | Low blood pressure |
| **infarction**<br>(ĭn-fărk′ shŭn) | infarct<br><br>-ion | R<br><br>S | infarct (necrosis of an area)<br>process | Process of development of an infarct, which is necrosis of tissue resulting from obstruction of blood flow |

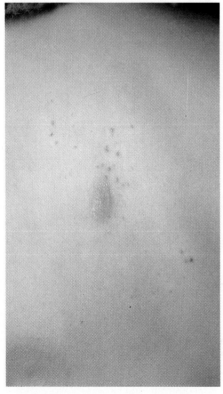

▶ **FIGURE 9–21**   Hemangioma. (Courtesy of Jason L. Smith, MD)

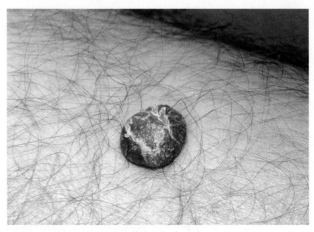

▶ **FIGURE 9–22**   Sclerosing hemangioma. (Courtesy of Jason L. Smith, MD)

| MEDICAL WORD | WORD PARTS (WHEN APPLICABLE) | | | DEFINITION |
|---|---|---|---|---|
| | **Part** | **Type** | **Meaning** | |
| **ischemia**<br>(ĭs-k ē′ mĭ-ă) | isch<br>-emia | R<br>S | to hold back<br>blood condition | Condition in which there is a lack of blood supply to a part of the body caused by constriction or obstruction of a blood vessel |
| **lipoprotein**<br>(lĭp-ō-prō′ tēn) | | | | Fat *(lipid)* and protein molecules that are bound together. They are classified as **VLDL**—very-low-density lipoproteins; **LDL**—low-density lipoproteins; and **HDL**—high-density lipoproteins. High levels of VLDL and LDL are associated with cholesterol and triglyceride deposits in arteries, which could lead to coronary heart disease, hypertension, and atherosclerosis. |
| **mitral stenosis (MS)**<br>(mī′ trăl stĕ-nō′ sĭs) | mitr<br>-al<br>sten<br>-osis | R<br>S<br>R<br>S | mitral valve<br>pertaining to<br>narrowing<br>condition (usually abnormal) | Condition of narrowing of the mitral valve (bicuspid valve) |
| **mitral valve prolapse (MVP)**<br>(mī′ trăl vălv prō-lăps′) | | | | Condition that occurs when the leaflets of the mitral valve (bicuspid valve) between the left atrium and left ventricle bulge into the atrium and permit backflow of blood into the atrium. The condition is often associated with progressive mitral regurgitation (blood flows back into the left atrium instead of moving forward into the left ventricle). |
| **murmur**<br>(mər′ mər) | | | | Soft blowing or rasping sound heard by auscultation of various parts of the body, especially in the region of the heart |
| **myocardial**<br>(mī″ ō-kăr′ dĭ-ăl) | my/o<br>card/i<br>-al | CF<br>CF<br>S | muscle<br>heart<br>pertaining to | Pertaining to the heart muscle |
| **myocardial infarction (MI)**<br>(mī″ ō-kăr′ dē-ăl ĭn-fă rk′ shŭn) | my/o<br>card/i<br>-al<br>infarct<br><br>-ion | CF<br>CF<br>S<br>R<br><br>S | muscle<br>heart<br>pertaining to<br>infarct (necrosis of an area)<br>process | Occurs when an area of heart muscle dies or is permanently damaged because of an inadequate supply of oxygen to that area; also known as a heart attack. ✱ See Pathology Spotlight: Heart Attack on page 270. |
| **myocarditis**<br>(mī″ ō-kăr-dī′ tĭs) | my/o<br>card<br>-itis | CF<br>R<br>S | muscle<br>heart<br>inflammation | Inflammation of the heart muscle |
| **occlusion**<br>(ŏ-kloo′ zhŭn) | occlus<br>-ion | R<br>S | to shut up<br>process | Process or state of being closed |

| MEDICAL WORD | WORD PARTS (WHEN APPLICABLE) | | | DEFINITION |
|---|---|---|---|---|
| | Part | Type | Meaning | |
| **oximetry**<br>(ŏk-sĭm′ ĕ-trē) | ox/i<br>-metry | CF<br>S | oxygen<br>measurement | Process of measuring the oxygen saturation of blood. A photoelectric device (oximeter) measures oxygen saturation of the blood by recording the amount of light transmitted or reflected by deoxygenated versus oxygenated hemoglobin. A *pulse oximetry* is a noninvasive method of indicating the arterial oxygen saturation of functional hemoglobin. See Figure 9–23 ▼. |
| **oxygen ($O_2$)**<br>(ŏk′ sĭ-jĕn) | oxy<br>-gen | R<br>S | sour, sharp, acid<br>formation, produce | Colorless, odorless, tasteless gas essential to respiration in animals |
| **palpitation**<br>(păl-pĭ-tā′ shŭn) | palpitat<br>-ion | R<br>S | throbbing<br>process | Rapid throbbing or fluttering of the heart that is usually perceptible only to the patient |
| **percutaneous transluminal coronary angioplasty (PTCA)**<br>(pĕr″ kū-tā′ nē-ŭs trăns-lū′ mĭ-năl kŏr′ ō-nă-rē ăn′ jĭ-ō-plăs″ te) | | | | Use of a balloon-tipped catheter to compress fatty plaques against an artery wall. When successful, the plaques remain compressed, which permits more blood to flow through the artery, thereby relieving the symptoms of heart disease. See Figure 9–24 ►. |

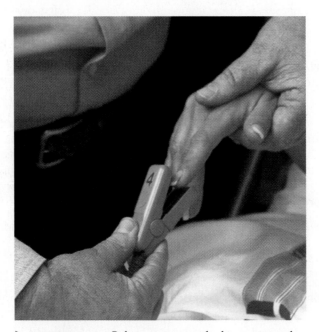

► **FIGURE 9–23** Pulse oximetry with the sensor probe applied securely, flush with skin, making sure that both sensor probes are aligned directly opposite each other.

| MEDICAL WORD | WORD PARTS (WHEN APPLICABLE) | | | DEFINITION |
|---|---|---|---|---|
| | **Part** | **Type** | **Meaning** | |
| **pericardial** (pěr″ ĭ-kăr′ dĭ-ăl) | peri- card/i -al | P CF S | around heart pertaining to | Pertaining to the pericardium, the sac surrounding the heart |
| **pericardiocentesis** (pěr″ ĭ-kăr″ dĭ-ō-sĕn-tē′ sĭs) | peri- cardi/o -centesis | P CF S | around heart surgical puncture | Surgical puncture of the pericardium to remove fluid from the pericardial sac for therapeutic or diagnostic purposes. See Figure 9–25 ▶. |
| **pericarditis** (pěr″ ĭ-kăr″ dĭ′tĭs) | peri- card -itis | P R S | around heart inflammation | Inflammation of the pericardium. A condition known as *cardiac tamponade* can result from pericarditis, a condition in which an accumulation of excess fluid in the pericardium decreases ventricular filling and cardiac output, resulting in cardiogenic shock and death if untreated. |
| **phlebitis** (flĕ-bĭ′ tĭs) | phleb -itis | R S | vein inflammation | Inflammation of a vein |
| **phlebotomy** (flĕ-bŏt′ ō-mē) | phleb/o -tomy | CF S | vein incision | Incision of a vein with a needle to withdraw blood for analysis |

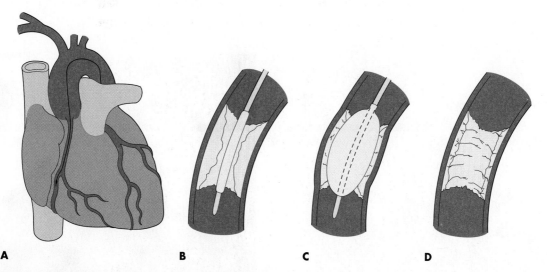

**A**        **B**        **C**        **D**

▶ **FIGURE 9–24** Balloon angioplasty. (A) The balloon catheter is threaded into the affected coronary artery. (B) The balloon is positioned across the area of obstruction. (C) The balloon is then inflated, flattening the plaque against the arterial wall (D).

| MEDICAL WORD | WORD PARTS (WHEN APPLICABLE) | | | DEFINITION |
|---|---|---|---|---|
| | **Part** | **Type** | **Meaning** | |
| **Raynaud's Phenomenon** (rā-nōz fĕ-nŏm' ĕ-nŏn) | | | | Disorder that generally affects the blood vessels in the fingers and toes; it is characterized by intermittent attacks that cause the blood vessels in the digits to narrow. The attack is usually due to exposure to cold or occurs during emotional stress. Once the attack begins, the patient can experience pallor, cyanosis, and/or rubor (redness) in the affected part. It is a type of peripheral vascular disease (PVD). See Figure 9–26 ▼. |
| **rheumatic heart disease** (rōō-măt' ĭk hart dĭ-zēz') | | | | Endocarditis or valvular heart disease that results from complications of acute rheumatic fever |
| **semilunar** (sĕm" ĭ-lū' năr) | semi- lun -ar | P R S | half moon pertaining to | Valves of the aorta and pulmonary artery |
| **septum** (sĕp' tŭm) | sept -um | R S | a partition tissue | Wall or partition that divides or separates a body space or cavity |
| **shock** | | | | State of disruption of oxygen supply to the tissues and a return of blood to the heart. In cardiogenic shock, there is failure to maintain the blood supply to the circulatory system and tissues because of inadequate cardiac output. See Figure 9–27 ▶. |

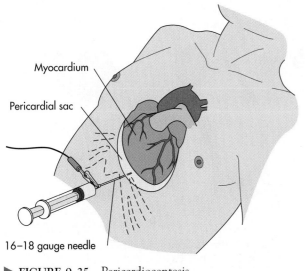

Myocardium

Pericardial sac

16–18 gauge needle

▶ **FIGURE 9–25** Pericardiocentesis.

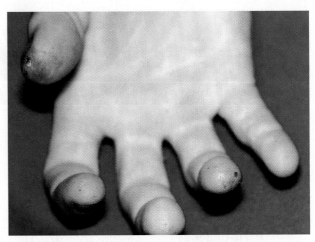

▶ **FIGURE 9–26** Raynaud's phenomenon. (Courtesy of Jason L. Smith, MD)

| MEDICAL WORD | WORD PARTS (WHEN APPLICABLE) | | | DEFINITION |
|---|---|---|---|---|
| | Part | Type | Meaning | |
| **sinoatrial (SA)**<br>(sīn″ ō-ā′ trĭ-ăl) | sin/o<br>atri<br>-al | CF<br>R<br>S | a curve<br>atrium<br>pertaining to | Pertaining to the sinus venosus and the atrium |
| **sphygmomano-meter**<br>(sfĭg″ mō -măn-ō mĕt-ĕr) | sphygm/o<br>man/o<br>-meter | CF<br>CF<br>S | pulse<br>thin<br>instrument<br>to measure | Instrument used to measure the arterial blood pressure. See Figure 9–9 on page 241. |
| **spider veins** | | | | Hemangioma in which numerous telangiectatic vessels radiate from a central point. |
| **stent**<br>(st′ēnt) | | | | Device made of expandable, metal mesh that is placed (by using a balloon catheter) at the site of a narrowing artery. The stent is then expanded and left in place to keep the artery open. See Figure 9–28 ▶. |
| **stethoscope**<br>(stĕth′ ō-skōp) | steth/o<br>-scope | CF<br>S | chest<br>instrument for examining | Instrument used to listen to the sounds of the heart, lungs, and other internal organs |

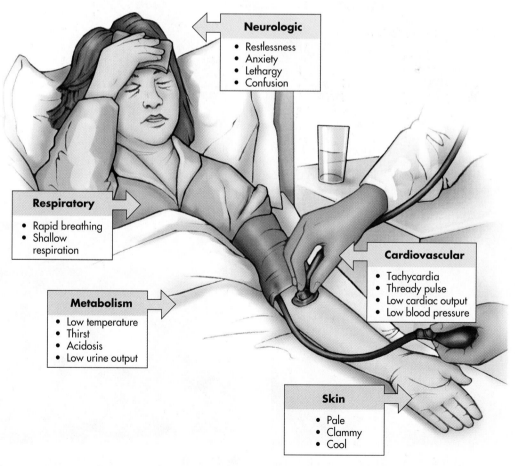

▶ **FIGURE 9–27** Symptoms of a patient in shock.

| MEDICAL WORD | WORD PARTS (WHEN APPLICABLE) | | | DEFINITION |
|---|---|---|---|---|
| | **Part** | **Type** | **Meaning** | |
| **systole**<br>(sĭs′ tō-lē) | | | | Contractive phase of the heart cycle during which blood is forced into the aorta and the pulmonary artery |
| **tachycardia**<br>(tăk″ ĭ-kăr′ dĭ-ă) | tachy-<br>card<br>-ia | P<br>R<br>S | fast<br>heart<br>condition | Abnormally fast heartbeat that is over 100 beats per minute |
| **telangiectasis**<br>(tĕl-ăn″ j ĕ-ĕk-tă′ sĭs) | tel<br>ang/i<br>-ectasis | R<br>CF<br>S | end<br>vessel<br>dilatation | Vascular lesion formed by dilatation of a group of small blood vessels; can appear as a birthmark or be caused by long-term exposure to the sun. See Figure 9–29 ▼. |
| **thrombophlebitis**<br>(thrŏm″ bō-flē-bī′ tĭs) | thromb/o<br>phleb<br>-itis | CF<br>R<br>S | clot of blood<br>vein<br>inflammation | Inflammation of a vein associated with the formation of a *thrombus* (blood clot). See Figure 9–30 ▼. |

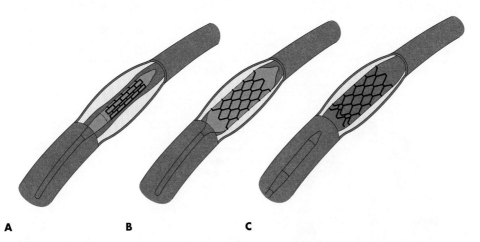

**A**    **B**    **C**

▶ **FIGURE 9–28**   Placement of a balloon expandable intracoronary stent. (A) The stainless steel stent is fitted over a balloon-tipped catheter. (B) The stent is positioned along the blockage and expanded. (C) The balloon is deflated and removed, leaving the stent in place.

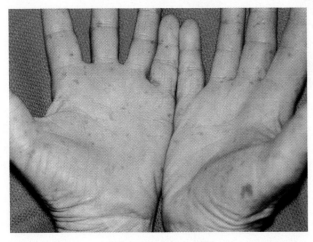

▶ **FIGURE 9–29**   Telangiectasis. (Courtesy of Jason L. Smith, MD)

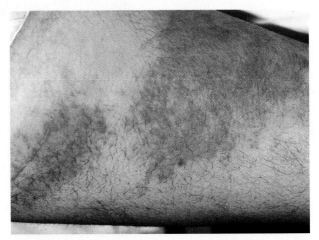

▶ **FIGURE 9–30**   Thrombophlebitis. (Courtesy of Jason L. Smith, MD)

| MEDICAL WORD | WORD PARTS (WHEN APPLICABLE) | | | DEFINITION |
|---|---|---|---|---|
| | **Part** | **Type** | **Meaning** | |
| **thrombosis**<br>(thrŏm-bō′ sĭs) | thromb<br>-osis | R<br>S | clot of blood<br>condition<br>(usually<br>abnormal) | Condition in which a blood clot is within the vascular system; *a stationary blood clot.* See Figure 9–31 ▼. |
| **tricuspid**<br>(trī-kŭs′ pĭd) | tri-<br>-cuspid | P<br>S | three<br>a point | Having three points; pertaining to the tricuspid valve |
| **triglyceride**<br>(trī-glĭs′ ĕr-īd) | tri-<br>glyc<br>-er<br>-ide | P<br>R<br>S<br>S | three<br>sweet, sugar<br>relating to<br>having a particular quality | Pertaining to a compound consisting of three molecules of fatty acids |
| **valve replacement surgery** | | | | Surgical replacement of diseased heart valve with an artificial one. There are two types of artificial valves: A mechanical heart valve is made of artificial materials and can usually last a lifetime; biological heart valves are made from tissue taken from animals or human cadavers and can wear out over time. |
| **valvuloplasty**<br>(văl′vū-lō-plăs″tē) | valvul/o<br>-plasty | CF<br>S | valve<br>surgical repair | Surgical repair of a valve, especially of a cardiac valve |

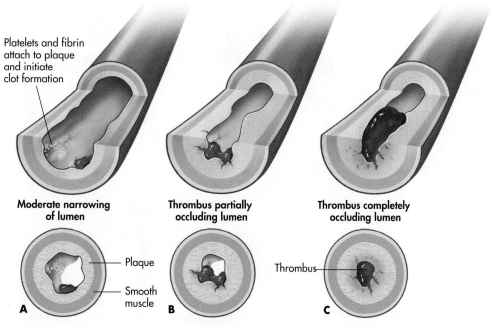

Platelets and fibrin attach to plaque and initiate clot formation

Moderate narrowing of lumen

Thrombus partially occluding lumen

Thrombus completely occluding lumen

Plaque

Smooth muscle

Thrombus

A

B

C

▶ **FIGURE 9–31**   Thrombus formation in an atherosclerotic vessel depicting: (A) the initial clot formation, and (B) and (C) the varying degrees of occlusion.

| MEDICAL WORD | WORD PARTS (WHEN APPLICABLE) | | | DEFINITION |
|---|---|---|---|---|
| | Part | Type | Meaning | |
| **varicose veins** (văr′ ĭ-kōs vāns) | | | | Swollen, distended, and knotted veins that usually occur in the lower leg(s). They result from a stagnated or sluggish flow of blood in combination with defective valves and weakened walls of the veins. See Figure 9–32 ▼. |
| **vasoconstrictive** (văs″ ō-kŏn-strĭk′ tĭv) | vas/o con- strict -ive | CF P R S | vessel together to draw, to bind nature of, quality of | Drawing together, as in the narrowing of a blood vessel |
| **vasodilator** (văs″ ō-dī-lā′ tor) | vas/o dilat -or | CF R S | vessel to widen one who, a doer | Nerve or agent that causes dilation of blood vessels |
| **vasospasm** (vās′ ō-spăzm) | vas/o -spasm | CF S | vessel contraction, spasm | Contraction of a blood vessel |
| **venipuncture** (věn′ ĭ-pŭnk″ chūr) | ven/i -puncture | CF S | vein to pierce | To pierce a vein with a needle for the removal of blood for analysis |
| **ventricular** (věn-trĭk′ ū-lăr) | ventricul -ar | R S | ventricle pertaining to | Pertaining to a ventricle |

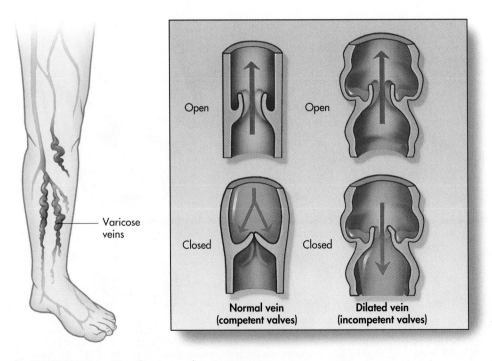

▶ **FIGURE 9–32**  Development of varicose veins.

# DRUG HIGHLIGHTS

| | |
|---|---|
| **Digitalis drugs** | Strengthen the heart muscle, increase the force and velocity of myocardial systolic contraction, slow the heart rate, and decrease conduction velocity through the atrioventricular (AV) node. These drugs are used in the treatment of congestive heart failure, atrial fibrillation, atrial flutter, and paroxysmal atrial tachycardia. The administration of digitalis can cause toxicity. The most common early symptoms of digitalis toxicity are anorexia, nausea, vomiting, and arrhythmias.<br><br>*Examples: Crystodigin (digitoxin), Lanoxin (digoxin), and Digitaline (digitoxin)* |
| **Antiarrhythmic agents** | Used in the treatment of cardiac arrhythmias (irregular heart rhythms).<br><br>*Examples: Tambocor (flecainide acetate), Tonocard (tocainide HCl), Inderal (propranolol HCl), Calan (verapamil), and Cordarone and Pacerone (amiodarone)* |
| **Vasopressors** | Cause contraction of the muscles associated with capillaries and arteries, thereby narrowing the space through which the blood circulates. This narrowing results in an elevation of blood pressure. Vasopressors are useful in the treatment of patients suffering from shock.<br><br>*Examples: Intropin (dopamine HCl), Aramine (metaraminol bitartrate), and Levophed Bitartrate (norepinephrine)* |
| **Vasodilators** | Cause relaxation of blood vessels and lower blood pressure. Coronary vasodilators are used for the treatment of angina pectoris.<br><br>*Examples: Sorbitrate (isosorbide dinitrate), nitroglycerin, amyl nitrate, and Peritrate (pentaerythritol tetranitrate)* |
| **Antihypertensive agents** | Used in the treatment of hypertension.<br><br>*Examples: Catapres (clonidine HCl), Aldomet (methyldopa), Lopressor (metoprolol tartrate), Capoten (captopril), and TOPROL–XL (metoprolol succinate)* |
| **Antihyperlipidemic agents** | Used to lower abnormally high blood levels of fatty substances (lipids) when other treatment regimens fail.<br><br>*Examples: Nicolar or Nicobid (niacin), Mevacor (lovastatin), Lopid (gemfibrozil), Lipitor (atorvastatin calcium), Pravachol (pravastatin), Zocor (simvastatin), Crestor (rosuvastatin calcium), Vytorin (ezetimibe/simvastatin), and Zetia (ezetimibe)* |
| **Antiplatelet drugs** | Help reduce the occurrence of and death from vascular events such as heart attacks and strokes. *Aspirin* is considered to be the reference standard antiplatelet drug and is recommended by the American Heart Association for use in patients with a wide range of cardiovascular disease. Aspirin helps keep platelets from sticking together to form clots. *Plavix (clopidogrel)* is approved by the Food and Drug Administration for many of the same indications as aspirin. It is recommended for patients for whom aspirin fails to achieve a therapeutic benefit. |
| **Thrombolytic agents** | Act to dissolve an existing thrombus when administered soon after its occurrence. They are often referred to as **tissue plasminogen activators** (tPA, TPA) and can reduce the chance of dying after a myocardial infarction by 50%. Unless contraindicated, the drug should be administered within 6 hours of the onset of chest pain. In some hospitals, the time period for administering thrombolytic agents has been extended to 12 and 24 hours. These agents dissolve the clot, reopen the artery, restore blood flow to the heart, and prevent further damage to the myocardium. Bleeding is the most common complication encountered during thrombolytic therapy.<br><br>*Examples: Kabikinase and Streptase (streptokinase), Eminase (anistreplase), Activase (alteplase), and Abbokinase (urokinase)* |

# DIAGNOSTIC AND LAB TESTS

| TEST | DESCRIPTION |
| --- | --- |
| **Angiography** (ăn″ jē-ŏg′ ră-fē) | X-ray recording of a blood vessel after the injection of a radiopaque substance. Used to determine the condition of the blood vessels, organ, or tissue being studied. Types: aortic, cardiac, cerebral, coronary, digital subtraction (use of a computer technique), peripheral, pulmonary, selective, and vertebral. |
| **Cardiac catheterization** (kăr′ dǐ-ăk kăth″ ĕ-tĕr-ǐ-z ā′ shŭn) | Test used to diagnose heart disorders. A tiny catheter is inserted into an artery in the arm or leg of the patient and is fed through this artery to the heart. Dye is then pumped through the catheter, enabling the physician to locate by x-ray any blockages in the arteries supplying the heart. See Figure 9–33 ▼. |
| **Cardiac enzymes** (kar′ dǐ-ăk ĕn′-zīmz)<br>    alanine aminotransferase (ALT)<br><br>    aspartate aminotransferase (AST)<br>    creatine phosphokinase (CPK)<br>    creatine kinase (CK)<br>    creatine kinase isoenzymes | Blood tests performed to determine cardiac damage in an acute myocardial infarction (AMI). Levels begin to rise 6 to 10 hours after an AMI and peak at 24 to 48 hours.<br><br>Levels begin to rise 6 to 10 hours after an AMI and peak at 24 to 48 hours.<br><br>Used to detect area of damage.<br><br>Level may be 5 to 8 times normal.<br>Used to indicate area of damage; CK-MB heart muscle, CK-MM skeletal muscle, and CK-BB brain |
| **Cholesterol** (kōl-lĕs′ tĕr-ŏl) | Blood test to determine the level of cholesterol in the serum. Elevated levels can indicate an increased risk of coronary heart disease. Any level more than 200 mg/dL is considered too high for good heart health. |
| **Echocardiography (ECHO)** (ĕk″ ō-kăr″ dē-ŏg′ rah-fē) | Used to analyze the size, shape, and movement of structures inside the heart.<br>Usually two echoes are taken: one of the heart at rest and another of the heart under stress. Comparison of the two images helps pinpoint abnormal valves or areas that are not receiving enough blood. |

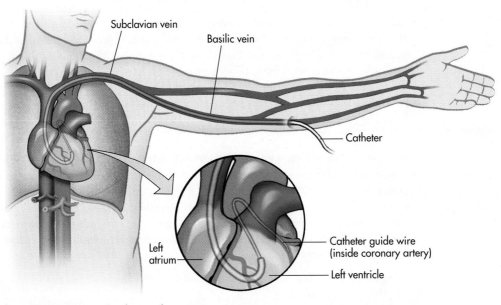

▶ **FIGURE 9–33**  Cardiac catheterization.

| TEST | DESCRIPTION |
|---|---|
| **Holter monitor**<br>(hōlt ər mŏn′ ĭ –tər) | Portable device small enough to be worn by the patient during normal activity to record a patient's ECG for 24 hours. |
| **Intracardiac electrophysiology study (EPS)**<br>(ĭn″tră-kăr′dē-ăk ē-lĕk″ trō-fĭz″ ĭ-ŏl′ ō-jē) | Invasive cardiac procedure that involves the placement of catheter-guided electrodes within the heart to evaluate and map the electrical conduction of cardiac arrhythmias. |
| **Lactic dehydrogenase (LD or LDH)**<br>(lăk′ tĭk dē-hī-drŏj′ ĕ-nās) | Intracellular enzyme present in nearly all metabolizing cells with the highest concentrations in the heart, skeletal muscles, RBCs, liver, kidney, lung, and brain. Used for diagnosing acute myocardial infarction (AMI). A high serum level occurs 12 to 24 hours after cardiac injury. |
| **Lipid profile**<br>(lĭp′ĭd) | Series of blood tests including cholesterol, high density lipoproteins, low density lipoproteins, and triglycerides. Used to determine levels of lipids and to assess risk factors of coronary heart disease. |
| **Magnetic resonance imaging (MRI)**<br>(măg-nĕt′ĭk rĕz′ŏ-năns) | Use of a magnet that sets the nuclei of atoms in the heart cells vibrating.<br>The oscillating atoms emit radio signals, which are converted by a computer into either still or moving 3-D images. The scan can reveal plaque-filled coronary arteries and the layer of fat that envelopes most hearts. MRI is also an ideal method for scanning children with congenital heart problems. Patients with pacemakers, stents, or other metal implants cannot have MRI. An MRI scan cannot pick up calcium deposits that could signal narrowed vessels. |
| **Stress test**<br>(strĕs tĕst) | Method of evaluating cardiovascular fitness, also called *exercise test, exercise stress test*, or *treadmill test*. The ECG is monitored while the patient is subjected to increasing levels of work using a treadmill or ergometer. It is a common test for diagnosing coronary artery disease, especially in patients who have symptoms of heart disease. The test helps doctors assess blood flow through coronary arteries in response to exercise, usually walking, at varied speeds and for various lengths of time on a treadmill. A stress test can include the use of electrocardiography, echocardiography, and injected radioactive substances. |
| **Thallium-201 stress test**<br>(thăl ē-ŭm strĕs tĕst | X-ray study that follows the path of radioactive potassium carried by the blood into heart muscle. Damaged or dead muscle can be defined, as can the extent of narrowing in an artery. |
| **Triglycerides**<br>(trī -glĭs′ ĕr-īds) | Blood test to determine the level of triglycerides in the serum. Elevated levels (more than 200 mg/dL) can indicate an increased risk of coronary heart disease and diabetes mellitus. |
| **Ultrasonography**<br>(ŭ l-tră-sŏn-ŏg′ ră-fē) | Test used to visualize an organ or tissue by using high-frequency sound waves; can be used as a screening test or as a diagnostic tool to determine abnormalities of the aorta, arteries, veins, and the heart. |
| **Ultrafast CT scan** | Ultrafast CT can take multiple images of the heart within the time of a single heartbeat, thus providing much more detail about the heart's function and structures while greatly decreasing the amount of time required for a study. It can detect very small amounts of calcium within the heart and the coronary arteries. This calcium has been shown to indicate that lesions, which can eventually block off one or more coronary arteries and cause chest pain or even a heart attack, are in the beginning stages of formation. Thus, many physicians are using ultrafast CT scanning as a means to diagnose early coronary artery disease in certain people, especially those who have no symptoms of the disease. |

# ABBREVIATIONS

| ABBREVIATION | MEANING | ABBREVIATION | MEANING |
|---|---|---|---|
| ACG | angiocardiography | Hgb | hemoglobin |
| AED | automated external defibrillator | H&L | heart and lungs |
| | | HTN | hypertension |
| AHD | arteriosclerotic heart disease | LA | left atrium |
| AMI | acute myocardial infarction | LBBB | left bundle branch block |
| ASHD | arteriosclerotic heart disease | LD or LDH | lactic dehydrogenase |
| AST | aspartate aminotransferase | LDL | low-density lipoprotein |
| A-V, AV | atrioventricular; arteriovenous | LV | left ventricle |
| BBB | bundle branch block | MI | myocardial infarction |
| BP | blood pressure | MRI | magnetic resonance imaging |
| CABG | coronary artery bypass graft | MS | mitral stenosis |
| CAD | coronary artery disease | MV | mitral valve |
| CC | cardiac catheterization | MVP | mitral valve prolapse |
| CCU | coronary care unit | $O_2$ | oxygen |
| CHD | coronary heart disease | OHS | open heart surgery |
| CHF | congestive heart failure | P | pulse |
| chol | cholesterol | PAD | peripheral artery disease |
| CK | creatine kinase | PAT | paroxysmal atrial tachycardia |
| CLI | critical limb ischemia | PMI | point of maximal impulse |
| CMP | cardiomyopathy | PTCA | percutaneous transluminal coronary angioplasty |
| CO | cardiac output | | |
| CPR | cardiopulmonary resuscitation | PVC | premature ventricular contraction |
| CV | cardiovascular | | |
| CVP | central venous pressure | PVD | peripheral vascular disease |
| DVT | deep vein thrombosis | R | respiration |
| ECC | extracorporeal circulation | RA | right atrium |
| ECG | electrocardiogram | RBCs | red blood cells |
| ECHO | echocardiography | RV | right ventricle |
| ECG, EKG | electrocardiogram | S-A, SA | sinoatrial (node) |
| EPS | electrophysiology study (intracardiac) | SCA | sudden cardiac arrest |
| | | SCD | sudden cardiac death |
| FFA | free fatty acids | SOB | shortness of breath |
| FHS | fetal heart sound | TOF | tetralogy of Fallot |
| HBP | high blood pressure | tPA, TPA | tissue plasminogen activator |
| HDL | high-density lipoprotein | VLDL | very-low-density lipoprotein |
| HF | heart failure | VSD | ventricular septal defect |
| Hg | mercury | | |

# PATHOLOGY SPOTLIGHTS

## ✳ Coronary Heart Disease

**Coronary heart disease** (CHD) is the most common form of heart disease. Also referred to as *coronary artery disease (CAD)*, it is the term for the narrowing of the coronary arteries that supply blood to the heart. It is a progressive disease that increases the risk of myocardial infarction (heart attack) and sudden death.

CHD usually results from the buildup of fatty material and plaque (**atherosclerosis**). See Figures 9–34 ▼ and 9–35 ▶. As the coronary arteries narrow, the flow of blood to the heart can slow or stop. Blockage can occur in one or many coronary arteries.

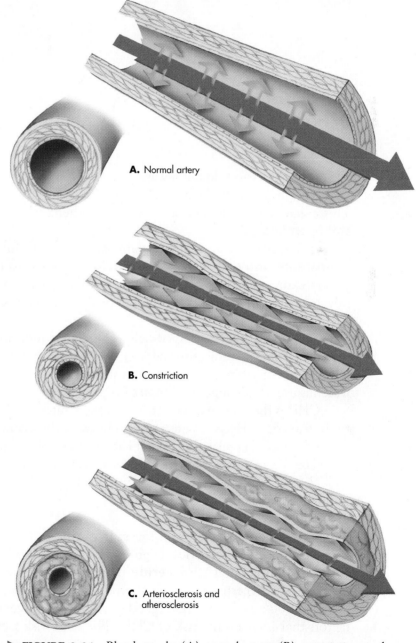

**A.** Normal artery

**B.** Constriction

**C.** Arteriosclerosis and atherosclerosis

▶ **FIGURE 9–34** Blood vessels: (A) normal artery, (B) constriction, and (C) arteriosclerosis and atherosclerosis.

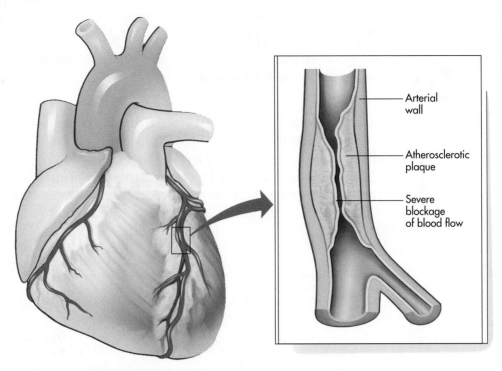

▶ **FIGURE 9–35**   Atherosclerotic artery.

Small blockages do not always affect the heart's performance. The person could have no symptoms until the heart needs more oxygen-rich blood than the arteries can supply. This commonly occurs during exercise or other activity. The pain that results is called **stable angina.**

If a blockage is large, angina pain can occur with little or no activity. This is known as **unstable angina.** In this case, the flow of blood to the heart is so limited that the person cannot do daily tasks without bringing on an angina attack. When the blood flow to an area of the heart is completely blocked, a myocardial infarction (heart attack) occurs.

Symptoms of CHD vary widely. The classic indicator of CHD is **angina,** or chest pain. The pain can radiate to the neck, jaw, or left arm. It is often described as a crushing, burning, or squeezing sensation. The person can also have shortness of breath (SOB), which is usually a symptom of **heart failure.**

CHD is the leading cause of death in the United States for men and women. According to the American Heart Association, about every 29 seconds someone in the United States suffers from a CHD-related event, and about every minute someone dies from such an event.

The lifetime risk of having coronary heart disease after age 40 is 49 percent for men and 32 percent for women. As women age, the risk increases almost to that of men. One in ten U.S. women 45 to 64 years of age has some form of heart disease, and this increases to one in four women over 65.

CHD affects people of all races. It can be caused by a combination of unhealthy lifestyle choices and genetics. High levels of VLDL and LDL lipoproteins are associated with **cholesterol** and **triglyceride** deposits in arteries, which could lead to coronary heart disease, hypertension, and atherosclerosis. A person's total cholesterol level should be below 200 mg/dL and HDL (good cholesterol) above 35 mg/dL. See Table 9–1 for risk factors that increase the risk of CHD. The more risk factors that one has, the higher is the possibility of developing coronary artery disease, a major cause of myocardial infarction.

**TABLE 9–1  Risk Factors Associated with Developing Coronary Heart Disease**

| | |
|---|---|
| Male age 45 or older | Diabetes mellitus |
| Female age 55 or older | High-density lipoprotein (HDL) below 35 mg/dL |
| Female under age 55 with premature menopause | Family history of early heart disease (parent or sibling; male less than 55, female less than 65) |
| Smoker | Obesity |
| Hypertension | |

## ＊ Peripheral Artery Disease

An estimated 12 million people in the U.S. have **peripheral artery disease** (PAD), a condition in which fatty deposits build up in the inner linings of the artery walls. These blockages restrict blood circulation, mainly in arteries leading to the kidneys, stomach, arms, legs, and feet. In its early stages, a common symptom is cramping or fatigue in the legs and buttocks during activity. Such cramping subsides when the person stands still. This is called *intermittent claudication*.

Symptoms of PAD can include, but are not limited to, the following:

- Claudication: dull, cramping pain in the hips, thighs, calves or buttocks.
- Numbness or tingling in the leg, foot, or toes.
- Changes in skin temperature: cold to the touch.
- Impotence.
- Sores or infections that do not heal.
- Weakness in legs or arms.

Techniques used to diagnose PAD include a medical history, physical exam, ultrasound, X-ray angiography, and magnetic resonance imaging (MRI). Peripheral artery disease can be treated with lifestyle changes, medications, or both. In certain cases, angioplasty or surgery is necessary. A stent is placed in the narrowed artery to expand it and lock it open. Another option is the SilverHawk™ Plaque Excision System. This system consists of two components, a low-profile catheter and a palm-size drive unit. It is the first technology of its kind to remove significant amounts of atherosclerotic tissue from long, diffusely diseased lesions.

If left untreated, PAD can progress to *critical limb ischemia* (CLI), which occurs when the oxygenated blood being delivered to the leg is not adequate to keep the tissue alive. An estimated 750,000 people in the United States suffer from CLI. This condition can cause constant pain and even lead to amputation of toes, feet, and/or part of the leg.

 ## ＊ Dysrhythmias

A **dysrhythmia** or **arrhythmia** of the heart is an abnormality of the rhythm or rate of the heartbeat. The dysrhythmia is caused by a disturbance of the normal electrical activity within the heart. Dysrhythmias can be divided into 2 main groups: **tachycardias** and **bradycardias.** Tachycardias cause a rapid heartbeat with more than 100 beats per minute. Bradycardias cause a slow heartbeat with less than 60 beats per minute. The rhythm of the heart could be regular during a dysrhythmia: Each beat of the atria, or upper chambers of the heart, is followed by one beat of the ventricles, or lower chambers of the heart. The beat could also be irregular and begin in an abnormal area of the heart.

Symptoms vary depending on the type of dysrhythmia but may include dizziness or light-headedness, palpitations, shortness of breath, fatigue, weakness, **angina,** and fainting.

Most dysrhythmias are caused by heart disease, including coronary heart disease and disease of the heart valves, from infections such as **endocarditis,** and **heart failure.**

Dysrhythmias can be life threatening if they cause a severe decrease in the pumping function of the heart. When the pumping function is severely decreased for more than a few seconds, blood circulation is essentially stopped, and organ damage (such as brain damage) can occur within a few minutes.

**Cardioversion** is the process of using an electrical shock to the heart to restore its rhythm to a normal pattern. The electrical energy can be delivered externally through electrodes placed on the chest or directly to the heart by placing paddles on the heart during an open chest surgery. The energy is synchronized to the ECG and is delivered during a critical part of the electrical sequence. It stops arrhythmias resulting from single or multiple reentry circuits in the atria or ventricles, such as atrial flutter, atrial fibrillation, atrioventricular nodal reentrant tachycardia, atrioventricular reentrant tachycardia, or monomorphic ventricular tachycardia. Arrhythmias that arise from multiple reentry circuits in the ventricles, specifically ventricular fibrillation, are terminated using a technique called **defibrillation,** which is the nonsynchronized delivery of an electric shock.

## ✳ Hypertension

Hypertension describes a blood pressure (BP) reading that is higher than normal. Approximately 50 million adults in the United States are believed to have hypertension (HTN). Hypertension can cause the blood vessels to become tight or constrict and the blood to press on the vessel walls with extra force. When this force exceeds a certain level and remains there, a person has high blood pressure (HBP). Hypertension can be controlled by a variety of methods, such as taking blood pressure medications as prescribed, seeing a physician on a regular basis, establishing healthy eating habits, exercising, avoiding stress, and making lifestyle changes.

Hypertension often has no symptoms and is frequently called *the silent killer* because, if left untreated, it can lead to kidney failure, stroke, heart attack, peripheral artery disease, and eye damage. See Figure 9–36 ▶.

Various factors can contribute to developing hypertension, and it is important to know these factors. See Table 9–2.

## ✳ Prehypertension

Individuals age 18 years and over with blood pressure ranging from 120/80 to 139/89 mm Hg belong to a new category designated as **prehypertension,** a high-risk precursor to hypertension, according to the Joint National Committee (JNC) Seventh Report.

According to the report, adults at the upper end of the prehypertension blood pressure range (130/80 to 139/89 mm Hg) are twice as likely to progress to hypertension as those with lower blood pressure levels. The reporting panel of experts recommended lifestyle modification for patients with prehypertension. Therapeutic behavior changes identified as critical in the prevention of high blood pressure included reducing dietary fat and sodium, increasing exercise, and limiting alcohol consumption.

## ✳ Heart Attack (Myocardial Infarction)

A **heart attack** (or **myocardial infarction**) occurs when the blood supply to part of the heart muscle (myocardium) is severely reduced or stopped. This occurs when one of the coronary arteries that supplies blood to the heart muscle is blocked. The blockage is usually from the buildup of plaque (deposits of fatlike substances) due to atherosclerosis. The plaque can eventually tear or rupture, triggering a blood clot that blocks the artery and leads to a heart attack. Such an event is called a *coronary thrombosis* or *coronary occlusion.*

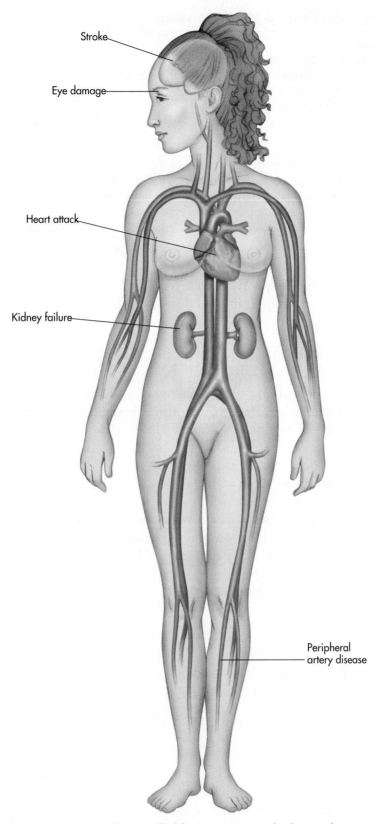

▶ **FIGURE 9–36** Uncontrolled hypertension can lead to stroke, eye damage, heart attack, kidney failure, and peripheral artery disease.

## TABLE 9–2 Factors Contributing to Hypertension

**Factors That One Can Control**

| | |
|---|---|
| Smoking | Avoid the use of tobacco products |
| Overweight | Maintain a proper weight for age and body size |
| Lack of exercise | Exercise regularly |
| Stress | Learn to manage stress |
| Alcohol | Limit intake of alcohol |

**Factors That One Cannot Control**

| | |
|---|---|
| Heredity | Family history of high blood pressure, heart attack, stroke, or diabetes |
| Race | Incidence of hypertension increases among African-Americans |
| Gender | Chance of developing hypertension increases for males |
| Age | Likelihood of hypertension increases with age |

If the blood supply is cut off severely or for a long time, muscle cells suffer irreversible injury and die, resulting in disability or death, depending on how much heart muscle is damaged.

A recent study indicates that having a large "pot belly" or "spare tire" around the middle is associated with an increased risk for atherosclerosis. Experts explain that in addition to the fat that can be seen bulging around the middle, fat deposits are also deep within the abdomen tucked around abdominal organs. The presence of this fat further increases the risk of having high cholesterol and insulin resistance, a precursor to diabetes.

The most common symptom of a heart attack is chest pain (**angina**), which is often described as a feeling of crushing, pressure, fullness, heaviness, or aching in the center of the chest. These sensations can extend into the neck, the jaw, and down the left arm. Angina is often associated with excessive sweating, feelings of apprehension, nausea, shortness of breath, and weakness.

Some heart attacks are sudden and intense, but most start slowly with mild pain or discomfort. Often the person affected is not sure what is happening and waits too long before getting help. Heart attack and stroke are life-and-death emergencies; every second counts.

The American Heart Association lists the following as warning signs of heart attack:

- Pressure, fullness, squeezing pain in the center of the chest that lasts 2 minutes or longer.
- Pain that spreads to the shoulders, neck, or arms.
- Dizziness, fainting, sweating, nausea, or shortness of breath.

Today heart attack and stroke victims can benefit from new medications and treatments. Clot-busting drugs can stop some heart attacks and strokes in progress, reducing disability and saving lives. To be effective, however, these drugs must be given relatively quickly after the heart attack or stroke symptoms first appear. It is said that the average heart attack victim waits 3 hours after symptoms first occur to seek help. Many times people try to ignore the symptoms or say "it's just indigestion." It is imperative to seek medical help immediately. Calling 911 is almost always the fastest way to get lifesaving treatment.

# ✔ PATHOLOGY CHECKPOINT

*Following is a concise list of the pathology-related terms that you have seen in the chapter. Review this checklist to make sure that you are familiar with the meaning of each term before moving to the next section.*

## Conditions and Symptoms

- ❏ aneurysm
- ❏ angina
- ❏ angina pectoris
- ❏ angioma
- ❏ angiostenosis
- ❏ arrhythmia
- ❏ arteriosclerosis
- ❏ arteritis
- ❏ atheroma
- ❏ atherosclerosis
- ❏ bradycardia
- ❏ bruit
- ❏ cardiac arrest
- ❏ cardiac tamponade
- ❏ cardiogenic shock
- ❏ cardiomegaly
- ❏ cardiomyopathy
- ❏ claudication
- ❏ congestive heart failure
- ❏ constriction
- ❏ coronary heart disease
- ❏ critical limb ischemia
- ❏ cyanosis
- ❏ diastolic failure
- ❏ dysrhythmia
- ❏ embolism
- ❏ endocarditis
- ❏ fibrillation
- ❏ flutter
- ❏ heart attack (myocardial infarction)

- ❏ heart failure
- ❏ hemangioma
- ❏ hyperlipidemia
- ❏ hypertension
- ❏ hypotension
- ❏ infarction
- ❏ ischemia
- ❏ mitral stenosis
- ❏ mitral valve prolapse
- ❏ murmur
- ❏ myocardial infarction
- ❏ myocarditis
- ❏ occlusion
- ❏ palpitation
- ❏ pericarditis
- ❏ peripheral artery disease
- ❏ phlebitis
- ❏ prehypertension
- ❏ pulmonary edema
- ❏ Raynaud's phenomenon
- ❏ rheumatic heart disease
- ❏ shock
- ❏ spider veins
- ❏ sudden cardiac arrest
- ❏ systolic failure
- ❏ tachycardia
- ❏ telangiectasis
- ❏ thrombophlebitis
- ❏ thrombosis
- ❏ vasoconstrictive
- ❏ vasospasm
- ❏ varicose veins

## Diagnosis and Treatment

- ❏ anastomosis
- ❏ angiocardiography
- ❏ angioplasty
- ❏ artificial pacemaker
- ❏ auscultation
- ❏ automated external defibrillator
- ❏ cardiac catheterization
- ❏ cardiometer
- ❏ cardiotonic
- ❏ cardioversion
- ❏ coronary bypass
- ❏ echocardiography
- ❏ electrocardiograph
- ❏ electrocardiophonograph
- ❏ endarterectomy
- ❏ extracorporeal circulation
- ❏ defibrillator
- ❏ heart-lung transplant
- ❏ heart transplant
- ❏ oximetry
- ❏ percutaneous transluminal coronary angioplasty
- ❏ pericardiocentesis
- ❏ phlebotomy
- ❏ sphygmomanometer
- ❏ stent
- ❏ stethoscope
- ❏ valvuloplasty
- ❏ vasodilator
- ❏ venipuncture

# STUDY AND REVIEW

## Anatomy and Physiology

*Write your answers to the following questions. Do not refer to the text.*

1. The cardiovascular system includes:

   a. _____    b. _____

   c. _____    d. _____

2. Name the three layers of the heart.

   a. _____    b. _____

   c. _____

3. The heart weighs approximately _____ grams.

4. The _____ or upper chambers of the heart are separated by the

   _____ septum.

5. The _____ or lower chambers of the heart are separated by the

   _____ septum.

6. By listing each cardiovascular part in the proper order, trace the flow of blood
   through the heart, to the lungs, back to the heart, and on to the various body parts.

   a. _____    b. _____

   c. _____    d. _____

   e. _____    f. _____

   g. _____    h. _____

   i. _____    j. _____

   k. _____    l. _____

   m. _____    n. _____

7. The _____ _____ _____ controls the heartbeat.

8. The _____ _____ is called the *pacemaker of the heart.*

9. The _____ _____ includes the bundle of His and the
   peripheral fibers.

10. Name the three primary pulse points and state their locations on the body.

    a. _____ located _____

b. _____  located _____

c. _____  located _____

11. Define the following terms:

   a. *Blood pressure* _____

   b. *Pulse pressure* _____

12. The average adult heart is about the size of a _____ and normally

   beats at a pulse rate of _____ to _____ beats per minute.

13. The average adult usually has a systolic pressure between _____ and

   _____ mm Hg and a diastolic pressure between _____ and

   _____ mm Hg.

14. Give the purpose and function of arteries.

   _____

   _____

   _____

15. Give the purpose and function of veins.

   _____

   _____

   _____

## Word Parts

1. In the spaces provided, write the definition of these prefixes, roots, combining forms, and suffixes. Do not refer to the listing of medical words. Leave blank those words you cannot define.

2. After completing as many as you can, refer to the medical word listings to check your work. For each word missed or left blank, write the word and its definition several times on the margins of these pages or on a separate sheet of paper.

3. To maximize the learning process, it is to your advantage to do the following exercises as directed. To refer to the word-building section before completing these exercises invalidates the learning process.

## PREFIXES

*Give the definitions of the following prefixes*

1. a- _____   2. bi- _____

3. brady- _____   4. con- _____

5. end- _____    6. endo- _____

7. extra- _____    8. hyper- _____

9. hypo- _____    10. peri- _____

11. dys- _____    12. semi- _____

13. tachy- _____    14. tri- _____

## ROOTS AND COMBINING FORMS

*Give the definitions of the following roots and combining forms.*

1. ang/i _____    2. angin _____

3. angi/o _____    4. anastom _____

5. aort/o _____    6. arter _____

7. arter/i _____    8. arteri/o _____

9. ather _____    10. ather/o _____

11. atri _____    12. atri/o _____

13. card _____    14. card/i _____

15. cardi/o _____    16. cyan _____

17. auscultat _____    18. dilat _____

19. electr/o _____    20. embol _____

21. glyc _____    22. hem _____

23. isch _____    24. chol/e _____

25. log _____    26. lun _____

27. man/o _____    28. mitr _____

29. my/o _____    30. circulat _____

31. oxy _____    32. phleb _____

33. phleb/o _____    34. phon/o _____

35. pulmonar _____    36. rrhythm _____

37. scler _____    38. sin/o _____

39. sphygm/o _____    40. sten _____

41. steth/o _____    42. strict _____

43. claudicat _____    44. tens _____

45. thromb _____    46. vascul _____

47. vas/o _____

48. ech/o _____

49. ven/i _____

50. corpor/e _____

51. ventricul _____

52. fibrillat _____

53. hem/o _____

54. dynam _____

55. infarct _____

56. occlus _____

57. ox/i _____

58. palpitat _____

59. sept _____

60. tel _____

61. thromb/o _____

62. sterol _____

63. pector _____

64. lipid _____

## SUFFIXES

*Give the definitions of the following suffixes.*

1. -ac _____

2. -al _____

3. -ar _____

4. -gram _____

5. -centesis _____

6. -cuspid _____

7. -metry _____

8. -ectasis _____

9. -ectomy _____

10. -emia _____

11. -er _____

12. -gen _____

13. -graph _____

14. -graphy _____

15. -ia _____

16. -ic _____

17. -ide _____

18. -ion _____

19. -ism _____

20. -ist _____

21. -itis _____

22. -ive _____

23. -logy _____

24. -malacia _____

25. -megaly _____

26. -meter _____

27. -oma _____

28. -or _____

29. -osis _____

30. -pathy _____

31. -plasty _____

32. -puncture _____

33. -scope _____

34. -spasm _____

35. -tomy _____

36. -um _____

37. -y _____

## Identifying Medical Terms

*In the spaces provided, write the medical terms for the following meanings.*

1. _____ Tumor of a blood vessel

2. _____ Germ cell from which blood vessels develop

3. _____ Surgical repair of a blood vessel or vessels

4. _____ Condition of narrowing of a blood vessel

5. _____ Incision into an artery

6. _____ Inflammation of an artery

7. _____ Having two points or cusps; pertaining to the mitral valve

8. _____ One who specializes in the study of the heart

9. _____ Enlargement of the heart

10. _____ Pertaining to the heart and lungs

11. _____ Process of drawing together as in the narrowing of a vessel

12. _____ Condition in which a blood clot obstructs a blood vessel

13. _____ Inflammation of a vein

14. _____ Fast heartbeat

15. _____ Widening of a blood vessel

## Spelling

*In the spaces provided, write the correct spelling of these misspelled terms.*

1. astomosis _____   2. athrosclerosis _____

3. atriventrcular _____   4. endcarditis _____

5. extracoporal _____   6. iscemia _____

7. mycardial _____   8. oyxgen _____

9. phelebitis _____   10. palpitaiton _____

## Matching

*Select the appropriate lettered meaning for each of the following words.*

_____ 1. cholesterol

_____ 2. claudication

_____ 3. dysrhythmia

_____ 4. diastole

_____ 5. fibrillation

_____ 6. lipoprotein

_____ 7. cardioversion

_____ 8. palpitation

_____ 9. percutaneous transluminal coronary angioplasty

_____ 10. systole

a. Used to treat different types of cardiac arrhythmias
b. Quivering of muscle fiber
c. Fat and protein molecules that are bound together
d. Waxy, fatlike substance in the bloodstream of all animals
e. Process of lameness, limping
f. Abnormal, difficult, or bad rhythm
g. Relaxation phase of the heart cycle
h. Contraction phase of the heart cycle
i. Rapid throbbing or fluttering of the heart
j. Use of a balloon-tipped catheter to compress fatty plaques against an artery wall
k. Process of being closed

## Abbreviations

*Place the correct word, phrase, or abbreviation in the space provided.*

1. acute myocardial infarction _____

2. atrioventricular _____

3. BP _____

4. CAD _____

5. cardiac catheterization _____

6. ECG, EKG _____

7. HDL _____

8. heart and lungs _____

9. MI _____

10. tPA, TPA _____

## Diagnostic and Laboratory Tests

*Select the best answer to each multiple choice question. Circle the letter of your choice.*

1. _____ is a cardiac procedure that maps the electrical activity of the heart from within the heart itself.
   a. Electrocardiogram
   b. Electrocardiomyogram
   c. Electrophysiology
   d. Cardiac catheterization

2. Blood tests performed to determine cardiac damage in an acute myocardial infarction.
   a. cardiac enzymes
   b. high density lipoproteins
   c. triglycerides
   d. low density lipoproteins

3. Method of recording a patient's ECG for 24 hours.
   a. stress test
   b. Holter monitor
   c. ultrasonography
   d. angiography

4. Test used to visualize an organ or tissue by using high-frequency sound waves.
   a. electrophysiology
   b. stress test
   c. ultrasonography
   d. cholesterol

5. X-ray recording of a blood vessel after the injection of a radiopaque contrast medium.
   a. ultrasonography
   b. angiography
   c. stress test
   d. cardiac catheterization

# PRACTICAL APPLICATION

## S O A P : Chart Note Analysis

*This exercise will make you aware of the information, abbreviations, and medical terminology typically found in a cardiology patient's chart.*

### Abbreviations Key

| | | | | |
|---|---|---|---|---|
| Abd | abdomen | | OTC | over-the-counter |
| BP | blood pressure | | P | pulse |
| CTA | clear to auscultation | | prn | as necessary |
| DOB | date of birth | | R | respiration |
| ECG, EKG | electrocardiogram | | ROM | range of motion |
| F | Fahrenheit | | SOAP | subjective, objective, assessment, plan |
| Ht | height | | | |
| HTN | hypertension | | T | temperature |
| lb | pound | | WNL | within normal limits |
| mg | milligram | | Wt | weight |
| MS | musculoskeletal | | y/o | year(s) old |
| NKDA | no known drug allergies | | | |

*Read the following chart note and then answer the questions that follow.*

**PATIENT:** Moore, William T.                                            **DATE:** 05/06/2007

**DOB:** 3/26/1962      **AGE:** 45      **SEX:** Male
**INSURANCE:** Reliant HealthCare

**Vital Signs:**
  T: 98.4 F
  P: 84
  R: 20
  BP: 138/90
  Ht: 5' 11"
  Wt: 196 lb

**Allergies:** NKDA

**Chief Complaint:** Tightness in chest, dyspnea, apprehension.

**S** | **Subjective:** 45 y/o Caucasian male describes experiencing "tightness" in his chest during a workout session. Noted patient clenching his fist while describing "shortness of breath" and how anxious he felt. He denies nausea, vomiting, or radiating pain to his left arm or jaw. The uncomfortable sensation "just went away" after he stopped exercising. He states that he has no prior history of cardiac disease.

**O** | **Objective:**

**General Appearance:** The patient appears apprehensive. Well-developed and muscular. No obvious signs of physical distress noted such as dyspnea, edema, pallor, or diaphoresis. Overall health appears WNL.

**Heart:** Rate at 84 beats per minute, rhythm regular, no extra sounds, no murmurs.

**Lungs:** CTA

**Abd:** Bowel sounds all 4 quadrants, no masses or tenderness.

**MS:** Joints and muscles symmetric; no swelling, masses, or deformity; normal spinal curvature. No tenderness to palpation of joints. Full ROM, movement smooth, no crepitant (crackling) sound heard, no tenderness. Muscle strength: able to maintain flexion against resistance and without tenderness.

**A**

**Assessment:** Angina pectoris (stable)

**P**

**Plan:**

1. After completing history and receiving results from a comprehensive physical examination, an EKG, and blood enzyme studies, a diagnosis of angina pectoris was made. Nitroglycerin (coronary vasodilator) sublingual tablets 0.4 mg prn was prescribed for chest pain.
2. Instruct patient to seek medical attention immediately if pain is not relieved by nitroglycerin tablets, taken one every 5 minutes over a 15-minute period.
3. Screen patient for personal cardiac risk factors such as nutrition, weight change, smoking, alcohol, exercise, drugs including prescription, OTC, or street. Encourage patient to avoid situations that precipitate angina attacks.
4. Discuss family cardiac history as related to HTN, obesity, diabetes, coronary artery disease, and sudden death of any family member occurring at a young age.
5. Educate patient that angina pectoris occurs due to myocardial ischemia that results when cardiac workload and myocardial oxygen demand exceed the ability of the coronary arteries to supply oxygenated blood. This commonly occurs during exercise or other activity.

**FYI:** Patients with acute chest pain frequently present with classical symptoms consisting of chest tightness and pain in the left arm. In the acute setting, if these symptoms are present, they heavily favor the diagnosis of unstable angina, and a cardiac work-up is indicated. However, in stable patients, chest pain may masquerade as indigestion, muscle spasm, or a myriad of other nonspecific complaints. In these patients, the object of imaging is to exclude myocardial ischemia as the etiology of the chest pain.

In unstable patients, myocardial infarction (MI) may be fatal, and establishing the diagnosis rapidly and accurately may be life saving. Thus the cardiac work-up usually consists of an electrocardiogram and serum markers, namely, creatine kinase isoenzymes. These studies are widely and rapidly available. Imaging studies are indicated when there is a question as to whether or not the chest pain is ischemic in origin.

*Note: This information is adapted from the National Guideline Clearinghouse: Acute Chest Pain at* www.guideline.gov.

## Chart Note Questions
*Place the correct answer in the space provided.*

1. Signs and symptoms of angina pectoris include tightness in the chest, apprehension and shortness of breath, which is also called _____.

2. A complete physical, an EKG, and _____ _____ studies are important in determining the diagnosis of angina pectoris.

3. Nitroglycerin 0.4 mg is a _____ medication placed under the tongue and is prescribed as needed for chest pain.

4. The abbreviation for *as necessary* is _____.

5. When chest pain is not relieved by nitroglycerin after the recommended dosage and time period, the patient should _____ seek medical attention.

6. Nitroglycerin sublingual tablets 0.4 mg should be taken for chest pain one every 5 minutes over a _____ -minute period.

7. Myocardial ischemia is a result of the body's inability to supply _____ blood.

8. EKG is an abbreviation for _____.

9. Nitroglycerin is a _____ _____ used to treat angina pectoris.

10. *Adventitious* means _____ _____ sounds.

# MULTIMEDIA PREVIEW

*Additional interactive resources and activities for this chapter can be found on the Companion Website. For videos, audio glossary, and review, access the accompanying CD-ROM in this book.*

 **CD-ROM HIGHLIGHTS**

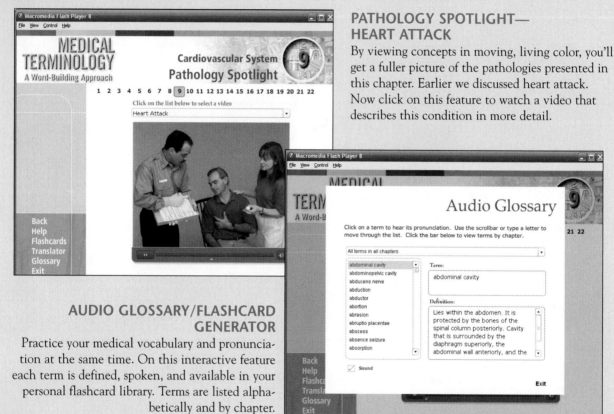

## PATHOLOGY SPOTLIGHT— HEART ATTACK

By viewing concepts in moving, living color, you'll get a fuller picture of the pathologies presented in this chapter. Earlier we discussed heart attack. Now click on this feature to watch a video that describes this condition in more detail.

## AUDIO GLOSSARY/FLASHCARD GENERATOR

Practice your medical vocabulary and pronunciation at the same time. On this interactive feature each term is defined, spoken, and available in your personal flashcard library. Terms are listed alphabetically and by chapter.

 **WEBSITE HIGHLIGHTS—www.prenhall.com/rice**

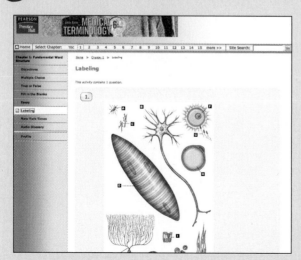

## LABELING EXERCISES

Click here and take advantage of the free-access online study guide that accompanies your textbook. You'll find a series of image labeling questions that correspond to the pictures in this chapter. By clicking on this URL you'll also access links to download mp3 audio reviews, current news articles, and an audio glossary.

# Blood and Lymphatic System

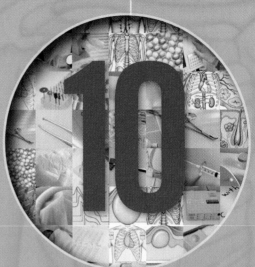

**10**

## ■ OUTLINE

## ■ OBJECTIVES

*On completion of this chapter, you will be able to:*

- Describe the blood.
- Describe the formed elements in blood.
- Name the four blood types.
- Describe and state the functions of the lymphatic system.
- Describe the accessory organs of the lymphatic system.
- Describe the immune system and the immune response.
- Analyze, build, spell, and pronounce medical words.
- Comprehend the drugs highlighted in this chapter.
- Describe diagnostic and laboratory tests related to blood and the lymphatic system.
- Identify and define selected abbreviations.
- Describe each of the conditions presented in the Pathology Spotlights.
- Review the Pathology Checkpoint.
- Complete the Study and Review section and the Chart Note Analysis.

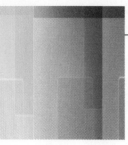

# Anatomy and Physiology Overview

Blood and lymph are two of the body's main fluids and are circulated through two separate but interconnected vessel systems. Blood is circulated by the action of the heart, through the circulatory system consisting largely of arteries, veins, and capillaries. Lymph does not actually circulate. It is propelled in one direction, away from its source, through increasingly larger lymph vessels, to drain into large veins of the circulatory system located in the neck region. Numerous valves within the lymph vessels permit one-directional flow, opening and closing as a consequence of pressure caused by the massaging action of muscles on the vessels and the fluid they contain. The various organs and components of blood and the lymphatic system this chapter describes.

## Blood and Lymphatic System

| Organ/Structure | Identification/Primary Functions |
| --- | --- |
| Blood | Fluid consisting of formed elements and plasma that transport respiratory gases (oxygen and carbon dioxide), chemical substances (foods, salts, hormones), and cells that act to protect the body from foreign substances |
| Lymphatic system | Vessel system composed of lymphatic capillaries, lymphatic vessels, lymphatic ducts, and lymph nodes that convey lymph from the tissue to the blood. The three main functions of the lymphatic system are to:<br>1. Transport proteins and fluids, lost by capillary seepage, back to the bloodstream<br>2. Protect the body against pathogens by phagocytosis and immune response<br>3. Serve as a pathway for the absorption of fats from the small intestines into the bloodstream |
| Spleen | Major site of erythrocyte destruction; serves as a reservoir for blood; acts as a filter, removing microorganisms from the blood |
| Tonsils | Filter bacteria and aid in the formation of white blood cells |
| Thymus | Plays essential role in the formation of antibodies and the development of the immune response in the newborn; manufactures infection-fighting T cells and helps distinguish normal T cells from those that attack the body's own tissue |

## BLOOD

**Blood** is a fluid consisting of formed elements and plasma, both of which are continuously produced by the body for the purpose of transporting respiratory gases (*oxygen and carbon dioxide*), chemical substances (*foods, salts, hormones*), and cells that act to protect the body from foreign substances. The blood volume within an individual depends on body weight. An individual weighing 154 lb (70 kg) has a blood volume of about 5 qt or 5 L.

### Formed Elements

The formed elements in blood are the erythrocytes (red blood cells), thrombocytes (platelets), and leukocytes (white blood cells). See Table 10–1. Formed elements constitute about 45% of the total volume of blood. Together, the plasma and formed elements constitute whole blood. These components can be separated for analysis and clinical purposes.

## TABLE 10–1  Types of Blood Cells and Functions

| Blood Cell | Function |
| --- | --- |
| Erythrocyte (red blood cell) | Transports oxygen and carbon dioxide |
| Thrombocyte (platelet) | Clots blood |
| Leukocyte (white blood cell) | Provides body's main defense against invasion of pathogens |
| Types of leukocytes | |
|   Neutrophil | Protects against infection; is readily attracted to foreign antigens and destroys them by phagocytosis (engulfing and eating of particulate substances) |
|   Eosinophil | Destroys parasitic organisms; plays a key role in allergic reactions |
|   Basophil | Plays a key role in releasing histamine and other chemicals that act on blood vessels; essential to nonspecific immune response to inflammation |
|   Monocyte | Provides one of the first lines of defense in the inflammatory process, phagocytosis |
| Lymphocyte | Provides immune capacity to the body |
|   B lymphocyte | Identifies foreign antigens and differentiates into antibody-producing plasma cells |
|   T lymphocyte | Plays essential role in the specific immune response of the body |

### Erythrocytes

**Erythrocytes,** commonly called **red blood cells** (RBC), are doughnut-shaped (biconcave) cells without nuclei. They transport oxygen (most of which is bound to hemoglobin contained in the cell) and carbon dioxide. There are approximately 5 million erythrocytes per cubic millimeter of blood, and they have a life span of 80 to 120 days. Erythrocytes are formed in the red bone marrow. See Figure 10–1 ▼.

### Thrombocytes

**Thrombocytes,** commonly called *platelets*, are disk-shaped cells about half the size of erythrocytes. They play an important role in the clotting process by releasing *thrombokinase*, which, in the presence of calcium, reacts with *prothrombin* to form *thrombin*. There are approximately 200,000 to 500,000 thrombocytes per cubic millimeter of blood. Thrombocytes are fragments of certain giant cells called *megakaryocytes*, which are formed in the red bone marrow. See Figure 10–1.

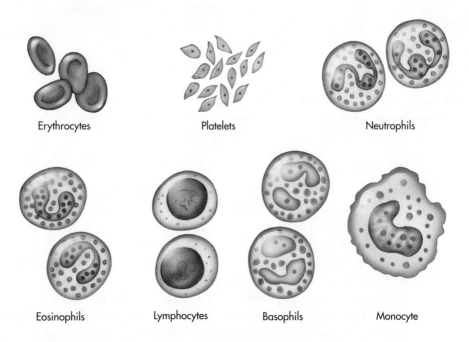

Erythrocytes   Platelets   Neutrophils

Eosinophils   Lymphocytes   Basophils   Monocyte

▶ **FIGURE 10–1**   Formed elements of blood: erythrocytes, leukocytes (neutrophils, eosinophils, basophils, lymphocytes, and monocytes), and thrombocytes (platelets).

### Leukocytes

**Leukocytes,** commonly called **white blood cells** (WBC), are sphere-shaped cells containing nuclei of varying shapes and sizes. See Figure 10–1. Leukocytes are the body's main defense against the invasion of **pathogens.** In a normal body state, when pathogens enter the tissue, the leukocytes leave the blood vessels through their walls and move in an amoebalike motion to the area of infection, where they ingest and destroy the invader. There are approximately 8,000 leukocytes per cubic millimeter of blood. The five types of leukocytes are **neutrophils, eosinophils, basophils, lymphocytes** (lymphs), and **monocytes.**

Neutophils, eosinophils, basophils, and monocytes contribute to the body's nonspecific defenses. These immune defenses are activated by a variety of stimuli. Lymphocytes are responsible for specific defenses against invading pathogens or foreign proteins.

## Blood Groups

A number of human blood systems are determined by a series of two or more genes closely linked on a single autosomal chromosome. The **ABO** system, which was discovered in 1901 by Karl Landsteiner, is of great significance in blood typing and blood transfusion. The four blood types identified in this system are types A, B, AB, and O. The differences in human blood are due to the presence or absence of certain protein molecules called *antigens* and *antibodies*. The antigens are located on the surface of the red blood cells, and the antibodies are in the blood plasma. Individuals have different types and combinations of these molecules. Individuals in the A group have the A antigen on the surface of their red blood cells and anti-B antibody in the blood plasma; B group has the B antigen and the anti-A antibody; AB group has both A and B antigens and no anti-A or anti-B antibodies; and group O has neither A or B antigens but has both anti-A and anti-B antibodies. Type AB blood is the universal donor of plasma and the universal recipient of cells, and type O is the universal donor of cells only. See Table 10–2 and Figure 10–2 ▶.

**TABLE 10–2  Blood Groups and Compatibilities**

| Type | Antigen | Plasma Antibody | Percentage/ Population | Compatible Donor Blood Groups | Incompatible Donor Blood Groups |
|------|---------|-----------------|------------------------|-------------------------------|---------------------------------|
| A | A | Anti-B | 41 | A, O | B, AB |
| B | B | Anti-A | 10 | B, O | A, AB |
| AB | Both A and B | No anti-A or anti-B | 4 | A, B, AB, O | None |
| O | No A and B | Both anti-A and anti-B | 45 | O | A, B, AB |

## Rh Factor

The presence of a substance called an **agglutinogen** in the red blood cells is responsible for what is known as the **Rh factor.** It was first discovered in the blood of the rhesus monkey from which the factor gets its name. About 85% of the population have the Rh factor and are called *Rh positive*. The other 15% lack the Rh factor and are designated *Rh negative*. More than 20 genetically determined blood group systems are known today, but the ABO and Rh systems are the most important ones used for blood transfusions. Not all blood groups are compatible with each other. Mixing incompatible blood groups leads to blood clumping, or agglutination, which is dangerous for individuals.

If an individual with Rh-negative blood receives a transfusion of Rh-positive blood, it causes the formation of anti-Rh agglutinin. Subsequent transfusions of Rh-positive blood can result in serious transfusion reactions (agglutination and hemolysis of red blood cells).

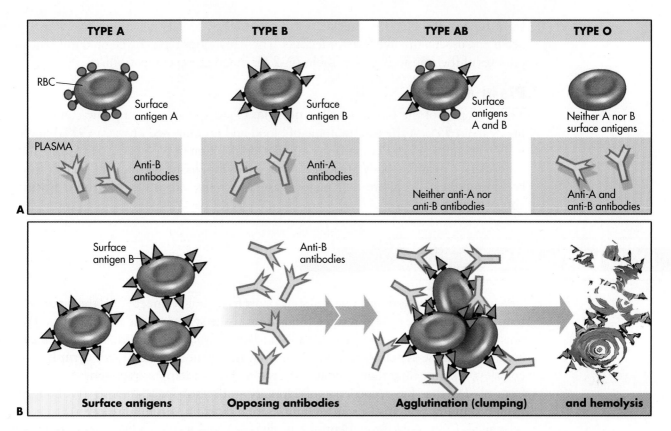

▶ FIGURE 10–2    Blood-typing and cross-reactions: The blood type depends on the presence of surface antigens (agglutinogens) on RBC surfaces. (A) The plasma antibodies (agglutinins) that will react with foreign surface antigens. (B) In a cross-reaction, antibodies that encounter their target antigens lead to agglutination and hemolysis of the affected RBCs.

A pregnant woman who is Rh-negative can become sensitized by blood of an Rh-positive fetus. Sensitization can also occur if an Rh-negative woman has had a previous miscarriage, induced abortion, or ectopic pregnancy. There is also a slight chance that a woman can develop antibodies after having amniocentesis done later in pregnancy. These are cases in which fetal blood (that might be Rh-positive) could mix with maternal blood, resulting in the production of antibodies that could complicate a subsequent pregnancy. In subsequent pregnancies, if the fetus is Rh-positive, Rh antibodies produced in maternal blood can cross the placenta and destroy fetal cells, producing hemolytic disease of the newborn (HDN).

Today, hemolytic disease can for the most part be prevented if the Rh-negative woman has not already made antibodies against the Rh factor from an earlier pregnancy or blood transfusion. Rh immunoglobulin (Rhogam) is a product that can safely prevent sensitization of an Rh-negative mother. It suppresses her ability to respond to Rh-positive red cells. It is given at 28 weeks of pregnancy, and a second dose is given within 72 hours after delivery if the baby is Rh-positive. With its use, sensitization can be prevented almost all of the time, although Rhogam is not helpful if the mother is already sensitized.

For a blood transfusion to be successful, ABO and Rh blood groups of the donor and the recipient must be compatible. If they are not, the red blood cells from the donated blood can agglutinate and cause clogging of blood vessels and slow and/or stop the circulation of blood to various parts of the body. The agglutinated red blood cells can also hemolyze (dissolve or be destroyed), and their contents leak out in the body. The red blood cells contain hemoglobin, which becomes toxic when outside the red blood cell, and this could lead to fatal consequences for the recipient. Before blood can be administered to a patient, a type and crossmatch must be performed. This means mixing the donor cells with the recipient's serum and watching for agglutination. If none occurs, the blood is considered compatible.

Even though the blood is checked for compatibility, blood transfusion reactions can still occur and usually involve fever and chills. These reactions typically begin during the first 15 minutes of the transfusion. See Table 10–2 for blood group compatibilities.

## Plasma

The fluid part of the blood is called **plasma.** Clear and somewhat straw-colored, it comprises about 55% of the total volume of blood and is composed of water (91%) and chemical compounds (9%). Plasma is the circulation medium of blood cells, providing nutritive substances to various body structures and removing waste products of metabolism from body structures. There are four major plasma proteins: **albumin, globulin, fibrinogen,** and **prothrombin.**

# LYMPHATIC SYSTEM

The **lymphatic system** is a vessel system apart from, but connected to, the circulatory system. The lymphatic system returns fluids from tissue spaces to the bloodstream. The lymphatic system is composed of *lymphatic capillaries, lymphatic vessels, lymphatic ducts,* and *lymph nodes.* The system conveys lymph from the tissues to the blood. **Lymph** is a clear, colorless, alkaline fluid that is about 95% water. The principal component of lymph is fluid from plasma that has seeped out of capillary walls into spaces among the body tissues. Lymph contains proteins (serum albumin, serum globulin, serum fibrinogen), salts, organic substances (urea, creatinine, neutral fats, glucose), and water. Cells present are principally lymphocytes, formed in the lymph nodes and other lymphatic tissues. Lymph from the intestines contains fats and other substances absorbed from the intestines. Figure 10–3 ▶ shows the major lymphatics of the body.

The three main functions of the lymphatic system are as follows:

1. Transports proteins and fluids, lost by capillary seepage, back to the bloodstream
2. Protects the body against pathogens by phagocytosis and immune response
3. Serves as the pathway for the absorption of fats from the small intestines into the bloodstream

# ACCESSORY ORGANS

The spleen, the tonsils, and the thymus are not actually part of the lymphatic system; however, they are closely related to it in their functions. See Figure 10–4 ▶.

## Spleen

The **spleen** is a soft, dark red oval body lying in the upper left quadrant of the abdomen. It is the major site of erythrocyte destruction. It serves as a reservoir for blood. The spleen plays an essential role in the immune response and acts as a filter, removing microorganisms from the blood.

## Tonsils

The **tonsils** are lymphoid masses located in depressions of the mucous membranes of the face and pharynx. They consist of the *palatine tonsil, pharyngeal tonsil* (adenoid), and the *lingual tonsil.* The tonsils filter bacteria and aid in the formation of white blood cells. See Figure 10–5 ▶.

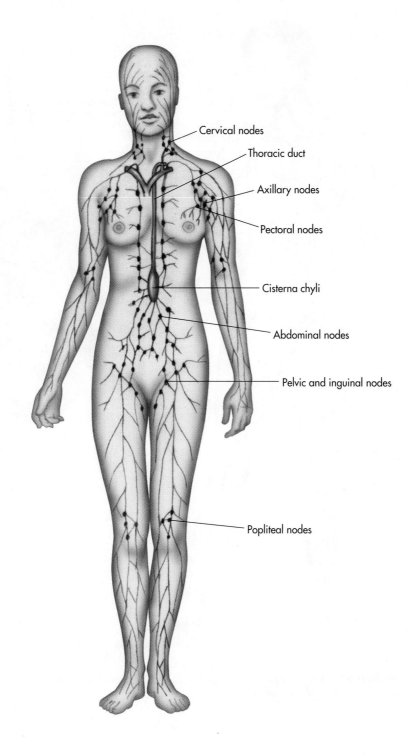

Cervical nodes

Thoracic duct

Axillary nodes

Pectoral nodes

Cisterna chyli

Abdominal nodes

Pelvic and inguinal nodes

Popliteal nodes

▶ **FIGURE 10–3**   Lymphatic system.

## Thymus

The **thymus** is considered to be one of the endocrine glands, but because of its function and appearance, it is a part of the lymphoid system. Located in the mediastinal cavity, the thymus plays an essential role in the formation of antibodies and the development of the immune response in the newborn. It manufactures infection-fighting **T cells** and helps distinguish normal T cells from those that attack the body's own tissue. T cells are important in the body's cellular immune response.

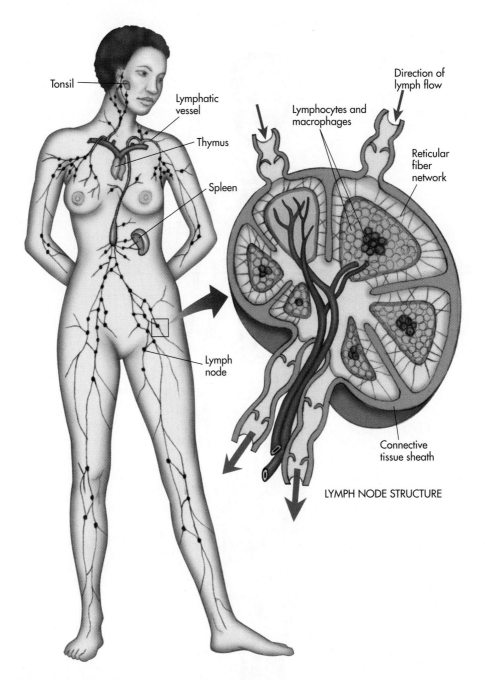

Tonsil

Lymphatic
vessel

Thymus

Spleen

Lymph
node

Direction of
lymph flow

Lymphocytes and
macrophages

Reticular
fiber
network

Connective
tissue sheath

LYMPH NODE STRUCTURE

▶ **FIGURE 10–4**   Tonsils, lymph nodes, thymus, spleen, and lymphatic vessels with an expanded view of a lymph node.

## Immune System

The **immune system** consists of the tissues, organs, and physiologic processes used by the body to identify abnormal cells, foreign substances, and foreign tissue cells that may have been transplanted into the body. Many of these tissues and organs are part of the lymphatic system.

Fortunately, the average, healthy human body is equipped with natural defenses that assist it in fighting off disease and cancer. These natural defenses are intact skin, the cleansing action of the body's secretions (such as tears, mucus), white blood cells, body chemicals (such as hormones, enzymes), and antibodies. As long as the immune system is

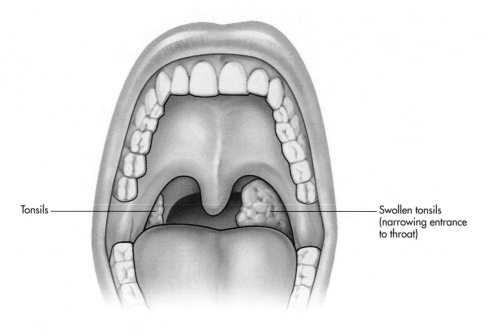

▶ **FIGURE 10–5**    Tonsils—normal and enlarged.

intact and functioning properly, it can defend the body against invading foreign substances and cancer.

## Immune Response Overview

The **immune response** is the reaction of the body to foreign substances and the means by which it protects the body. The following is an overview of this response.

The immune response can be described as humoral immunity or antibody-mediated immunity and cellular immunity or cell-mediated immunity.

**Humoral** (pertaining to body fluids or substances contained in them) **immunity** or **antibody-mediated immunity** involves the production of plasma lymphocytes (B cells) in response to antigen exposure with subsequent formation of antibodies. Humoral immunity is a major defense against bacterial infections.

An **antigen** is a substance such as bacteria, toxins, or certain allergens that induces the formation of antibodies. **Antibodies** are protein substances that are developed in response to a specific antigen. An antibody is also referred to as an *immunoglobulin;* it is a complex glycoprotein produced by B lymphocytes in response to the presence of an antigen. Antibodies neutralize or destroy antigens in several ways. They can initiate destruction of the antigen by activating the complement system, neutralizing toxins released by bacteria, opsonizing (coating) the antigen, or forming a complex to stimulate phagocytosis, promoting antigen clumping or preventing the antigen from adhering to host cells. See Table 10–3 for the five classes of antibodies: IgG, IgM, IgA, IgE, and IgD.

**Cellular immunity** or **cell-mediated immunity** involves the production of lymphocytes (T cells) that respond to any form of injury and NK (natural killer) cells that attack foreign cells, normal cells infected with viruses, and cancer cells. Cellular immunity constitutes a major defense against infections caused by viruses, fungi, and a few bacteria, such as the tubercle bacillus that causes tuberculosis. It also helps defend against the formation of tumors, especially cancer.

TABLE 10–3  **Antibodies/Immunoglobulins**

| Antibody | Functions |
|---|---|
| IgG | Crosses placenta to provide passive immunity for the newborn; opsonizes (coats) microorganisms to enhance phagocytosis; activates complement system (a group of proteins in the blood) <br> *Components of complement are labeled C1 through C9. Complement acts by directly killing organisms; by opsonizing an antigen; and by stimulating inflammation and the B-cell-mediated immune response* |
| IgM | Activates complement; is first antibody produced in response to bacterial and viral infections |
| IgA | Protects epithelial surfaces; activates complement; is passed to breast-feeding newborn via the colostrum (first milk after birth) |
| IgE | Responds to allergic reactions and some parasitic infections; triggers mast cells to release histamine, serotonin, kinins, slow-reacting substance of anaphylaxis, and the neutrophil factor, mediators that produce allergic skin reaction, asthma, and hay fever |
| IgD | Possibly influences B lymphocyte differentiation, but role not clear |

Four general phases are associated with the body's immune response to a foreign substance:

1. The first phase recognizes the foreign substance or the invader (enemy).

2. The second phase activates the body's defenses by producing more white blood cells that are designed to seek and destroy the invader(s), especially the macrophages that eat and engulf the foreign substances and lymphocytes, B cells, and T cells (see Table 10–4).

   • T cells of the helper type identify the enemy and rush to the spleen and lymph nodes, where they stimulate the production of other cells to aid in the fight of the foreign substance.

   • T cells of the natural killer (NK) type are large granular lymphocytes that also specialize in killing cells of the body that have been invaded by foreign substances and fighting cells that have turned cancerous.

   • B cells reside in the spleen or lymph nodes and produce antibodies for specific antigens.

3. The third phase is the attack phase during which the preceding defenders of the body produce antibodies and/or seek out to kill and/or remove the foreign invader. They do this by phagocytosis in which the macrophages squeeze out between the cells in the capillaries and crawl into the tissue to the site of the infection. Here they surround and eat the foreign substances that caused the infection. Other white blood cells respond to infection by producing antibodies, which are released into the bloodstream and carried to the site of the infection where they surround and immobilize the invaders. Later, the phagocytes can eat both antibody and invader.

4. The fourth phase is the slowdown phase in which the number of defenders returns to normal, following victory over the foreign invader.

TABLE 10–4  **Summary of Functions of Lymphocytes**

| Type of Cell | Functions |
|---|---|
| T cells (thymus-dependent) | Provide cellular immunity |
| B cells (bone marrow-derived) | Provide humoral immunity |
| NK cells (natural killers) | Attack foreign cells, normal cells infected with viruses, and cancer cells |

# LIFE SPAN CONSIDERATIONS

## ■ THE CHILD

In the embryo, plasma and blood cells are formed about the second week of life. At approximately the fifth week of development, blood formation occurs in the liver and later in the spleen, thymus, lymphatic system, and bone marrow. At 12 weeks, the fetus is 11.5 cm (4.5 inches) from the crown (or top) of the head to the rump (or bottom) and weighs 45 g (1.6 oz). The fetal **liver** is the chief producer of red blood cells, and the gallbladder secretes **bile.** At 16 weeks, blood vessels are visible through the now-transparent skin. Fetal circulation provides oxygenation and nutrition to the fetus and disposes of carbon dioxide and other waste products.

The **thymus gland** plays an important role in the development of the immune response in the newborn. At birth, the average weight of the thymus is 10 to 15 g. It attains a weight of 40 g at puberty, after which it begins to undergo involution which replaces the thymus with adipose and connective tissue.

## ■ THE OLDER ADULT

With advancing age, lymphatic tissue shrinks, the bone marrow becomes less productive, and the walls of peripheral vessels stiffen. The peripheral vessels also lose elasticity, which causes increases in peripheral resistance, impairs the flow of blood, and results in an increase in the workload of the left ventricle. As a result of these changes in the peripheral vascular system, the transportation of oxygen and nutrients to the tissues and the removal of wastes from the tissues are affected adversely. The transportation of oxygen can also be compromised by the decrease of **hemoglobin** in some older adults.

Immune response declines with age, limiting the body's ability to identify and fight foreign substances such as bacteria and viruses. With aging comes the loss of the thymus cortex, which leads to a reduced production of T lymphocytes, including T cells, natural killer cells, and B lymphocytes. Persons at the extremes of the life span are more likely to develop immune response problems than those in their middle years. Frequency and severity of infections generally increase in elderly persons because of a decreased ability of the immune system to respond adequately to invading microorganisms. The incidence of **autoimmune diseases** also increases with aging, most likely due to a decreased ability of antibodies to differentiate between self and nonself. Failure of the immune response system to recognize mutant, or abnormal, cells could be the reason for the high incidence of cancer associated with increasing age.

# BUILDING YOUR MEDICAL VOCABULARY

This section provides the foundation for learning medical terminology. Review the following alphabetized word list. Note how common prefixes and suffixes are repeatedly applied to word roots and combining forms to create different meanings.

| | |
|---|---|
| P | Prefix |
| R | Root |
| CF | Combining form |
| S | Suffix |

| | |
|---|---|
| Pink words | Terms not built from word parts. |
| * | Indicates words covered in the Pathology Spotlights section. |
|  | Check the CD-ROM for more information. |

| MEDICAL WORD | WORD PARTS (WHEN APPLICABLE) | | | DEFINITION |
|---|---|---|---|---|
| | Part | Type | Meaning | |
| **acquired immuno-deficiency syndrome (AIDS)** (ă-kwīrd ĭm″ ū-nō dĕ-fĭsh′ ĕn-sē sĭn-drōm)  | | | | AIDS is a disease caused by the human immunodeficiency virus (HIV), which is transmitted through sexual contact, exposure to infected blood or blood components, and perinatally from mother to infant. The HIV virus invades the T4 lymphocytes, and, as the disease progresses, the body's immune system becomes paralyzed. See Figure 10–6 ▶. The patient becomes severely weakened and potentially fatal infections can occur. *Pneumocystis carinii* pneumonia (PCP) and Kaposi's sarcoma (KS) account for many of the deaths of AIDS patients. ✴ See Pathology Spotlight: AIDS on page 311. |
| **agglutination** (ă-glōō″ tĭ-nā′ shŭn) | agglutinat -ion | R S | clumping process | Process of clumping together, as of blood cells that are incompatible |
| **albumin** (ăl-bū′ mĭn) | | | | One of a group of simple proteins found in blood plasma and serum |
| **allergy** (ăl′ ĕr-jē)  | all -ergy | R S | other work | Individual hypersensitivity to a substance that is usually harmless. ✴ See Pathology Spotlight: Allergic Rhinitis on page 312 and Figure 10–19. |
| **anaphylaxis** (ăn″ ă-fĭ-lăk′ sĭs) | ana- -phylaxis | P S | up protection | Unusual or exaggerated allergic reaction to foreign proteins or other substances. ✴ See Pathology Spotlight: Anaphylaxis on page 312 and Figure 10–20. |
| **anemia** (ă-nē′ mĭ-ă)  | an- -emia | P S | lack of blood condition | Literally *a lack of red blood cells,* it is a reduction in the number of circulating red blood cells, the amount of the hemoglobin, or the volume of packed red cells (hematocrit). ✴ See Pathology Spotlight: Anemia on page 314 and Figures 10–21, 10–22, and 10–23. |

| MEDICAL WORD | WORD PARTS (WHEN APPLICABLE) | | | DEFINITION |
|---|---|---|---|---|
| | Part | Type | Meaning | |
| **anisocytosis**<br>(ăn-ī″ sō-sī-tō′ sĭs) | anis/o<br>cyt<br>-osis | CF<br>R<br>S | unequal<br>cell<br>condition (usually<br>abnormal) | Condition in which the erythrocytes are<br>unequal in size and shape |

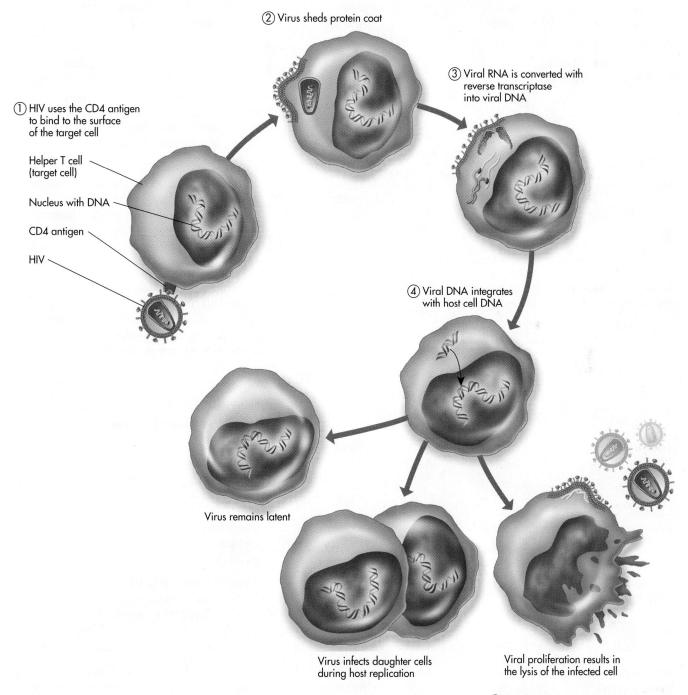

② Virus sheds protein coat

③ Viral RNA is converted with reverse transcriptase into viral DNA

① HIV uses the CD4 antigen to bind to the surface of the target cell

Helper T cell (target cell)

Nucleus with DNA

CD4 antigen

HIV

④ Viral DNA integrates with host cell DNA

Virus remains latent

Virus infects daughter cells during host replication

Viral proliferation results in the lysis of the infected cell

⑤ The net result of an HIV infection is decreased cellular immunity

▶ **FIGURE 10–6**   Human immunodeficiency virus gains entry into helper T cells, uses the cell DNA to replicate, interferes with normal function of the T cells, and destroys the normal cells.

| MEDICAL WORD | WORD PARTS (WHEN APPLICABLE) | | | DEFINITION |
|---|---|---|---|---|
| | Part | Type | Meaning | |
| **antibody**<br>(ăn′ tǐ-bŏd″ ē) | anti-<br>-body | P<br>S | against<br>body | Protein substance produced in the body in response to an invading foreign substance (antigen) |
| **anticoagulant**<br>(ăn″ tǐ-kō-ăg′ ū-lănt) | anti-<br>coagul<br>-ant | P<br>R<br>S | against<br>clots<br>forming | Agent that works against the formation of blood clots |
| **antigen**<br>(ăn′ tǐ-jĕn) | anti-<br>-gen | P<br>S | against<br>formation, produce | Invading foreign substance that induces the formation of antibodies |
| **autoimmune disease**<br>(aw″ tō-ǐm-mūn dǐ-zēz) | | | | Condition in which the body's immune system becomes defective and produces antibodies against itself. Hemolytic anemia, rheumatoid arthritis, myasthenia gravis, and scleroderma are considered to be autoimmune diseases. |
| **autotransfusion**<br>(aw″ tō-trăns-fū′ zhŭn) | auto-<br>trans-<br>fus<br>-ion | P<br>P<br>R<br>S | self<br>across<br>to pour<br>process | Process of reinfusing a patient's own blood. Methods used include *harvesting* the blood 1 to 3 weeks before elective surgery; *salvaging* intraoperative blood; and collecting blood from trauma or selected surgical patients for reinfusion within 4 hours. |
| **basophil (baso)**<br>(bā′ sō-fǐl) | bas/o<br>-phil | CF<br>S | base<br>attraction | Cell that has an attraction for a base dye; a circulating granulocyte (white blood cell) that is essential to the nonspecific immune response to inflammation because of its role in releasing histamine and other chemicals that act on blood vessels |
| **blood** | | | | Fluid that circulates through the heart, arteries, veins, and capillaries |
| **coagulable**<br>(kō-ăg′ ū-lăb-l) | coagul<br>-able | R<br>S | to clot<br>capable | Capable of forming a clot |
| **corpuscle**<br>(kŏr′ pŭs-ĕl) | | | | Blood cell |
| **creatinemia**<br>(krē″ ă-tǐn-ē′ mǐ-ă) | creatin<br>-emia | R<br>S | flesh, creatine<br>blood condition | Condition of excess creatine (nitrogenous compound produced by metabolic processes) in the blood |
| **embolus**<br>(ĕm′ bō-lŭs) | | | | Blood clot carried in the bloodstream. A mass of undissolved matter present in a blood or lymphatic vessel and brought there by the blood or lymph current. Emboli can be solid, liquid, or gaseous. |
| **eosinophil**<br>**(eos, eosin)**<br>(ē″ ŏ-sǐn′ ō-fǐl) | eosin/o<br>-phil | CF<br>S | rose-colored<br>attraction | Cell that stains readily with an acid stain; attraction for the rose-colored stain; type of granulocytic white blood cell that destroys parasitic organisms and plays a major role in allergic reactions |

| MEDICAL WORD | WORD PARTS (WHEN APPLICABLE) | | | DEFINITION |
|---|---|---|---|---|
| | **Part** | **Type** | **Meaning** | |
| **erythroblast**<br>(ĕ-rĭth′ rō-blăst) | erythr/o<br>-blast | CF<br>S | red<br>immature cell,<br>germ cell | Immature red blood cell |
| **erythrocyte**<br>(ĕ-rĭth′ rō-sīt) | erythr/o<br>-cyte | CF<br>S | red<br>cell | Red blood cell |
| **erythrocytosis**<br>(ĕ-rĭth″ rō-sī-tō′ sĭs) | erythr/o<br>cyt<br>-osis | CF<br>R<br>S | red<br>cell<br>condition (usually<br>abnormal) | Abnormal condition in which there is an increase in red blood cells |
| **erythropoiesis**<br>(ĕ-rĭth″ rō-poy-ē′ sĭs) | erythr/o<br>-poiesis | CF<br>S | red<br>formation | Formation of red blood cells |
| **erythropoietin**<br>(ĕ-rĭth″ rō-poy′ ĕ′-tĭn) | erythr/o<br>poiet<br>-in | CF<br>R<br>S | red<br>formation<br>chemical | Glyco-protein hormone secreted by the kidneys in the adult and by the liver in the fetus, which acts on stem cells of the bone marrow to stimulate the production of red blood cells |
| **extravasation**<br>(ĕks-tră″ vă-sā′ shŭn) | extra-<br>vas(at)<br>-ion | P<br>R<br>S | beyond<br>vessel<br>process | Process by which fluids and/or medications (IVs) escape into surrounding tissue |
| **fibrin**<br>(fī′ brĭn) | fibr<br>-in | R<br>S | fiber<br>chemical | Insoluble protein formed from fibrinogen by the action of thrombin in the blood-clotting process |
| **fibrinogen**<br>(fī-brĭn′ ō-gĕn) | fibrin/o<br>-gen | CF<br>S | fiber<br>formation,<br>produce | Blood protein converted to fibrin by the action of thrombin in the blood-clotting process |
| **globulin**<br>(glŏb′ ū-lĭn) | globul<br>-in | R<br>S | globe<br>chemical | Plasma protein found in body fluids and cells |
| **granulocyte**<br>(grăn′ ū-lō-sīt″) | granul/o<br><br>-cyte | CF<br><br>S | little grain,<br>granular<br>cell | Granular leukocyte (white blood cell containing granules); a polymorpho-nuclear white blood cell (includes neutrophils, eosinophils, or basophils) |
| **hematocrit (Hct, HCT)**<br>(hē-măt′ ō-krĭt) | hemat/o<br>-crit | CF<br>S | blood<br>to separate | Blood test that separates solids from plasma in the blood by centrifuging the blood sample |
| **hematologist**<br>(hē″ mă-tŏl′ ō-jĭst) | hemat/o<br>log<br>-ist | CF<br>R<br>S | blood<br>study of<br>one who<br>specializes | Physician who specializes in the study of the blood |
| **hematology**<br>(hē″ mă-tŏl′ ō-jē) | hemat/o<br>-logy | CF<br>S | blood<br>study of | Study of the blood |
| **hematoma**<br>(hē″ mă-tō′ mă) | hemat<br>-oma | R<br>S | blood<br>mass, fluid<br>collection | Collection of blood that has escaped from a vessel into the surrounding tissues; results from trauma or incomplete hemostasis after surgery. See Figure 10–7 ▶. |

| MEDICAL WORD | WORD PARTS (WHEN APPLICABLE) | | | DEFINITION |
|---|---|---|---|---|
| | Part | Type | Meaning | |
| **hemochromatosis** (hē″ mō-krō″ mă-tō′ sǐs) | hem/o chromat -osis | CF R S | blood color condition (usually abnormal) | Genetic disease condition in which iron is not metabolized properly and accumulates in body tissues. The skin has a bronze hue, the liver becomes enlarged, and diabetes and cardiac failure can occur. |
| **hemoglobin (Hb, Hgb, HGB)** (hē″ mō-glō′ bǐn) | hem/o -globin | CF S | blood globe, protein | Blood protein; the iron-containing pigment of red blood cells that carries oxygen from the lungs to the tissues |
| **hemolysis** (hē-mŏl′ ǐ-sǐs) | hem/o -lysis | CF S | blood destruction | Destruction of red blood cells |
| **hemophilia** (hē″ mō-fǐl′ ǐ-ă) | hem/o -philia | CF S | blood attraction | Hereditary blood disease characterized by prolonged coagulation and tendency to bleed |
| **hemorrhage** (hĕm′ ĕ-rǐj) | hem/o -rrhage | CF S | blood bursting forth | Excessive bleeding; bursting forth of blood. See Figure 10–8 ▼. |

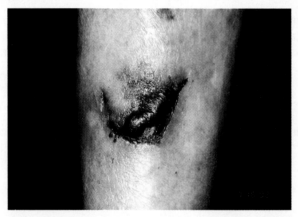

▶ **FIGURE 10–7** Traumatic hematoma. (Courtesy of Jason L. Smith, MD)

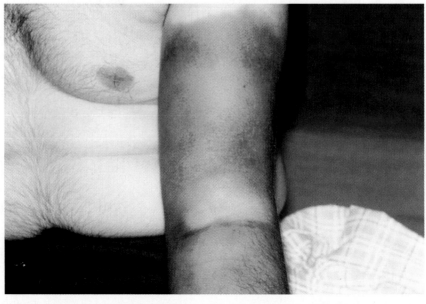

▶ **FIGURE 10–8** Hemorrhage, vein. (Courtesy of Jason L. Smith, MD)

| MEDICAL WORD | WORD PARTS (WHEN APPLICABLE) | | | DEFINITION |
|---|---|---|---|---|
| | Part | Type | Meaning | |
| **hemostasis**<br>(hē-mŏs′ tā-sĭs) | hem/o<br>-stasis | CF<br>S | blood<br>control, stop,<br>stand still | Control or stopping of bleeding. See Figure 10–9 ▼. |
| **heparin**<br>(hĕp′ ă-rĭn) | | | | Substance found in the liver, lungs, and other body tissues that inhibits blood clotting (anticoagulant). Clinically, heparin is used during certain types of surgery and in the treatment of deep venous thrombosis or pulmonary infarction. It can be administered by either subcutaneous or intravenous injection. |
| **hypercalcemia**<br>(hī″ pĕr-kăl-sē′ mĭ-ă) | hyper-<br>calc<br>-emia | P<br>R<br>S | excessive<br>lime, calcium<br>blood condition | Condition of excessive amounts of calcium in the blood |
| **hyperglycemia**<br>(hī″ pĕr-glī-sē′ mĭ-ă) | hyper-<br>glyc<br>-emia | P<br>R<br>S | excessive<br>sweet, sugar<br>blood condition | Condition of excessive amounts of sugar in the blood |
| **hyperlipemia**<br>(hī″ pĕr-lĭp-ē′ mĭ-ă) | hyper-<br>lip<br>-emia | P<br>R<br>S | excessive<br>fat<br>blood condition | Condition of excessive amounts of fat in the blood |
| **hypoglycemia**<br>(hī″ pō-glī-sē′ mĭ-ă) | hypo-<br>glyc<br>-emia | P<br>R<br>S | deficient<br>sweet, sugar<br>blood condition | Condition of deficient amounts of sugar in the blood |

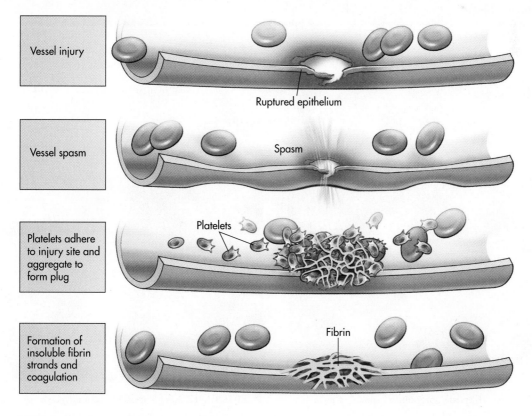

Vessel injury — Ruptured epithelium

Vessel spasm — Spasm

Platelets adhere to injury site and aggregate to form plug — Platelets

Formation of insoluble fibrin strands and coagulation — Fibrin

▶ **FIGURE 10–9** Basic steps in hemostasis.

| MEDICAL WORD | WORD PARTS (WHEN APPLICABLE) | | | DEFINITION |
|---|---|---|---|---|
| | Part | Type | Meaning | |
| **hypoxia**<br>(hī″ pŏks′ē-ă) | hyp-<br>-oxia | P<br>S | deficient<br>oxygen | Deficient amount of oxygen in the blood, cells, and tissues; also known as *anoxia* and *hypoxemia* |
| **immunoglobulin (Ig)**<br>(ĭm″ ū-nō-glŏb′ ū-lĭn) | immun/o<br>globul<br>-in | CF<br>R<br>S | immunity<br>globe<br>chemical | Blood protein capable of acting as an antibody. The five major types are IgA, IgD, IgE, IgG, and IgM. |
| **Kaposi's sarcoma (KS)**<br>(kăp′ ō-sēz săr-kō′ mă) | | | | Malignant neoplasm that causes violaceous (violet-colored) vascular lesions and general lymphadenopathy (diseased lymph nodes); it is the most common AIDS-related tumor. See Figures 10–10 ▼ and 10–11 ▼. |
| **leukapheresis**<br>(loo″ kă-fĕ-rē′ sĭs) | leuk/a<br>-pheresis | CF<br>S | white<br>removal | Separation of white blood cells from the blood, which are then transfused back into the patient |
| **leukemia**<br>(loo-kē′ mē-ă) | leuk<br>-emia | R<br>S | white<br>blood condition | Disease of the blood characterized by overproduction of leukocytes. See Figure 10–12 ▶. The disease may be malignant, acute, or chronic. ✶ See Pathology Spotlight: Leukemia on page 315 and Figure 10–24. |
| **leukocyte**<br>(loo′ kō-sīt) | leuk/o<br>-cyte | CF<br>S | white<br>cell | White blood cell |
| **leukocytopenia**<br>(loo″ kō-sī″ tō-pē′ nĭ-ă) | leuk/o<br>cyt/o<br>-penia | CF<br>CF<br>S | white<br>cell<br>lack of | Lack of white blood cells |
| **lymph**<br>(lĭmf) | | | | Clear, colorless, alkaline fluid found in the lymphatic vessels |
| **lymphadenitis**<br>(lĭm-făd″ ĕn-ī′ tĭs) | lymph<br>aden<br>-itis | R<br>R<br>S | lymph<br>gland<br>inflammation | Inflammation of the lymph glands |

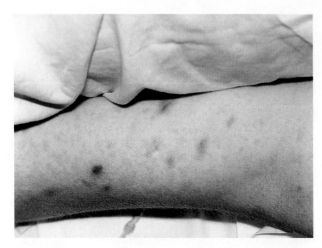

▶ **FIGURE 10–10**  Kaposi's sarcoma. (Courtesy of Jason L. Smith, MD)

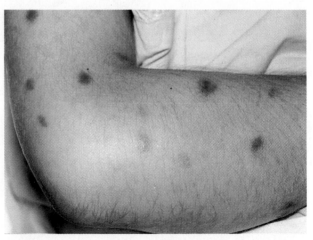

▶ **FIGURE 10–11**  Kaposi's sarcoma. (Courtesy of Jason L. Smith, MD)

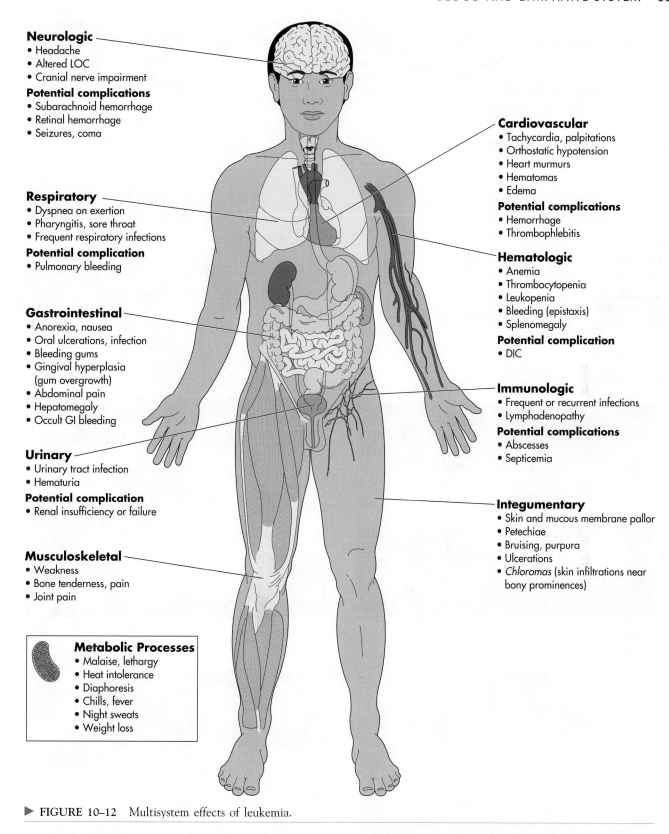

**Neurologic**
- Headache
- Altered LOC
- Cranial nerve impairment

**Potential complications**
- Subarachnoid hemorrhage
- Retinal hemorrhage
- Seizures, coma

**Respiratory**
- Dyspnea on exertion
- Pharyngitis, sore throat
- Frequent respiratory infections

**Potential complication**
- Pulmonary bleeding

**Gastrointestinal**
- Anorexia, nausea
- Oral ulcerations, infection
- Bleeding gums
- Gingival hyperplasia (gum overgrowth)
- Abdominal pain
- Hepatomegaly
- Occult GI bleeding

**Urinary**
- Urinary tract infection
- Hematuria

**Potential complication**
- Renal insufficiency or failure

**Musculoskeletal**
- Weakness
- Bone tenderness, pain
- Joint pain

**Metabolic Processes**
- Malaise, lethargy
- Heat intolerance
- Diaphoresis
- Chills, fever
- Night sweats
- Weight loss

**Cardiovascular**
- Tachycardia, palpitations
- Orthostatic hypotension
- Heart murmurs
- Hematomas
- Edema

**Potential complications**
- Hemorrhage
- Thrombophlebitis

**Hematologic**
- Anemia
- Thrombocytopenia
- Leukopenia
- Bleeding (epistaxis)
- Splenomegaly

**Potential complication**
- DIC

**Immunologic**
- Frequent or recurrent infections
- Lymphadenopathy

**Potential complications**
- Abscesses
- Septicemia

**Integumentary**
- Skin and mucous membrane pallor
- Petechiae
- Bruising, purpura
- Ulcerations
- *Chloromas* (skin infiltrations near bony prominences)

▶ FIGURE 10–12   Multisystem effects of leukemia.

| MEDICAL WORD | WORD PARTS (WHEN APPLICABLE) | | | DEFINITION |
|---|---|---|---|---|
| | **Part** | **Type** | **Meaning** | |
| **lymphadenotomy**<br>(lĭm-făd″ ĕ-nō tō-mē) | lymph<br>aden/o<br>-tomy | R<br>CF<br>S | lymph<br>gland<br>incision | Incision into a lymph gland |
| **lymphangiology**<br>(lĭm-făn″ jē-ŏl′ ō-jē) | lymph<br>angi/o<br>-logy | R<br>CF<br>S | lymph<br>vessel<br>study of | Study of the lymphatic vessels |
| **lymphangitis**<br>(lĭm″ făn-jī′ tĭs) | lymph<br>ang<br>-itis | R<br>R<br>S | lymph<br>vessel<br>inflammation | Inflammation of lymphatic vessels. See Figure 10–13 ▼. |
| **lymphedema**<br>(lĭmf-ĕ-dē′ mă) | lymph<br>-edema | R<br>S | lymph<br>swelling | Abnormal accumulation of lymph in the interstitial spaces. See Figure 10–14 ▼. |
| **lymphoma**<br>(lĭm-fō′ mă) | lymph<br>-oma | R<br>S | lymph<br>mass, fluid collection | Lymphoid neoplasm, usually malignant. See Figures 10–15 ▼ and 10–16 ▼. Lymphomas are identified as Hodgkin's disease or non-Hodgkin's lymphomas. Radiation therapy is the primary treatment for early stage Hodgkin's disease. |

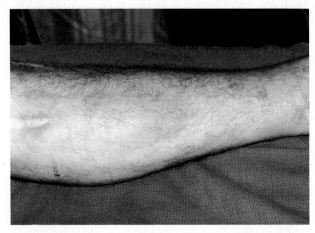

▶ **FIGURE 10–13** Lymphangitis. (Courtesy of Jason L. Smith, MD)

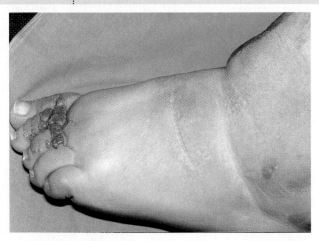

▶ **FIGURE 10–14** Chronic lymphedema. (Courtesy of Jason L. Smith, MD)

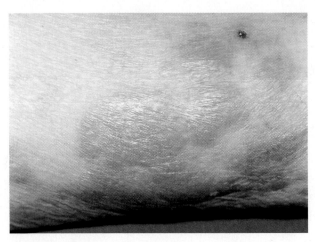

▶ **FIGURE 10–15** Lymphoma. (Courtesy of Jason L. Smith, MD)

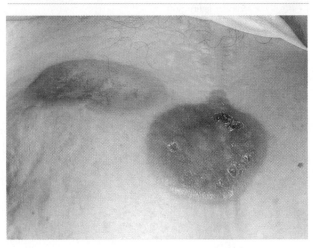

▶ **FIGURE 10–16** Cutaneous T cell lymphoma. (Courtesy of Jason L. Smith, MD)

| MEDICAL WORD | WORD PARTS (WHEN APPLICABLE) | | | DEFINITION |
|---|---|---|---|---|
| | **Part** | **Type** | **Meaning** | |
| **lymphostasis**<br>(lĭm-fō′ stā-sĭs) | lymph/o<br>-stasis | CF<br>S | lymph<br>control, stop,<br>stand still | Control or stopping of the flow of lymph |
| **macrocyte**<br>(măk′ rō-sīt) | macr/o<br>-cyte | CF<br>S | large<br>cell | Abnormally large erythrocyte |
| **monocyte (mono)**<br>(mŏn′ ō-sīt) | mono-<br>-cyte | P<br>S | one<br>cell | Largest leukocyte, which has one nucleus |
| **mononucleosis**<br>(mŏn″ ō-nū″ klē-ō′ sĭs) | mono-<br>nucle<br>-osis | P<br>R<br>S | one<br>kernel, nucleus<br>condition (usually<br>abnormal) | Condition of excessive amounts of mononuclear leukocytes in the blood |
| **neutrophil**<br>(nū′ trō-fĭl) | neutr/o<br>-phil | CF<br>S | neither<br>attraction | Leukocyte that stains with neutral dyes |
| **opportunistic infection**<br>(ŏp″ ŏr-too-nĭs′ tĭk ĭn-fĕk′ shŭn) | | | | Protozoal (PCP or toxoplasmosis), fungal/yeast (candidiasis), viral (herpes simplex), or bacterial (TB) infection that occurs when the immune system is compromised. AIDS patients are very vulnerable to these types of infections. |
| **pancytopenia**<br>(păn″ sī-tō-pē′ nĭ-ă) | pan-<br>cyt/o<br>-penia | P<br>CF<br>S | all<br>cell<br>lack of | Lack of the cellular elements of the blood |
| **phagocytosis**<br>(făg″ ō-sī-tō′ sĭs) | phag/o<br>cyt<br>-osis | CF<br>R<br>S | eat, engulf<br>cell<br>condition (usually<br>abnormal) | Engulfing and eating of particulate substances such as bacteria, protozoa, cells and cell debris, dust particles, and colloids by phagocytes (leukocytes or macrophages) |
| **plasma**<br>(plăz′ ma) | | | | Fluid part of the blood |
| **plasmapheresis**<br>(plăz″ mă-fĕr-ē′ sĭs) | plasma<br><br>-pheresis | R<br><br>S | a thing formed,<br>plasma<br>removal | Removal of blood from the body and centrifuging it to separate the plasma from the blood and reinfusing the cellular elements back into the patient |
| ***Pneumocystis carinii***<br>(nū″ mō-sĭs′ tĭs kă-rī′ nē-ī) | | | | Protozoan that causes *Pneumocystis carinii* pneumonia |
| ***Pneumocystis carinii* pneumonia (PCP)**<br>(nū″ mō-sĭs′ tĭs kă-rī′ nē-ī nū-mō′ nē-ă) | | | | Opportunistic infection that is prevalent in AIDS patients; has high mortality rate if not treated |
| **polycythemia**<br>(pŏl″ ē-sī-thē′ mĭ-ă) | poly-<br>cyt<br>hem<br>-ia | P<br>R<br>R<br>S | many<br>cell<br>blood<br>condition | Condition of too many red blood cells |
| **prothrombin**<br>(prō-thrŏm′ bĭn) | pro-<br>thromb<br>-in | P<br>R<br>S | before<br>clot<br>chemical | Chemical substance that interacts with calcium salts to produce thrombin |

| MEDICAL WORD | WORD PARTS (WHEN APPLICABLE) | | | DEFINITION |
|---|---|---|---|---|
| | **Part** | **Type** | **Meaning** | |
| **radioimmunoassay (RIA)** (rā″ dē-ō-ĭm″ ū-nō-ăs′ ā) | | | | Method of determining the concentration of protein-bound hormones in the blood plasma |
| **reticulocyte** (rĕ-tĭk′ ū-lō-sīt) | reticul/o -cyte | CF S | net cell | Red blood cell containing a network of granules; the last immature stage of a red blood cell |
| **retrovirus** (rĕt″rō-vī′rŭs) | | | | Virus that contains a unique enzyme called *reverse transcriptase* that allows it to replicate within new host cells. HIV is a retrovirus; once it enters the cell, it can replicate and kill the cells, some lymphocytes directly, and disrupt the functioning of the remaining CD4 cells. |
| **septicemia** (sĕp″ tĭ-sē′ mĭ-ă) | septic -emia | R S | putrefying blood condition | Condition in which pathogenic bacteria are present in the blood |
| **seroculture** (sē′ rō-kŭl″ chūr) | ser/o -culture | CF S | whey, serum cultivation | Bacterial culture of blood serum |
| **serum** (sē′ rŭm) | ser(a) -um | R S | whey, serum tissue | Clear, yellowish fluid that separates from the clot when blood clots |
| **sideropenia** (sĭd″ ĕr-ō-pē′ nĭ-ă) | sider/o -penia | CF S | iron lack of | Lack of iron in the blood |
| **splenomegaly** (splē″ nō-mĕg′ ă-lē) | splen/o -megaly | CF S | spleen enlargement | Enlargement of the spleen |
| **stem cell** (stĕm sĕl) | | | | Cell in the bone marrow that gives rise to various types of blood cells |
| **thalassemia** (thăl-ă-sē′ mĭ-ă) | thalass -emia | R S | sea blood condition | Hereditary anemias occurring in populations bordering the Mediterranean Sea and in Southeast Asia |
| **thrombectomy** (thrŏm-bĕk′ tō-mē) | thromb -ectomy | R S | clot surgical excision | Surgical excision of a blood clot |
| **thrombin** (thrŏm′ bĭn) | thromb -in | R S | clot chemical | Blood enzyme that causes clotting by forming fibrin |
| **thrombocyte** (thrŏm′ bō-sīt) | thromb/o -cyte | CF S | clot cell | Clotting cell; *a blood platelet* |
| **thromboplastin** (thrŏm″ bō-plăs′ tĭn) | thromb/o plast -in | CF R S | clot a developing chemical | Essential factor in the production of thrombin and blood clotting |

| MEDICAL WORD | WORD PARTS (WHEN APPLICABLE) | | | DEFINITION |
|---|---|---|---|---|
| | **Part** | **Type** | **Meaning** | |
| **thrombosis**<br>(thrŏm-bō' sĭs) | thromb<br>-osis | R<br>S | clot<br>condition<br>(usually abnormal) | Formation, development, or existence of a blood clot (thrombus) within the vascular system. In venous thrombosis (thrombophlebitis), a thrombus forms on the wall of a vein, accompanied by inflammation and obstructed blood flow. Thrombi can form in either superficial or deep veins. Deep vein thrombosis (DVT) is generally a complication of hospitalization, surgery, and immobilization. See Figure 10–17 ▼. |
| **thymoma**<br>(thī-mō' mă) | thym<br>-oma | R<br>S | thymus<br>mass, fluid<br>collection | Tumor of the thymus |

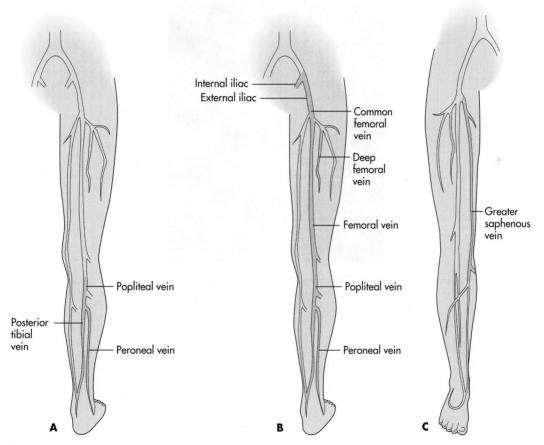

▶ **FIGURE 10–17**   Common locations of venous thrombosis. (A) The most common sites of deep vein thrombosis. (B) DVT extending from the calf to the iliac veins. (C) superficial venous thrombosis.

| MEDICAL WORD | WORD PARTS (WHEN APPLICABLE) | | | DEFINITION |
|---|---|---|---|---|
| | Part | Type | Meaning | |
| **tonsillectomy** (tŏn″ sĭl-ĕk′ tō-mē) | tonsill -ectomy | R S | tonsil surgical excision | Surgical excision of the tonsil. *Note that the root tonsill has two l's for tonsil. This is to form the correct spelling of the word tonsillectomy or other such words that relate to the tonsil.* |
| **transfusion** (trăns-fū″ zhŭn) | trans- fus -ion | P R S | across to pour process | Process by which blood is transferred from one individual to the vein of another |
| **vasculitis** (văs″ kŭ-lī′ tĭs) | vascul -itis | R S | small vessel inflammation | Inflammation of a lymph or blood vessel. See Figure 10–18 ▼. |

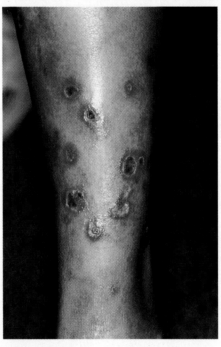

▶ **FIGURE 10–18** Vasculitis. (Courtesy of Jason L. Smith, MD)

# DRUG HIGHLIGHTS

| | |
|---|---|
| **Anticoagulants** | Used in inhibiting or preventing a blood clot formation. Hemorrhage can occur at almost any site in patients on anticoagulant therapy.<br><br>*Examples: heparin sodium, Coumadin (warfarin sodium), and Lovenox (enoxaparin)* |
| **Hemostatic agents** | Used to control bleeding; can be administered systemically or topically.<br><br>*Examples: Proplex (factor IX complement), Amicar (aminocaproic acid), vitamin K, and Surgicel (oxidized cellulose)* |
| **Antianemic agents (*irons*)** | Used to treat iron deficiency anemia. Oral iron preparations interfere with the absorption of oral tetracycline antibiotics. These products should not be taken within 2 hours of each other.<br><br>*Examples: Femiron (ferrous fumarate), Fergon, Fertinic (ferrous gluconate), and Feosol (ferrous sulfate)* |
| **Epoetin alfa (*EPO, Procrit*)** | Genetically engineered hemopoietin that stimulates the production of red blood cells. It is a recombinant version of erythropoietin and is indicated for treating anemia in patients with chronic renal failure and HIV-infected patients taking zidovudine (AZT). |
| **Other agents** | Agents used in treating folic acid deficiency including *Folvite (folic acid)*. Agents used in treating vitamin B$_{12}$ deficiency include *vitamin B$_{12}$ (cyanocobalamin)* injection. |

# DIAGNOSTIC AND LAB TESTS

| TEST | DESCRIPTION |
|---|---|
| **Antinuclear antibodies (ANA)**<br>(ăn″ tĭ-nū′ klē-ăr ăn′ tĭ-bŏd″ ēs) | Blood test to identify antigen–antibody reactions. ANA antibodies are present in a number of autoimmune diseases. |
| **Bleeding time**<br>(blēd′ ĭng tīm) | Puncture of the ear lobe or forearm to determine the time required for blood to stop flowing. With the Duke method (ear lobe), 1 to 3 minutes is the normal time, and with the Ivy (forearm), 1 to 9 minutes is the normal time for the flow of blood to cease. Times longer than these can indicate thrombocytopenia, aplastic anemia, leukemia, decreased platelet count, hemophilia, and potential hemorrhage. Anticoagulant drugs delay the bleeding time. |
| **Blood typing (ABO groups and Rh factor)**<br>(blod tīp′ ĭng) | Blood test to determine an individual's blood type (A, B, AB, and O) and Rh factor (can be negative [Rh−] or positive [Rh+]). |
| **Bone marrow aspiration**<br>(bōn măr′ ō ăs-pĭ-rā′ shŭn) | Removal of bone marrow for examination; can be performed to determine aplastic anemia, leukemia, certain cancers, and polycythemia. |
| **CD4 cell count**<br>(sēl kount) | Most widely used serum blood test to monitor the progress of AIDS. CD4 count of less than 200/mm$^3$ confirms AIDS diagnosis. CD4 is a protein on the surface of cells that normally helps the body's immune system fight disease. The HIV attaches itself to the protein to attack WBC, causing a failure of the patient's defense system. |

| **Complete blood count (CBC)** (kom-plēt′ blod kount) | Blood test that includes a hematocrit, hemoglobin, red and white blood cell count, and differential; usually part of a complete physical examination and a good indicator of hematologic system functioning. |
|---|---|
| **Enzyme-linked immuno-sorbent assay (ELISA)** (ĕn′zīm-lĭnk′ĕd ĭm″ū-nō-sŏr-bĕnt′ ă-sā) | Most widely used screening test for HIV. The latest generation of ELISA tests are 99.5% sensitive to HIV. Occasionally, the ELISA test will be positive for a patient without symptoms of AIDS from a low-risk group. Because this result is likely to be a false positive, the ELISA must be repeated *on the same sample of the patient's blood.* If the second ELISA is positive, the result should be confirmed by the Western blot test. |
| **Hematocrit (Hct, HCT)** (hē-măt′ ō-krĭt) | Blood test performed on whole blood to determine the percentage of red blood cells in the total blood volume. |
| **Hemoglobin (Hb, Hgb, HGB)** (hē″ mō-glō′ bĭn) | Blood test to determine the amount of iron-containing pigment of the red blood cells. |
| **Immunoglobulins (Ig)** (ĭm″ ŭ-nō-glŏb′ ū-lĭns) | Serum blood test to determine the presence of IgA, IgD, IgE, IgG, and/or IgM. Lymphocytes and plasma cells produce immunoglobulins in response to antigen exposure. Increased and/or decreased values can indicate certain disease conditions. |
| **Partial thromboplastin time (PTT)** (păr′ shāl thrŏm″ bō-plăs′ tĭn tīm) | Test performed on blood plasma to determine how long it takes for fibrin clots to form; used to regulate heparin dosage and to detect clotting disorders. |
| **Platelet count** (plāt′ lĕt kount) | Test performed on whole blood to determine the number of thrombocytes present. Increased and/or decreased amounts can indicate certain disease conditions. |
| **Prothrombin time (PT)** (prō-thrŏm′ bĭn tīm) | Test performed on blood plasma to determine the time needed for oxalated plasma to clot; used to regulate anticoagulant drug therapy and to detect clotting disorders. |
| **Red blood count (RBC)** (red blod kount) | Test performed on whole blood to determine the number of erythrocytes present; increased and/or decreased amounts can indicate certain disease conditions. |
| **Sedimentation rate (ESR)** (sĕd″ -ĭmĕn-tā′ shŭn rāt) | Blood test to determine the rate at which red blood cells settle in a long, narrow tube. The distance the RBCs settle in 1 hour is the rate. Higher or lower rate can indicate certain disease conditions. |
| **Viral load** (vī′ ral lōd) | Blood test that measures the amount of HIV in the blood. Results can range from 50 to more than 1 million copies per milliliter (mL) of blood. Two tests that are used to measure viral load are bDNA and PCR. |
| **Western blot test or immunoblot test** (Wĕst-ĕrn blōt or ĭm″ū-nō-blōt) | Used as a reference procedure to confirm the diagnosis of AIDS. In Western blot testing, HIV antigen is purified by electrophoresis (large protein molecules are suspended in a gel and separated from one another by running an electric current through the gel). If antibodies to HIV are present, a detectable antigen-antibody response occurs and a positive result is noted. |
| **White blood count (WBC)** (wīt blod kount) | Blood test to determine the number of leukocytes present. Increased level indicates infection and/or inflammation and decreased level indicates aplastic anemia, pernicious anemia, and malaria. |

# ABBREVIATIONS

| ABBREVIATION | MEANING |
|---|---|
| ABO | blood groups |
| AIDS | acquired immunodeficiency syndrome |
| ALL | acute lymphocytic leukemia |
| ANA | antinuclear antibodies |
| AZT | zidovudine |
| baso | basophil |
| CBC | complete blood count |
| CLL | chronic lymphocytic leukemia |
| CPR | cardiopulmonary resuscitation |
| diff | differential count |
| DVT | deep vein thrombosis |
| ELISA | enzyme-linked immunosorbent assay |
| eos, eosin | eosinophil |
| HAART | highly active antiretroviral therapy |
| Hb, Hgb, HGB | hemoglobin |
| Hct, HCT | hematocrit |

| ABBREVIATION | MEANING |
|---|---|
| HDN | hemolytic disease of the newborn |
| HIV | human immunodeficiency virus |
| Ig | immunoglobulin |
| IV | intravenous |
| KS | Kaposi's sarcoma |
| lymphs | lymphocytes |
| mL | milliliter |
| mono | monocyte |
| NK | natural killer (cells) |
| PCP | *Pneumocystis carinii* pneumonia |
| PT | prothrombin time |
| PTT | partial thromboplastin time |
| RBC | red blood cell (count) |
| Rh | Rhesus (factor) |
| RIA | radioimmunoassay |
| SOB | shortness of breath |
| TB | tuberculosis |
| WBC | white blood cell (count) |

# PATHOLOGY SPOTLIGHTS

## ✳ Acquired Immunodeficiency Syndrome

**Acquired immunodeficiency syndrome** (AIDS) is caused by the human immunodeficiency virus (HIV) and is the final stage of HIV disease. The virus attacks the immune system and leaves the body vulnerable to a variety of life-threatening illnesses and cancers.

The Centers for Disease Control and Prevention (CDC) defines AIDS as beginning when a person with HIV infection has a CD4 cell (also called a *T cell*, which is a type of immune cell) count below 200/mm³. AIDS is also defined by the opportunistic infections and cancers that occur in someone with HIV infection

Initial manifestation of HIV infection presents symptoms of a mononucleosis-type illness. It can take as little as a few weeks for minor symptoms to appear or as long as 10 years or more for more serious symptoms. Symptoms can include headache, chronic cough, diarrhea, swollen glands, lack of energy, loss of appetite and weight loss, frequent fevers and sweats, frequent yeast infections, skin rashes, pelvic and abdominal cramps, sores on certain parts of the body, and short-term memory loss. People age 50 and older might not recognize HIV symptoms in themselves because they think what they are feeling and experiencing is part of normal aging.

Anyone can get HIV and AIDS, regardless of age, particularly if any of the following is true:

- **Sexually active and does not properly use a latex condom.** Anyone can get HIV/AIDS from having sex with someone who is infected with the HIV virus. The virus passes from the infected person to another through the exchange of body fluids such as blood, semen, and vaginal fluid. HIV can get into the body during sex through any opening, such as a tear or cut in the lining of the vagina, vulva, penis, rectum, or mouth.

- **Ignorant of partner's sexual and drug history.** Has the partner been tested for HIV/AIDS? Has he or she had a number of different sex partners? Does the partner inject drugs?
- **Injects drugs and shares needles or syringes with other people.** Drug users are not the only people who share needles. People with diabetes, for example, who inject insulin or draw blood to test glucose levels, could share needles.
- **Had blood transfused between 1978 and 1985 or a blood transfusion or operation in a developing country at any time.**

One in ten persons with AIDS is 50 years of age or older. Approximately 4% of all AIDS cases are among those age 65 or older. Incidence of AIDS among older adults appear to be rising faster than in younger age groups. Immune function diminishes with age, and AIDS infection usually progresses more quickly in older adults.

The main form of treatment of AIDS is with antiviral therapy that suppresses the replication of the HIV virus. This treatment involves a combination of several antiretroviral agents, called *highly active antiretroviral therapy (HAART)*, and has been highly effective in reducing the number of HIV particles in the blood stream (as measured by a blood test called the *viral load*). This can help the immune system recover and improve the T cell count.

Medications are also used to prevent opportunistic infections (such as *Pneumocystis carinii* pneumonia) and can keep AIDS patients healthier for longer periods of time. Opportunistic infections are treated as they occur.

## ✱ Allergic Rhinitis

**Allergic rhinitis** is a collection of symptoms that typically occur in the nose and eyes after exposure to airborne particles of dust, dander, or the pollens of certain seasonal plants in people who are allergic to these substances. Symptoms include coughing, headache, sneezing, and itching nose, mouth, and eyes.

When the symptoms are caused by pollens, the allergic rhinitis is commonly known as *hay fever*. See Figure 10–19 ▶. This same reaction occurs with allergy to mold, animal dander, dust, and similar inhaled allergens.

To diagnose allergic rhinitis, the history of the person's symptoms is important, including whether the symptoms vary according to time of day or the season, exposure to pets or other allergens, and diet. Allergy testing can reveal the specific allergens to which the person is reacting. Skin testing, the most common method of allergy testing, can include intradermal, scratch, patch, or other tests.

The goal of treatment is to reduce the inflammation that causes allergy symptoms. The most effective treatment is avoidance of the allergens or reducing exposure to allergens. Medication options include over-the-counter and prescription antihistamines, nasal corticosteroid sprays, and decongestants.

Allergy shots (immunotherapy) can be administered if the allergen cannot be avoided and if symptoms are difficult to control. Immunotherapy includes regular injections of the allergen, given in increasing doses (each dose is slightly larger than the previous dose) that can help the body adjust to the allergen.

## ✱ Anaphylaxis

**Anaphylaxis** is a type of allergic reaction that is sudden (within seconds or minutes) and severe (can be life threatening) and affects the whole body. It is a response to a substance to which a person has become very sensitive.

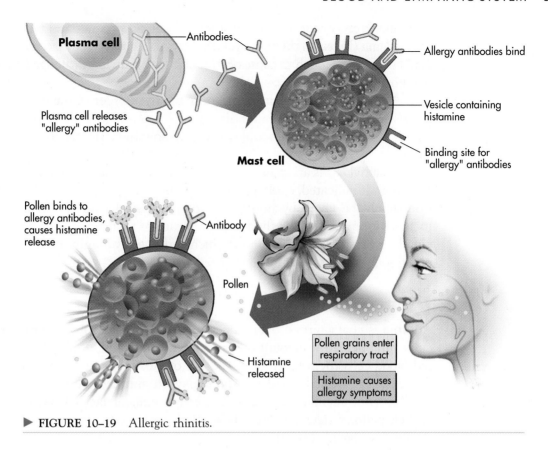

▶ **FIGURE 10–19**  Allergic rhinitis.

During an anaphylactic allergic reaction, tissues in different parts of the body release histamine and other substances. This causes constriction of the airways, resulting in wheezing, difficulty breathing, and gastrointestinal symptoms such as abdominal pain, cramps, vomiting, and diarrhea. See Figure 10–20 ▼.

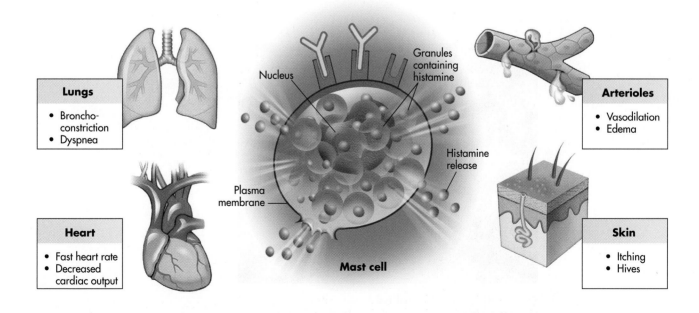

▶ **FIGURE 10–20**  Symptoms of anaphylaxis.

Shock can occur as a result of lowered blood pressure and blood volume. Hives and angioedema (hives on the lips, eyelids, throat, and/or tongue) often occur, and angioedema could be severe enough to cause obstruction of the airway. Prolonged anaphylaxis can cause heart arrhythmias.

Anaphylaxis can occur in response to any allergen. Common causes include insect bites/stings, food allergies, and drug allergies. Risks include prior history of any type of allergic reaction. Some people have an anaphylactic reaction with no identifiable cause.

Anaphylaxis is an emergency condition that requires immediate professional medical attention. If indicated, cardiopulmonary resuscitation (CPR) should be initiated. Epinephrine should be given by injection without delay. If the person is in shock, treatment includes intravenous (IV) fluids and medications that support the actions of the heart and circulatory system. Antihistamines (such as diphenhydramine) and corticosteroids (such as prednisone) can be given to further reduce symptoms.

 ## ✶ Anemia

**Anemia** is characterized by a reduction in the number of circulating red blood cells per cubic millimeter, the amount of hemoglobin per 100 mL of blood, or the volume of packed red blood cells (hematocrit) per 100 mL of blood. A normal red blood cell is doughnut-shaped with no nuclei and transports oxygen and carbon dioxide. See Figure 10–21 ▼. Symptoms of anemia are due to tissue **hypoxia,** or lack of oxygen. General symptoms include pallor, fatigue, dizziness, headaches, decreased exercise tolerance, tachycardia, and shortness of breath (SOB).

There are many types and causes of anemia. Iron deficiency anemia (see Figure 10–22 ▶) occurs when there is an increased iron requirement, impaired absorption of iron, or hemorrhage. Iron requirements are greatest during the first two years of life. During adolescence, girls and boys can become iron deficient due to inadequate dietary iron and increased growth requirements; and in girls at the onset of menses. Supplemental iron is usually required during this time and during pregnancy. Decrease in iron absorption occurs with malabsorption syndromes and chronic disease. Hemorrhage causes a loss of blood

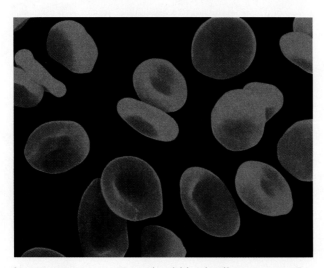

▶ **FIGURE 10–21** Normal red blood cells. (Source: Dr. Gopal Murti/Science Photo Library/Custom Medical Stock Photo, Inc.)

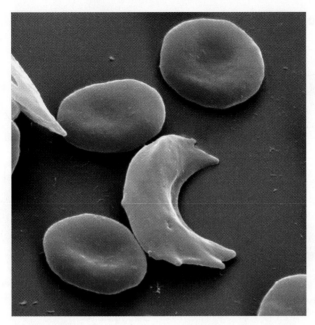

► **FIGURE 10–22**   Iron deficiency anemia blood cells.
(Source: Oliver Meckes & Nicole Ottawa/Photo Researchers, Inc.)

that could result in anemia. Other types of anemias include hemolytic, pernicious, vitamin $B_{12}$ deficiency, folic acid deficiency, sickle cell (see Figure 10–23 ► ), and thalassemia.

Treatment is according to the type of anemia and can include supplemental iron preparations, iron-rich foods, injections of iron, injections of vitamin $B_{12}$, folic acid supplementation, blood transfusions, or medications such as epoetin alfa.

## ✷ Leukemia

**Leukemia** is any of a group of diseases of the blood involving uncontrolled increase of white blood cells (leukocytes). Common types include chronic lymphocytic leukemia (CLL) and acute lymphocytic leukemia (ALL).

CLL is a malignancy (cancer) of the white blood cells (lymphocytes) characterized by a slow, progressive increase of these cells in the blood and the bone marrow.

Usually the symptoms develop gradually (see Figure 10–24 ►). The incidence of CLL is about 2 per 100,000 and increases with age; 90% of cases are found in people over 50 years old. Many cases are detected by routine blood tests in people with no symptoms. The cause of CLL is unknown.

ALL is a cancer of the lymph cells. It is characterized by large numbers of immature white blood cells that resemble lymphoblasts. These cells can be found in the blood, the bone marrow, the lymph nodes, the spleen, and other organs. ALL causes the blood cell to lose its ability to mature and specialize (differentiate) its function. These malignant cells multiply rapidly and replace the normal cells. Bone marrow failure occurs as malignant cells replace normal bone marrow elements. The person becomes susceptible to bleeding and infection because the normal blood cells are reduced in number.

ALL is responsible for 80% of the acute leukemias of childhood with the peak incidence occurring between ages 3 and 7, and comprises 20% of all adult leukemias. Most cases of ALL seem to have no apparent cause. However, radiation, some toxins such as benzene, and some chemotherapy agents are thought to contribute to this type of leukemia. Abnormalities in chromosomes can also play a role in the development of ALL.

## Hemoglobin S and Red Blood Cell Sickling

Sickle cell anemia is caused by an inherited autosomal recessive defect in Hb synthesis. Sickle cell hemoglobin (HbS) differs from normal hemoglobin only in the substitution of the amino acid valine for glutamine in both beta chains of the hemoglobin molecule.

When HbS is oxygenated, it has the same globular shape as normal hemoglobin. However, when HbS loses its oxygen, it becomes insoluble in intracellular fluid and crystallizes into rodlike structures. Clusters of rods form polymers (long chains) that bend the erythrocyte into the characteristic crescent shape of the sickle cell.

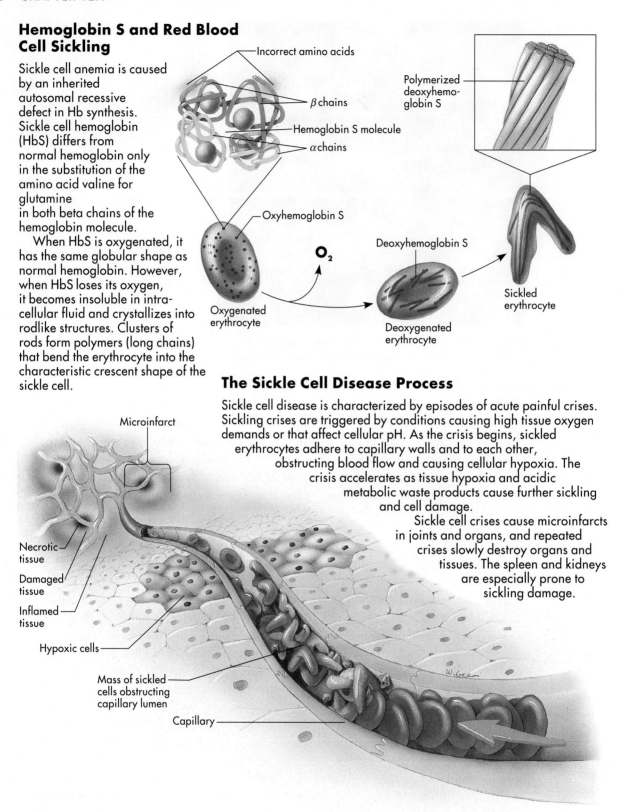

## The Sickle Cell Disease Process

Sickle cell disease is characterized by episodes of acute painful crises. Sickling crises are triggered by conditions causing high tissue oxygen demands or that affect cellular pH. As the crisis begins, sickled erythrocytes adhere to capillary walls and to each other, obstructing blood flow and causing cellular hypoxia. The crisis accelerates as tissue hypoxia and acidic metabolic waste products cause further sickling and cell damage.

Sickle cell crises cause microinfarcts in joints and organs, and repeated crises slowly destroy organs and tissues. The spleen and kidneys are especially prone to sickling damage.

▶ **FIGURE 10–23** Sickle cell anemia. The clinical manifestations of sickle cell anemia result from pathologic changes to structures and systems throughout the body.

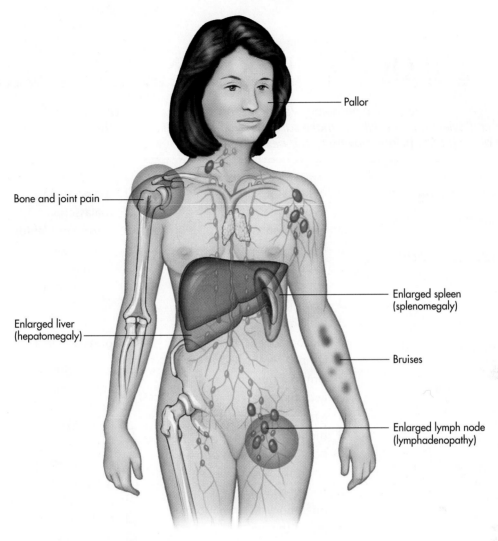

Pallor

Bone and joint pain

Enlarged spleen
(splenomegaly)

Enlarged liver
(hepatomegaly)

Bruises

Enlarged lymph node
(lymphadenopathy)

▶ **FIGURE 10–24**  Signs and symptoms of leukemia.

# ✔ PATHOLOGY CHECKPOINT

*Following is a concise list of the pathology-related terms that you have seen in the chapter. Review this checklist to make sure that you are familiar with the meaning of each term before moving to the next section.*

## Conditions and Symptoms

- ❑ acquired immunodeficiency syndrome
- ❑ acute lymphocytic leukemia
- ❑ allergy
- ❑ anaphylaxis
- ❑ anemia
- ❑ anisocytosis
- ❑ anoxia
- ❑ autoimmune disease
- ❑ chronic lymphocytic leukemia
- ❑ creatinemia
- ❑ deep vein thrombosis
- ❑ embolus
- ❑ erythrocytosis
- ❑ extravasation
- ❑ hematoma
- ❑ hemochromatosis
- ❑ hemophilia
- ❑ hemorrhage
- ❑ Hodgkin's disease

- ❑ hypercalcemia
- ❑ hyperglycemia
- ❑ hyperlipemia
- ❑ hypoglycemia
- ❑ hypoxemia
- ❑ hypoxia
- ❑ Kaposi's sarcoma
- ❑ leukemia
- ❑ leukocytopenia
- ❑ lymphadenitis
- ❑ lymphangitis
- ❑ lymphedema
- ❑ lymphoma
- ❑ mononucleosis
- ❑ non-Hodgkin's lymphoma
- ❑ opportunistic infection
- ❑ pancytopenia
- ❑ pneumocystis pneumonia
- ❑ polycythemia
- ❑ septicemia
- ❑ sickle cell anemia
- ❑ sideropenia

- ❑ splenomegaly
- ❑ thalassemia
- ❑ thrombophlebitis
- ❑ thrombosis
- ❑ thymoma
- ❑ tonsillectomy
- ❑ vasculitis

## Diagnosis and Treatment

- ❑ anticoagulant
- ❑ autotransfusion
- ❑ hematocrit
- ❑ hemostasis
- ❑ leukapheresis
- ❑ lymphadenotomy
- ❑ lymphostasis
- ❑ plasmapheresis
- ❑ radioimmunoassay
- ❑ seroculture
- ❑ thrombectomy
- ❑ transfusion

# STUDY AND REVIEW

## Anatomy and Physiology

*Write your answers to the following questions. Do not refer to the text.*

1. Name the three formed elements of blood.

   a. _____    b. _____

   c. _____

2. State the function of erythrocytes. _____

   _____

3. There are approximately _____ million erythrocytes per cubic millimeter of blood.

4. The life span of an erythrocyte is _____.

5. State the function of leukocytes. _____

   _____

6. There are approximately _____ thousand leukocytes per cubic millimeter of blood.

7. Name the five types of leukocytes.

   a. _____    b. _____

   c. _____    d. _____

   e. _____

8. State the function of thrombocytes. _____

   _____

9. There are approximately _____ thrombocytes per cubic millimeter of blood.

10. Name the four blood types.

    a. _____    b. _____

    c. _____    d. _____

11. State the three main functions of the lymphatic system.

    a. _____

    b. _____

    c. _____

12. Name the three accessory organs of the lymphatic system.

a. _____

b. _____

c. _____

## Word Parts

1. In the spaces provided, write the definition of these prefixes, roots, combining forms, and suffixes. Do not refer to the listings of medical words. Leave blank those words you cannot define.

2. After completing as many as you can, refer to the medical word listings to check your work. For each word missed or left blank, write the word and its definition several times on the margins of these pages or on a separate sheet of paper.

3. To maximize the learning process, it is to your advantage to do the following exercises as directed. To refer to the word-building section before completing these exercises invalidates the learning process.

## PREFIXES

*Give the definitions of the following prefixes.*

1. an- _____     2. anti- _____

3. auto- _____    4. ana- _____

5. extra- _____    6. hyper- _____

7. hypo- _____     8. mono- _____

9. pan- _____    10. poly- _____

11. pro- _____    12. trans- _____

13. hyp _____

## ROOTS AND COMBINING FORMS

*Give the definitions of the following roots and combining forms.*

1. aden _____     2. aden/o _____

3. agglutinat _____    4. all _____

5. angi/o _____    6. anis/o _____

7. bas/o _____    8. calc _____

9. chromat _____

10. fus _____

11. coagul _____

12. creatin _____

13. cyt _____

14. hem _____

15. cyt/o _____

16. eosin/o _____

17. erythr/o _____

18. globul _____

19. granul/o _____

20. hemat _____

21. hemat/o _____

22. hem/o _____

23. leuk _____

24. leuk/o _____

25. lip _____

26. log _____

27. lymph _____

28. lymph/o _____

29. macr/o _____

30. neutr/o _____

31. nucle _____

32. phag/o _____

33. plasma _____

34. reticul/o _____

35. septic _____

36. ser/o _____

37. sider/o _____

38. fibr _____

39. splen/o _____

40. thalass _____

41. thromb _____

42. thromb/o _____

43. thym _____

44. fibrin/o _____

45. tonsill _____

46. poiet _____

47. immun/o _____

48. ang _____

49. ser (a) _____

50. plast _____

51. vas (at) _____

52. vascul _____

## Suffixes

*Give the definitions of the following suffixes.*

1. -able _____

2. -ant _____

3. -blast _____

4. -body _____

5. -edema _____

6. -crit _____

7. -culture _____

8. -cyte _____

9. -ectomy _____

10. -emia _____

11. -ergy _____

12. -gen _____

13. -phylaxis _____

14. -globin _____

15. -um _____

16. -ic _____

17. -in _____

18. -ion _____

19. -ist _____

20. -itis _____

21. -logy _____

22. -lysis _____

23. -megaly _____

24. -oma _____

25. -osis _____

26. -penia _____

27. -pheresis _____

28. -phil _____

29. -philia _____

30. -poiesis _____

31. -rrhage _____

32. -stasis _____

33. -tomy _____

34. -ia _____

35. –oxia _____

## Identifying Medical Terms

*In the spaces provided, write the medical terms for the following meanings.*

1. _____ Process of clumping together, as of blood cells that are incompatible

2. _____ Individual hypersensitivity to a substance that is usually harmless

3. _____ Protein substance produced in the body in response to an invading foreign substance

4. _____ Agent that works against the formation of blood clots

5. _____ Invading foreign substance that induces the formation of antibodies

6. _____ Base cell, leukocyte

7. _____ Capable of forming a clot

8. _____ Excess of creatine in the blood

9. _____ Cell that readily stains with the acid stain

10. _____ Granular leukocyte

11. _____ One who specializes in the study of the blood

12. _____ Blood protein

13. _____ Excessive amounts of sugar in the blood

14. _____ Excessive amounts of fat in the blood

15. _____ White blood cell

16. _____ Control or stopping of the flow of lymph

17. _____ Condition of excessive amounts of mononuclear leukocytes in the blood

18. _____ Chemical substance that interacts with calcium salts to produce thrombin

19. _____ Surgical fixation of a movable spleen

20. _____ Clotting cell; blood platelet

## Spelling

*In the spaces provided, write the correct spelling of these misspelled terms.*

1. allregy _____

2. cretinemia _____

3. etravasation _____

4. erythcytosis _____

5. thrombplastin _____

6. hemacrit _____

7. hemorhage _____

8. lukemia _____

9. lymphadnotomy _____

10. anphylaxis _____

## Matching

*Select the appropriate lettered meaning for each of the following word.*

_____ 1. autotransfusion

_____ 2. erythrocyte

_____ 3. erythropoietin

_____ 4. extravasation

_____ 5. hemorrhage

_____ 6. immunoglobulin

_____ 7. hemochromatosis

_____ 8. radioimmunoassay

_____ 9. reticulocyte

_____ 10. thrombectomy

a. Method of determining the concentration of protein-bound hormones in the blood plasma

b. Disease condition in which iron is not metabolized properly and accumulates in body tissues

c. Blood protein capable of acting as an antibody

d. Red blood cell

e. Hormone that stimulates the production of red blood cells

f. Excessive bleeding

g. Process by which fluids and/or medications escape into surrounding tissue

h. Process of reinfusing a patient's own blood

i. Surgical excision of a blood clot

j. Red blood cell containing a network of granules

k. White blood cell

## Abbreviations

*Place the correct word, phrase, or abbreviation in the space provided.*

1. acquired immunodeficiency syndrome _____

2. body systems isolation _____

3. CML _____

4. hemoglobin _____

5. Hct _____

6. human immunodeficiency virus _____

7. PCP _____

8. PT _____

9. RBC _____

10. radioimmunoassay _____

## Diagnostic and Laboratory Tests

*Select the best answer to each multiple choice question. Circle the letter of your choice.*

1. Blood test to identify antigen–antibody reactions.
   a. sedimentation rate
   b. hematocrit
   c. immunoglobulins
   d. antinuclear antibodies

2. Blood test that includes a hematocrit, hemoglobin, red and white blood cell count, and differential.
   a. blood typing
   b. sedimentation rate
   c. CBC
   d. Hb, Hgb

3. Blood test performed on whole blood to determine the percentage of red blood cells in the total blood volume.
   a. RBC
   b. WBC
   c. Hct
   d. PTT

4. Blood test to determine the number of leukocytes present.
   a. RBC
   b. WBC
   c. Hct
   d. PTT

5. Puncture of the ear lobe or forearm to determine the time required for blood to stop flowing.
   a. bleeding time
   b. platelet count
   c. prothrombin time
   d. PTT

# PRACTICAL APPLICATION

## SOAP: Chart Note Analysis

*This exercise will make you aware of information, abbreviations, and medical terminology typically found in a family practice patient's chart.*

### Abbreviations Key

| | | | |
|---|---|---|---|
| **Abd** | abdomen | **NKDA** | no known drug allergies |
| **AIDS** | acquired immunodeficiency syndrome | **P** | pulse |
| | | **PCP** | *Pneumocystis carinii* pneumonia |
| **bid** | twice a day | | |
| **BP** | blood pressure | **PE** | physical examination |
| **CDC** | Centers for Disease Control and Prevention | **PERRLA** | pupils equal round and react to light and accommodation |
| **c/o** | complains of | | |
| **CTA** | clear to auscultation | **PO** | orally, by mouth |
| **DOB** | date of birth | **q4h** | every 4 hours |
| **F** | Fahrenheit | **R** | respiration |
| **GI** | gastrointestinal | **ROM** | range of motion |
| **Ht** | height | **SOAP** | subjective, objective, assessment, plan |
| **HEENT** | head, eyes, ears, nose, throat | **T** | temperature |
| **HIV** | human immunodeficiency virus | **Tab** | tablet |
| | | **TB** | tuberculosis |
| **lb** | pound | **TM** | tympanic membrane |
| **mg** | milligram | **Wt** | weight |
| **MS** | musculoskeletal | **y/o** | year(s) old |
| **Neuro** | neurology | | |

*Read the following chart note and then answer the questions that follow.*

**PATIENT:** Callins, Cora M.                                                      **DATE:** 8/1/2007

**DOB:** 7/21/55     **AGE:** 52     **SEX:** Female

**INSURANCE:** Millennia Health Insurance

**Vital Signs:**

T: 99.8 F

P: 88

R: 18

BP: 138/86

Ht: 5' 5"

Wt: 164 lb

**Allergies:** NKDA

**Chief Complaint:** Night sweats, weight loss, fatigue, diarrhea, swollen lymph nodes, and unusual confusion

**S | Subjective:** 52 y/o African American female presents with c/o night sweats, weight loss, fatigue, diarrhea, swollen lymph nodes, and unusual confusion. "It was months after the death of my husband when I began dating a younger man. We became sexually involved," she anxiously explained. She states that they did not use condoms because they were not concerned about pregnancy, and she didn't think to ask him about his previous sexual activities. "I am so afraid. Bill has just told me that he is HIV positive and could have AIDS."

**O | Objective:**

**General Appearance:** Middle-aged female, appears weary and anxious. Dark circles under both eyes.

**HEENT:** Normocephalic, PERRLA without exudate, conjunctivae clear, TM pearly gray in color with light reflex and landmarks intact, no perforations, no discharge or swelling, no lesions or exudate. Uvula midline and rises with phonation. Tonsils removed. Gag reflex present.

**Lymphatic:** Enlarged right parotid gland, painful to palpation. No other lymphadenopathy.

**Lungs:** CTA

**Heart:** Normal rate and rhythm. No murmurs or extra sounds. History of hypertension for past 6 years. Controlled with medication.

**Abd:** Bowel sounds all 4 quadrants. Soft, nontender. No palpable masses.

**MS:** Joints and muscles symmetric. Normal spinal curvature. No tenderness or palpation of joints. Full ROM.

**Neuro:** Oriented to person, place and time. Reflexes intact.

**Skin:** Warm and dry. No rashes or lesions.

**A | Assessment:** Acquired immunodeficiency syndrome (AIDS)

**P | Plan:**

1. Following a medical history, social history, complete PE, and receiving laboratory results: CD4 count of 180 cells/mm$^3$ and Western blot tests—positive, prescribed was a combination of antiretroviral drugs. The three drug regimen included AZT (zidovudine) 100 mg q4h; 3TC (lamiudine) 150 mg bid; and Norvir (ritonavir) 600 mg bid. Patient is to continue on Tenormin (atenolol) 50 mg Tab PO daily and Demadex (torsemide) 20 mg Tab PO daily for hypertension.
2. Monitor patient's response to antiretroviral drug therapy.
3. Instruct to notify physician if adverse reactions such as skin rash, fever, GI disturbances, headache, and malaise occur.
4. Schedule follow-up visits for clinical evaluation and laboratory monitoring every 3 to 6 months or more frequently if indicated.
5. Teach the patient about her condition. Provide brochures and written material on HIV infection, general effects of AIDS on the body, precautions that should be used during sexual intercourse, and opportunistic infections (such as TB, PCP, candidiasis, toxoplasmosis, and herpes simplex). Describe methods to avoid direct contact with microorganisms that can cause disease. One such method is proper handwashing, especially after urination, defecation, handling raw meat and/or pets, changing pet litter, gardening, or working with soil. Advise the patient to try to stay away from individuals who have contagious diseases because of risk of becoming infected due to her compromised immune system.
6. Stress the importance of appropriate nutrition, suitable sleep, proper personal hygiene, and getting regular exercise.
7. Inform the patient of the CDC's AIDS Hotline at 1-800-342-AIDS and web site resources for AIDS/HIV information: http://hivinsite.ucsf.edu; www.hopkins-aids.edu; and www.medscape.com.

**FYI:** Although the HIV virus can remain inactive in infected cells for years, antibodies are produced to its proteins, a process known as **seroconversion.** These antibodies are usually detectable 6 weeks to 6 months after the initial infection. Helper T or CD4 cells are the primary cells infected by HIV; these cells are involved in cellular immunity and the body's immune response in fighting off infection and disease. The loss of these CD4 cells leads to immunodeficiencies and developing opportunistic infections. A normal CD4 lymphocyte count is 1,000 to 1,300 cells/mm$^3$ and this patient's CD4 count was 180 cells/mm$^3$.

## Chart Note Questions
*Place the correct answer in the space provided.*

1. Signs and symptoms of AIDS include night sweats, weight loss, fatigue, _____ , swollen lymph nodes, and confusion.

2. The diagnosis of AIDS was determined by a complete physical examination and receiving laboratory results: CD4 count of 180 cells/mm$^3$ and Western blot tests, which was _____.

3. The three-drug regimen prescribed for this patient included AZT (zidovudine) 100 mg q4h; 3TC (lamiudine) 150 mg bid; and _____ 600 mg bid.

4. The patient is to continue on Tenormin (atenolol) 50 mg Tab PO daily and Demadex (torsemide) 20 mg Tab PO daily for _____.

5. The patient is instructed to notify the physician if adverse reactions such as skin rash, fever, GI disturbances, _____, and malaise occur.

6. Why did the patient not use condoms? _____

7. Why should the patient try to stay away from individuals who have contagious diseases? _____

8. What does the abbreviation *bid* mean? _____

9. Was the patient's blood pressure within normal limits? _____

10. _____ is one method that can be used to help avoid direct contact with microorganisms.

# MULTIMEDIA PREVIEW

*Additional interactive resources and activities for this chapter can be found on the Companion Website. For videos, audio glossary, and review, access the accompanying CD-ROM in this book.*

 **CD-ROM HIGHLIGHTS**

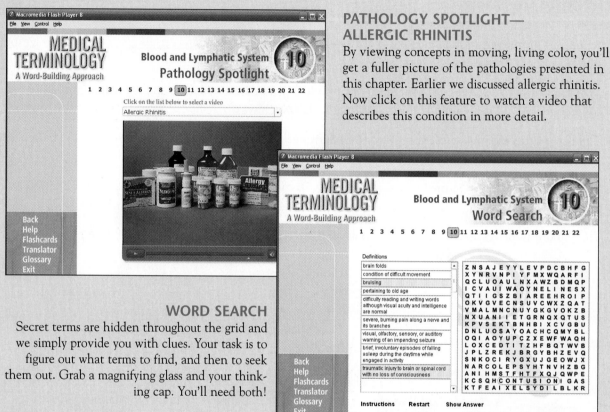

## PATHOLOGY SPOTLIGHT— ALLERGIC RHINITIS

By viewing concepts in moving, living color, you'll get a fuller picture of the pathologies presented in this chapter. Earlier we discussed allergic rhinitis. Now click on this feature to watch a video that describes this condition in more detail.

## WORD SEARCH

Secret terms are hidden throughout the grid and we simply provide you with clues. Your task is to figure out what terms to find, and then to seek them out. Grab a magnifying glass and your thinking cap. You'll need both!

 **WEBSITE HIGHLIGHTS—www.prenhall.com/rice**

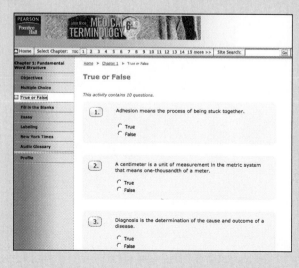

## TRUE/FALSE QUIZ

Take advantage of the free-access on-line study guide that accompanies your textbook. You'll find a true/false quiz that provides instant feedback, allowing you to check your score and see what you got right or wrong. By clicking on this URL you'll also access links to download mp3 audio reviews, current news articles, and an audio glossary.

# Respiratory System

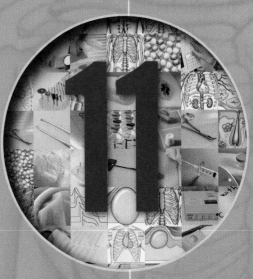

**11**

## ■ OBJECTIVES

*On completion of this chapter, you will be able to:*

- Describe the organs of the respiratory system.
- State the functions of the organs of the respiratory system.
- Define terms that physiologists and respiratory specialists use to describe the volume of air exchanged in breathing.
- State the vital function of respiration.
- Describe respiratory differences of the child and the older adult.
- Analyze, build, spell, and pronounce medical words.
- Comprehend the drugs highlighted in this chapter.
- Describe diagnostic and laboratory tests related to the respiratory system.
- Identify and define selected abbreviations.
- Describe each of the conditions presented in the Pathology Spotlights.
- Review the Pathology Checkpoint.
- Complete the Study and Review section and Chart Note Analysis.

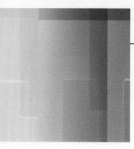

# Anatomy and Physiology Overview

The respiratory system consists of the nose, pharynx, larynx, trachea, bronchi, and lungs. Its primary function is to furnish oxygen ($O_2$) for individual tissue cells to use and to take away their gaseous waste product, carbon dioxide ($CO_2$). See Figure 11–1 ►. This process is accomplished through the act of **respiration** (R), which consists of external and internal processes. **External respiration** is the process by which the lungs are ventilated and oxygen and carbon dioxide are exchanged between the air in the lungs and the blood within capillaries of the alveoli. **Internal respiration** is the process by which oxygen and carbon dioxide are exchanged between the blood in tissue capillaries and the cells of the body.

## The Respiratory System

| Organ/Structure | Primary Functions |
|---|---|
| Nose | Serves as an air passageway; warms and moistens inhaled air; its cilia and mucous membrane trap dust, pollen, bacteria, and other foreign matter; contains olfactory receptors, which sort out odors; aids in phonation and the quality of voice |
| Pharynx | Serves as a passageway for air and for food; aids in phonation by changing its shape |
| Larynx | Produces vocal sounds |
| Trachea | Provides an open passageway for air to the lungs |
| Bronchi | Provide a passageway for air to and from the lungs |
| Lungs | Bring air into intimate contact with blood so that oxygen and carbon dioxide can be exchanged in the alveoli |

# NOSE

The **nose** is the projection in the center of the face; it consists of an external and internal portion. The *external portion* is a triangle of cartilage and bone that is covered with skin and lined with mucous membrane. The external entrance of the nose is known as the **nostrils** or **anterior nares**. The *internal portion* of the nose is divided into two chambers by a partition, the **septum,** separating it into a right and a left cavity. These cavities are divided into three air passages: the *superior, middle,* and *inferior conchae.* These passages lead to the pharynx and are connected with the paranasal sinuses by openings, with the ears by the eustachian tube, and with the region of the eyes by the nasolacrimal ducts.

The *palatine bones* and *maxillae* separate the nasal cavities from the mouth cavity. When the palatine bones fail to unite during fetal development, a congenital defect known as **cleft palate** occurs; it can be corrected by surgery. The nose is lined with mucous membrane, which is covered with *cilia.* The nasal mucosa produces about 946 mL or 1 qt of mucus per day. Four pairs of paranasal sinuses drain into the nose. These are the *frontal, maxillary, ethmoidal,* and *sphenoidal* sinuses. See Figure 11–2 ►.

## Functions of the Nose

Five functions have been attributed to the nose:

1. It serves as an air passageway.
2. It warms and moistens inhaled air.
3. Its cilia and mucous membrane trap dust, pollen, bacteria, and other foreign matter.

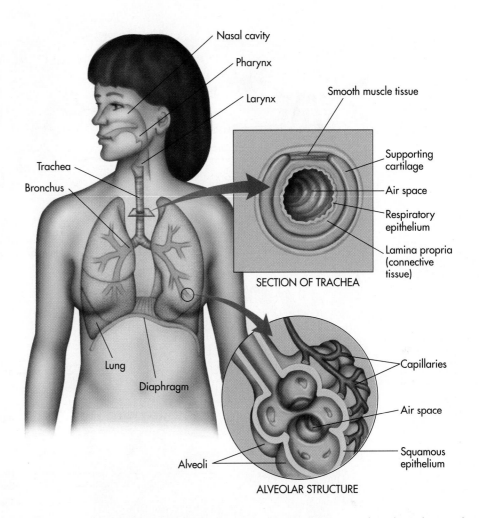

Nasal cavity
Pharynx
Larynx
Smooth muscle tissue
Supporting cartilage
Air space
Respiratory epithelium
Lamina propria (connective tissue)
SECTION OF TRACHEA
Trachea
Bronchus
Capillaries
Air space
Squamous epithelium
Lung
Diaphragm
Alveoli
ALVEOLAR STRUCTURE

▶ **FIGURE 11–1**   The respiratory system: nasal cavity, pharynx, larynx, trachea, bronchus, and lung with expanded views of the trachea and alveolar structure.

**4.** It contains olfactory receptors, which sort out odors.

**5.** It aids in phonation and the quality of voice.

# PHARYNX

The **pharynx** or throat is a musculomembranous tube about 5 inches long that extends from the base of the skull, lies anterior to the cervical vertebrae, and becomes continuous with the esophagus. It is divided into three portions: the *nasopharynx* located behind the nose, the *oropharynx* located behind the mouth, and the *laryngopharynx* located behind the larynx. Seven openings are found in the pharynx: two openings from the eustachian tubes, two openings from the posterior nares into the nasopharynx, the fauces or opening from the mouth into the oropharynx, and the openings from the larynx and the esophagus into the laryngopharynx. See Figure 11–2. Associated with the pharynx are three pairs of lymphoid tissues, which are the **tonsils.** The nasopharynx contains the *adenoids* or *pharyngeal* tonsils. The oropharynx contains the *faucial* or *palatine* tonsils and the *lingual* tonsils. The tonsils are accessory organs of the lymphatic system and aid in filtering bacteria and other foreign substances from the circulating lymph.

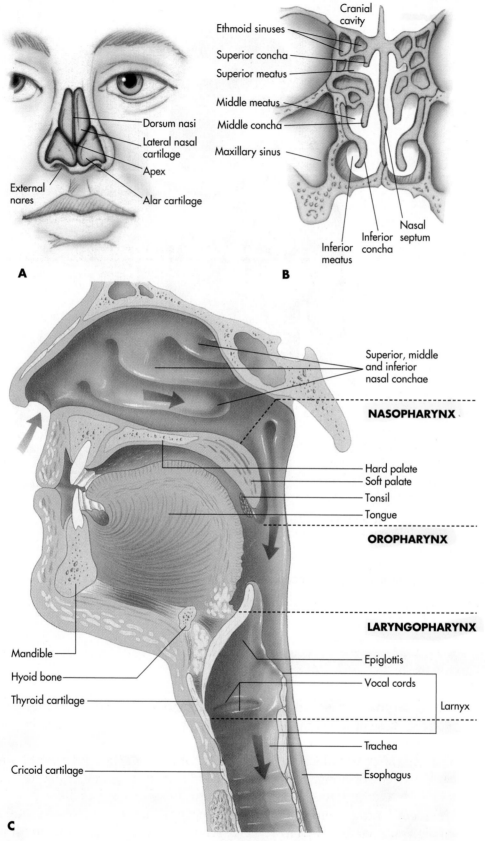

**A**

- Dorsum nasi
- Lateral nasal cartilage
- Apex
- External nares
- Alar cartilage

**B**

- Cranial cavity
- Ethmoid sinuses
- Superior concha
- Superior meatus
- Middle meatus
- Middle concha
- Maxillary sinus
- Inferior meatus
- Inferior concha
- Nasal septum

**C**

- Superior, middle and inferior nasal conchae

**NASOPHARYNX**

- Hard palate
- Soft palate
- Tonsil
- Tongue

**OROPHARYNX**

**LARYNGOPHARYNX**

- Mandible
- Hyoid bone
- Thyroid cartilage
- Epiglottis
- Vocal cords
- Larnyx
- Trachea
- Cricoid cartilage
- Esophagus

▶ **FIGURE 11–2**   Nose, nasal cavity, and pharynx: (A) nasal cartilages and external structure; (B) meatus and positions of the entrance to the ethmoid and maxillary sinuses; and (C) sagittal section of the nasal cavity and pharynx.

## Functions of the Pharynx

The following three functions are associated with the pharynx:

1. Serves as a passageway for air.
2. Serves as a passageway for food.
3. Aids in phonation by changing its shape.

# LARYNX

The **larynx** or voicebox is a muscular, cartilaginous structure lined with mucous membrane. It is the enlarged upper end of the trachea below the root of the tongue and hyoid bone. See Figures 11–1 and 11–2.

## Cartilages of the Larynx

The larynx is composed of nine cartilages bound together by muscles and ligaments. The three unpaired cartilages, each of which is described in following sections, are the *thyroid, cricoid,* and *epiglottis,* and the three paired cartilages are the *arytenoid, cuneiform, and corniculate.*

### Thyroid Cartilage

The **thyroid cartilage** is the largest cartilage in the larynx and forms the structure commonly called the *Adam's apple.* This structure is usually larger and more prominent in men than in women and contributes to the deeper male voice.

### Epiglottis

The **epiglottis** covers the entrance of the larynx, and during swallowing, it acts as a lid to prevent aspiration of food into the trachea. When the epiglottis fails to cover the entrance to the larynx, food or liquid intended for the esophagus can enter the trachea, causing irritation, coughing, or, in extreme cases, choking.

### Cricoid Cartilage

The **cricoid cartilage** is the lowermost cartilage of the larynx. It is shaped like a signet ring with the broad portion being posterior and the anterior portion forming the arch and resembling the ring's band.

The cavity of the larynx contains a pair of *ventricular folds* (false vocal cords) and a pair of vocal folds or true vocal cords (see Figure 11–3 ▶). The cavity is divided into three regions: vestibule, ventricle, and entrance to the glottis. The **glottis** is a narrow slit at the opening between the true vocal folds.

## Function of the Larynx

The function of the larynx is to produce vocal sounds. High notes are formed by short, tense vocal cords. Low notes are produced by long, relaxed vocal cords. The nose, mouth, pharynx, and bony sinuses aid in phonation.

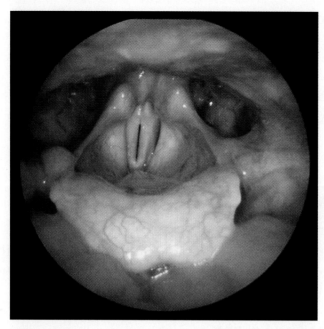

▶ **FIGURE 11–3**   Vocal cords. (CNRI/Phototake NYC)

## TRACHEA

The **trachea** or windpipe is a cylindrical cartilaginous tube that is the air passageway extending from the pharynx and larynx to the main bronchi. It is about 1 inch wide and 4½ inches (11.3 cm) long. It is composed of smooth muscle that is reinforced at the front and sides by C-shaped rings of cartilage. Mucous membrane lining the trachea contains **cilia,** which sweep foreign matter out of the passageway. The function of the trachea is to provide an open passageway for air to the lungs. See Figure 11–1.

## BRONCHI

The **bronchi** are the two main branches of the trachea, which provide the passageway for air to the lungs. The trachea divides into the **right bronchus** and the **left bronchus.** The right bronchus is larger and extends down in a more vertical direction than the left bronchus. When a foreign body is inhaled or aspirated, it frequently lodges in the right bronchus or enters the right lung. Each bronchus enters the lung at a depression, the **hilum.** The bronchi then subdivide into the bronchial tree composed of smaller bronchi, bronchioles, and alveolar ducts. The bronchial tree terminates in the *alveoli*, which are tiny air sacs supporting a network of capillaries from pulmonary blood vessels. The function of the bronchi is to provide a passageway for air to and from the lungs. See Figure 11–1.

## LUNGS

The **lungs** are cone-shaped, spongy organs of respiration lying on either side of the heart within the pleural cavity of the thorax. They occupy a large portion of the thoracic cavity and are enclosed in the **pleura,** a serous membrane composed of several layers. The six layers of the pleura are the *costal, parietal, pericardiaca, phrenica, pulmonalis,* and *visceral.* The *parietal pleura* extends from the roots of the lungs and lines the walls of the thorax and the superior surface of the diaphragm. The *visceral pleura* covers the surface of the lungs and enters into and lines the interlobar fissures. The pleural cavity is a space between the parietal and visceral pleura and contains a serous fluid that lubricates and prevents friction caused by the rubbing together of the two layers. The thoracic cavity is separated from the abdominal cavity by a musculomembranous wall, the **diaphragm.** The central portion of the thoracic cavity, between the lungs, is a space called the **mediastinum,** containing the heart and other structures.

The lungs consist of elastic tissue filled with interlacing networks of tubes and sacs that carry air and with blood vessels carrying blood. The broad inferior surface of the lung is the **base,** which rests on the diaphragm, while the **apex,** or pointed upper margin, rises from 2.5 to 5.0 cm above the sternal end of the first rib. The lungs are divided into **lobes,** with the right lung having three lobes and the left lung having two lobes. The left lung has an indentation, the **cardiac depression,** for the normal placement of the heart. In an average adult male, the right lung weighs approximately 625 g and the left about 570 g. In an average adult male, the total lung capacity (TLC) is 3.6 to 9.4 L, whereas in an average adult female it is 2.5 to 6.9 L. The lungs contain around 300 million **alveoli,** which are the air cells where the exchange of oxygen and carbon dioxide takes place. The main function of the lungs is to bring air into intimate contact with blood so that oxygen and carbon dioxide can be exchanged in the alveoli. See Figure 11–4 ▶.

## RESPIRATION

### Volume

The following terms are used by physiologists and respiratory specialists to describe the volume of air exchanged in breathing:

**Tidal volume (TV).** Amount of air in a single inspiration and expiration. In the average adult male, about 500 mL of air enters the respiratory tract during normal quiet breathing.

**Supplemental air.** Amount of air that can be forcibly expired after a normal quiet respiration. This is also the *expiratory reserve volume* and measures approximately 1200 mL.

**Complemental air.** Amount of air that can be forcibly inspired over and above a normal inspiration. This is known as the *inspiratory reserve volume* (IRV) and measures approximately 3600 mL.

**Residual volume (RV).** Amount of air remaining in the lungs after maximal expiration, about 1500 mL.

**Minimal air.** Small amount of air that remains in the alveoli. After death, if the thorax is opened and the lungs collapse, the minimal air pressure allows the lungs to float.

**Vital capacity (VC).** Volume of air that can be exhaled after a maximal inspiration. This amount equals the sum of the tidal air, complemental air, and the supplemental air.

**Functional residual capacity.** Volume of air that remains in the lungs at the end of a normal expiration.

**Total lung capacity (TLC).** Maximal volume of air in the lungs after a maximal inspiration.

### Vital Function of Respiration

**Temperature, pulse, respiration,** and **blood pressure** are the vital signs that are essential elements for determining an individual's state of health. A deviation from normal of one or all of the vital signs denotes a state of illness. Evaluation of an individual's response

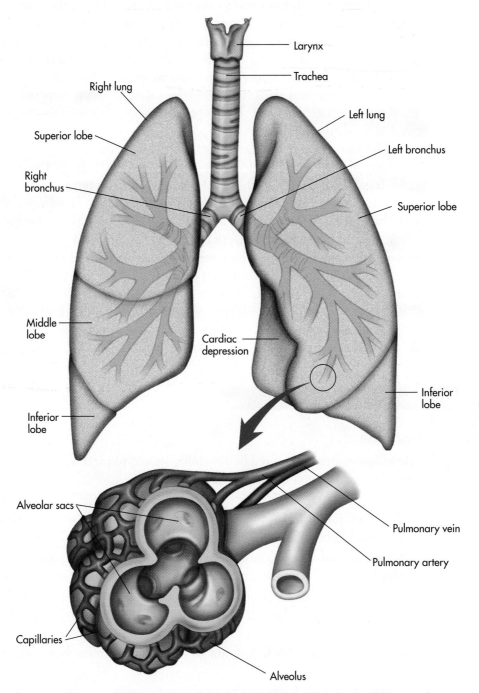

Larynx

Trachea

Right lung

Left lung

Superior lobe

Left bronchus

Right
bronchus

Superior lobe

Middle
lobe

Cardiac
depression

Inferior
lobe

Inferior
lobe

Alveolar sacs

Pulmonary vein

Pulmonary artery

Capillaries

Alveolus

▶ **FIGURE 11–4** Larynx, trachea, bronchi, and lungs with an expanded view showing the structures of an alveolus and the pulmonary blood vessels.

to changes occurring within the body can be measured by taking the vital signs. Through careful analysis of these changes in the vital signs, a physician can determine a diagnosis, a prognosis, and a plan of treatment for the patient. The variations of certain vital signs signify a typical disease process and its stages of development. For example, in a patient who has pneumonia, the temperature is elevated to 101° to 106°F, and pulse and respiration increase to almost twice their normal rates. When the temperature falls, the patient will perspire profusely and the pulse and respiration will begin to return to normal rates.

The process of *respiration* is interrelated with other systems of the body. The *medulla oblongata* and the *pons* of the central nervous system regulate and control respiration. The rate, rhythm, and depth of respiration are controlled by nerve impulses from the medulla oblongata and the pons via the spinal cord and nerves to the muscles of the diaphragm, abdomen, and rib cage.

## Respiratory Rate

Individuals of different ages breathe at different respiratory rates. The **respiratory rate** is regulated by the respiratory center located in the medulla oblongata. The following are respiratory rates for some different age groups:

| | |
|---|---|
| Newborn | 30 to 80 per minute |
| 1st year | 20 to 40 per minute |
| 5th year | 20 to 25 per minute |
| 15th year | 15 to 20 per minute |
| Adult | 15 to 20 per minute |

# LIFE SPAN CONSIDERATIONS

### ■ THE CHILD

At 12 weeks gestation, the lungs of the fetus have a definite shape. At 20 weeks, the fetus is able to suck its thumb and swallow amniotic fluid. The cellular structure of the **alveoli** of the lungs is complete. At 24 weeks, the nostrils open and respiratory movements occur. At 28 to 32 weeks, **surfactant** is produced. This is a substance formed in the lung that regulates the amount of surface tension of the fluid lining the alveoli. In preterm infants, the lack of surfactant contributes to respiratory distress syndrome.

During fetal life, gaseous exchange occurs at the placental interface. The lungs do not function until birth. The respiratory rate of the newborn is 30 to 80 per minute. During the first year, it is 20 to 40 per minute, and at age 5 it is 20 to 25 per minute. Around the 15th year, the respiratory rate is 15 to 20, the same as the average, healthy adult rate. Diaphragmatic abdominal breathing is common in infants. Accessory muscles of respiration are not as strong in infants as in older children and adults.

Oxygen consumption and metabolic rate are higher in children than in adults. Airway diameter is smaller in children, thereby increasing the potential for airway obstruction. The mucous membranes of children are vascular and susceptible to trauma, edema, and spasm.

### ■ THE OLDER ADULT

With advancing age, the respiratory system is vulnerable to injuries caused by infections, environmental pollutants, and allergic reactions. Age-related changes include a decline in the protection normally provided by intact mucous barrier, a decrease in the effectiveness of the bronchial cilia, and changes in the composition of the connective tissues of the lungs and chest. Older adults generally rely more on the **diaphragm** for inspiration, and when lying down, breathing requires more effort. **Vital capacity** declines with age; there is a decline in the elastic recoil of the lungs and an increase in the stiffness of the chest wall. This makes it more difficult for the older adult to inspire or expire air.

In the pharynx and larynx muscle, atrophy can occur with slackening of the vocal cords and loss of elasticity of the laryngeal muscles and cartilages. These changes can cause a gravelly, softer voice with a rise in pitch, making communication more difficult, especially if there is impaired hearing.

# BUILDING YOUR MEDICAL VOCABULARY

This section provides the foundation for learning medical terminology. Review the following alphabetized word list. Note how common prefixes and suffixes are repeatedly applied to word roots and combining forms to create different meanings.

| | |
|---|---|
| P | Prefix |
| R | Root |
| CF | Combining form |
| S | Suffix |

| | |
|---|---|
| Pink words | Terms not built from word parts. |
| * | Indicates words covered in the Pathology Spotlights section. |
| (CD) | Check the CD-ROM for more information. |

| MEDICAL WORD | WORD PARTS (WHEN APPLICABLE) | | | DEFINITION |
|---|---|---|---|---|
| | Part | Type | Meaning | |
| **alveolus** (ăl-vē′ ō-lŭs) | alveol | R | small, hollow air sac | Pertaining to a small air sac in the lungs |
| | -us | S | pertaining to | |
| **anthracosis** (ăn″ thră-kō′ sĭs) | anthrac | R | coal | Black lung, a lung condition caused by inhalation of coal dust and silica |
| | -osis | S | condition (usually abnormal) | |
| **apnea** (ăp′ -nē ă)  | a- | P | lack of | Temporary cessation of breathing. * See Pathology Spotlight: Apnea on page 353. |
| | -pnea | S | breathing | |
| **asphyxia** (ăs-fĭk′ sĭ-ă) | a- | P | lack of | Condition in which there is a depletion of oxygen in the blood with an increase of carbon dioxide in the blood and tissues; symptoms include dyspnea, cyanosis, and rapid pulse |
| | sphyx | R | pulse | |
| | -ia | S | condition | |
| **aspiration** (ăs″ pĭ-rā′ shŭn) | aspirat | R | to draw in | Process of drawing in or out by suction; can draw foreign bodies into the nose, throat, or lungs on inspiration |
| | -ion | S | process | |
| **asthma** (ăz′ mă) | | | | Disease of the bronchi characterized by wheezing, dyspnea, and a feeling of constriction in the chest. See Figure 11–5 ▶. * See Pathology Spotlight: Asthma on page 353. |
| **atelectasis** (ăt″ ĕ-lĕk′ tă-sĭs) | atel | R | imperfect | Condition of imperfect dilation of the lungs; the collapse of an alveolus, a lobule, or a larger lung unit |
| | -ectasis | S | dilation, expansion | |
| **bronchiectasis** (brŏng″ kĭ-ĕk′ tă-sĭs) | bronch/i | CF | bronchi | Chronic dilation of a bronchus or bronchi, with a secondary infection that usually involves the lower portion of a lung |
| | -ectasis | S | dilation, expansion | |

| MEDICAL WORD | WORD PARTS (WHEN APPLICABLE) | | | DEFINITION |
|---|---|---|---|---|
| | Part | Type | Meaning | |
| **bronchiolitis**<br>(brŏng″ kĭ-ō-lī′ tĭs) | bronchiol<br>-itis | R<br>S | bronchiole<br>inflammation | Inflammation of the bronchioles. |
| **bronchitis**<br>(brŏng-kī′ tĭs) | bronch<br>-itis | R<br>S | bronchi<br>inflammation | Inflammation of the bronchi |
| **bronchoscope**<br>(brŏng′ kō-skōp) | bronch/o<br>-scope | CF<br>S | bronchi<br>instrument for<br>examining | Instrument used to examine the bronchi.<br>See Figure 11–6 ▶. |
| **carbon dioxide (CO₂)**<br>(kăr bən dī-ŏk′ sīd) | | | | Colorless, odorless gas produced by the oxidation of carbon, it is a waste gas from metabolism that needs to be exhaled |
| **Cheyne-Stokes respiration**<br>(chān′ stōks′ rĕs″ pĭr-ā′ shŭn) | | | | Rhythmic cycle of breathing with a gradual increase in respiration followed by apnea (which may last from 10 to 60 sec), then a repeat of the same cycle |
| **cough**<br>(kawf) | | | | Sudden, forceful expulsion of air from the lungs; an essential protective response that clears irritants, secretions, or foreign objects from the trachea, bronchi, and/or lungs |
| **croup**<br>(croop) | | | | Acute respiratory disease (ARD) characterized by obstruction of the larynx, a barking cough, dyspnea, hoarseness, and stridor. See Figure 11–7 ▶. |

COPB – CHRONIC

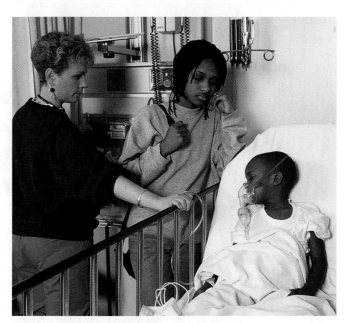

▶ FIGURE 11–5  Acute exacerbations of asthma can require management in the emergency department. The child is placed in a semisitting position to facilitate respiratory effort.

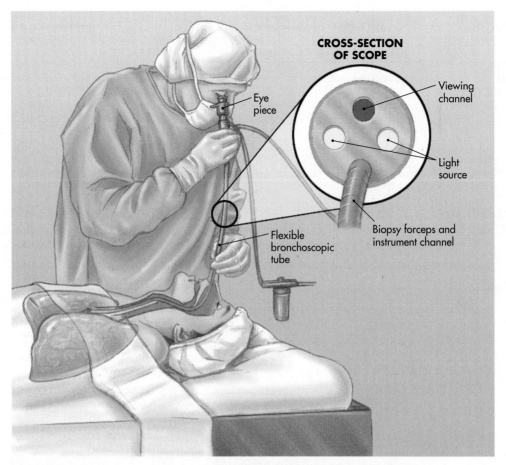

**CROSS-SECTION OF SCOPE**

Eye piece

Viewing channel

Light source

Flexible bronchoscopic tube

Biopsy forceps and instrument channel

▶ **FIGURE 11–6** Use of a bronchoscope during a bronchoscopy.

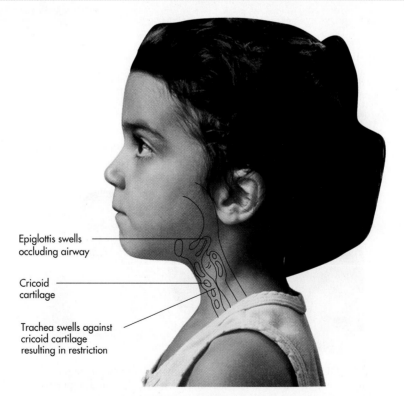

Epiglottis swells occluding airway

Cricoid cartilage

Trachea swells against cricoid cartilage resulting in restriction

▶ **FIGURE 11–7** Two important changes occur in the upper airway in croup: The epiglottis swells, thereby occluding the airway, and the trachea swells against the cricoid cartilage, causing restriction.

| MEDICAL WORD | WORD PARTS (WHEN APPLICABLE) | | | DEFINITION |
|---|---|---|---|---|
| | Part | Type | Meaning | |
| **cyanosis**<br>(sī″ ăn-ō′ -sĭs) | cyan<br>-osis | R<br>S | dark blue<br>condition (usually abnormal) | Abnormal condition of the skin and mucous membrane caused by oxygen deficiency in the blood. The skin, fingernails, and mucous membranes can appear slightly bluish or grayish. |
| **cystic fibrosis (CF)**<br>(sĭs′ tĭk fī-brō′ sĭs) | cyst<br>-ic<br>fibr<br>-osis | R<br>S<br>R<br>S | sac<br>pertaining to<br>fiber<br>condition (usually abnormal) | Inherited disease that affects the pancreas, respiratory system, and sweat glands. The gene responsible for this condition has been identified, and persons carrying the gene can be determined through genetic testing. See Figure 11–8 ▶. |
| **diaphragmatocele**<br>(dī″ ă-frăg-măt′ ō-sēl) | diaphrag-mat/o<br>-cele | CF<br>S | diaphragm, partition<br>hernia, tumor, swelling | Hernia of the diaphragm |
| **dysphonia**<br>(dĭs-fō′ nĭ-ă) | dys-<br>phon<br>-ia | P<br>R<br>S | difficult<br>voice<br>condition | Condition of difficulty in speaking; *hoarseness* |
| **dyspnea**<br>(dĭsp-nē′ ă) | dys<br>-pnea | P<br>S | difficult<br>breathing | Difficulty in breathing |
| **emphysema**<br>(ĕm″ fĭ-sē′ mă) | | | | Chronic pulmonary disease in which the alveoli become distended and the alveolar walls become damaged or destroyed, making it difficult to exhale air from the lungs. See Figure 11–9 ▶. |
| **empyema**<br>(ĕm″ pī-ē′ mă) | | | | Pus in a body cavity, especially the pleural cavity |
| **endotracheal (ET)**<br>(ĕn″ dō-trā′ kē-ăl) | endo-<br>trach/e<br>-al | P<br>CF<br>S | within<br>trachea<br>pertaining to | Within the trachea |
| **epistaxis**<br>(ĕp″ ĭ-stăk′ sĭs) | epi-<br>-staxis | P<br>S | upon<br>dripping | Nosebleed; usually results from traumatic or spontaneous rupture of blood vessels in the mucous membranes of the nose |
| **eupnea**<br>(ūp-nē′ ă) | eu-<br>-pnea | P<br>S | good, normal<br>breathing | Good or normal breathing |
| **exhalation**<br>(ĕks″ hə-lā′ shŭn) | ex-<br>halat<br>-ion | P<br>R<br>S | out<br>breathe<br>process | Process of breathing out |

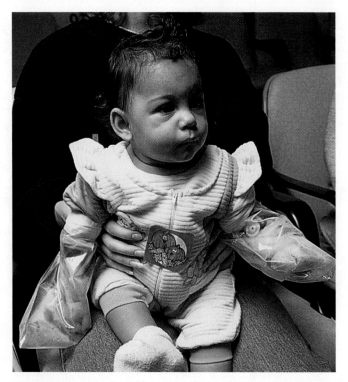

► FIGURE 11–8 Evaluation of a child for cystic fibrosis with a sweat chloride test. Sweat is being collected under the wrappings for later analysis of the amount of sodium and chloride.

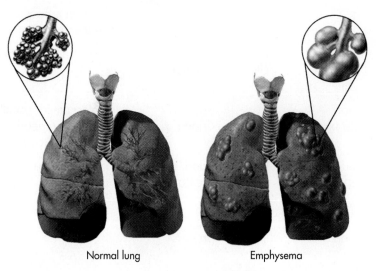

Normal lung                    Emphysema

► FIGURE 11–9 Normal lung and one with emphysema.

| MEDICAL WORD | WORD PARTS (WHEN APPLICABLE) | | | DEFINITION |
|---|---|---|---|---|
| | Part | Type | Meaning | |
| **expectoration**<br>(ĕk-spĕk″ tə′ rā′ shŭn) | ex-<br>pectorat<br>-ion | P<br>R<br>S | out<br>breast, chest<br>process | Process of coughing up and spitting out material (sputum) from the lungs, bronchi, and trachea |
| **Heimlich maneuver**<br>(hīm′ lĭk mă-nōō′ văr) | | | | Technique for removing a foreign body (usually a bolus of food) that is blocking the trachea. See Figure 11–10 ▼. |
| **hemoptysis**<br>(hē-mŏp′ tĭ-sĭs) | hem/o<br>-ptysis | CF<br>S | blood<br>to spit | Spitting up blood |
| **hyperpnea**<br>(hī″ pĕrp-nē′ ă) | hyper-<br>-pnea | P<br>S | excessive<br>breathing | Excessive or rapid breathing |
| **hyperventilation**<br>(hī″ pĕr-vĕn″ tĭ-lā′ shŭn) | hyper-<br>ventilat<br>-ion | P<br>R<br>S | excessive<br>to air<br>process | Process of excessive ventilating, thereby increasing the air in the lungs beyond the normal limit |
| **hypoxia**<br>(hī-pŏks′ ĭ-ă) | hyp-<br>ox<br>-ia | P<br>R<br>S | below, deficient<br>oxygen<br>condition | Condition of deficient amounts of oxygen in the inspired air |
| **influenza**<br>(ĭn″ floo-ĕn′ ză) | | | | Acute, contagious respiratory infection caused by a virus. Onset is usually sudden, and symptoms are fever, chills, headache, myalgia, cough, and sore throat. |
| **inhalation**<br>(ĭn″ hă-lă′ shŭn) | in-<br>halat<br>-ion | P<br>R<br>S | in<br>breathe<br>process | Process of breathing in |
| **laryngeal**<br>(lăr-ĭn′ jĭ-ăl) | laryng/e<br>-al | CF<br>S | larynx, voice box<br>pertaining to | Pertaining to the larynx (voice box) |

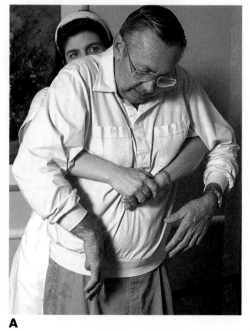
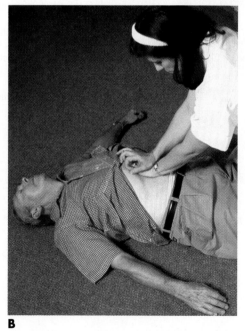

**A**    **B**

▶ FIGURE 11–10   Administration of abdominal thrusts (the Heimlich maneuver) to (A) a conscious victim and (B) an unconscious victim.

| MEDICAL WORD | WORD PARTS (WHEN APPLICABLE) | | | DEFINITION |
|---|---|---|---|---|
| | **Part** | **Type** | **Meaning** | |
| **laryngitis**<br>(lăr″ ĭn-jī′ tĭs) | laryng<br>-itis | R<br>S | larynx, voice box<br>inflammation | Inflammation of the larynx (voice box).<br>See Figure 11–11 ▼. |
| **laryngoscope**<br>(lăr-ĭn′ gō-skōp) | laryng/o<br>-scope | CF<br>S | larynx, voice box<br>instrument for<br>examining | Instrument used to examine the larynx<br>(voice box) |
| **Legionnaires' disease**<br>(lē jə naerz′ dĭ-zēz′) | | | | Severe pulmonary pneumonia caused by<br>*Legionella pneumophilia* |
| **lobectomy**<br>(lō-běk′ tō-mē) | lob<br>-ectomy | R<br>S | lobe<br>surgical excision | Surgical excision of a lobe of any organ<br>or gland, such as the lung |
| **mesothelioma**<br>(měs″ ō-thē″ lĭ-ō′ mă) | mes/o<br>thel/i<br>-oma | CF<br>CF<br>S | middle<br>nipple<br>tumor | Malignant tumor of mesothelium (serous<br>membrane of the pleura) caused by the<br>inhalation of asbestos |
| **nasopharyngitis**<br>(nā″ zō-făr′ ĭn-jī′ tĭs) | nas/o<br>pharyng<br>-it is | CF<br>R<br>S | nose<br>pharynx, throat<br>inflammation | Inflammation of the nose and pharynx<br>(throat) |
| **olfaction**<br>(ŏl-făk′ shŭn) | olfact<br>-ion | R<br>S | smell<br>process | Process of smelling |
| **oropharynx**<br>(or″ ō-făr′ ĭnks) | or/o<br>pharynx | CF<br>R | mouth<br>pharynx, throat | Central portion of the throat that lies<br>between the soft palate and upper<br>portion of the epiglottis |

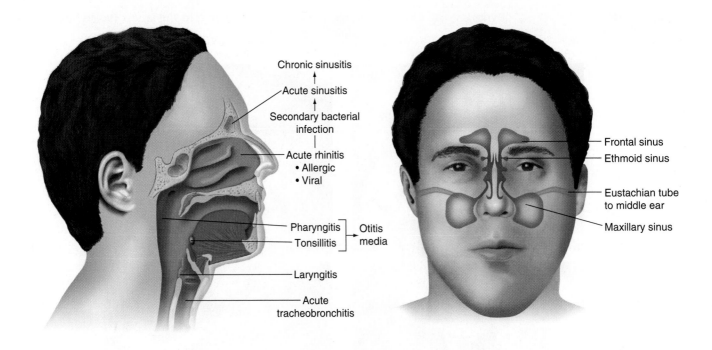

▶ **FIGURE 11–11** Paranasal sinuses are part of the upper respiratory system. From here, infections can spread via the nasopharynx to the middle ear or bronchi. Note locations of laryngitis, pharyngitis, sinusitis, and tonsillitis.

| MEDICAL WORD | WORD PARTS (WHEN APPLICABLE) | | | DEFINITION |
|---|---|---|---|---|
| | **Part** | **Type** | **Meaning** | |
| **orthopnea** (or″ thŏp-nē′ ă) | orth/o -pnea | CF S | straight breathing | Inability to breathe unless in an upright or straight position |
| **palatopharyngo- plasty** (păl″ ăt-ō-făr″ ĭn′ gō- plăs″ tē) | palat/o pharyng/o -plasty | CF CF S | palate pharynx, throat surgical repair | Type of surgery that relieves snoring and sleep apnea by removing the uvula and the tonsils and reshaping the lining at the back of the throat to enlarge the air passageway |
| **pertussis** (pĕr-tŭs′ ĭs) | | | | Acute, infectious disease caused by a bacterium *Bordetella pertussis*; characterized by a peculiar paroxysmal cough ending in a "crowing" or "whooping" sound; also called *whooping cough* |
| **pharyngitis** (făr″ ĭn-jī′ tĭs) | pharyng -itis | R S | pharynx, throat inflammation | Inflammation of the pharynx (throat). See Figure 11–11 on page 344. |
| **pleurisy** (ploo′ rĭsē) | | | | Inflammation of the pleura caused by injury, infection, or a tumor |
| **pleuritis** (ploo-rī′ tĭs) | pleur -itis | R S | pleura inflammation | Inflammation of the pleura |
| **pleurodynia** (ploo″ rō-dĭn′ ĭ-ă) | pleur/o -dynia | CF S | pleura pain | Pain in the pleura |
| **pneumoconiosis** (nū″ mō-kō″ nĭ-ō′ sĭs) | pneum/o con/i -osis | CF CF S | lung, air dust condition (usually abnormal) | Abnormal condition of the lung caused by the inhalation of dust particles such as coal dust (anthracosis), stone dust (chalicosis), iron dust (siderosis), and asbestos (asbestosis). Fiberotic tissue surrounding the alveoli limit their ability to stretch, thereby restricting the intake of air. |
| **pneumonia** (nū-mō′ nĭ-ă) | pneumon -ia | R S | lung, air condition | Inflammation of the lung caused by bacteria, viruses, fungi, or chemical irritants. See Figure 11–12 ▶. ✳ See Pathology Spotlight: Pneumonia on page 355. |
| **pneumonitis** (nū″ mō-nī′ tĭs) | pneumon -itis | R S | lung inflammation | Inflammation of the lung |
| **pneumothorax** (nū″ mō-thō′ răks) | pneum/o thorax | CF R | air chest | Collection of air in the chest cavity. See Figure 11–13 ▶. |
| **polyp** (pŏl′ ĭp) | | | | Tumor with a stem; can occur where there are mucous membranes, such as the nose, ears, mouth, uterus, and intestines |
| **pulmonectomy** (pŭl″ mō-nĕk′ tō-mē) | pulmon -ectomy | R S | lung surgical excision | Surgical excision of the lung or a part of a lung |

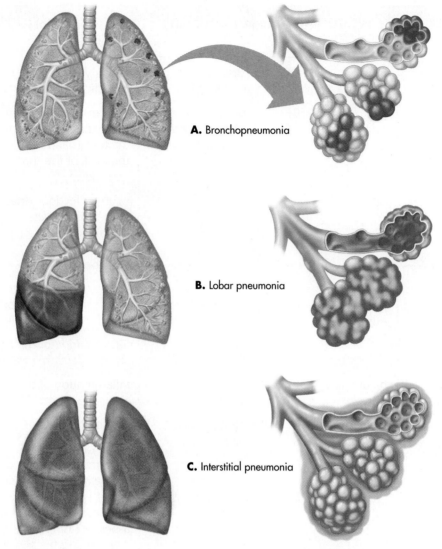

**A.** Bronchopneumonia

**B.** Lobar pneumonia

**C.** Interstitial pneumonia

▶ **FIGURE 11–12** (A) Bronchopneumonia with localized pattern. (B) Lobar pneumonia with a diffuse pattern within the lung lobe. (C) Interstitial pneumonia is typically diffuse and bilateral.

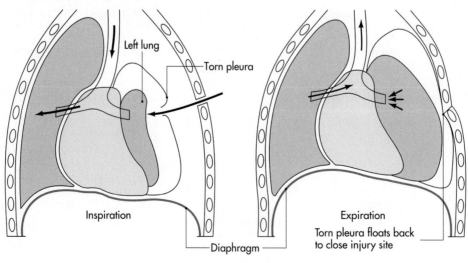

Left lung

Torn pleura

Inspiration

Diaphragm

Expiration

Torn pleura floats back to close injury site

▶ **FIGURE 11–13** Sucking chest wound (pneumothorax).

| MEDICAL WORD | WORD PARTS (WHEN APPLICABLE) | | | DEFINITION |
|---|---|---|---|---|
| | Part | Type | Meaning | |
| **pyothorax**<br>(pī″ ō-thō′ răks) | py/o<br>thorax | CF<br>R | pus<br>chest | Pus in the chest cavity |
| **rale**<br>(rahl) | | | | Abnormal sound heard on auscultation of the chest; a crackling, rattling, or bubbling sound |
| **respirator**<br>(rĕs′ pĭ-rā″ tor) | respirat<br>-or | R<br>S | breathing<br>a doer | Type of machine used for prolonged artificial respiration |
| **respiratory distress syndrome (RDS)**<br>(rĕs′ pĭ-ră-tō″ rē dĭs-trĕs′ sĭn′ drōm) | | | | Condition that can occur in a premature infant in which the lungs are not matured to the point of manufacturing lecithin, a pulmonary surfactant, resulting in collapse of the alveoli, which leads to cyanosis and hypoxia; also called *hyaline membrane disease (HMD)* |
| **respiratory syncytial virus (RSV) infection**<br>(rĕs′ pĭ-ră-tō″ rē sĭn″sĭ′shăl vī′rŭs) | | | | Most common cause of bronchiolitis and pneumonia among infants and children under 1 year of age. Illness begins with fever, runny nose, cough, and sometimes wheezing. Most children recover from illness in 8 to 15 days. It is contagious and is spread from respiratory secretions through close contact with infected persons or contact with contaminated surfaces or objects. |
| **rhinoplasty**<br>(rī′ nō-plăs″ tē) | rhin/o<br>-plasty | CF<br>S | nose<br>surgical repair | Surgical repair of the nose |
| **rhinorrhea**<br>(rī″ nō-rē′ ă) | rhin/o<br>-rrhea | CF<br>S | nose<br>flow, discharge | Discharge from the nose |
| **rhinovirus**<br>(rī″ nō-vī′ rŭs) | rhin/o<br>vir<br>-us | CF<br>R<br>S | nose<br>virus<br>pertaining to | One of a subgroup of viruses that cause the common cold (*coryza*) in humans |
| **rhonchus**<br>(rŏng′ kŭs) | rhonch<br>-us | R<br>S | snore<br>pertaining to | Rale or rattling sound in the throat or bronchial tubes caused by a partial obstruction |
| **sarcoidosis**<br>(sar″ koyd-ō′ sĭs) | sarc<br>-oid<br>-osis | R<br>S<br>S | flesh<br>resemble<br>condition (usually abnormal) | Chronic granulomatous condition that can involve almost any organ system of the body, usually involves the lungs, causing dyspnea on exertion |
| **severe acute respiratory syndrome (SARS)**<br>(si-vir′ ă-kūt′ rĕs′ pĭ-ră-tō″ -rē sin′ drōm) | | | | Contagious respiratory infection that was first described in February 2003; serious form of pneumonia resulting in acute respiratory distress and sometimes death |
| **sinusitis**<br>(sī″ nūs-ī′ tĭs) | sinus<br>-itis | R<br>S | a curve, hollow<br>inflammation | Inflammation of a sinus. See Figure 11–11 on page 344. |

| MEDICAL WORD | WORD PARTS (WHEN APPLICABLE) | | | DEFINITION |
|---|---|---|---|---|
| | Part | Type | Meaning | |
| **spirometer** (spī-rŏm' ĕt-ĕr) | spir/o -meter | CF S | breath instrument to measure | Instrument used to measure the volume of respired air |
| **sputum** (spū' tŭm) | | | | Substance coughed up from the lungs; can be watery, thick, purulent, clear, or bloody and can contain microorganisms |
| **stridor** (strī' dōr) | | | | High-pitched sound caused by obstruction of the air passageway |
| **tachypnea** (tăk" ĭp-nē' ă) | tachy- -pnea | P S | fast breathing | Fast breathing |
| **thoracocentesis** (thō" răk-ō-sĕn-tē' sĭs) | thorac/o -centesis | CF S | chest surgical puncture | Surgical puncture of the chest for removal of fluid; also called *thoracentesis*. See Figure 11–14 ▼. |
| **thoracoplasty** (thō' ră-kō-plăs" tē) | thorac/o -plasty | CF S | chest surgical repair | Surgical repair of the chest |
| **thoracotomy** (thō" răk- ŏt' ō-mē) | thorac/o -tomy | CF S | chest incision | Incision into the chest |
| **tonsillectomy** (tŏn" sĭl-ĕk' tō-mē) | tonsil -ectomy | R S | almond, tonsil surgical excision | Surgical excision of the tonsils |

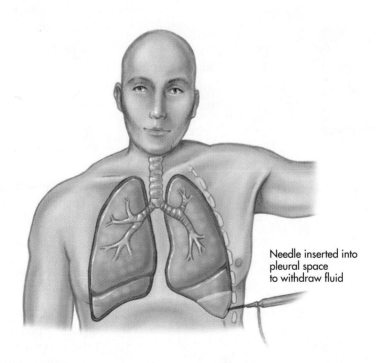

Needle inserted into pleural space to withdraw fluid

▶ FIGURE 11–14  Thoracocentesis (thoracentesis).

| MEDICAL WORD | WORD PARTS (WHEN APPLICABLE) | | | DEFINITION |
|---|---|---|---|---|
| | **Part** | **Type** | **Meaning** | |
| **tonsillitis**<br>(tŏn″ sĭl-ī′ tĭs) | tonsil<br>-itis | R<br>S | almond, tonsil<br>inflammation | Inflammation of the tonsils. See Figure 11–11 on page 344. |
| **tracheal**<br>(trā′ kē-ăl) | trach/e<br>-al | CF<br>S | trachea, windpipe<br>pertaining to | Pertaining to the trachea (windpipe) |
| **trachealgia**<br>(trā″ kē-ăl′ jĭ-ă) | trach/e<br>-algia | CF<br>S | trachea, windpipe<br>pain | Pain in the trachea (windpipe) |
| **tracheolaryn-**<br>**gotomy**<br>(trā″ kē-ō-lăr″ ĭn-gŏt′ ō-mē) | trache/o<br>laryng/o<br>-tomy | CF<br>CF<br>S | trachea, windpipe<br>larynx, voice box<br>incision | Incision into the larynx (voice box) and trachea (windpipe) |
| **tracheostomy**<br>(trā″ kē-ŏs′ tō-mē) | trache/o<br>-stomy | CF<br>S | trachea, windpipe<br>new opening | New opening into the trachea (windpipe). See Figure 11–15 ▼. |
| **tuberculosis (TB)**<br>(tū-bĕr″ kū-lō′ sĭs) | tubercul<br>-osis | R<br>S | a little swelling<br>condition (usually abnormal) | Infectious disease caused by the tubercle bacillus, *Mycobacterium tuberculosis.*<br>★ See Pathology Spotlight: Tuberculosis on page 355. |
| **wheeze**<br>(hwēz) | | | | Whistling sound caused by obstruction of the air passageway |

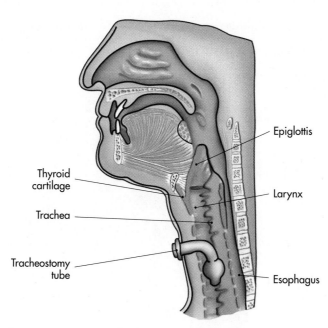

▶ **FIGURE 11–15**  Tracheostomy tube in place.

# DRUG HIGHLIGHTS

| | |
|---|---|
| **Antihistamines** | Act to counter the effects of histamine by blocking histamine 1 ($H_1$) receptors. They are used to treat allergy symptoms, prevent or control motion sickness, and in combination with cold remedies to decrease mucus secretion and produce bedtime sedation. See Figure 11–16 ▼.<br><br>*Examples: Benadryl (diphenhydramine HCl), Dimetane (brompheniramine maleate), Allegra (fexofenadine), Claritin (loratadine), and Zyrtec (cetirizine)* |
| **Decongestants** | Act to constrict dilated arterioles in the nasal mucosa. These agents are used for the temporary relief of nasal congestion associated with the common cold, hay fever, other upper respiratory allergies, and sinusitis. See Figure 11–16.<br><br>*Examples: Sudafed (pseudoephedrine HCl), Coricidin (phenylephrine HCl), Sinutab Long-Lasting Sinus Spray (xylometazoline HCl), and Afrin (oxymetazoline HCl)* |
| **Antitussives** | Can be classified as non-narcotic and narcotic. See Figure 11–16. |
|   Non-narcotic agents | Anesthetize the stretch receptors located in the respiratory passages, lungs, and pleura by dampening their activity and thereby reducing the cough reflex at its source.<br><br>*Examples: Tessalon (benzonatate), Benylin (diphenhydramine HCl), and dextromethorphan hydrobromide* |
|   Narcotic agents | Depress the cough center located in the medulla, thereby raising its threshold for incoming cough impulse.<br><br>*Examples: codeine and Codimal (hydrocodone bitartrate)* |
| **Expectorants** | Promote and facilitate the removal of mucus from the lower respiratory tract. See Figure 11–16.<br><br>*Examples: Robitussin (guaifenesin) and SSKI (saturated solution of potassium iodide)* |
| **Mucolytics** | Break chemical bonds in mucus, thereby lowering its thickness. See Figure 11–16.<br><br>*Example: Mucomyst (acetylcysteine)* |

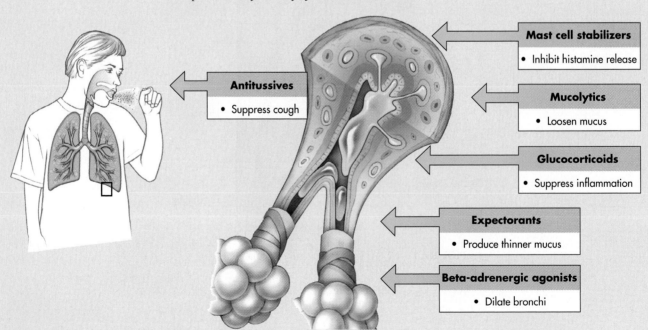

▶ **FIGURE 11–16** Drugs used to treat respiratory disorders.

| Bronchodilators | Used to improve pulmonary airflow by dilating air passages. See Figure 11–16. |
| | *Examples: Adrenalin (epinephrine), Proventil (albuterol), ephedrine sulfate, aminophylline, and Theo-24 (theophylline)* |
| Inhalational glucocorticoids | Used in the treatment of bronchial asthma and in seasonal or perennial allergic conditions when other forms of treatment are not effective. See Figure 11–16. |
| | *Examples: Beclovent (beclomethasone dipropionate), Azmacort (triamcinolone acetonide), Flovent (fluticasone), and Aerobid (flunisolide)* |
| Antituberculosis agents | Used in the long-term treatment of tuberculosis (9 months to 1 year). They are often used in combination of two or more drugs and the primary drug regimen for active tuberculosis combines the drugs *Myambutol (ethambutol HCl)*; *INH, Nydrazid (isoniazid)*; *and Rifadin, Rimactane (rifampin)* |

# DIAGNOSTIC AND LAB TESTS

| TEST | DESCRIPTION |
|---|---|
| **Acid-fast bacilli (AFB)** (ăs ĭd-făst" bă-sĭl' ī) | Test performed on sputum to detect the presence of *Mycobacterium tuberculosis*, an acid-fast bacilli. Positive results indicate tuberculosis. |
| **Antistreptolysin O (ASO)** (ăn" tĭ-strĕp-tŏl' ī-sĭn) | Test performed on blood serum to detect the presence of streptolysin enzyme O, which is secreted by beta-hemolytic streptococcus. Positive results indicate streptococcal infection. |
| **Arterial blood gases (ABGs)** (ăr-tē' rē-ăl blod găs' ĕs) | Series of tests performed on arterial blood to establish acid–base balance. Important in determining respiratory acidosis and/or alkalosis, metabolic acidosis, and/or alkalosis. |
| **Bronchoscopy** (brŏng-kŏs' kō-pē) | Visual examination of the larynx, trachea, and bronchi via a flexible bronchoscope. With the use of biopsy forceps, tissues and secretions can be removed for further analysis. |
| **Culture, sputum** (kŭl tūr, spū tŭm) | Examination of the sputum to determine the presence of microorganisms. Abnormal results can indicate tuberculosis, bronchitis, pneumonia, bronchiectasis, and other infectious respiratory diseases (RD). |
| **Culture, throat** (kŭl' tūr, thrōt) | Test that identifies the presence of microorganisms in the throat, especially beta-hemolytic streptococci. |
| **Laryngoscopy** (lăr" ĭn-gŏs' kō-pē) | Visual examination of the larynx via a laryngoscope. |
| **Nasopharyngography** (nā" zō-făr-ĭn-ŏg' ră-fē) | X-ray examination of the nasopharynx. |
| **Pulmonary function test** (pŭl' mō-nĕ-rē fŭng' shŭn test) | Series of tests performed to determine the diffusion of oxygen and carbon dioxide across the cell membrane in the lungs, including tidal volume (TV), vital capacity (VC), expiratory reserve volume (ERV), inspiratory capacity (IC), residual volume (RV), forced inspiratory volume (FIV), functional residual capacity (FRC), maximal voluntary ventilation (MVV), total lung capacity (TLC), and flow volume loop (F-V loop). Abnormal results can indicate various respiratory diseases and conditions. |
| **Rhinoscopy** (rī-nŏs' kō-pē) | Visual examination of the nasal passages. |

# ABBREVIATIONS

| ABBREVIATION | MEANING |
|---|---|
| ABGs | arterial blood gases |
| AFB | acid-fast bacilli |
| AIDS | acquired immunodeficiency syndrome |
| ARD | acute respiratory disease |
| ARDS | adult respiratory distress syndrome |
| ASO | antistreptolysin O |
| CF | cystic fibrosis |
| $CO_2$ | carbon dioxide |
| COLD | chronic obstructive lung disease |
| COPD | chronic obstructive pulmonary disease |
| CXR | chest x-ray |
| ENT | ear, nose, throat (otorhinolaryngology) |
| ERV | expiratory reserve volume |
| ET | endotracheal |
| FEF | forced expiratory flow |
| FEV | forced expiratory volume |
| FIV | forced inspiratory volume |
| FRC | functional residual capacity |
| F-V loop | flow volume loop |
| HBOT | hyperbaric oxygen therapy |
| HIV | human immunodeficiency virus |
| HMD | hyaline membrane disease |
| IC | inspiratory capacity |
| IPPB | intermittent positive-pressure breathing |

| ABBREVIATION | MEANING |
|---|---|
| IRDS | infant respiratory distress syndrome |
| IRV | inspiratory reserve volume |
| MBC | maximal breathing capacity |
| MV | minute volume |
| MVV | maximal voluntary ventilation |
| NSAIDs | nonsteroidal anti-inflammatory drugs |
| $O_2$ | oxygen |
| PE | pulmonary embolism |
| PEEP | positive end-expiratory pressure |
| PND | postnasal drip, paroxysmal nocturnal dyspnea |
| PPD | purified protein derivative |
| R | respiration |
| RD | respiratory disease |
| RDS | respiratory distress syndrome |
| RSV | respiratory syncytial virus |
| RV | residual volume |
| SARS | severe acute respiratory syndrome |
| SIDS | sudden infant death syndrome |
| SOB | shortness of breath |
| T & A | tonsillectomy and adenoidectomy |
| TLC | total lung capacity |
| TV | tidal volume |
| URI | upper respiratory infection |
| VC | vital capacity |

# PATHOLOGY SPOTLIGHTS

 **\* Apnea**    *STOP BREATHING*

**Apnea** is defined as a temporary cessation of breathing. **Sleep apnea** is cessation of breathing during sleep. The disruption of sleep patterns due to an obstruction of airways affects about 18 million Americans. To be so classified, the apnea must last for at least 10 seconds and occur 30 or more times during a 7-hour period of sleep. This definition cannot apply to older adults in whom periods of sleep apnea are increased. Sleep apnea is classified according to the mechanisms involved.

- **Obstructive apnea** is caused by obstruction to the upper airway. This condition generally occurs in middle-aged men who are obese and have a history of excessive daytime sleepiness. It is associated with loud snorting, snoring, and gasping sounds.
- **Central apnea** is marked by absence of respiratory muscle activity. A person with this type of apnea can exhibit excessive daytime sleepiness, but the snorting and gasping sounds during sleep are absent.

Sleep deprivation can make a person tired, sluggish, irritable, prone to accidents, and less productive. Although the amount of sleep needed is different for every person, adults need at least 7 hours of sleep in a 24-hour period, children under the age of 10 need 11 to 13 hours of sleep, and teenagers need 10 to 12 hours of sleep.

 **\* Asthma**

**Asthma** is an inflammatory disease of the bronchi characterized by **wheezing, dyspnea,** and a feeling of **constriction** in the chest. Inflammation of the airways causes airflow into and out of the lungs to be restricted. During an asthma attack, the muscles of the bronchial tree constrict and the lining of the air passages swells, reducing airflow and producing the characteristic wheezing sound. See Figure 11–17 ▼.

Asthma occurs in 3% to 5% of adults and 7% to 10% of children. Most people with asthma develop it before age 30 and half develop it before age 10. Generally, people with asthma experience periodic wheezing attacks as well as symptom-free periods. Specific symptoms can vary. Some asthmatics have chronic shortness of breath (SOB). Other

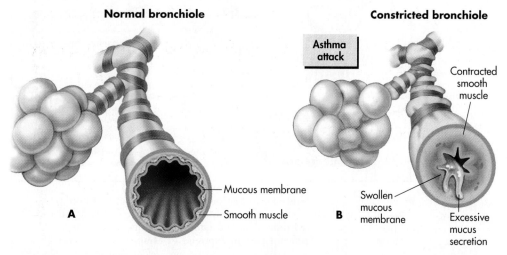

▶ **FIGURE 11–17**   Changes in bronchioles during an asthma attack: (A) normal bronchiole and (B) in asthma attack.

asthmatics have cough as the predominant symptom. The duration of asthma attacks varies from minutes to days. The attack can become dangerous if the airflow becomes severely restricted.

In asthma-prone individuals, symptoms can be triggered by inhaled allergens, such as pet dander, dust mites, cockroach allergens, molds, or pollens. A variety of other situations can also trigger symptoms, including respiratory infections, exercise, cold air, tobacco smoke and other pollutants, stress, and food or drug allergies. Aspirin and other non-steroidal anti-inflammatory drugs (NSAIDs) provoke asthma in some patients. See Figure 11–18 ▼.

The goal of treatment is to avoid known allergens and respiratory irritants and control symptoms and airway inflammation through medication. Two basic types of medication are used to treat asthma. The first type, long-term control medications such as inhaled

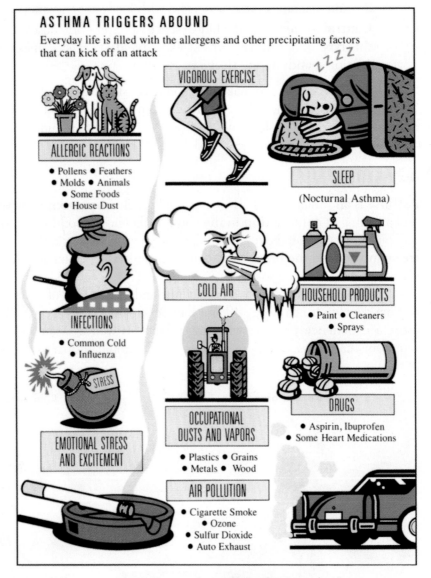

▶ **FIGURE 11–18**  This educational piece from the American Lung Association explains what triggers an asthmatic episode. The required lifestyle changes for the affected individual and family are significant. Culture sometimes plays a significant part in exposure to lifestyle triggers. (Reprinted with permission © 2006 American Lung Association.) For more information about the American Lung Association or to support the work it does, call 1-800-LUNG-USA (1-800-586-4872) or log on to www.lungusa.org.

glucocorticoids, are used on a regular basis to prevent attacks (not for treatment during an attack). The second type, quick relief (rescue) medications such as short-acting bronchodilators, are used to relieve symptoms during an attack.

## ✳ Pneumonia

**Pneumonia** is an inflammation of the lung (or lungs) caused by many different organisms such as bacteria, viruses, fungi, and chemical irritants. Bacterial pneumonias tend to be the most serious. In adults, bacteria are the most common cause of pneumonia, and of these, *Streptococcus pneumoniae* (pneumococcus) is the most common. In some people, particularly the elderly and those who are debilitated, pneumonia can follow influenza.

Pneumonia affects 3 to 4 million people each year in the United States. Symptoms include a cough with greenish mucus or puslike sputum, chills, fever, fatigue, chest pain, and muscle aches. Initial diagnosis is made through auscultation of the chest with a stethoscope. In patients with pneumonia, rales and other abnormal breathing sounds can be heard. Tests that are used to confirm the diagnosis include a chest x-ray (See Figure 11–19 ▼) and a sputum culture.

Treatment of pneumonia is determined by the organism that caused it. If the cause is bacterial, the infection is treated with antibiotics. However, if the pneumonia is caused by a virus, antibiotics are not effective. Supportive therapy includes oxygen and respiratory treatments to remove secretions, if needed.

## ✳ Tuberculosis

**Tuberculosis** (TB) is a contagious disease caused by the bacillus *Mycobacterium tuberculosis,* which is carried in airborne particles known as **droplets.** An infected person releases large and small droplets through talking, coughing, sneezing, laughing, or singing. The

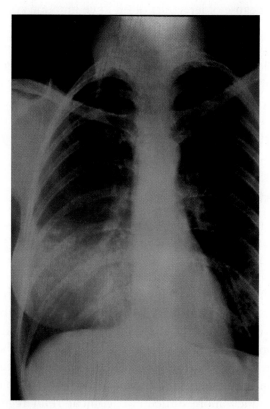

▶ **FIGURE 11–19** Lobar pneumonia. (Source: Photo Researchers, Inc.)

large droplets settle while the small droplets remain suspended in the air and can be inhaled by a susceptible person. Virtually anyone who comes in contact with an infected person is at risk of contracting TB. An estimated 10 million people in the United States are infected with the TB bacterium, and it is still a major cause of death worldwide, killing 2 million people each year.

Symptoms of TB depend on where in the body the TB bacteria are growing. The disease is characterized by the development of granulomas (granular tumors) in the infected tissues. TB bacteria usually grow in the lungs; symptoms include a chronic cough, hemoptysis, and—in the early stages—scanty, whitish or grayish-yellow frothy sputum. Other symptoms are fatigue, low-grade fever, night sweats, weakness, chills, anorexia, and weight loss.

Diagnosis includes examination of the lungs by stethoscope (auscultation), which can reveal rales or crackles. Enlarged or tender lymph nodes can be present in the neck or other areas. Fluid can be detected around a lung (pleural effusion). Tests to confirm diagnosis often include a chest x-ray, sputum cultures, a tuberculin skin test, and bronchoscopy. Treatment of TB requires long-term drug therapy (9 to 12 months), often using a regimen that includes a combination of antituberculosis agents (generally *rifampin, isoniazid,* and *ethambutol*). A balanced diet and rest are also important aspects of the treatment plan.

Factors contributing to the spread of tuberculosis in the United States include these:

- Infection with HIV, which suppresses the immune system, making it difficult for the body to control TB bacteria. As a result, most HIV-positive people who are newly infected with tuberculosis progress to active TB. About one-third of the 38 million people living with AIDS also have tuberculosis.

- Crowded living conditions, such as in prisons, juvenile detention centers, homeless shelters, and other cramped, poorly ventilated spaces. TB bacteria also can flourish in nursing homes because older adults often have immune systems weakened by illness or aging.

- Increased number of foreign-born immigrants and travelers to the United States appears to be an element in the spread of TB. Although tuberculosis rates for people born in the United States are declining, the incidence among people from other parts of the world, especially Africa, Asia, and Latin America, is increasing. It is reported that nearly half the TB cases in the United States occur in people born outside the country. These numbers point to the global nature of the disease and the need to combat it on a worldwide scale.

## ✷ Multidrug-Resistant TB

The development of drug-resistant strains of bacteria is one of the most alarming trends in health care. The problem is particularly serious with regard to TB bacteria that have developed strains resistant to treatment with one of each of the major tuberculosis medications. Even more dangerous are strains that are resistant to at least two anti-TB drugs, leading to a condition called **multidrug-resistant TB** (MDR TB). People with untreated MDR TB are highly contagious and can transmit this serious type of tuberculosis to others. Multidrug-resistant TB bacteria can develop when people either do not complete the entire course of medication or fail to take their medications as prescribed, when health care professionals prescribe the wrong kinds of treatment, or when the drug supply is inconsistent—a particular problem in impoverished or war-torn areas. Although MDR TB can be treated successfully, it is much more difficult to combat than regular tuberculosis and requires long-term therapy—up to two years—with drugs that can cause serious side effects.

# ✓ PATHOLOGY CHECKPOINT

*Following is a concise list of the pathology-related terms that you have seen in the chapter. Review this checklist to make sure that you are familiar with the meaning of each term before moving to the next section.*

## Conditions and Symptoms

- ❏ anthracosis
- ❏ apnea
- ❏ asphyxia
- ❏ asthma
- ❏ atelectasis
- ❏ bronchiectasis
- ❏ bronchiolitis
- ❏ bronchitis
- ❏ Cheyne-Stokes respiration
- ❏ cough
- ❏ croup
- ❏ cyanosis
- ❏ cystic fibrosis
- ❏ diaphragmatocele
- ❏ dysphonia
- ❏ dyspnea
- ❏ emphysema
- ❏ empyema
- ❏ epistaxis
- ❏ eupnea
- ❏ hemoptysis
- ❏ hyperpnea
- ❏ hyperventilation
- ❏ hypoxia
- ❏ influenza
- ❏ laryngitis
- ❏ Legionnaires' disease
- ❏ mesothelioma
- ❏ multidrug-resistant TB
- ❏ nasopharyngitis
- ❏ orthopnea
- ❏ pertussis
- ❏ pharyngitis
- ❏ pleurisy
- ❏ pleuritis
- ❏ pleurodynia
- ❏ pneumoconiosis
- ❏ pneumonia
- ❏ pneumonitis
- ❏ pneumothorax
- ❏ polyp
- ❏ pyothorax
- ❏ rale
- ❏ respiratory distress syndrome (hyaline membrane disease)
- ❏ respiratory syncytial virus infection
- ❏ rhinorrhea
- ❏ rhonchus
- ❏ sarcoidosis
- ❏ severe acute respiratory syndrome
- ❏ sinusitis
- ❏ sputum
- ❏ stridor
- ❏ tachypnea
- ❏ tonsillitis
- ❏ trachealgia
- ❏ tuberculosis
- ❏ wheeze

## Diagnosis and Treatment

- ❏ bronchoscope
- ❏ culture, sputum
- ❏ laryngoscope
- ❏ lobectomy
- ❏ palatopharyngoplasty
- ❏ pulmonectomy
- ❏ respirator
- ❏ rhinoplasty
- ❏ spirometer
- ❏ thoracocentesis
- ❏ thoracoplasty
- ❏ thoracotomy
- ❏ tonsillectomy
- ❏ tracheolaryngotomy
- ❏ tracheostomy

# STUDY AND REVIEW

## Anatomy and Physiology

*Write your answers to the following questions. Do not refer to the text.*

1. List the organs of the respiratory system.

   a. _____     b. _____

   c. _____     d. _____

   e. _____     f. _____

2. State the primary function of the respiratory system. _____

   _____

3. Define *external respiration*. _____

4. Define *internal respiration*. _____

5. List the five functions of the nose.

   a. _____

   b. _____

   c. _____

   d. _____

   e. _____

6. Name the three divisions of the pharynx.

   a. _____     b. _____

   c. _____

7. List the three functions of the pharynx.

   a. _____

   b. _____

   c. _____

8. State the function of the epiglottis. _____

9. Define *glottis*. _____

10. State the function of the larynx. _____

11. State the function of the trachea. _____

12. The trachea divides into the _____ _____

    and the _____ _____.

13. State the function of the bronchi. _____

14. Give a brief description of the lungs. _____

    _____

15. Define *pleura.* _____

16. The thoracic cavity is separated from the abdominal cavity by a musculomem-

    branous wall commonly known as the _____.

17. The central portion of the thoracic cavity between the lungs is a space called the

    _____.

18. The right lung has _____ lobes and the left lung has _____
    lobes.

19. The air cells of the lungs are the _____.

20. State the main function of the lungs. _____

    _____.

21. The vital signs, which are essential elements for determining an individual's state

    of health, are _____, _____, _____, and

    _____.

22. Define the following terms:

    a. *Tidal volume* _____

    b. *Residual volume* _____

    c. *Vital capacity* _____

23. The _____ _____ and the _____ of the central ner-
    vous system regulate and control respiration.

24. The respiratory rate for a newborn is _____ to _____ breaths
    per minute.

25. The respiratory rate for an adult is _____ to _____ breaths
    per minute.

## Word Parts

1. In the spaces provided, write the definition of these prefixes, roots, combining
   forms, and suffixes. Do not refer to the listings of medical words. Leave blank
   those words you cannot define.

2. After completing as many as you can, refer to the medical word listings to check your work. For each word missed or left blank, write the word and its definition several times on the margins of these pages or on a separate sheet of paper.

3. To maximize the learning process, it is to your advantage to do the following exercises as directed. To refer to the word-building section before completing these exercises invalidates the learning process.

## PREFIXES

*Give the definitions of the following prefixes.*

1. a- _____

2. epi- _____

3. dys- _____

4. endo- _____

5. eu- _____

6. ex- _____

7. hyp- _____

8. hyper- _____

9. in- _____

10. tachy- _____

## ROOTS AND COMBINING FORMS

*Give the definitions of the following roots and combining forms.*

1. aspirat _____

2. alveol _____

3. anthrac _____

4. atel _____

5. bronch _____

6. bronch/i _____

7. bronchiol _____

8. bronch/o _____

9. con/i _____

10. cyan _____

11. halat _____

12. hem/o _____

13. laryng _____

14. larynge _____

15. laryng/o _____

16. lob _____

17. cyst _____

18. fibr _____

19. nas/o _____

20. orth/o _____

21. mes/o _____

22. tubercul _____

23. palat/o _____

24. pectorat _____

25. pharyng _____

26. pharyng/o _____

27. thel/i _____

28. phragmat/o _____

29. pleur _____

30. pleura _____

31. pleur/o _____

32. pneum/o _____

33. pneumon _____

34. pulm/o _____

35. pulmon _____    36. py/o _____

37. rhin/o _____    38. sinus _____

39. spir/o _____    40. respirat _____

41. thorac/o _____    42. ventilat _____

43. tonsill _____    44. trach/e _____

45. trache/o _____    46. rhonch _____

47. sarc _____    48. diaphragmat/o _____

## SUFFIXES

*Give the definitions of the following suffixes.*

1. -al _____    2. -algia _____

3. -cele _____    4. -centesis _____

5. -dynia _____    6. -ectasis _____

7. -ectomy _____    8. -ic _____

9. -ia _____    10. -ion _____

11. -itis _____    12. -meter _____

13. -osis _____    14. -oma _____

15. -staxis _____    16. -plasty _____

17. -or _____    18. -pnea _____

19. -ptysis _____    20. -rrhea _____

21. -scope _____    22. -stomy _____

23. -tomy _____    24. -us _____

## Identifying Medical Terms

*In the spaces provided, write the medical terms for the following meanings.*

1. _____ Pertaining to a small air sac in the lungs

2. _____ Dilation of the bronchi

3. _____ Inflammation of the bronchi

4. _____ Difficulty in speaking

5. _____ Good or normal breathing

6. _____ Spitting up of blood

7. _____ Process of breathing in

8. _____ Inflammation of the larynx

9. _____ Collection of air in the chest cavity

10. _____ Surgical repair of the nose

11. _____ Discharge from the nose

12. _____ Inflammation of a sinus

## Spelling

*In the spaces provided, write the correct spelling of these misspelled words.*

1. bronchscope _____

2. diaphramatcele _____

3. expectorion _____

4. laryngal _____

5. orthpnea _____

6. peluritis _____

7. pulmnectomy _____

8. rhoncus _____

9. trachypnea _____

10. trachal _____

## Matching

*Select the appropriate lettered meaning for each of the following words.*

_____ 1. cough

_____ 2. cystic fibrosis

_____ 3. influenza

_____ 4. inhalation

_____ 5. olfaction

_____ 6. pleurodynia

_____ 7. rhinovirus

_____ 8. sputum

_____ 9. tachypnea

_____ 10. thoracocentesis

a. Substance coughed up from the lungs
b. Pain in the pleura
c. Process of smelling
d. One of a subgroup of viruses that causes the common cold in humans
e. Fast breathing
f. Process of breathing in
g. Surgical puncture of the chest for removal of fluid
h. Sudden, forceful expulsion of air from the lungs
i. Inherited disease that affects the pancreas, respiratory system, and sweat glands
j. Slow breathing
k. Acute, contagious respiratory infection caused by a virus

## Abbreviations

*Place the correct word, phrase, or abbreviation in the space provided.*

1. acid-fast bacilli _____

2. CF _____

3. Chest x-ray _____

4. chronic obstructive lung disease _____

5. ET _____

6. PND _____

7. respiration _____

8. SIDS _____

9. shortness of breath _____

10. TB _____

## Diagnostic and Laboratory Tests

*Select the best answer to each multiple choice question. Circle the letter of your choice.*

1. Test performed on sputum to detect the presence of *Mycobacterium tuberculosis*.
   a. antistreptolysin O
   b. acid-fast bacilli
   c. pulmonary function test
   d. bronchoscopy

2. Visual examination of the nasal passages.
   a. bronchoscopy
   b. laryngoscopy
   c. rhinoscopy
   d. nasopharyngography

3. _____ is/are important in determining respiratory acidosis
   and/or alkalosis, metabolic acidosis and/or alkalosis.
   a. Acid-fast bacilli
   b. Antistreptolysin O
   c. Arterial blood gases
   d. Pulmonary function test

4. Series of tests to determine the diffusion of oxygen and carbon dioxide across the
   cell membrane in the lungs.
   a. acid-fast bacilli
   b. antistreptolysin O
   c. arterial blood gases
   d. pulmonary function test

5. Visual examination of the larynx, trachea, and bronchi via a flexible scope.
   a. bronchoscopy
   b. laryngoscopy
   c. nasopharyngography
   d. rhinoscopy

# PRACTICAL APPLICATION

## S O A P : Chart Note Analysis

*This exercise will make you aware of information, abbreviations, and medical terminology typically found in a patient's chart from a walk-in clinic.*

### Abbreviations Key

| | | | | |
|---|---|---|---|---|
| **Abd** | abdomen | | **MS** | musculoskeletal |
| **BP** | blood pressure | | **NKDA** | no known drug allergies |
| **CDC** | Centers for Disease Control and Prevention | | **Neuro** | neurology |
| | | | **P** | pulse |
| **CTA** | clear to auscultation | | **R** | respiration |
| **DOB** | date of birth | | **ROM** | range of motion |
| **DOT** | directly observed therapy | | **SOAP** | subjective, objective, assessment, plan |
| **F** | Fahrenheit | | **T** | temperature |
| **HEENT** | head, eyes, ears, nose, throat | | **TB** | tuberculosis |
| | | | **TM** | tympanic membrane |
| **Ht** | height | | **Wt** | weight |
| **lb** | pound | | **y/o** | year(s) old |
| **MDR TB** | multidrug-resistant tuberculosis | | | |

*Read the following chart note and then answer the questions that follow.*

**PATIENT:** Sanchez, Wilmer                                      **DATE:** 5/2/07

**DOB:** 2/15/79      **AGE:** 28      **SEX:** Male

**INSURANCE:** none

    **Vital Signs:**
        T: 99.8 F
        P: 88
        R: 20
        BP: 132/86
        Ht: 5' 5"
        Wt: 140 lb

    **Allergies:** NKDA

    **Chief Complaint:** Chronic cough, fatigue, night sweats, weakness, anorexia, and weight loss

**S** | **Subjective:** 28 y/o male migrant worker presents with feelings of being "very tired." He has a recent weight loss of 8 lb and no appetite. He reports " bad coughing for the past 3 weeks" and waking up at night "soaked with sweat."

**O** **Objective:**

**General Appearance:** Appeared exhausted, apprehensive. Had dark circles under eyes, bilateral. Noted lack of color around lips, "washed out" look.

**Heent:** Head: normocephalic. Eyes: pupils equal round react to light, no lesions. Ears: TM pearly gray with landmarks intact. Nose: symmetric, no discharge, mucosa pink, no swelling.

**Throat:** Pharyngeal wall red, no lesions or exudate.

**Lungs:** Rales noted in upper lobe of the right lung and persisted following full expiration and cough.

**Heart:** Regular rate and rhythm. No murmurs, gallops, or rubs.

**Abd:** Bowel sounds all 4 quadrants. No masses or tenderness.

**MS:** ROM within normal limits.

**Neuro:** Oriented to person, place, and time.

**Skin:** Moist, warm, and pale around lips.

**A** **Assessment:** Pulmonary tuberculosis.

**P** **Plan:** Because of a positive sputum culture for *Mycobacterium tuberculosis* and a chest x-ray revealing lesions in the upper lobe of the right lung, ordered was a three-drug regimen of isoniazid, rifampin, and ethambutol. Rest and a balanced diet are also important parts of the treatment plan. Note: Family members and close contacts must be tested for *Mycobacterium tuberculosis* and if anyone tests positive, treatment regimen must be started immediately.

1. Explain that TB is spread by airborne particles known as droplets and that he is contagious until his sputum converts from positive to negative. Advise patient to stay home from work and to avoid close contact with others; to cover mouth with tissue during sneezing, coughing, laughing, or singing; and to dispose of tissue in a designated container and then wash his hands.

2. Explain that it takes at least six months (of taking the medication as ordered) to kill the TB bacteria. If drug therapy is not properly followed, multidrug-resistant TB (MDR TB) can occur.

3. To assist in medication compliance, inform the patient of the use of incentives and enablers that are given each time the patient appears at the clinic or doctor's office for treatment. Incentives and enablers are combined with the use of directly observed therapy (DOT). Check to see if the patient would like to participate in the DOT system of treatment. The medication will be administered by a nurse or health worker, and he will be observed taking the medication.

4. Teach the patient about the adverse effects of the medication regimen and to call the doctor immediately if any of the following symptoms occur:
   - Abdominal pain
   - Blurred vision
   - Continued loss of appetite
   - Dark (coffee-colored) urine
   - Fever
   - Nausea
   - Rash or itching
   - Tingling or burning feeling in your hands or feet
   - Tiredness without reason
   - Vomiting
   - Yellow color of eyes or skin

   The following are less serious side effects that the patient should be aware of:
   - Rifampin can turn urine, saliva, or tears orange.
   - Rifampin can make one more sensitive to the sun.

5. Monitor response to medication regimen including sputum culture at least monthly until conversion to negative and then recheck of sputum at completion of therapy.

6. Explain that follow-up care is essential. A liver function test should be performed monthly.

7. Instruct to avoid alcohol and not to take acetaminophen (Tylenol) while on antituberculosis medications.

**FYI:** A sputum culture is essential to confirming a diagnosis, determining the organisms' susceptibility to drugs, and assessing response to treatment. For more information on tuberculosis go to the Centers for Disease Control and Prevention (CDC) website: www.cdc.gov or call 1-800-458-5231.

## Chart Note Questions

*Place the correct answer in the space provided.*

1. Tuberculosis was diagnosed by a positive _____ _____ indicating *Mycobacterium tuberculosis* and a chest x-ray revealing lesions in the upper lobe of the right lung.

2. During the objective examination, the skin was noted to appear moist, _____, and pale around the lips.

3. _____ were noted in the upper lobe of the right lung and persisted following full expiration and cough.

4. Treatment for this patient included a balanced diet, rest, and a three-drug regimen of isoniazid, rifampin, and _____.

5. What does the abbreviation MDR TB mean? _____

6. How long does it take for antituberculosis medication to kill the TB bacteria? _____

7. The patient is "contagious" until the sputum culture converts from _____ to _____.

8. What is DOT? _____

9. TB is spread by _____.

10. A sputum culture is essential to confirming a diagnosis, determining the organisms' susceptibility to drugs, and assessing response to _____.

# MULTIMEDIA PREVIEW

*Additional interactive resources and activities for this chapter can be found on the Companion Website. For videos, audio glossary, and review, access the accompanying CD-ROM in this book.*

 **CD-ROM HIGHLIGHTS**

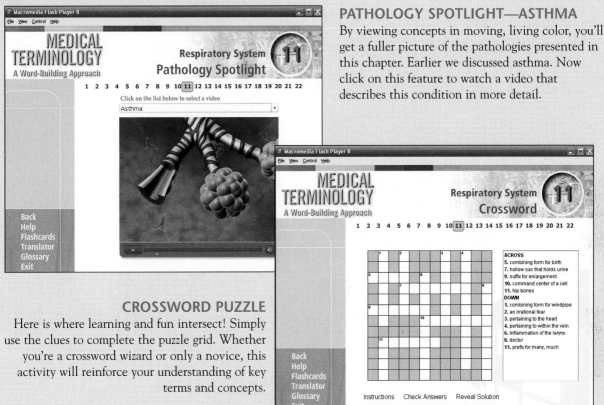

## PATHOLOGY SPOTLIGHT—ASTHMA

By viewing concepts in moving, living color, you'll get a fuller picture of the pathologies presented in this chapter. Earlier we discussed asthma. Now click on this feature to watch a video that describes this condition in more detail.

## CROSSWORD PUZZLE

Here is where learning and fun intersect! Simply use the clues to complete the puzzle grid. Whether you're a crossword wizard or only a novice, this activity will reinforce your understanding of key terms and concepts.

 **WEBSITE HIGHLIGHTS—www.prenhall.com/rice**

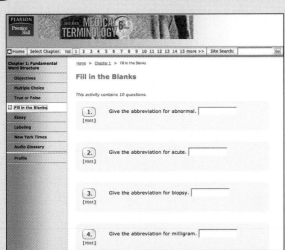

## FILL-IN-THE-BLANKS EXERCISE

Take advantage of the free-access on-line study guide that accompanies your textbook. You'll find a fill-in-the-blank quiz that provides instant feedback, allowing you to check your score and see what you got right or wrong. By clicking on this URL you'll also access links to download mp3 audio reviews, current news articles, and an audio glossary.

# Urinary System

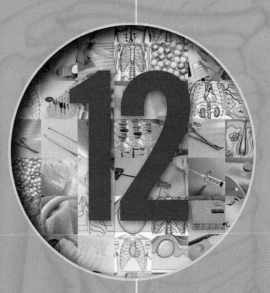

## OUTLINE

## OBJECTIVES

*On completion of this chapter, you will be able to:*

- Describe the organs of the urinary system.
- State the vital function of the urinary system.
- Describe the formation of urine.
- Describe urinalysis.
- Identify the normal constituents of urine.
- Identify abnormal constituents of urine.
- Analyze, build, spell, and pronounce medical words.
- Describe each of the conditions presented in the Pathology Spotlights.
- Comprehend the drugs highlighted in this chapter.
- Describe diagnostic and laboratory tests related to the urinary system.
- Identify and define selected abbreviations.
- Review the Pathology Checkpoint.
- Complete the Study and Review section and the Chart Note Analysis.

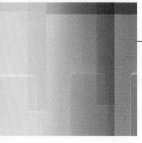

# Anatomy and Physiology Overview

The urinary system consists of two kidneys, two ureters, one bladder, and one urethra (see Figures 12–1 ▼ and 12–2 ▶). It is also called the excretory, genitourinary (GU), or urogenital (UG) system. The vital function of the urinary system is to extract certain wastes from the bloodstream, convert these materials to urine, transport the urine from the kidneys via the ureters to the bladder, and eliminate it at appropriate intervals via the urethra. Through this vital function, homeostasis of body fluids is maintained.

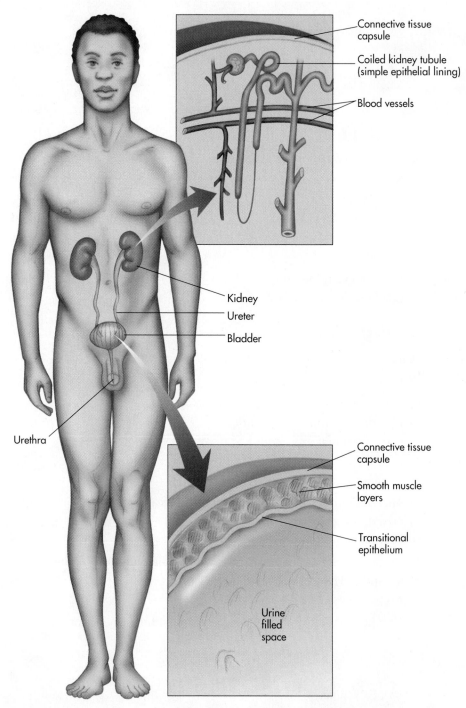

▶ FIGURE 12–1   The urinary system: kidneys, ureters, bladder, and urethra with expanded view of a nephron and the urine-filled space within a bladder.

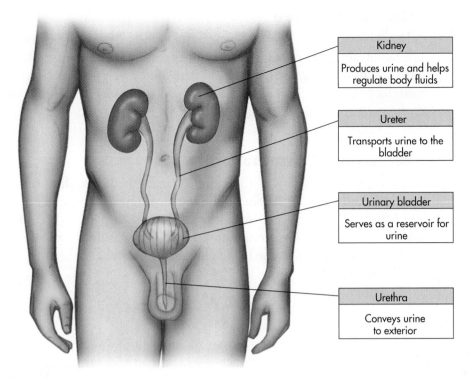

| Kidney |
|---|
| Produces urine and helps regulate body fluids |

| Ureter |
|---|
| Transports urine to the bladder |

| Urinary bladder |
|---|
| Serves as a reservoir for urine |

| Urethra |
|---|
| Conveys urine to exterior |

▶ **FIGURE 12–2** Organs of the urinary system with major functions.

## The Urinary System

| Organ/Structure | Primary Functions |
|---|---|
| Kidneys | Produce urine and help regulate body fluids |
| Ureters | Transport urine from the kidneys to the bladder |
| Urinary bladder | Serves as a reservoir for urine |
| Urethra | Conveys urine to the outside of the body; in the male conveys both urine and semen |

# KIDNEYS

The **kidneys** are purplish-brown, bean-shaped organs located at the back of the abdominal cavity (*retroperitoneal area*). They lie, one on each side of the spinal column, just above the waistline, against the muscles of the back. Each kidney is surrounded by three capsules; the **true capsule,** the **perirenal fat,** and the **renal fascia.** The true capsule is a smooth, fibrous connective membrane that loosely adheres to the surface of the kidney. The perirenal fat is the adipose capsule that embeds each kidney in fatty tissue. The renal fascia is a sheath of fibrous tissue that helps to anchor the kidney to the surrounding structures and helps to maintain its normal position.

## External Structure

Each kidney has a *concave* border and a *convex* border. The center of the concave border opens into a notch called the **hilum.** The renal artery and vein, nerves, and lymphatic vessels enter and leave through the hilum. The ureter enters the kidney through the hilum into a saclike collecting portion called the *renal pelvis.*

### Internal Structure

When a cross section is made through the kidney, its anterior can be seen to comprise two distinct areas: the **cortex,** which is the outer layer, and the **medulla** or inner portion. The cortex contains the arteries, veins, convoluted tubules, and glomerular capsules. The medulla contains the renal pyramids, conelike masses with papillae projecting into calyces of the pelvis.

### Microscopic Anatomy

Microscopic examination of the kidney reveals about 1 million **nephrons,** which are the structural and functional units of the organ. Each nephron consists of a **renal corpuscle** and **tubule.** The renal corpuscle or malpighian body consists of a **glomerulus** and a Bowman's capsule. Extending from each **Bowman's capsule** is a tubule consisting of the proximal convoluted portion, the loop of Henle, and a distal convoluted portion that opens into a collecting tubule.

### Nephron

The vital function of the **nephron** is to remove the waste products of metabolism from the blood plasma. These waste products are urea, uric acid, and creatinine, as well as any excess sodium, chloride, and potassium ions and ketone bodies. The nephron plays a vital role in the maintenance of normal fluid balance in the body by allowing for reabsorption of water and some electrolytes back into the blood. Approximately 1000 to 1200 milliliter (mL) of blood flows through the kidney per minute. At a rate of 1000 mL of blood per minute, about 1.5 million mL flows through the kidney in each 24-hour day. See Figure 12–3 ▶.

## URETERS

Each kidney has a **ureter.** They are narrow, muscular tubes that transport urine from the kidneys to the bladder. They are from 28 to 34 centimeters (cm) long and vary in diameter from 1 millimeter (mm) to 1 centimeter (cm). The walls of the ureters consist of three layers: an inner coat of mucous membrane, a middle coat of smooth muscle, and an outer coat of fibrous tissue.

## URINARY BLADDER

The **urinary bladder** is the muscular, membranous sac that serves as a reservoir for urine. It is located in the anterior portion of the pelvic cavity and consists of a lower portion, the **neck,** which is continuous with the urethra, and an upper portion, the **apex,** which is connected with the umbilicus by the median umbilical ligament. The **trigone** is a small triangular area near the base of the bladder. The wall of the bladder consists of four layers: an inner layer of epithelium, a muscular coat of smooth muscle, an outer layer composed of longitudinal muscle (*detrusor urinae*), and a fibrous layer. An empty bladder feels firm as the muscular wall becomes thick. As the bladder fills with urine, the muscular wall becomes thinner and distends according to the amount of urine present.

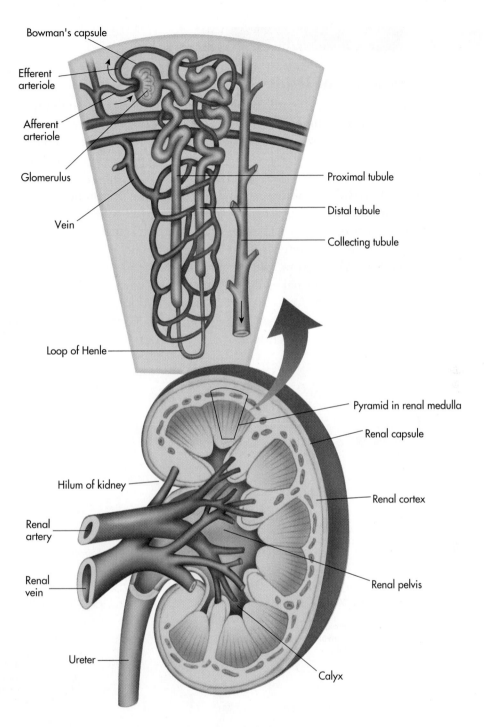

Bowman's capsule

Efferent arteriole

Afferent arteriole

Glomerulus

Vein

Proximal tubule

Distal tubule

Collecting tubule

Loop of Henle

Pyramid in renal medulla

Renal capsule

Hilum of kidney

Renal cortex

Renal artery

Renal vein

Renal pelvis

Ureter

Calyx

▶ **FIGURE 12–3**  Kidney with an expanded view of a nephron.

## URETHRA

The **urethra** is the musculomembranous tube extending from the bladder to the outside of the body. The external urinary opening is the **urinary meatus.** The male urethra is approximately 20 cm long and is divided into three sections: *prostatic*, *membranous*, and *penile*. It conveys both urine and semen. The female urethra is approximately 3 cm long. The urinary meatus is situated between the clitoris and the opening of the vagina. The female urethra conveys only urine.

## URINE

### Formation of Urine

**Urine** is formed by the process of *filtration* and *reabsorption* in the nephron. Blood enters the nephron via the afferent arteriole. As it passes through the glomerulus, water and dissolved substances are filtered through the glomerular membrane and collect in the Bowman's capsule. The glomerular filtrate passes through the proximal tubule into the loop of Henle, the distal tubule, and then the collecting tubule. Water and some selected substances are reabsorbed into the capillaries surrounding the tubules. Substances such as uric acid and hydrogen ions, through the process of secretion, may be added to the fluid now known as *urine*, which consists of 95% water and 5% solid substances. It is secreted by the kidneys and transported by the ureters to the bladder, where it is stored before being discharged from the body via the urethra. See Figure 12–4 ▼.

An average normal adult feels the need to void when the bladder contains around 300 to 350 mL of urine. An average of 1000 to 1500 mL of urine is voided daily. Normal urine is clear and yellow to amber in color and has a faintly aromatic odor, a specific gravity of 1.003 to 1.030, and a slightly acid pH (hydrogen ion concentration).

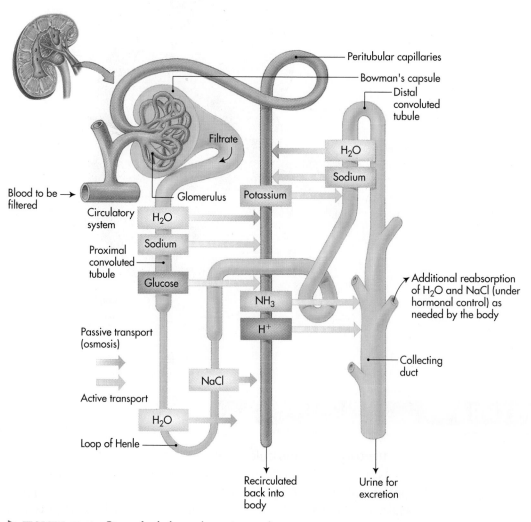

▶ **FIGURE 12–4** Sites of tubular reabsorption and secretion.

## Urinalysis

**Urinalysis** (UA) is a laboratory procedure that can involve the physical, chemical, and microscopic examination of urine. A freshly voided urine specimen provides for more accurate test results because certain changes may occur in urine that is left standing. If the urinalysis cannot be performed on the specimen within 1 hour of the time voided, it should be refrigerated, with the time of collection written on the label of the container. Urine should be collected in a clean, dry container. A disposable container is preferred. When a bacteriologic culture is to be done on urine, the specimen is collected by **catheterization.**

Urinalysis is a valuable diagnostic tool. Abnormal conditions or diseases can be quickly and easily detected because of the fact that the physical and chemical constituents of normal urine are constant. See Table 12–1.

### TABLE 12–1  Normal and Abnormal Constituents of Urine

| Constituent | Normal | Abnormal/Significance |
| --- | --- | --- |
| Color | Yellow to amber | Red or reddish—presence of hemoglobin<br>Orange—due to Pyridium<br>Greenish-brown or black—caused by bile pigments.<br>*The color of urine darkens upon standing.* |
| Appearance | Clear | Milky—fat globules, pus, bacteria<br>Smoky—blood cells<br>Hazy—refrigeration |
| Reaction | Between 4.6 to 8.0 pH, with an average of 6.0 | High acidity—diabetic acidosis, fever, diarrhea, dehydration<br>Alkaline—chronic cystitis, urinary tract infection, renal failure |
| Specific gravity (sp. gr.) | Between 1.003 and 1.030 | Low (1.001 to 1.002)—diabetes insipidus<br>High (over 1.030)—diabetes mellitus, hepatic disease, congestive heart failure |
| Odor | Faintly aromatic | Fruity sweet—acetone, associated with diabetes mellitus<br>Unpleasant—decomposition of drugs, foods, alcohol |
| Quantity | Around 1000 to 1500 mL per day | High—diabetes mellitus, diabetes insipidus, nervousness, diuretics, excessive intake<br>Low—acute neprhritis, heart disease, diarrhea, vomiting<br>None—uremia, renal failure |
| Protein | Negative | Positive—renal disease, pyelonephritis |
| Glucose | Negative | Positive—diabetes mellitus, pain, excitement, liver damage |
| Ketones | Negative | Positive—uncontrolled diabetes mellitus, high-protein, low-carbohydrate diet |
| Bilirubin | Negative | Positive—liver disease, biliary obstruction, congestive heart failure |
| Blood | Negative | Positive—renal disease or disorders, trauma |
| Nitrites | Negative | Positive—bacteriuria |
| Urobilinogen | 0.1 to 1.0 | Absent—biliary obstruction<br>Reduced—antibiotic therapy<br>Increased—early warning of hepatic or hemolytic disease |

# LIFE SPAN CONSIDERATIONS

## ■ THE CHILD

Soon after implantation, the embryonic mass differentiates into three distinct layers of cells: the **ectoderm, mesoderm,** and **endoderm.** The urinary and reproductive organs originate from the mesoderm. At 10 weeks, urine forms and enters the bladder. At about the third month of gestation, the fetal kidneys begin to secrete urine. The amount increases gradually as the fetus matures. The newborn's kidneys are immature and lack the ability to concentrate urine. Glomerular filtration and absorption are relatively low until the child is 1 or 2 years of age. In the child, the kidneys are more susceptible to trauma because they usually do not have as much fat padding as in the adult. Infants are more prone to fluid volume changes, excess, and/or dehydration.

**Urinary tract infections** (UTIs) are common in children. The microorganisms *Escherichia coli, Klebsiella,* and *Proteus* cause most urinary tract infections seen in children. The signs and symptoms of urinary tract infection are age related. See Table 12–2.

**TABLE 12–2  Signs and Symptoms of Urinary Tract Infection in Children**

| | |
|---|---|
| Infants | Fever, loss of weight, nausea, vomiting, increased urination, foul-smelling urine, persistent diaper rash, failure to thrive |
| Older child | Increased urination (frequency), pain during urination, abdominal pain, hematuria, fever, chills, bedwetting in a "trained" child |

## ■ THE OLDER ADULT

With advancing age, the kidneys may lose mass as blood vessels degenerate. The loss of glomerular capillaries causes a decrease in glomerular filtration, and the kidneys lose their ability to conserve water and sodium. Additionally, the tubules of the aging kidneys diminish in their capacity for conserving base and ridding the body of excess hydrogen ions. Because the renal system helps to regulate acid–base balance, fluid and electrolyte imbalances can occur quickly in the older adult. Additional changes noted in the urinary system of the older adult are loss of muscle tone in the ureters, bladder, and urethra. Bladder capacity can be reduced by half, and the older adult could have to make frequent trips to the bathroom. **Urge incontinence** (or the inability to retain urine voluntarily) is a concern for older adults.

During the fourth decade, the kidneys begin to decrease in size and function. By the eighth decade, the kidneys have generally shrunk 30% and have lost a proportionate amount of function. If stressed, kidneys respond more slowly to changes in a person's internal environment. Some causes of stressful situations that can cause the kidneys to respond more slowly and contribute to fluid and electrolyte imbalance follow:

- Vomiting and diarrhea
- Surgery
- Diuretics
- Decreased fluid intake
- Fever
- Renal damage from medications

# BUILDING YOUR MEDICAL VOCABULARY

This section provides the foundation for learning medical terminology. Review the following alphabetized word list. Note how common prefixes and suffixes are repeatedly applied to word roots and combining forms to create different meanings.

| | |
|---|---|
| **P** | Prefix |
| **R** | Root |
| **CF** | Combining form |
| **S** | Suffix |

| | |
|---|---|
| **Pink words** | Terms not built from word parts. |
| **\*** | Indicates words covered in the Pathology Spotlights section. |
| 💿 | Check the CD-ROM for more information. |

| MEDICAL WORD | WORD PARTS (WHEN APPLICABLE) | | | DEFINITION |
|---|---|---|---|---|
| | **Part** | **Type** | **Meaning** | |
| **albuminuria** (ăl-bū″ mĭn-oo′ rĭ-ă) | albumin -uria | R S | protein urine | Presence of serum protein in the urine |
| **antidiuretic** (ăn″ tĭ-dī″ ū-rĕt′ ĭk) | anti- di(a)- uret -ic | P P R S | against complete, through urine pertaining to | Pertaining to a medication that decreases urine secretion |
| **anuria** (ăn-ū′ rĭ-ă) | an- -uria | P S | without urine | Without the formation of urine |
| **bacteriuria** (băk-tē″ rĭ-ū′ rĭ-ă) | bacter/i -uria | CF S | bacteria urine | Presence of bacteria in the urine |
| **calciuria** (kăl″ sĭ-ū′ rĭ-ă) | calc/i -uria | CF S | calcium urine | Presence of calcium in the urine |
| **calculus** (kăl′ kū-lŭs) | | | | Pebble; any abnormal concretion (*stone*); plural: calculi. See Figure 12–5 ▼. |

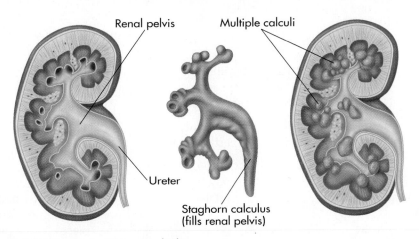

Renal pelvis    Multiple calculi

Ureter

Staghorn calculus (fills renal pelvis)

▶ **FIGURE 12–5** Urinary calculi.

| MEDICAL WORD | WORD PARTS (WHEN APPLICABLE) | | | DEFINITION |
|---|---|---|---|---|
| | **Part** | **Type** | **Meaning** | |
| **catheter**<br>(kăth′ ĕ-tĕr) | | | | Tube of elastic, elastic web, rubber, glass, metal, or plastic that is inserted into a body cavity to remove fluid or to inject fluid. See Figure 12–6 ▶. |
| **cystectomy**<br>(sĭs-tĕk′ tō-mē) | cyst<br>-ectomy | R<br>S | bladder<br>surgical excision | Surgical excision of the bladder or part of the bladder |
| **cystitis**<br>(sĭs-tī′ tĭs) | cyst<br>-itis | R<br>S | bladder<br>inflammation | Inflammation of the bladder. ✳ See Pathology Spotlight: Cystitis on page 390. |
| **cystocele**<br>(sĭs′ tō-sēl) | cyst/o<br>-cele | CF<br>S | bladder<br>hernia | Hernia of the bladder that protrudes into the vagina |
| **cystodynia**<br>(sĭs″ tō-dĭn′ ĭ-ă) | cyst/o<br>-dynia | CF<br>S | bladder<br>pain | Pain in the bladder; commonly called *cystalgia* |
| **cystogram**<br>(sĭs′ tō-grăm) | cyst/o<br>-gram | CF<br>S | bladder<br>a mark, record | X-ray record of the bladder |
| **cystolithectomy**<br>(sĭs″ tō-lĭ-thĕk′ tō-mē) | cyst/o<br>-lith<br>-ectomy | CF<br>S<br>S | bladder<br>stone<br>surgical excision | Surgical excision of a stone from the bladder |
| **cystoscope**<br>(sĭst′ ō-skōp) | cyst/o<br>-scope | CF<br>S | bladder<br>instrument for examining | Instrument used for examination of the bladder |
| **dialysis**<br>(dī-ăl′ ĭ-sĭs) | dia-<br><br>-lysis | P<br><br>S | complete, through<br>destruction, to separate | Procedure to separate waste material from the blood and to maintain fluid, electrolyte, and acid–base balance in impaired kidney function or in the absence of the kidney |
| **diuresis**<br>(dī″ ū-rē′ sĭs) | di(a)-<br><br>ur<br>-esis | P<br><br>R<br>S | complete, through<br>urinate<br>condition | Condition of increased or excessive flow of urine; occurs in conditions such as diabetes mellitus, diabetes insipidus, and acute renal failure. Diuretics also produce diuresis. |
| **dysuria**<br>(dĭs-ū′ rĭ-ă) | dys-<br>-uria | P<br>S | difficult, painful<br>urine | Difficult or painful urination |
| **edema**<br>(ĕ-dē′ mă) | | | | Abnormal condition in which the body tissues contain an accumulation of fluid |
| **enuresis**<br>(ĕn″ ū-rē′ sĭs) | en-<br>ur<br>-esis | P<br>R<br>S | within<br>urinate<br>condition | Condition of involuntary emission of urine; *bedwetting* |
| **excretory**<br>(ĕks′ krə-tō-rē) | excretor<br>-y | R<br>S | sifted out<br>pertaining to | Pertaining to the elimination of waste products from the body |
| **extracorporeal shock wave lithotriptor (ESWL)**<br>(ĕks″ tră-kor-por′ ē-ăl lĭth′ ō-trip″ tor) | extra-<br>corpor/e<br>-al | P<br>CF<br>S | outside, beyond<br>body<br>pertaining to | Device used to crush kidney stones (*renal calculi*). The patient is sedated and immersed in a water bath while shock waves pound the stones until they crumble into small pieces. These pieces are flushed out with urine. ✳ See Pathology Spotlight: Kidney Stones on page 390 and Figure 12–16. |

| MEDICAL WORD | WORD PARTS (WHEN APPLICABLE) | | | DEFINITION |
|---|---|---|---|---|
| | Part | Type | Meaning | |
| **glomerular** (glō-měr′ ū-lăr) | glomerul | R | glomerulus, little ball | Pertaining to the glomerulus. See Figure 12–7 ▼. |
| | -ar | S | pertaining to | |
| **glomerulitis** (glō-měr″ ū-lī′tĭs) | glomerul/o | CF | glomerulus, little ball | Inflammation of the renal glomeruli |
| | -itis | S | inflammation | |
| **glomerulonephritis** (glō-měr″ ū-lō-ně-frī′ tĭs) | glomerul/o | CF | glomerulus, little ball | Inflammation of the kidney involving primarily the glomeruli. There are three types: acute glomerulonephritis (AGN), chronic glomerulonephritis (CGN), and subacute glomerulonephritis. See Figure 12–8 ▶. |
| | nephr | R | kidney | |
| | -itis | S | inflammation | |
| **glycosuria** (glī″ kō-soo′ rĭ-ă) | glycos | R | glucose, sugar | Presence of glucose in the urine |
| | -uria | S | urine | |
| **hematuria** (hē″ mă-tū′ rĭ-ă) | hemat | R | blood | Presence of blood in the urine |
| | -uria | S | urine | |
| **hemodialysis (HD)** (hē″ mō-dī-ăl′ ĭ-sĭs) | hem/o | CF | blood | Use of an artificial kidney to separate waste from the blood. The blood is circulated through tubes made of semipermeable membranes, and these tubes are continually bathed by solutions that remove waste. See Figure 12–9 ▶. |
| | dia- | P | through, complete | |
| | -lysis | S | separation, loosening, dissolution | |

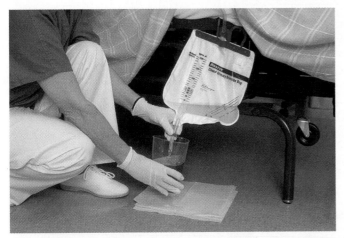

▶ **FIGURE 12–6** Closed urinary drainage system. Urine being measured after it leaves patient's body via catheter.

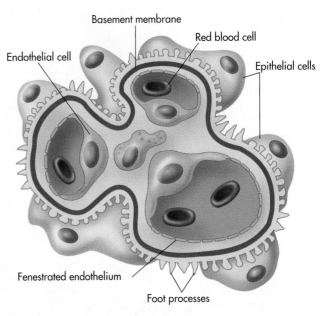

Basement membrane

Red blood cell

Endothelial cell

Epithelial cells

Fenestrated endothelium

Foot processes

▶ **FIGURE 12–7** Normal glomerulus.

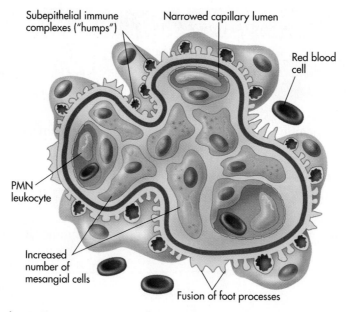

Subepithelial immune complexes ("humps")

Narrowed capillary lumen

Red blood cell

PMN leukocyte

Increased number of mesangial cells

Fusion of foot processes

▶ **FIGURE 12–8**  Acute glomerulonephritis.

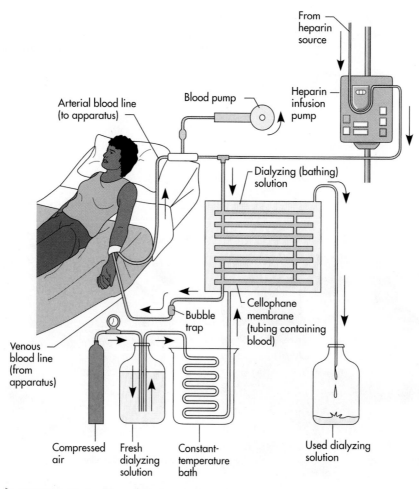

From heparin source

Arterial blood line (to apparatus)

Blood pump

Heparin infusion pump

Dialyzing (bathing) solution

Cellophane membrane (tubing containing blood)

Bubble trap

Venous blood line (from apparatus)

Compressed air

Fresh dialyzing solution

Constant-temperature bath

Used dialyzing solution

▶ **FIGURE 12–9**  Hemodialysis system.

| MEDICAL WORD | WORD PARTS (WHEN APPLICABLE) | | | DEFINITION |
|---|---|---|---|---|
| | **Part** | **Type** | **Meaning** | |
| **hydronephrosis** (hī″ drō-něf-rō′ sĭs) | hydro- nephr -osis | P R S | water kidney condition (usually abnormal) | Condition in which urine collects in the renal pelvis because of an obstructed outflow, thereby forming distention and atrophy of the kidney; can be caused by renal calculi, tumor, or hyperplasia of the prostate gland. See Figure 12–10 ▼. |
| **hypercalciuria** (hī″ pĕr-kăl sĭ-ū′ rĭ-ă) | hyper- calci -uria | P R S | excessive calcium urine | Excessive amount of calcium in the urine |
| **incontinence** (ĭn-kən′ tĭn-əns) | in- continence | P R | not to hold | Inability to hold or control urination or defecation |
| **interstitial cystitis (IC)** (ĭn″ ter-stĭsh′ al sĭs-tī′ tĭs) | | | | Chronically irritable and painful inflammation of the bladder wall |
| **ketonuria** (kē″ tō-nū′ rĭ-ă) | keton -uria | R S | ketone urine | Presence of ketones in the urine resulting from breakdown of fats due to faulty carbohydrate metabolism. It occurs primarily as a complication of diabetes mellitus; also called *ketoacidosis.* |
| **lithotripsy** (lĭth′ ō trĭp″ sē) | lith/o -tripsy | CF S | stone crushing | Crushing of a kidney stone. ✳ See Pathology Spotlight: Kidney Stones on page 390 and Figure 12–16. |
| **meatotomy** (mē″ ă-tŏt′ ō-mē) | meat/o -tomy | CF S | passage incision | Incision of the urinary meatus to enlarge the opening |
| **meatus** (mē-ā′ tŭs) | | | | Opening or passage; the external opening of the urethra |

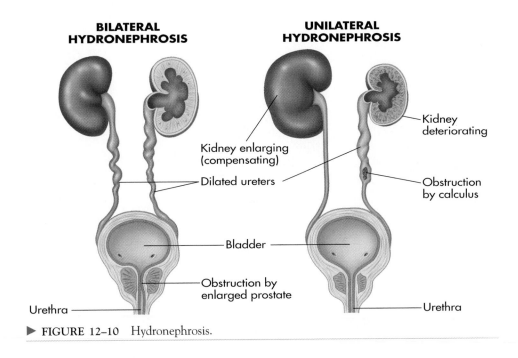

**BILATERAL HYDRONEPHROSIS**  **UNILATERAL HYDRONEPHROSIS**

Kidney enlarging (compensating)

Dilated ureters

Bladder

Obstruction by enlarged prostate

Urethra

Kidney deteriorating

Obstruction by calculus

Urethra

▶ FIGURE 12–10  Hydronephrosis.

| MEDICAL WORD | WORD PARTS (WHEN APPLICABLE) | | | DEFINITION |
|---|---|---|---|---|
| | **Part** | **Type** | **Meaning** | |
| **micturition**<br>(mĭk' tū-rĭ' shŭn) | micturit<br>-ion | R<br>S | to urinate<br>process | Process of urination |
| **nephrectomy**<br>(nĕ-frĕk' tō-mē) | nephr<br>-ectomy | R<br>S | kidney<br>surgical excision | Surgical excision of a kidney. See Figure 12–11 ▼. |
| **nephritis**<br>(nĕf-rī' tĭs) | nephr<br>-itis | R<br>S | kidney<br>inflammation | Inflammation of the kidney |
| **nephrocystitis**<br>(nĕf" rō-sĭs' tĭ' tĭs) | nephr/o<br>cyst<br>-itis | CF<br>R<br>S | kidney<br>bladder<br>inflammation | Inflammation of the bladder and the kidney |
| **nephrolith**<br>(nĕf' rō-lĭth) | nephr/o<br>-lith | CF<br>S | kidney<br>stone, calculus | Kidney stone, calculus. A condition characterized by the presence of a kidney stone is *nephrolithiasis.* ✳ See Pathology Spotlight: Kidney Stones on page 390. |
| **nephrology**<br>(nĕ-frŏl' ō-jē) | nephr/o<br>-logy | CF<br>S | kidney<br>study of | Study of the kidney |
| **nephroma**<br>(nĕ-frō' mă) | nephr<br>-oma | R<br>S | kidney<br>tumor | Kidney tumor |
| **nephron**<br>(nĕf' rŏn) | | | | Structural and functional unit of the kidney |
| **nephropathy**<br>(nē-frŏp' ă-thē) | nephr/o<br>-pathy | CF<br>S | kidney<br>disease | Disease of the kidney |
| **nephrosclerosis**<br>(nĕf" rō-sklē-rō' sĭs) | nephr/o<br>scler<br>-osis | CF<br>R<br>S | kidney<br>hardening<br>condition (usually abnormal) | Condition of hardening of the kidney |

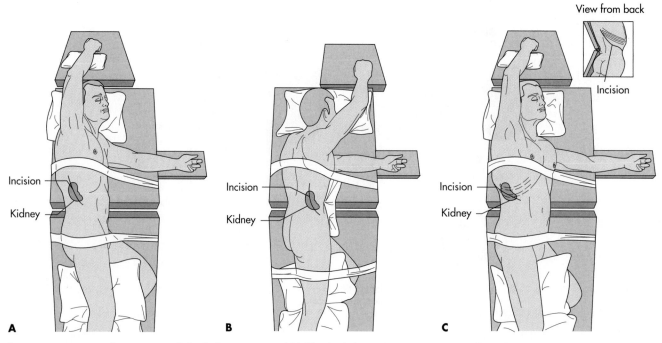

View from back

Incision

Incision
Kidney

Incision
Kidney

Incision
Kidney

A          B          C

► **FIGURE 12–11**   Incisions used for kidney surgery. (A) Flank. (B) Lumbar. (C) Thoracoabdominal.

| MEDICAL WORD | WORD PARTS (WHEN APPLICABLE) | | | DEFINITION |
|---|---|---|---|---|
| | Part | Type | Meaning | |
| **nocturia** (nŏk-tū′ rĭ-ă) | noct -uria | R S | night urine | Excessive urination during the night |
| **oliguria** (ŏl-ĭg-ū′ rĭ-ă) | olig- -uria | P S | scanty urine | Scanty urination |
| **percutaneous ultrasonic lithotripsy (PUL)** (pĕr″ kū-tā′ nē-ŭs) (ŭl-tră-sōn′ ĭk) (lĭth′ ō-trĭp″ sē) | per- cutan/e -ous ultra- son -ic lith/o -tripsy | P CF S P R S CF S | through skin pertaining to beyond sound pertaining to stone crushing | Crushing of a kidney stone by using ultrasound. This is an invasive surgical procedure performed by using a nephroscope or fluoroscopy. See Figure 12–12 ▼. |
| **peritoneal dialysis (PD)** (pĕr″ ĭ-tō-nē′ ăl dī-ăl′ ĭ-sĭs) | periton/e -al dia- -lysis | CF S P S | peritoneum pertaining to complete, through to separate | Separation of waste from the blood by using a peritoneal catheter and dialysis. Fluid is introduced into the peritoneal cavity, and wastes from the blood pass into this fluid. The fluid and waste are then removed from the body. Types of peritoneal dialysis are IPD—intermittent and CAPD—continuous ambulatory. See Figure 12–13 ▼. |

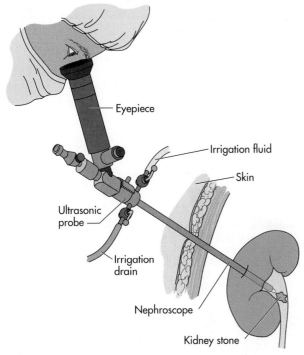

▶ **FIGURE 12–12**   Percutaneous ultrasonic lithotripsy. A nephroscope is inserted into the renal pelvis, and ultrasound waves are used to fragment the stones. The fragments then are removed through the nephroscope.

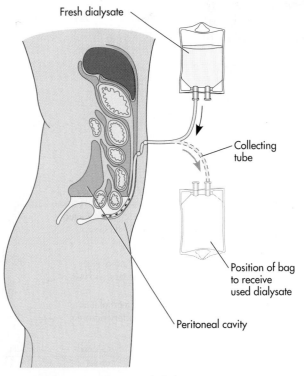

▶ **FIGURE 12–13**   Peritoneal dialysis.

| MEDICAL WORD | WORD PARTS (WHEN APPLICABLE) | | | DEFINITION |
|---|---|---|---|---|
| | **Part** | **Type** | **Meaning** | |
| **periurethral**<br>(pĕr″ ĭ-ū-rē′ thrăl) | peri-<br>urethr<br>-al | P<br>R<br>S | around<br>urethra<br>pertaining to | Pertaining to around the urethra |
| **polyuria**<br>(pŏl″ ē-ū′ rĭ-ă) | poly-<br>-uria | P<br>S | excessive<br>urine | Excessive urination |
| **pyelocystitis**<br>(pī″ ĕ-lō-sĭs-tī′ tĭs) | pyel/o<br>cyst<br>-itis | CF<br>R<br>S | renal pelvis<br>bladder<br>inflammation | Inflammation of the bladder and renal pelvis |
| **pyelolithotomy**<br>(pī″ ĕ-lō-lĭth-ŏt′ ō-mē) | pyel/o<br>lith/o<br>-tomy | CF<br>CF<br>S | renal pelvis<br>stone<br>incision | Surgical incision into the renal pelvis for removal of a stone |
| **pyelonephritis**<br>(pī″ ĕ-lō-nĕ-frī′ tĭs) | pyel/o<br>nephr<br>-itis | CF<br>R<br>S | renal pelvis<br>kidney<br>inflammation | Inflammation of the kidney and renal pelvis. ✶ See Pathology Spotlight: Pyelonephritis on page 390. |
| **pyuria**<br>(pī-ū′ rĭ-ă) | py<br>-uria | R<br>S | pus<br>urine | Pus in the urine |
| **renal**<br>(rē′ năl) | ren<br>-al | R<br>S | kidney<br>pertaining to | Pertaining to the kidney |
| **renal colic**<br>(rē′ năl kŏl′ ĭk) | | | | Acute pain that occurs in the kidney area caused by blockage during the passage of a stone |
| **renal failure**<br>(rē′ năl fāl′ yŭr) | | | | Cessation of proper functioning of the kidney. ✶ See Pathology Spotlight: Renal Failure on page 392. |
| **renal transplant**<br>(rē′ năl trăns′ plănt) | | | | Surgical procedure to implant a donor kidney into a recipient. See Figure 12–14 ▼. |

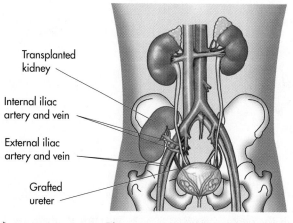

▶ **FIGURE 12–14**   Placement of transplanted kidney.

| MEDICAL WORD | WORD PARTS (WHEN APPLICABLE) | | | DEFINITION |
|---|---|---|---|---|
| | **Part** | **Type** | **Meaning** | |
| **renin**<br>(rĕn′ ĭn) | | | | Enzyme produced by the kidney that is elevated in some types of hypertension |
| **residual urine**<br>(rē-zĭd′ ŭ-ăl ū′ rĭn) | | | | Urine that is left in the bladder after urination |
| **sediment**<br>(sĕd′ ĭ-mĕnt) | | | | Substance that settles at the bottom of a liquid; a precipitate |
| **specific gravity (sp. gr.)**<br>(spĕ-sĭf′ ĭk grăv′ ĭ-tē) | | | | Weight of a substance compared with an equal amount of water. Urine has a specific gravity of 1.003 to 1.030. |
| **specimen**<br>(spĕs′ ĭ-mĕn) | | | | Sample of tissue, blood, urine, or other material intended to show the nature of the whole |
| **sterile**<br>(stĕr′ ĭl) | | | | State of being free from living microorganisms; *asepsis* |
| **stricture**<br>(strĭk′ chŭr) | strict<br><br>-ure | R<br><br>S | to tighten, contraction<br>process | Abnormal narrowing of a duct or passage such as the esophagus, ureter, or urethra |
| **trigonitis**<br>(trĭg″ ō-nī′ tĭs) | trigon<br>-itis | R<br>S | trigone<br>inflammation | Inflammation of the trigone of the bladder |
| **urea**<br>(ū-rē′ ă) | | | | Chief nitrogenous constituent of urine |
| **uremia**<br>(ū-rē′ mĭ-ă) | ur<br>-emia | R<br>S | urine<br>blood condition | Excess of urea, creatinine, and other nitrogenous end products of protein and amino acid metabolism accumulated in the blood; also referred to as *azotemia*. In current usage, it refers to the syndrome associated with end-stage renal failure.<br>✳ See Pathology Spotlight: Renal Failure on page 392. |
| **ureterocolostomy**<br>(ū-rē″ tĕr-ō-kō-lŏs′ tō-mē) | ureter/o<br>col/o<br>-stomy | CF<br>CF<br>S | ureter<br>colon<br>new opening | Surgical implantation of the ureter into the colon |
| **ureteropathy**<br>(ū-rē″ tĕr-ŏp′ ă-thē) | ureter/o<br>-pathy | CF<br>S | ureter<br>disease | Disease of the ureter |
| **ureteroplasty**<br>(ū-rē′ tĕr-ō-plăs″ tē) | ureter/o<br>-plasty | CF<br>S | ureter<br>surgical repair | Surgical repair of the ureter |
| **urethralgia**<br>(ū-rē-thrăl′ jĭ-ă) | urethr<br>-algia | R<br>S | urethra<br>pain | Pain in the urethra |
| **urethral stricture**<br>(ū-rē′ thrăl strĭk′ chŭr) | urethr<br>-al<br>strict<br><br><br>-ure | R<br>S<br>R<br><br><br>S | urethra<br>pertaining to<br>to tighten, contraction<br>process | Narrowing or constriction of the urethra |
| **urethroperineal**<br>(ū-rē″ thrō-pĕr″ ĭ nē′ ăl) | urethr/o<br>perine<br>-al | CF<br>R<br>S | urethra<br>perineum<br>pertaining to | Pertaining to the urethra and perineum |

| MEDICAL WORD | WORD PARTS (WHEN APPLICABLE) | | | DEFINITION |
|---|---|---|---|---|
| | Part | Type | Meaning | |
| **urgency**<br>(ŭr-jěn' sē) | | | | Sudden need to void, urinate |
| **uric acid**<br>(ū' rĭk ăs' ĭd) | | | | End product of purine metabolism; common component of urinary and renal stones |
| **urinal**<br>(ū' rĭn-ăl) | urin<br>-al | R<br>S | urine<br>pertaining to | Container, toilet, or bathroom fixture into which one urinates |
| **urinalysis (UA)**<br>(ū' rĭ-năl' ĭ-sĭs) | urin<br>a-<br>-lysis | R<br>P<br>S | urine<br>apart<br>destruction,<br>to separate | Analysis of urine; separating of the urine for examination to determine the presence of abnormal elements |
| **urination**<br>(ū" rĭ-nā' shŭn) | urinat<br>-ion | R<br>S | urine<br>process | Process of voiding urine |
| **urine**<br>(ū' rĭn) | | | | Waste product of fluid and dissolved substances secreted by the kidneys, stored in the bladder, and excreted through the urethra. See Figure 12–15 ▼. |
| **urinometer**<br>(ū" rĭ-nŏm' ĕ-tĕr) | urin/o<br>-meter | CF<br>S | urine<br>instrument | Instrument used to measure the specific gravity of urine |

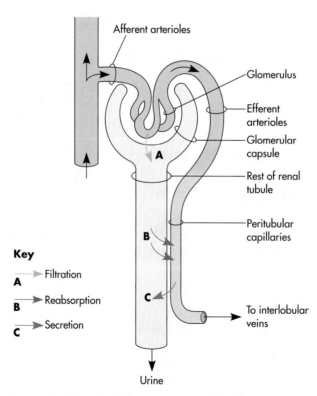

▶ **FIGURE 12–15** Schematic view of the three stages of urine production: (A) filtration; (B) reabsorption; and (C) secretion.

| MEDICAL WORD | WORD PARTS (WHEN APPLICABLE) | | | DEFINITION |
|---|---|---|---|---|
| | **Part** | **Type** | **Meaning** | |
| **urobilin**<br>(ū″ rō-bī′ lǐn) | ur/o<br>bil<br>-in | CF<br>R<br>S | urination<br>bile<br>chemical | Brown pigment formed by the oxidation of urobilinogen; may be formed in the urine after exposure to air |
| **urochrome**<br>(ū′ rō-krōm) | | | | Pigment that gives urine the normal yellow color |
| **urologist**<br>(ū-rǒl′ ō-jǐst) | ur/o<br>log<br>-ist | CF<br>R<br>S | urination<br>study of<br>one who specializes | Physician who specializes in the study of the urinary system |
| **urology**<br>(ū-rǒl′ ō-jē) | ur/o<br>-logy | CF<br>S | urination<br>study of | Study of the urinary system |
| **void**<br>(voyd) | | | | To empty the bladder |

# DRUG HIGHLIGHTS

**Diuretics**
Decrease reabsorption of sodium chloride by the kidneys, thereby increasing the amount of salt and water excreted in the urine. This action reduces the amount of fluid retained in the body and prevents edema. Diuretics are classified according to site and mechanism of action.

Thiazide
Appears to act by inhibiting sodium and chloride reabsorption in the early portion of the distal tubule.

*Examples: Diuril (chlorothiazide), HydroDiuril (hydrochlorothiazide), and Lozol (indapamide)*

Loop
Acts by inhibiting the reabsorption of sodium and chloride in the ascending loop of Henle.

*Examples: Bumex (bumetanide) and Lasix (furosemide)*

Potassium sparing
Acts by inhibiting the exchange of sodium for potassium in the distal tubule; inhibits potassium excretion.

*Examples: Aldactone (spironolactone) and Dyrenium (triamterene)*

Osmotic
Is capable of being filtered by the glomerulus but has a limited capability of being reabsorbed into the bloodstream.

*Example: Osmitrol (mannitol)*

Carbonic anhydrase inhibitor
Acts to increase the excretion of bicarbonate ($HCO_3$) ion, which carries out sodium (Na), water ($H_2O$), and potassium (K).

*Example: Diamox (acetazolamide)*

**Urinary tract antibacterials**
Sulfonamides are generally the drugs of choice for treating acute, uncomplicated urinary tract infections, especially those caused by *Escherichia coli* and *Proteus mirabilis* bacterial strains. They exert a bacteriostatic effect against a wide range of gram-positive and gram-negative microorganisms.

*Examples: Gantrisin (sulfisoxazole), Gantanol (sulfamethoxazole), Microsulfon (sulfadiazine), and Bactrim and Septra, which are mixtures of trimethoprim and sulfamethoxazole*

| | |
|---|---|
| **Urinary tract antiseptics** | May inhibit the growth of microorganisms by bactericidal, bacteriostatic, anti-infective, and/or antibacterial action.<br><br>*Examples: NegGram (nalidixic acid), Furadanton and Macrodantin (nitrofurantoin), Mandelamine and Hiprex (methenamine), and Cipro (ciprofloxacin HCl)* |
| **Other drugs** | Treat disorders of the lower urinary tract by either stimulating or inhibiting smooth muscle activity, thereby improving urinary bladder functions. These functions are the storage of urine and its subsequent excretion from the body.<br><br>*Examples: Cystospaz-M and Levsin (hyoscyamine sulfate), Urispas (flavoxate HCl), and Urecholine (bethanechol chloride)* |
| Rimso-50 (dimethyl sulfoxide) | Used in the treatment of interstitial cystitis. |
| Pyridium (phenazopyridine HCl) | Analgesic, anesthetic action on the urinary tract mucosa, causes the urine to turn an orange color and can stain clothing. The patient should be informed of this. |
| Urispas (flavoxate HCl) | Reduces dysuria, nocturia, and urinary frequency. |
| Tofranil (imipramine HCl) | Treats nocturnal enuresis in children. |
| Ditropan XL (oxybutynin chloride) | Relaxes the muscles in the bladder, thereby decreasing the occurrence of wetting accidents. |
| Detrol (tolterodine tartrate) | Helps control involuntary contractions of the bladder muscle. |

# DIAGNOSTIC AND LAB TESTS

| TEST | DESCRIPTION |
|---|---|
| **Blood urea nitrogen (BUN)** (blod ū-rē′ ă nĭ′ trō-jěn) | Blood test to determine the amount of urea excreted by the kidneys. Abnormal results indicate urinary tract disease. |
| **Creatinine** (krē′ ă-tĭn ēn) | Blood test to determine the amount of creatinine present. Abnormal results indicate kidney disease. |
| **Creatinine clearance** (krē′ ă-tĭn ēn klir′ ăns) | Urine test to determine the glomerular filtration rate (GFR). Abnormal results indicate kidney disease. |
| **Culture, urine** (kūl′ tūr, ū′ rĭn) | Urine test to determine the presence of microorganisms. Abnormal results indicate urinary tract infection. |
| **Cystoscopy (cysto)** (sĭs-tŏs′ kə-pē) | Visual examination of the bladder and urethra via a lighted cystoscope. Abnormal results can indicate the presence of renal calculi, a tumor, prostatic hyperplasia, and/or bleeding. |
| **Intravenous pyelography (pyelogram) (IVP)** (ĭn-tră-vē′ nŭs pī″ ĕ-lŏg′ ră-fē) | Test to visualize the kidneys, ureters, and bladder. A radiopaque substance is intravenously injected, and x-rays are taken. Abnormal results can indicate renal calculi, kidney or bladder tumors, and kidney disease. |

| Kidney, ureter, bladder (KUB) (kĭd′ nē, ū′ rĕ-tĕr, blăd′ dĕr) | Flat-plate x-ray is taken of the abdomen to indicate the size and position of the kidneys, ureters, and bladder. |
|---|---|
| Renal biopsy (rē′ năl bī′ ŏp-sē) | Removal of tissue from the kidney. Abnormal results can indicate kidney cancer, kidney transplant rejection, and glomerulonephritis. |
| Retrograde pyelography (RP) (rĕt′rō-grād pī″ ĕ-lŏg′ ră-fē) | X-ray recording of the kidneys, ureters, and bladder following the injection of a contrast medium through a urinary catheter into the ureters and the calyces of the pelves of the kidneys. Useful in locating urinary stones and obstructions. |
| Ultrasonography, kidneys (ŭl-tră-sŏn-ŏg′ ră-fē, kĭd′ nēs) | Use of high-frequency sound waves to visualize the kidneys. The sound waves (echoes) are recorded on an oscilloscope and film. Abnormal results can indicate kidney tumors, cysts, abscess, and kidney disease. |

# ABBREVIATIONS

| ABBREVIATION | MEANING | ABBREVIATION | MEANING |
|---|---|---|---|
| AGN | acute glomerulonephritis | IVP | intravenous pyelogram |
| ARF | acute renal failure | K | potassium |
| BUN | blood urea nitrogen | KUB | kidney, ureter, bladder |
| CAPD | continuous ambulatory peritoneal dialysis | LOC | level of consciousness |
| | | mL | milliliter |
| CGN | chronic glomerulonephritis | mm | millimeter |
| | | Na | sodium |
| cm | centimeter | NaCl | sodium chloride |
| CRF | chronic renal failure | NH$_3$ | ammonia |
| cysto | cystoscopy | PD | peritoneal dialysis |
| ESRD | end-stage renal disease | pH | hydrogen ion concentration |
| ESWL | extracorporeal shock wave lithotripsy | PKU | phenylketonuria |
| GFR | glomerular filtration rate | PUL | percutaneous ultrasonic lithotripsy |
| GU | genitourinary | | |
| H | hydrogen | RP | retrograde pyelography |
| HCO$_3$ | bicarbonate | sp. gr. | specific gravity |
| HD | hemodialysis | UA | urinalysis |
| H$_2$O | water | UG | urogenital |
| IC | interstitial cystitis | UTI | urinary tract infection |
| IPD | intermittent peritoneal dialysis | | |

# PATHOLOGY SPOTLIGHTS

## * Cystitis

**Cystitis** is an inflammation of the bladder, usually occurring secondarily to ascending urinary tract infections. It occurs when the lower urinary tract (urethra and bladder) is infected by bacteria and becomes irritated and inflamed and can be acute or chronic. More than 85% of cases of cystitis are caused by *Escherichia coli*, a bacillus found in the lower gastrointestinal tract.

Cystitis is very common and occurs in more than 6 million Americans a year. The condition frequently affects sexually active women ages 20 to 50 but can also occur in those who are not sexually active or in young girls and older adults. During sexual activity, bacteria can be introduced into the bladder through the urethra. Once bacteria enter the bladder, they normally are removed through urination. When bacteria multiply faster than they are removed by urination, infection results.

Females are more prone to cystitis because of their shorter urethra (bacteria do not have to travel as far to enter the bladder) and because of the short distance between the opening of the urethra and the anus. Cystitis in men is usually secondary to some other type of infection such as epididymitis, prostatitis, gonorrhea, syphilis, and/or kidney stones.

The most common symptom is frequent, painful urination. Other symptoms include a burning sensation during urination, chills, and fever. With chronic cystitis, pyuria may be the only symptom.

**Interstitial cystitis** (IC) is a painful inflammation of the bladder wall. Approximately 450,000 people suffer from this condition, and, of those, 90% are women. Symptoms can vary from mild to severe. The cause is unknown, and IC does not respond to antibiotic therapy.

## * Kidney Stones

**Kidney stones** (**nephroliths**) are deposits of mineral salts, called *calculi*, in the kidney. These stones can pass into the ureter, irritate kidney tissue, and block urine flow. Kidney stones occur when the urine has a high level of minerals (usually calcium) that form stones.

Kidney stones are one of the most common and painful disorders of the urinary tract. Men tend to be affected more frequently than women. Most kidney stones pass out of the body without any intervention by a physician. Stones that cause lasting symptoms or other complications can be treated by various techniques, most of which do not involve major surgery. Some of these techniques include **extracorporeal shock wave lithotripsy** (ESWL)(see Figure 12–16 ▶) and **percutaneous ultrasonic lithotripsy** (PUL). (See Figure 12–12 on page 383.)

Usually, the first symptom of a kidney stone is extreme pain, which begins suddenly when a stone moves in the urinary tract, causing irritation or blockage. A sharp, cramping pain in the back and side in the area of the kidney or in the lower abdomen is felt; nausea and vomiting may occur. If the stone is too large to pass easily, pain continues, and blood may appear in the urine.

## * Pyelonephritis

**Pyelonephritis** is an infection of the kidney and renal pelvis. It is usually caused by bacteria entering the kidneys from the bladder. *Escherichia coli* is a bacillus that is normally found in the large intestine. It causes about 90% of kidney infections. These infections usually spread from the genital area through the ureters to the bladder. See Figure 12–17 ▶.

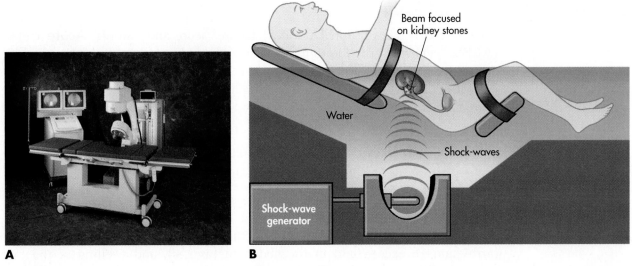

**A**  **B**

▶ **FIGURE 12–16** (A) Dornier Compact Delta® lithotripsy system. Acoustic shock waves generated by the shock-wave generator travel through soft tissue to shatter the renal stone into fragments, which are then eliminated in the urine. (Source: Courtesy of Dornier Medical Products, Inc.) (B) Illustration of water immersion lithotripsy procedure.

In a healthy urinary tract, the infection is prevented from going to the kidneys by the flow of urine, which washes organisms out. When bacteria enter the normally sterile urinary tract, they can cause pyelonephritis. Other possible causes of infection include the use of a catheter to drain urine from the bladder, use of a **cystoscope** to examine the bladder and urethra, and conditions such as prostate enlargement and kidney stones that prevent the efficient flow of urine from the bladder.

Symptoms include back, side, and groin pain; urgent, frequent urination; pain or burning during urination; fever; nausea and vomiting; and pus and blood in the urine.

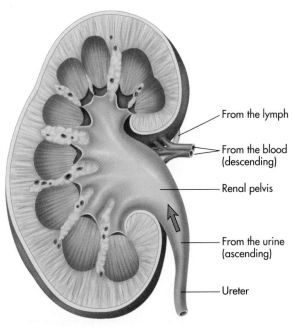

▶ **FIGURE 12–17** Routes of infection for pyelonephritis.

**✳ Renal Failure**

There are two types of renal (kidney) failure: acute and chronic. **Acute renal failure** (ARF) occurs when the filtering function of the kidneys changes so that the kidneys are not able to maintain healthy body function. People who have preexisting kidney disease or damage are at higher risk for acute renal failure. The following conditions can also lead to acute renal failure:

- A blockage of urine flow out of the kidneys and into the bladder.
- Exposure to certain drugs and/or toxic substances.
- Significant loss of blood or sudden drop in blood flow to the kidneys.

At first, acute renal failure causes no specific signs or symptoms, but as the disease progresses, urine output can decrease. As a result, fluid builds up in the body tissues and organs. Some common symptoms of acute renal failure include irregular heartbeats (arrhythmias), excess fluid in the abdomen (ascites), and swelling of the extremities (edema).

In **chronic renal failure** (CRF), there is a gradual and progressive loss of kidney function. It most often results from any disease that causes gradual loss of kidney function. Chronic renal failure affects more than 2 of 1,000 people in the United States. Diabetes and hypertension are the two most common causes and account for approximately two-thirds of the cases of chronic renal failure.

Chronic renal failure often is not identified until its final, uremic stage is reached. **Uremia** refers to the syndrome or group of symptoms associated with end-stage renal disease (ESRD). In uremia, clinical and metabolic abnormalities of fluid, electrolyte, and hormonal imbalances develop in parallel with deterioration of renal function. The regulatory and endocrine functions of the kidney are impaired, and accumulated metabolic waste products affect essentially every organ system of the body. See Figure 12–18 ▶.

The goal of treatment of acute and chronic renal failure is to identify and treat any reversible causes of the kidney failure. Treatment also focuses on preventing excess accumulation of fluids and wastes while allowing the kidneys to heal and gradually resume their normal function.

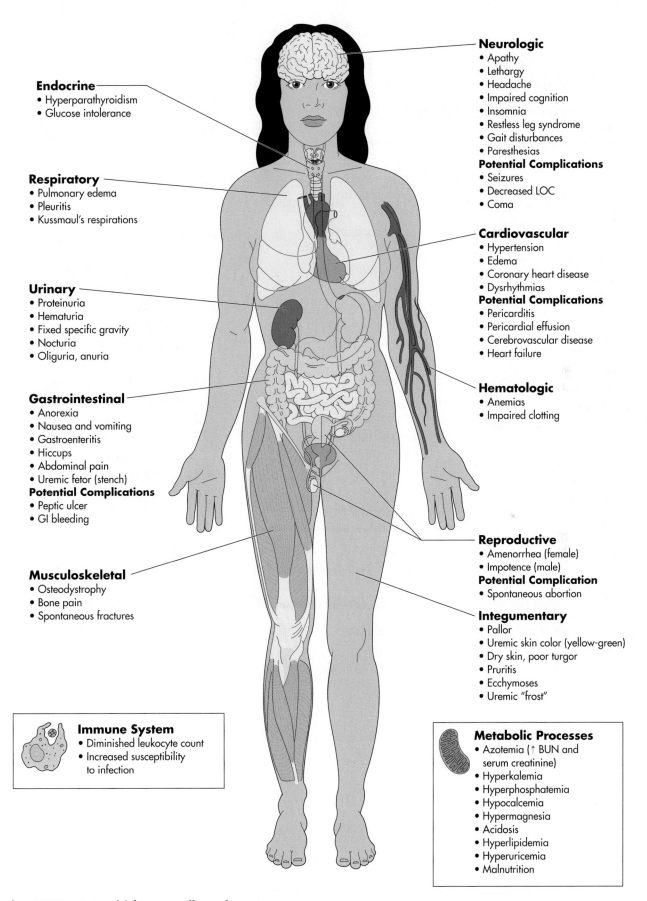

**Neurologic**
- Apathy
- Lethargy
- Headache
- Impaired cognition
- Insomnia
- Restless leg syndrome
- Gait disturbances
- Paresthesias

**Potential Complications**
- Seizures
- Decreased LOC
- Coma

**Endocrine**
- Hyperparathyroidism
- Glucose intolerance

**Respiratory**
- Pulmonary edema
- Pleuritis
- Kussmaul's respirations

**Cardiovascular**
- Hypertension
- Edema
- Coronary heart disease
- Dysrhythmias

**Potential Complications**
- Pericarditis
- Pericardial effusion
- Cerebrovascular disease
- Heart failure

**Urinary**
- Proteinuria
- Hematuria
- Fixed specific gravity
- Nocturia
- Oliguria, anuria

**Hematologic**
- Anemias
- Impaired clotting

**Gastrointestinal**
- Anorexia
- Nausea and vomiting
- Gastroenteritis
- Hiccups
- Abdominal pain
- Uremic fetor (stench)

**Potential Complications**
- Peptic ulcer
- GI bleeding

**Reproductive**
- Amenorrhea (female)
- Impotence (male)

**Potential Complication**
- Spontaneous abortion

**Musculoskeletal**
- Osteodystrophy
- Bone pain
- Spontaneous fractures

**Integumentary**
- Pallor
- Uremic skin color (yellow-green)
- Dry skin, poor turgor
- Pruritis
- Ecchymoses
- Uremic "frost"

**Immune System**
- Diminished leukocyte count
- Increased susceptibility to infection

**Metabolic Processes**
- Azotemia (↑ BUN and serum creatinine)
- Hyperkalemia
- Hyperphosphatemia
- Hypocalcemia
- Hypermagnesia
- Acidosis
- Hyperlipidemia
- Hyperuricemia
- Malnutrition

▶ FIGURE 12–18  Multisystem effects of uremia.

# ✔PATHOLOGY CHECKPOINT

*Following is a concise list of the pathology-related terms that you have seen in the chapter. Review this checklist to make sure that you are familiar with the meaning of each term before moving to the next section.*

## Conditions and Symptoms

- ❏ albuminuria
- ❏ anuria
- ❏ bacteriuria
- ❏ calciuria
- ❏ calculus
- ❏ cystitis
- ❏ cystocele
- ❏ cystodynia (cystalgia)
- ❏ diuresis
- ❏ dysuria
- ❏ edema
- ❏ end-stage renal disease
- ❏ enuresis
- ❏ glomerulitis
- ❏ glomerulonephritis
- ❏ glycosuria
- ❏ hematuria
- ❏ hydronephrosis
- ❏ hypercalciuria
- ❏ incontinence
- ❏ interstitial cystitis
- ❏ ketonuria
- ❏ micturition
- ❏ nephritis
- ❏ nephrocystitis

- ❏ nephrolith
- ❏ nephroma
- ❏ nephropathy
- ❏ nephrosclerosis
- ❏ nocturia
- ❏ oliguria
- ❏ polyuria
- ❏ pyelocystitis
- ❏ pyelonephritis
- ❏ pyuria
- ❏ renal colic
- ❏ renal failure
- ❏ residual urine
- ❏ stricture
- ❏ trigonitis
- ❏ uremia
- ❏ ureteropathy
- ❏ urethralgia
- ❏ urethral stricture
- ❏ urgency
- ❏ uric acid

## Diagnosis and Treatment

- ❏ antidiuretic
- ❏ catheter
- ❏ cystectomy

- ❏ cystogram
- ❏ cystolithectomy
- ❏ cystoscope
- ❏ dialysis
- ❏ extracorporeal shock wave lithotripsy
- ❏ hemodialysis
- ❏ lithotripsy
- ❏ meatotomy
- ❏ nephrectomy
- ❏ percutaneous ultrasonic lithotripsy
- ❏ peritoneal dialysis
- ❏ pyelolithotomy
- ❏ renal transplant
- ❏ specific gravity
- ❏ specimen
- ❏ ureterocolostomy
- ❏ urinometer
- ❏ ureteroplasty
- ❏ urinalysis

# STUDY AND REVIEW

## Anatomy and Physiology

*Write your answers to the following questions. Do not refer to the text.*

1. List the organs of the urinary system.

   a. _____    b. _____

   c. _____    d. _____

2. State the vital function of the urinary system. _____
   _____

3. Name the three capsules that surround each kidney.

   a. _____    b. _____

   c. _____

4. Define *hilum.* _____

5. Define *renal pelvis.* _____

6. The cortex of the kidney contains the _____, _____,
   _____ _____, and _____ _____.

7. The medulla is the _____ portion of the kidney.

8. Define *nephron.* _____

9. Each nephron consists of a _____ _____ and a
   _____.

10. The malpighian corpuscle consists of _____ and _____
    _____.

11. State the vital function of the nephron.

    _____

12. Urine is formed by the process of _____ and _____ in the
    nephron.

13. Urine consists of _____ percent water and _____ percent
    solid substances.

14. An average of _____ to _____ mL of urine is voided daily.

15. Describe the ureters and state their function. _____
    _____

16. Describe the urinary bladder and state its function. _____

_____

17. Define *trigone.* _____

18. State the function of the male urethra. _____

19. State the function of the female urethra. _____

20. The external urinary opening is the _____.

21. Define *urinalysis.* _____

_____

22. Give the normal constituents for the physical examination of urine.

    a. Color _____        b. Appearance _____

    c. Reaction _____        d. Specific gravity _____

    e. Odor _____        f. Quantity _____

23. Name the three types of epithelial cells that can be found in urine.

    a. _____        b. _____

    c. _____

24. A urine that has a fruity, sweet odor can indicate _____

_____.

25. Under chemical examination, the presence of protein in urine is an important

    sign of _____.

## Word Parts

1. In the spaces provided, write the definition of these prefixes, roots, combining forms, and suffixes. Do not refer to the listings of medical words. Leave blank those words you cannot define.

2. After completing as many as you can, refer to the medical word listings to check your work. For each word missed or left blank, write the word and its definition several times on the margins of these pages or on a separate sheet of paper.

3. To maximize the learning process, it is to your advantage to do the following exercises as directed. To refer to the word-building section before completing these exercises invalidates the learning process.

## PREFIXES

*Give the definitions of the following prefixes.*

1. an- _____

2. anti- _____

3. di(a)- _____

4. dia- _____

5. dys- _____

6. en- _____

7. hydro- _____

8. extra- _____

9. in- _____

10. olig- _____

11. per- _____

12. ultra- _____

13. poly- _____

## ROOTS AND COMBINING FORMS

*Give the definitions of the following roots and combining forms.*

1. excretor _____

2. albumin _____

3. bacter/i _____

4. bil _____

5. calc/i _____

6. col/o _____

7. continence _____

8. cyst _____

9. corpor/e _____

10. cyst/o _____

11. cutan/e _____

12. glomerul _____

13. glomerul/o _____

14. glycos _____

15. hemat _____

16. keton _____

17. lith/o _____

18. log _____

19. hem/o _____

20. meat/o _____

21. micturit _____

22. nephr _____

23. nephr/o _____

24. noct _____

25. periton/e _____

26. perine _____

27. son _____

28. strict _____

29. py _____

30. pyel/o _____

31. ren _____

32. scler _____

33. trigon _____

34. ur _____

35. uret _____

36. ureter/o _____

37. urethr _____

38. urethr/o _____

39. urin _____

40. urinat _____

41. urin/o _____

42. ur/o _____

## SUFFIXES

*Give the definitions of the following suffixes.*

1. -al _____
2. -algia _____
3. -ar _____
4. -cele _____
5. -dynia _____
6. -y _____
7. -ous _____
8. -ectomy _____
9. -emia _____
10. -gram _____
11. -ic _____
12. -in _____
13. -ion _____
14. -ist _____
15. -itis _____
16. -lith _____
17. -logy _____
18. -lysis _____
19. -tripsy _____
20. -ure _____
21. -meter _____
22. -oma _____
23. -osis _____
24. -pathy _____
25. -plasty _____
26. -scope _____
27. -esis _____
28. -stomy _____
29. -tomy _____
30. -uria _____

## Identifying Medical Terms

*In the spaces provided, write the medical terms for the following meanings.*

1. _____ Pertaining to a medication that decreases urine secretion

2. _____ Surgical excision of the bladder or part of the bladder

3. _____ Inflammation of the bladder

4. _____ Difficult or painful urination

5. _____ Inflammation of the renal glomeruli

6. _____ Excessive amount of calcium in the urine

7. _____ Process of urinating

8. _____ Kidney stone

9. _____ Pertaining to around the urethra

10. _____ Pus in the urine

11. _____ Disease of the ureter

12. _____ Pain in the urethra

13. _____ Physician who specializes in the study of the urinary system

## Spelling

*In the spaces provided, write the correct spelling of these misspelled words.*

1. excreteory _____

2. euresis _____

3. glycouria _____

4. hemauria _____

5. incontence _____

6. nephrcysitis _____

7. nocuria _____

8. ueteroplasty _____

9. urinalsis _____

10. urbilin _____

## Matching

*Select the appropriate lettered meaning for each of the following words.*

_____ 1. lithotriptor

_____ 2. hemodialysis

_____ 3. lithotripsy

_____ 4. peritoneal dialysis

_____ 5. renal colic

_____ 6. urethral stricture

_____ 7. urgency

_____ 8. urination

_____ 9. urochrome

_____ 10. urinometer

a. Acute pain that occurs in the kidney area and is caused by blockage during the passage of a stone

b. Crushing of a kidney stone

c. Process of voiding urine

d. Device used to crush kidney stones

e. Use of an artificial kidney to separate waste from the blood

f. Separation of waste from the blood by using a peritoneal catheter and dialysis

g. Narrowing or constriction of the urethra

h. Pigment that gives urine its normal yellow color

i. Instrument used to measure the specific gravity of urine

j. Sudden need to void, urinate

k. Analysis of the urine

## Abbreviations

*Place the correct word, phrase, or abbreviation in the space provided.*

1. acute renal failure _____

2. BUN _____

3. chronic renal failure _____

4. cysto _____

5. GU _____

6. HD _____

7. intravenous pyelogram _____

8. PD _____

9. pH _____

10. urinalysis _____

## Diagnostic and Laboratory Tests

*Select the best answer to each multiple choice question. Circle the letter of your choice.*

1. Urine test to determine the glomerular filtration rate.
   a. BUN
   b. creatinine
   c. creatinine clearance
   d. KUB

2. Urine test to determine the presence of microorganisms.
   a. BUN
   b. creatinine
   c. urine culture
   d. KUB

3. Test to visualize the kidneys, ureters, and bladder.
   a. cystoscopy
   b. intravenous pyelography
   c. KUB
   d. renal biopsy

4. Use of high-frequency sound waves to visualize the kidneys.
   a. retrograde pyelography
   b. intravenous pyelography
   c. ultrasonography
   d. cystoscopy

5. Flat-plate x-ray of the abdomen to indicate the size and position of the kidneys, ureters, and bladder.
   a. cystoscopy
   b. KUB
   c. BUN
   d. retrograde pyelography

# PRACTICAL APPLICATION

## S O A P : Chart Note Analysis

*This exercise will make you aware of information, abbreviations, and medical terminology typically found in a family practice patient's chart.*

### Abbreviations Key

| | | | |
|---|---|---|---|
| Abd | abdomen | NSSC | normal size, shape, and consistency |
| bid | twice a day | OTC | over-the-counter |
| BP | blood pressure | P | pulse |
| CTA | clear to auscultation | PO | orally, by mouth |
| DOB | date of birth | R | respiration |
| DS | double strength | SOAP | subjective, objective, assessment, plan |
| F | Fahrenheit | T | temperature |
| GYN | gynecology | Tab | tablet |
| Ht | height | tid | three times a day |
| Hx | history | UTI | urinary tract infection |
| lb | pound | Wt | weight |
| mg | milligram | y/o | year(s) old |
| N&V | nausea & vomiting | | |

*Read the following chart note and then answer the questions that follow.*

**PATIENT:** Hall, Christie M.                                  **DATE:** 5/21/07
**DOB:** 4/30/86        **AGE:** 21        **SEX:** Female
**INSURANCE:** Excel HealthCare

**Vital Signs:**
   T: 99.8 F
   P: 86
   R: 18
   BP: 120/72
   Ht: 5′ 7″
   *Wt:* 142 lb

**Allergies:** Penicillin

**Chief Complaint:** Increased frequency, burning sensation and pain during urination, chills, and fever.

**S** | **Subjective:** 21 y/o white female presents complaining that for the past two days she has needed to go "to the bathroom a lot" and that "it burns and hurts" when she urinates. She also has had chills and fever. She denies N&V, and Hx of previous UTI. States she is sexually active.

**O** | **Objective:**
**General Appearance:** Patient appears uncomfortable, having difficulty sitting still. She displays a sense of urgency
**Abd:** Bowel sounds all 4 quadrants. Suprapubic tenderness noted upon palpation. No costovertebral tenderness

**Heart:** Regular rate and rhythm. No murmurs, gallops, or rubs

**Lungs:** CTA

**Skin:** Warm and moist

**GYN:** Breast: Symmetrical, no palpable masses or tenderness, no dimpling or skin changes.

External genitalia: Noted signs of inflammation: redness, swelling, and heat around urinary meatus, apparent pain upon touch.

Cervix: Pink, smooth, no cervical motion tenderness

Uterus: NSSC

Pregnancies: Gravida 0 Para 0 Abortions 0

**A | Assessment:** Acute cystitis

**P | Plan:**

1. Upon receiving the results of a complete urinalysis that revealed red blood cells, white blood cells, and bacteria, the patient was placed on Bactrim DS 160mg/800mg (trimethoprim-sulfamethoxazole ) 1 Tab PO bid × 14 days and Pyridium (phenazopyridine HCl) 200mg 1 Tab PO tid × 2 days.
2. Explain to the patient that urine will turn orange while taking Pyridium and that it can stain her clothing.
3. Teach the patient about her medication, especially to take it with 8 ounces of water; take every 12 hours around the clock; and take as ordered for the full period; to avoid direct sunlight because she could be more sensitive to burns and photosensitivity while taking sulfonamides; not to take OTC medications that contain aspirin and vitamin C that could interact with sulfonamides; that sulfonamides could decrease the effectiveness of oral contraceptives and about signs of serious adverse reactions, such as itching, skin rash, aching of joints and muscles, and yellow eyes or skin.
4. Schedule a follow-up visit for one week.
5. Provide the patient with a copy of *Guidelines to Help Avoid Cystitis.* Review the guidelines with the patient and allow time for discussion.
6. Teach the patient that cystitis is most often caused by an ascending infection from the urethra and is more common in females due to the short length of their urethra, which promotes the transmission of bacteria from the skin and genitals to the bladder.

**FYI:** The most common type of bacteria that causes cystitis in females is *Escherichia coli* (*E. coli*), the colon bacillus. *Note:* 75% to 90% of infections are due to gram negative bacilli, *E. coli.* Only 5% to 15% of infections are caused by gram positive cocci such as *Staphylococcus saprophyticus* (a newly classified species that can cause urinary tract infections).

**Guidelines to Help Avoid Cystitis**

- Drink 8 glasses or more of water daily.
- Females should wipe themselves from front to back after bowel movements to avoid contamination of the urinary meatus.
- Have partner wear a condom to help prevent the sexual transmission of bacteria during intercourse. Bacteria can be introduced into the bladder through the urethra.
- Do not use vaginal deodorants, bubble baths, colored toilet paper, and other substances that could cause irritation to the urinary meatus.
- To help prevent infection, wear cotton underclothes and keep the genital area dry.
- Urinate immediately after intercourse to help flush out bacteria.

## Chart Note Questions
*Place the correct answer in the space provided.*

1.  Burning, _____ frequency, and pain during urination, chills, and fever are all symptoms that can present with cystitis.

2.  The diagnosis of acute cystitis was determined after combining a history of symptoms and a complete

    _____ revealing red blood cells, white blood cells, and bacteria.

3.  Treatment for acute cystitis included _____, an antibacterial, and Pyridium, an analgesic.

4.  What is the anatomic reasoning for an increased occurrence of cystitis in females? _____

5.  What is the most common bacillus that causes cystitis in females? _____

6.  To avoid contamination of the urinary meatus after a bowel movement, a female should _____.

7.  Having a partner wear a condom helps to prevent _____.

8.  The signs of an inflammation include redness, swelling, heat, and _____.

9.  Vaginal deodorants, bubble baths, colored toilet paper, and other substances could cause

    _____ to the urinary meatus.

10. Why is it important for the patient to avoid direct sunlight while taking sulfonamides?

    _____

# MULTIMEDIA PREVIEW

*Additional interactive resources and activities for this chapter can be found on the Companion Website. For videos, audio glossary, and review, access the accompanying CD-ROM in this book.*

 **CD-ROM HIGHLIGHTS**

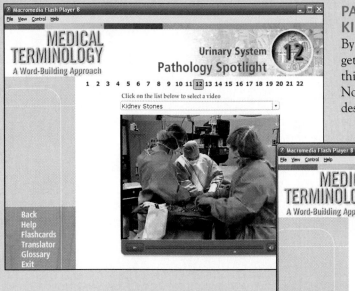

## PATHOLOGY SPOTLIGHT—KIDNEY STONES

By viewing concepts in moving, living color, you'll get a fuller picture of the pathologies presented in this chapter. Earlier we discussed kidney stones. Now click on this feature to watch a video that describes this condition in more detail.

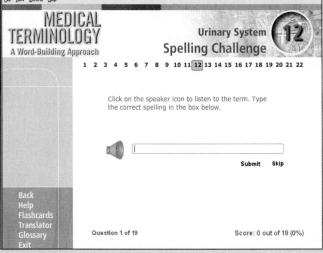

## SPELLING CHALLENGE

Maybe you're not ready for the National Spelling Bee, but you can be an expert speller of medical terms. Listen as each word is pronounced and then type it correctly in the space provided. Choose your letters carefully!

 **WEBSITE HIGHLIGHTS—www.prenhall.com/rice**

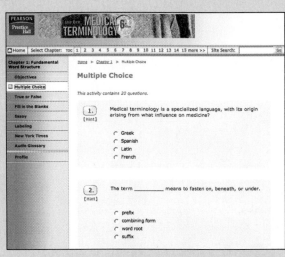

## MULTIPLE CHOICE QUIZ

Take advantage of the free-access on-line study guide that accompanies your textbook. You'll find a multiple choice quiz that provides instant feedback, allowing you to check your score and see what you got right or wrong. By clicking on this URL you'll also access links to download mp3 audio reviews, current news articles, and an audio glossary.

# Endocrine System

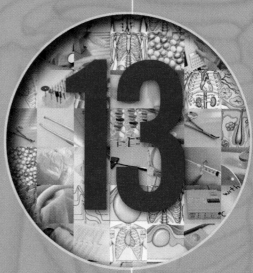

13

## ◼ OUTLINE

## ◼ OBJECTIVES

*On completion of this chapter, you will be able to:*

- Describe the primary glands of the endocrine system.
- State the vital function of the endocrine system.
- Identify and state the functions of the various hormones secreted by the endocrine glands.
- Analyze, build, spell, and pronounce medical words.
- Comprehend the drugs highlighted in this chapter.
- Describe diagnostic and laboratory tests related to the endocrine system.
- Identify and define selected abbreviations.
- Describe each of the conditions presented in the Pathology Spotlights.
- Review the Pathology Checkpoint.
- Complete the Study and Review section and the Chart Note Analysis.

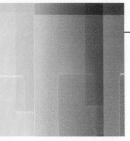

# Anatomy and Physiology Overview

The endocrine system is made up of glands and the hormones they secrete. Although the endocrine glands are the body's main hormone producers, some other organs such as the brain, heart, lungs, liver, skin, thymus, and the gastrointestinal mucosa as well as the placenta during pregnancy produce and release hormones. The primary glands of the endocrine system are the pituitary, pineal, thyroid, parathyroid, islets of Langerhans, adrenals, ovaries in the female, and testes in the male. See Figure 13–1 ▼.

The vital function of the endocrine system involves the production and regulation of chemical substances called *hormones*. A hormone is a chemical transmitter that is released in small amounts and transported via the bloodstream to a target organ or other cells. The word *hormone* is derived from the Greek language and means *to excite* or *to urge on*. As the

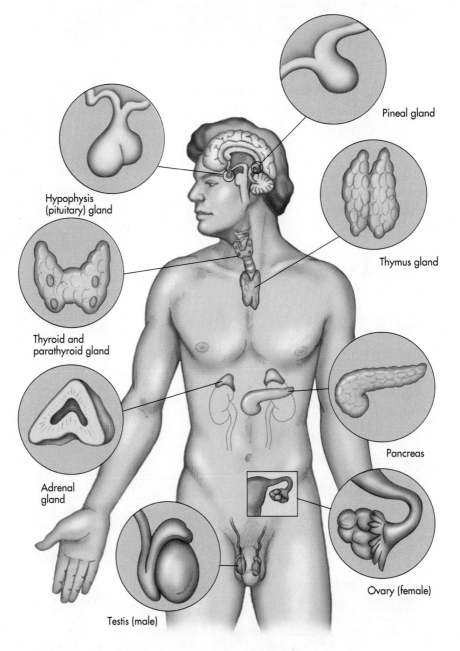

▶ **FIGURE 13–1**  Primary glands of the endocrine system.

body's chemical messengers, hormones transfer information and instructions from one set of cells to another. They regulate growth, development, mood, tissue function, metabolism, and sexual function in the male and female.

## The Endocrine System

| Gland | Primary Functions |
|---|---|
| Pituitary (hypophysis) | Master gland; has regulatory effects on other endocrine glands |
| *Anterior lobe* | Influences growth and sexual development, thyroid function, adrenocortical function; regulates skin pigmentation |
| *Posterior lobe* | Stimulates the reabsorption of water and elevates blood pressure; stimulates the uterus to contract during labor, delivery, and parturition; stimulates the release of milk during suckling |
| Pineal | Helps regulate the release of gonadotropin and controls body pigmentation |
| Thyroid | Plays vital role in metabolism; regulates the body's metabolic processes; influences bone and calcium metabolism; helps maintain plasma calcium homeostasis |
| Parathyroid | Maintains normal serum calcium level; plays a role in the metabolism of phosphorus |
| Pancreas (islets of Langerhans) | Regulates blood glucose levels; plays a vital role in metabolism of carbohydrates, proteins, and fats |
| Adrenals (suprarenals) | |
| *Adrenal cortex* | Regulates carbohydrate metabolism, anti-inflammatory effect; helps body cope during stress; regulates electrolyte and water balance; promotes development of male characteristics |
| *Adrenal medulla* | Synthesizes, secretes, and stores catecholamines (dopamine, epinephrine, norepinephrine) |
| Ovaries | Promote growth, development, and maintenance of female sex organs |
| Testes | Promote growth, development, and maintenance of male sex organs |

Hyposecretion or hypersecretion of specific hormones of the endocrine system cause or are associated with many pathological conditions. Too much or too little of any hormone can be harmful to the body. Controlling the production of or replacing specific hormones can treat many hormonal disorders and/or conditions.

The endocrine system and the nervous system work closely together to help maintain homeostasis. The **hypothalamus,** a collection of specialized cells that are located in the lower central part of the brain, is the primary link between the endocrine and nervous system. Nerve cells in the hypothalamus control the pituitary gland by producing chemicals that either stimulate or suppress hormone secretions from the pituitary.

The hypothalamus synthesizes and secretes releasing hormones such as thyrotropin-releasing hormone (TRH) and gonadotropin-releasing hormone (GnRH) and releasing factors such as corticotropin-releasing factor (CRF), growth hormone-releasing factor (GHRF), prolactin-releasing factor (PRF), and melanocyte-stimulating hormone-releasing factor (MRF). The hypothalamus also synthesizes and secretes release-inhibiting hormones such as growth hormone release-inhibiting hormone. It also produces release-inhibiting factors such as prolactin release-inhibiting factor (PIF) and melanocyte-stimulating hormone release-inhibiting factor (MIF). The hypothalamus also exerts direct nervous control over the anterior pituitary and the adrenal medulla and controls the secretion of the hormones epinephrine and norepinephrine. See Table 13–1 for an overview of the endocrine glands, hormones, and hormonal function.

TABLE 13–1 **Summary of the Endocrine Glands, Hormones, and Hormonal Functions**

| Endocrine Glands | Hormones | Hormonal Functions |
| --- | --- | --- |
| Pituitary gland | | |
| *Anterior lobe* | Growth hormone (GH) | Promotes growth and development of bones, muscles, and other organs |
| | Adrenocorticotropin hormone (ACTH) | Stimulates growth and development of the adrenal cortex |
| | Thyroid-stimulating hormone (TSH) | Stimulates growth and development of the thyroid gland |
| | Follicle-stimulating hormone (FSH) | Stimulates the growth of ovarian follicles in the female and sperm in the male |
| | Luteinizing hormone (LH) | Stimulates the development of the corpus luteum in the female and the production of testosterone in the male |
| | Prolactin hormone (PRL) | Stimulates the development and growth of the mammary glands. It is important in the initiation and maintenance of milk production during pregnancy. Following childbirth, the act of suckling provides the stimulus for prolactin synthesis and release. When suckling ceases, prolactin secretion slows and milk production decreases and then stops. |
| | Melanocyte-stimulating hormone (MSH) | Regulates skin pigmentation and promotes the deposit of melanin in the skin after exposure to sunlight |
| *Posterior lobe* | Antidiuretic hormone (ADH) | Stimulates the reabsorption of water by the renal tubules and has a pressor effect that elevates the blood pressure |
| | Oxytocin | Acts on the mammary glands to stimulate the uterus to contract during labor, delivery, and parturition; stimulates the release of milk during suckling |
| Pineal gland | Melatonin | Helps regulate the release of gonadotropin and influences the body's internal clock |
| | Serotonin | Stimulates neurotransmitter, vasoconstrictor, and smooth muscle; acts to inhibit gastric secretion |
| Thyroid gland | Thyroxine (T4) | Maintains and regulates the basal metabolic rate (BMR) |
| | Triiodothyronine (T3) | Influences the basal metabolic rate |
| | Calcitonin | Influences calcium metabolism |
| Parathyroid glands | Parathyroid hormone (PTH); also called *parathormone hormone* | Plays a role in maintenance of a normal serum calcium level and in the metabolism of phosphorus |
| Islets of Langerhans | Glucagon | Facilitates the breakdown of glycogen to glucose |
| | Insulin | Plays a role in maintenance of normal blood sugar |
| | Somatostatin | Suppresses the release of glucagon and insulin |
| Adrenal glands | | |
| *Cortex* | Cortisol | Principal steroid hormone; regulates carbohydrate, protein, and fat metabolism; gluconeogenesis; increases blood sugar level; provides anti-inflammatory effect; helps body cope during times of stress |
| | Corticosterone | Steroid hormone; is essential for normal use of carbohydrates, the absorption of glucose, and gluconeogenesis; also influences potassium (K) and sodium (Na) metabolism |
| | Aldosterone | Principal mineralocorticoid; is essential in regulating electrolyte and water balance |
| | Testosterone | Influences development of male secondary sex characteristics |
| | Androsterone | Influences development of male secondary sex characteristics |

**TABLE 13–1  Summary of the Endocrine Glands, Hormones, and Hormonal Functions (*cont.*)**

| Endocrine Glands | Hormones | Hormonal Functions |
|---|---|---|
| *Medulla* | Dopamine | Dilates systemic arteries, elevates systolic blood pressure, increases cardiac output, increases urinary output |
| | Epinephrine (adrenaline) | Acts as vasoconstrictor, vasopressor, cardiac stimulant, antispasmodic, and sympathomimetic |
| | Norepinephrine | Acts as vasoconstrictor, vasopressor, and neurotransmitter |
| Ovaries | Estrogens (estradiol, estrone, and estriol) | Female sex hormones, are essential for the growth, development, and maintenance of female sex organs and secondary sex characteristics, promote the development of the mammary glands, and play a vital role in a woman's emotional well-being and sexual drive |
| | Progesterone | Prepares the uterus for pregnancy |
| Testes | Testosterone | Is essential for normal growth and development of the male accessory sex organs; plays a vital role in the erection process of the penis and, thus, is necessary for the sexual act, *copulation* (sexual intercourse) |
| Thymus gland | Thymosin | Promotes the maturation process of T lymphocytes |
| | Thymopoietin | Influences the production of lymphocyte precursors and aids in their process of becoming T lymphocytes |
| Gastrointestinal mucosa | Gastrin | Stimulates gastric acid secretion |
| | Secretin | Stimulates pancreatic juice, bile, and intestinal secretion |
| | Pancreozymin | Stimulates the pancreas to produce pancreatic juice |
| | Cholecystokinin | Causes contraction and emptying of the gallbladder |
| | Enterogastrone | Regulates gastric secretions |

# PITUITARY GLAND (HYPOPHYSIS)

The **pituitary gland** is a small gray gland located at the base of the brain. It lies or rests in a shallow depression of the sphenoid bone known as the *sella turcica*. It is attached by the infundibulum stalk to the hypothalamus. The pituitary is approximately 1 centimeter (cm) in diameter and weighs approximately 0.6 gram (g). It is divided into the anterior lobe (adenohypophysis) and the posterior lobe (neurohypophysis). The pituitary is also called the **master gland** of the body because of its regulatory effects on the other endocrine glands.

## Anterior Lobe

The *adenohypophysis* or **anterior lobe** secretes several hormones that are essential for the growth and development of bones, muscles, other organs, sex glands, the thyroid gland, and the adrenal cortex. The hormones secreted by the anterior lobe and their functions are described in the following sections (see Figure 13–2 ▶).

### Growth Hormone (GH)

**Growth hormone,** also called *somatotropin hormone* (STH), is essential for the growth and development of bones, muscles, and other organs. It also enhances protein synthesis, decreases the use of glucose, and promotes fat destruction (lipolysis). Hyposecretion of this hormone can result in **dwarfism** and **Simmonds' disease.** Hypersecretion of the hormone can result in **gigantism** during early life and **acromegaly** in adults.

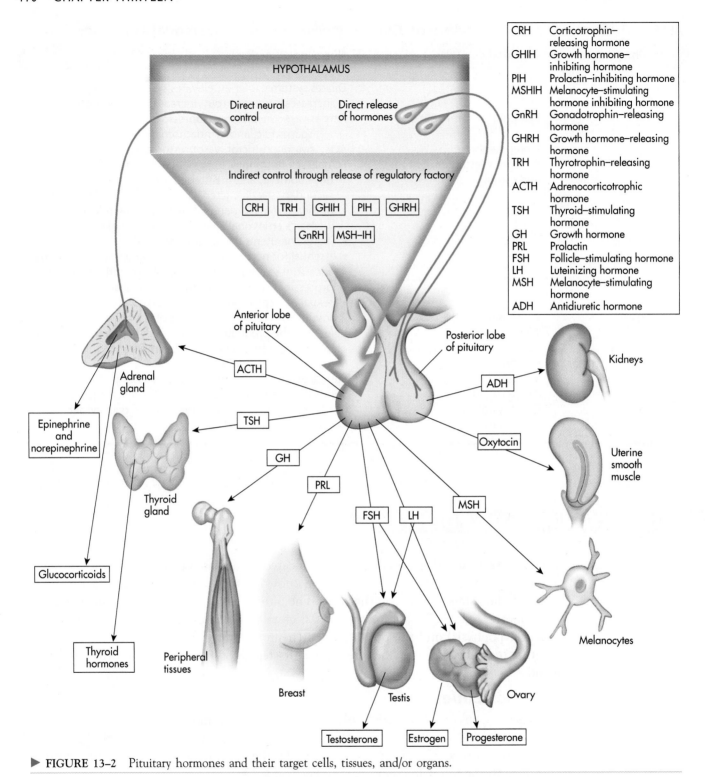

| CRH | Corticotrophin–releasing hormone |
|---|---|
| GHIH | Growth hormone–inhibiting hormone |
| PIH | Prolactin–inhibiting hormone |
| MSHIH | Melanocyte–stimulating hormone inhibiting hormone |
| GnRH | Gonadotrophin–releasing hormone |
| GHRH | Growth hormone–releasing hormone |
| TRH | Thyrotrophin–releasing hormone |
| ACTH | Adrenocorticotrophic hormone |
| TSH | Thyroid–stimulating hormone |
| GH | Growth hormone |
| PRL | Prolactin |
| FSH | Follicle–stimulating hormone |
| LH | Luteinizing hormone |
| MSH | Melanocyte–stimulating hormone |
| ADH | Antidiuretic hormone |

▶ FIGURE 13–2  Pituitary hormones and their target cells, tissues, and/or organs.

### Adrenocorticotropin (ACTH)

**Adrenocorticotropin** is essential for growth and development of the middle and inner zones of the adrenal cortex. The adrenal cortex secretes the glucocorticoids cortisol and corticosterone.

### Thyroid-Stimulating Hormone (TSH)

**Thyroid-stimulating hormone** is essential for the growth and development of the thyroid gland. It stimulates the production of thyroxine and triiodothyronine. It also influences the body's metabolic processes and plays an important role in metabolism.

### Follicle-Stimulating Hormone (FSH)

**Follicle-stimulating hormone** is a gonadotropic hormone that is essential in stimulating the growth of ovarian follicles in the female and the production of sperm in the male.

### Luteinizing Hormone (LH)

*Luteinizing hormone* is a gonadotropic hormone that is essential in the maturation process of the ovarian follicles and stimulates the development of the corpus luteum in the female and the production of testosterone in the male.

### Prolactin (PRL)

**Prolactin** is also known as *lactogenic hormone* (LTH). It is a gonadotropic hormone that stimulates the development and growth of the mammary glands. It is important in the initiation and maintenance of milk production during pregnancy. Following childbirth, the act of suckling provides the stimulus for prolactin synthesis and release. When suckling ceases, prolactin secretion slows and milk production decreases and then stops.

### Melanocyte-Stimulating Hormone (MSH)

**Melanocyte-stimulating hormone** regulates skin pigmentation and promotes the deposit of melanin in the skin after exposure to sunlight.

## Posterior Lobe

The *neurohypophysis* or **posterior lobe** stores and secretes two important hormones that are synthesized in the hypothalamus: antidiuretic hormone and oxytocin (see Figure 13–2). The following sections describe the functions of these hormones.

### Antidiuretic Hormone (ADH)

**Antidiuretic hormone** is also known as *vasopressin* (VP). It stimulates the reabsorption of water by the renal tubules and has a pressor effect that elevates blood pressure. Hyposecretion of this hormone can result in **diabetes insipidus** (DI).

### Oxytocin

**Oxytocin** acts on the mammary glands to stimulate the release of milk during suckling and stimulates the uterus to contract during labor, delivery, and parturition.

## PINEAL GLAND (BODY)

The **pineal gland** is a small, pine cone–shaped gland located near the posterior end of the corpus callosum. It is less than 1 cm in diameter and weighs approximately 0.1 g (see Figure 13–1). The pineal gland secretes **melatonin** and **serotonin.** Melatonin is a hormone that can be released at night to help regulate the release of gonadotropin. Serotonin is a hormone that is a neurotransmitter, vasoconstrictor, and smooth muscle stimulant and acts to inhibit gastric secretion.

## THYROID GLAND

The **thyroid gland** is a large, bilobed gland located in the neck. It is anterior to the trachea and just below the thyroid cartilage. The thyroid is approximately 5 cm long and 3 cm wide and weighs approximately 30 g (see Figure 13–1 and Figure 13–3 ▼). It plays a vital role in metabolism and regulates the body's metabolic processes. The hormones in the following sections are stored and secreted by the thyroid gland.

### Thyroxine (T4)

**Thyroxine** is essential to the maintenance and regulation of the *basal metabolic rate* (BMR). It contains four iodine atoms, which are attached to its nucleus. Thyroxine influences growth and development, both physical and mental, and the metabolism of fats, proteins, carbohydrates, water, vitamins, and minerals. It can be synthetically produced or extracted from animal thyroid glands in crystalline form to be used in the treatment of thyroid dysfunction, especially cretinism, myxedema, and Hashimoto's disease.

### Triiodothyronine (T3)

**Triiodothyronine** is an effective thyroid hormone (TH) that contains three iodine atoms. It influences the basal metabolic rate and is more biologically active than thyroxine.

### Calcitonin

**Calcitonin,** also known as thyrocalcitonin, is a thyroid hormone that influences bone and calcium metabolism. It helps maintain plasma calcium homeostasis.

Hyposecretion of the thyroid hormones T3 and T4 results in **cretinism** during infancy, **myxedema** during adulthood, and **Hashimoto's disease,** which is a chronic thyroid disease. Hypersecretion of the thyroid hormones T3 and T4 results in **hyperthyroidism,** which is also called **thyrotoxicosis,** and **Graves' disease, exophthalmic goiter, toxic goiter,** or **Basedow's disease.** Simple or **endemic goiter** is an enlargement of the thyroid gland caused by a deficiency of iodine in the diet. See Figure 13–18 on page 435.

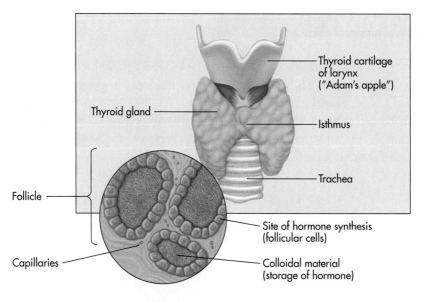

▶ **FIGURE 13–3** Thyroid gland.

# PARATHYROID GLANDS

The **parathyroid glands** are small, yellowish-brown bodies occurring as two pairs located on the dorsal surface and lower aspect of the thyroid gland. Each parathyroid gland is approximately 6 mm in diameter and weighs approximately 0.033 g (see Figure 13–1 and Figure 13–4 ▼). The hormone secreted by the parathyroids is *parathyroid (PTH)*, which is also called *parathormone hormone*. This hormone is essential for the maintenance of a normal serum calcium level. It also plays a role in the metabolism of phosphorus. Hyposecretion of PTH can result in **hypoparathyroidism,** which can result in **tetany** (intermittent cramp or tonic muscular contractions). See Figure 13–5 ▼. Hypersecretion of PTH can result in **hyperparathyroidism,** which may result in **osteoporosis, kidney stones,** and **hypercalcemia.**

# PANCREAS (ISLETS OF LANGERHANS)

The **islets of Langerhans** are small clusters of cells located within the pancreas (see Figure 13–1 and Figure 13–6 ▶). They are composed of three major types of cells: **alpha, beta,** and **delta.** The alpha cells secrete the hormone glucagon (see Figure 13–7 ▶), which facilitates the breakdown of glycogen to glucose, thereby elevating blood sugar.

The beta cells secrete the hormone insulin (see Figure 13–7), which is essential for the maintenance of normal blood sugar (70–110 mg/100 mL of blood). Insulin is essential to life. It acts to regulate the metabolism of glucose and the process necessary for the intermediary metabolism of carbohydrates, fats, and proteins. It promotes the use of glucose in cells, thereby lowering the blood glucose (BG) level. Insulin can be synthetically produced in various types and was first discovered and used successfully by Sir F. G. Banting in the early 1920s. Hyposecretion or inadequate use of insulin may result in **diabetes mellitus** (DM). Hypersecretion of insulin may result in **hyperinsulinism.** The delta cells secrete a hormone, *somatostatin*, which suppresses the release of glucagon and insulin.

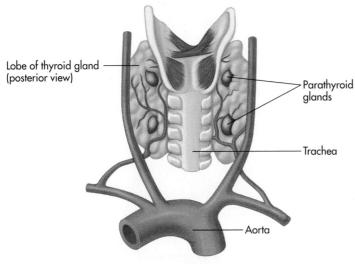

Lobe of thyroid gland (posterior view)

Parathyroid glands

Trachea

Aorta

▶ **FIGURE 13–4**   Parathyroid glands.

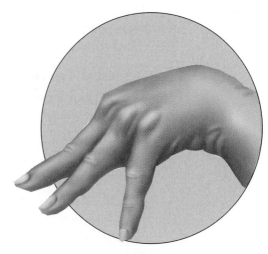

▶ **FIGURE 13–5**   Tetany of the hand in hypoparathyroidism.

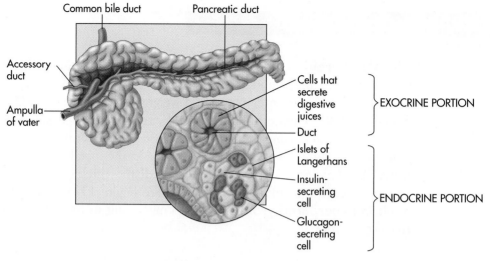

**FIGURE 13–6** Pancreas—an endocrine and exocrine gland.

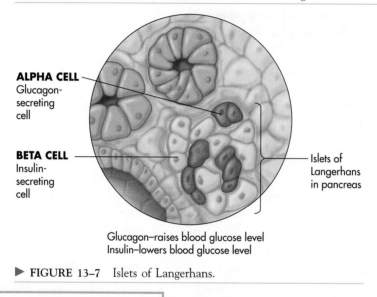

**FIGURE 13–7** Islets of Langerhans.

# ADRENAL GLANDS (SUPRARENALS)

The **adrenal glands** are two small, triangular-shaped glands located on top of each kidney. Each gland weighs about 5 g and consists of an outer portion or *cortex* and an inner portion called the *medulla* (see Figure 13–1 and Figure 13–8 ▶).

## Adrenal Cortex

The **cortex** is essential to life for secreting a group of hormones, the glucocorticoids, the mineralocorticoids, and the androgens. These hormones and their effects on the body are described next.

### Glucocorticoids

The two glucocorticoid hormones are *cortisol* and *corticosterone*.

Cortisol. Cortisol (hydrocortisone) is the principal steroid hormone secreted by the cortex. The following are some of the known influences and functions of cortisol:

- Regulates carbohydrate, protein, and fat metabolism.
- Stimulates output of glucose from the liver (**gluconeogenesis**).
- Increases the blood sugar level.

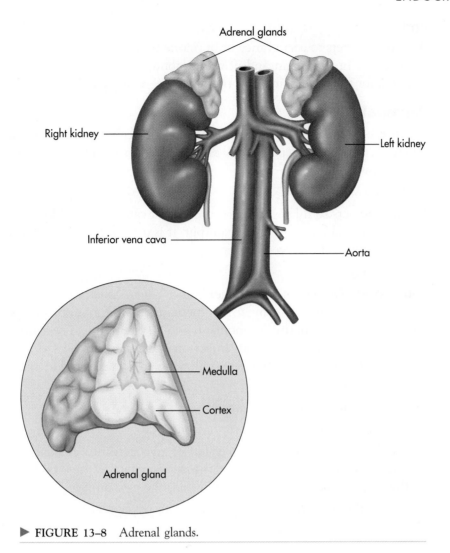

► FIGURE 13–8   Adrenal glands.

- Regulates other physiologic body processes.
- Promotes the transport of amino acids into extracellular tissue, thereby making them available for energy.
- Influences the effectiveness of catecholamines such as dopamine, epinephrine, and norepinephrine.
- Has an anti-inflammatory effect.
- Helps the body cope during times of stress.

Hyposecretion of cortisol can result in **Addison's disease;** hypersecretion can result in **Cushing's disease.**

Corticosterone.   Corticosterone is a steroid hormone secreted by the adrenal cortex. It is essential for the normal use of carbohydrates, the absorption of glucose, and the formation of glycogen in the liver and tissues. It also influences potassium and sodium metabolism.

### Mineralocorticoids
**Aldosterone** is the principal **mineralocorticoid** secreted by the adrenal cortex. It is essential in regulating electrolyte and water balance by promoting sodium and chloride retention and potassium excretion. Hyposecretion of this hormone can result in a **reduced plasma volume,** and hypersecretion can result in a condition known as **primary aldosteronism.**

### Androgens

**Androgen** refers to a substance or hormone that promotes the development of male characteristics. The two main androgen hormones are *testosterone* and *androsterone*. They are essential for the development of the male secondary sex characteristics.

## Adrenal Medulla

The **medulla** synthesizes, secretes, and stores catecholamines, specifically, dopamine, epinephrine, and norepinephrine. A discussion of these substances and their effects on the body follows.

### Dopamine

**Dopamine** acts to dilate systemic arteries, elevates systolic blood pressure, increases cardiac output, and increases urinary output. It is used in the treatment of shock and is a neurotransmitter in the nervous system.

### Epinephrine

**Epinephrine** *(Adrenalin, adrenaline)* acts as a vasoconstrictor, vasopressor, cardiac stimulant, antispasmodic, and sympathomimetic. Its main function is to assist in regulating the sympathetic branch of the autonomic nervous system. It can be synthetically produced and administered *parenterally* (by an injection), *topically* (on a local area of the skin), or by *inhalation* (by nose or mouth). The following are some of the known influences and functions of epinephrine:

- Elevates the systolic blood pressure.
- Increases the heart rate and cardiac output.
- Increases glycogenolysis (conversion of glycogen into glucose), thereby hastening the release of glucose from the liver; this action elevates the blood sugar level and provides the body a spurt of energy; referred to as the *fight-or-flight syndrome*.
- Dilates the bronchial tubes and relaxes air passageways.
- Dilates the pupils to see more clearly.

### Norepinephrine

**Norepinephrine** *(noradrenaline)* acts as a vasoconstrictor, vasopressor, and neurotransmitter. It elevates systolic and diastolic blood pressure, increases the heart rate and cardiac output, and increases glycogenolysis.

## OVARIES

The **ovaries** produce *estrogens (estradiol, estrone,* and *estriol)* and *progesterone.* Estrogen is the female sex hormone secreted by the graafian follicles of the ovaries. Progesterone is a steroid hormone secreted by the corpus luteum. These hormones are essential for promoting the growth, development, and maintenance of secondary female sex organs and characteristics. They also prepare the uterus for pregnancy, promote development of the mammary glands, and play a vital role in a woman's emotional well-being and sexual drive (see Figure 13–1).

## TESTES

The **testes** produce the male sex hormone *testosterone,* which is essential for normal growth and development of the male accessory sex organs. Testosterone plays a vital role in the erection process of the penis and, thus, is necessary for the sexual act, copulation (see Figure 13–1).

# PLACENTA

During pregnancy, the **placenta,** a spongy structure joining mother and child, serves as an endocrine gland. It produces chorionic gonadotropin hormone, estrogen, and progesterone.

# GASTROINTESTINAL MUCOSA

The **mucosa** of the pyloric area of the stomach secretes the hormone *gastrin*, which stimulates gastric acid secretion. Gastrin also affects the gallbladder, pancreas, and small intestine secretory activities.

The mucosa of the duodenum and jejunum secretes the hormone *secretin*, which stimulates pancreatic juice, bile, and intestinal secretion. The mucosa of the duodenum also secretes *pancreozymin-cholecystokinin*, which stimulates the pancreas. *Enterogastrone*, a hormone that regulates gastric secretions, is also secreted by the duodenal mucosa.

# THYMUS

The **thymus** is a bilobed body located in the mediastinal cavity in front of and above the heart (see Figure 13–9 ▼). It is composed of lymphoid tissue and is a part of the lymphatic system. It is a ductless glandlike body and secretes the hormones *thymosin* and *thymopoietin*. Thymosin promotes the maturation process of T lymphocytes (thymus dependent). Thymopoietin is a hormone that influences the production of lymphocyte precursors and aids in their process of becoming T lymphocytes.

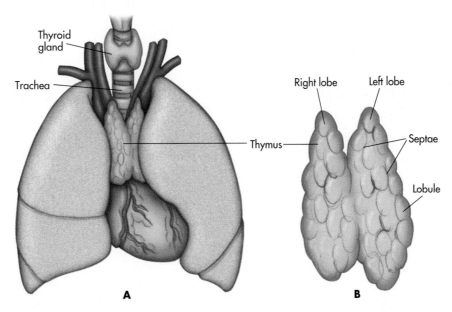

▶ **FIGURE 13–9**    Thymus gland. (A) Appearance and position; (B) with anatomic structures.

# LIFE SPAN CONSIDERATIONS

## ■ THE CHILD

Most of the structures and glands of the endocrine system develop during the first 3 months of pregnancy. The endocrine system of the newborn is supplemented by hormones that cross the placental barrier. Both male and female newborns may have swelling of the breast and genitalia from maternal hormones.

Either excessively high or insufficient production of growth hormone (GH) by the anterior lobe of the pituitary gland can cause abnormal growth patterns. Excessive production of GH can cause **gigantism.** Insufficient production of GH can cause **dwarfism.**

**Diabetes mellitus** (DM) is the most common endocrine system disorder of childhood. The rate of occurrence is highest among 5- to 7-year-olds and 11- to 15-year-olds. The classic symptoms of diabetes mellitus—**polyuria** (frequent urination), **polydipsia** (excessive thirst), and **polyphagia** (extreme hunger)—appear more rapidly in children. Other symptoms seen during childhood are weakness, loss of weight, lethargy, anorexia, irritability, dry skin, vaginal yeast infections in the female child and/or recurrent infections, and abdominal cramps. The management of diabetes mellitus during childhood is very difficult because diet, exercise, and medication have to be adjusted and regulated according to the various stages of growth and development of the child.

## ■ THE OLDER ADULT

With aging, **hormonal changes** vary with each individual. Generally, the number of tissue receptors decreases, thus diminishing the body's response to hormones. This is especially the case with older adults who develop **Type 2 diabetes mellitus.** In this condition, sufficient insulin is produced, but because the number of cell receptors is reduced, glucose does not enter the cells.

An older adult may not be diagnosed with diabetes until he or she goes in for a regular eye exam, and the ophthalmologist discovers a problem, and/or goes in for a physical examination and the blood test indicates an elevated blood glucose level. The multiple risk factors associated with the older adult and the development of diabetes follow:

- Age-related decreased insulin production.
- Age-related insulin resistance.
- Heredity.
- Decreased physical activity.
- Multiple diseases.
- Polypharmacy (the use of many drugs together).
- Obesity.
- New stressors in life.

# BUILDING YOUR MEDICAL VOCABULARY

This section provides the foundation for learning medical terminology. Review the following alphabetized word list. Note how common prefixes and suffixes are repeatedly applied to word roots and combining forms to create different meanings.

| P | Prefix |
|---|---|
| R | Root |
| CF | Combining form |
| S | Suffix |

| Pink words | Terms not built from word parts. |
|---|---|
| * | Indicates words covered in the Pathology Spotlights section. |
| 💿 | Check the CD-ROM for more information. |

| MEDICAL WORD | Part | Type | Meaning | DEFINITION |
|---|---|---|---|---|
| **acidosis**<br>(ăs″ ĭ-dō′ sĭs) | acid<br>-osis | R<br>S | acid<br>condition (usually abnormal) | Condition of excessive acidity of body fluids |
| **acromegaly**<br>(ăk″ rō-mĕg′ ă-lē) | acr/o<br>-megaly | CF<br>S | extremity<br>enlargement, large | Chronic disease characterized by a gradual marked enlargement and elongation of the bones of the face, jaw, and extremities. It is caused by overproduction of growth hormone and is treated by x-ray or surgery. |
| **Addison's disease**<br>(ăd′ ĭ-sŭns dĭ-zēz) | | | | Results from a deficiency in the secretion of adrenocortical hormones; also called *hypoadrenocorticism.* * See Pathology Spotlight: Addison's Disease on page 431. |
| **adenectomy**<br>(ăd″ ĕn-ĕk′ tō-mē) | aden<br>-ectomy | R<br>S | gland<br>surgical excision | Surgical excision of a gland |
| **adenoma**<br>(ăd″ ĕ-nō′ mă) | aden<br>-oma | R<br>S | gland<br>tumor | Tumor of a gland |
| **adenosis**<br>(ăd″ ĕ-nō′ sĭs) | aden<br>-osis | R<br>S | gland<br>condition (usually abnormal) | Any disease condition of a gland |
| **adrenal**<br>(ăd-rē′ năl) | adren<br>-al | R<br>S | adrenal gland<br>pertaining to | Pertaining to the adrenal glands, triangular bodies that cover the superior surface of the kidneys; also called *suprarenal glands* |
| **adrenalectomy**<br>(ăd-rē″ năl-ĕk′ tō-mē) | adren<br>-al<br>-ectomy | R<br>S<br>S | adrenal gland<br>pertaining to<br>surgical excision | Surgical excision of an adrenal gland |
| **adrenopathy**<br>(ăd″ rĕn-ŏp′ ă-thē) | adren/o<br>-pathy | CF<br>S | adrenal gland<br>disease | Any disease of an adrenal gland |
| **aldosterone**<br>(ăl-dŏs′ tĕr-ōn) | | | | Mineralocorticoid hormone secreted by the adrenal cortex that helps regulate metabolism of sodium, chloride, and potassium |

| MEDICAL WORD | WORD PARTS (WHEN APPLICABLE) | | | DEFINITION |
|---|---|---|---|---|
| | **Part** | **Type** | **Meaning** | |
| **androgen**<br>(ăn' drō-jĕn) | andr/o<br>-gen | CF<br>S | man<br>formation,<br>produce | Hormones that produce or stimulate the development of male characteristics. The two major androgens are testosterone and androsterone. |
| **catecholamines**<br>(kăt" ĕ-kōl' ăm-ēns) | | | | Biochemical substances, epinephrine, norepinephrine, and dopamine |
| **cortisone**<br>(kŏr' tĭ-sōn) | cortis<br>-one | R<br>S | cortex<br>hormone | Glucocorticoid hormone that is isolated from the adrenal cortex; used as an anti-inflammatory agent |
| **cretinism**<br>(krē' tĭn-ĭzm) | cretin<br>-ism | R<br>S | cretin<br>condition | Congenital condition caused by deficiency in secretion of the thyroid hormones and characterized by arrested physical and mental development. Treatment consist of appropriate thyroid replacement therapy. See Figure 13–10 ▼. |
| **Cushing's disease**<br>(koosh' ĭngs dĭ-zēz) | | | | Results from hypersecretion of cortisol; symptoms include fatigue, muscular weakness, and changes in body appearance. Prolonged administration of large doses of ACTH can cause Cushing's syndrome. A *buffalo hump* and a *moon face* are characteristic signs of this condition. See Figure 13–11 ▶. |

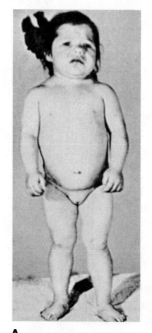 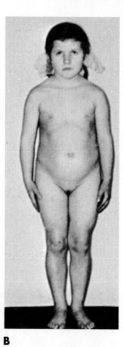

**A**                    **B**

▶ **FIGURE 13–10**   (A) A 6-year-old child with congenital hypothyroidism, cretinism, exhibiting marked mental and physical retardation. (B) The same patient after 3 years of thyroxine therapy, which resulted in a spurt of growth and regression of pathological manifestations. Mental retardation is delayed.

| MEDICAL WORD | WORD PARTS (WHEN APPLICABLE) | | | DEFINITION |
|---|---|---|---|---|
| | **Part** | **Type** | **Meaning** | |
| **diabetes** (dī″ ă-bē′ tēz) | dia- -betes | P S | through to go | General term used to describe diseases characterized by excessive discharge of urine. FYI: In the second century, Aretaeus the Cappadocian, an Alexandrian physician, was confronted with a patient who had excessive urination. He chose a Greek word, *diabetes* (that which passes through), to define what he considered to be the most dominant clinical sign in his patient. Later the word diabetes was combined with *mellitus,* a word of Latin origin that means honey. In 1670, in those suffering from polyuria, a distinction was made between those patients who had a sweet tasting urine (diabetes mellitus) and those patients whose urine had no taste (diabetes insipidus). ✱ See Pathology Spotlight: Diabetes Mellitus on page 432. |

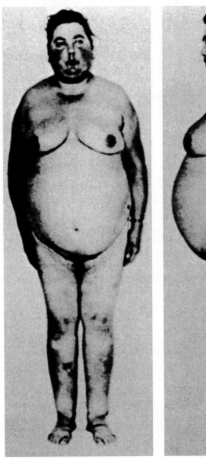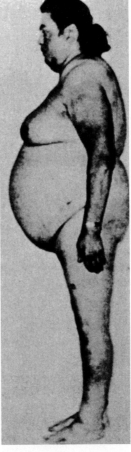

▶ **FIGURE 13–11**  Cushing's syndrome patient showing round, red face; stocky neck; and marked obesity of the trunk with protruding abdomen. Note bruises on trunk and legs and stretch marks and fat pads above the collar bone and on the back of the neck, which produces the *buffalo hump*.

| MEDICAL WORD | WORD PARTS (WHEN APPLICABLE) | | | DEFINITION |
|---|---|---|---|---|
| | Part | Type | Meaning | |
| dopamine<br>(dō′ pă-mēn) | | | | Intermediate substance in the synthesis of norepinephrine; used in the treatment of shock because it acts to elevate blood pressure and increase urinary output |
| dwarfism<br>(dwar′ fizm) | dwarf<br>-ism | R<br>S | small<br>condition | Condition of being abnormally small |
| endocrine<br>(ĕn′ dō-krĭn) | endo-<br>crine | P<br>R | within<br>to secrete | Ductless gland that produces an internal secretion |
| endocrinologist<br>(ĕn″ dō-krĭn-ŏl′ ō-gĭst) | endo-<br>crin/o<br>log<br>-ist | P<br>CF<br>R<br>S | within<br>to secrete<br>study of<br>one who specializes | Physician who specializes in the study of the endocrine glands |
| endocrinology<br>(ĕn″ dō-krĭn-ŏl′ ō-jē) | endo-<br>crin/o<br>-logy | P<br>CF<br>S | within<br>to secrete<br>study of | Study of the endocrine glands |
| epinephrine<br>(ĕp″ ĭ-nĕf′ rĭn) | epi-<br>nephr<br>-ine | P<br>R<br>S | upon<br>kidney<br>substance | Hormone produced by the adrenal medulla; used as a vasoconstrictor and cardiac stimulant to relax bronchospasm and to relieve allergic symptoms; also called *adrenaline, Adrenalin* |
| estrogen<br>(ĕs′ trō-jĕn) | estr/o<br>-gen | CF<br>S | mad desire<br>formation, produce | Hormones produced by the ovaries, including estradiol, estrone, and estriol, female sex hormones important in the development of secondary sex characteristics and regulation of the menstrual cycle |
| euthyroid<br>(ū-thī′ royd) | eu-<br>thyr<br>-oid | P<br>R<br>S | good, normal<br>thyroid, shield<br>resemble | Normal activity of the thyroid gland |
| exocrine<br>(ĕks′ ō-krĭn) | exo-<br>crine | P<br>R | out, away from<br>to secrete | External secretion of a gland |
| exophthalmic<br>(ĕks″ ŏf-thăl′ mĭk) | ex-<br>ophthalm<br>-ic | P<br>R<br>S | out, away from<br>eye<br>pertaining to | Pertaining to an abnormal protrusion of the eye as often seen in exophthalmic goiter or exophthalmos seen in Graves' disease. See Figure 13–12 ▶. |
| galactorrhea<br>(gă-lăk″ tō-rĭ′ ă) | galact/o<br>-rrhea | CF<br>S | milk<br>flow, discharge | Excessive secretion of milk after cessation of nursing |
| gigantism<br>(ji′ găn-tĭzm) | gigant<br>-ism | R<br>S | giant<br>condition | Condition of being abnormally large |
| glandular<br>(glăn′ dū-lăr) | glandul<br>-ar | R<br>S | little acorn<br>pertaining to | Pertaining to a gland |
| glucocorticoid<br>(glū″ kō-kŏrt′ ĭ-koyd) | gluc/o<br>cortic<br>-oid | CF<br>R<br>S | sweet, sugar<br>cortex<br>resemble | General classification of the adrenal cortical hormones |

| MEDICAL WORD | WORD PARTS (WHEN APPLICABLE) | | | DEFINITION |
|---|---|---|---|---|
| | Part | Type | Meaning | |
| **hirsutism** (hŭr′ sūt-ĭzm) | hirsut -ism | R S | hairy condition | Abnormal condition characterized by excessive growth of hair, especially in women. See Figure 13–13 ▼. |
| **hormone** (hor′ mōn) | | | | Chemical substance produced by the endocrine glands |
| **hydrocortisone** (hĭ″ drō-kŏr′ tĭ-sōn) | hydro cortis -one | R R S | water cortex hormone | Glucocorticoid hormone produced by the adrenal cortex; used as an anti-inflammatory agent |
| **hypergonadism** (hī″ pĕr-gō′ năd-ĭzm) | hyper- gonad -ism | P R S | excessive seed condition | Condition of excessive secretion of the sex glands |
| **hyperinsulinism** (hī″ pĕr-ĭn′ sū-lĭn-ĭzm) | hyper- insulin -ism | P R S | excessive insulin condition | Condition of excessive amounts of insulin in the blood |

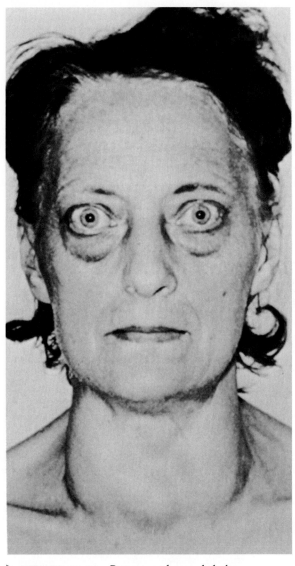

▶ **FIGURE 13–12**  Patient with exophthalmos.

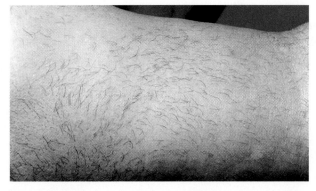

▶ **FIGURE 13–13**  Hirsutism. (Courtesy Jason L. Smith, MD)

| MEDICAL WORD | WORD PARTS (WHEN APPLICABLE) | | | DEFINITION |
|---|---|---|---|---|
| | Part | Type | Meaning | |
| **hyperkalemia** <br> (hī″ pĕr-kă-lē′ mĭ-ă) | hyper- <br> kal <br> -emia | P <br> R <br> S | excessive <br> potassium (K) <br> blood <br> condition | Condition of excessive amounts of potassium in the blood |
| **hyperthyroidism** <br> (hī″ pĕr-thī′ royd-ĭzm) | hyper- <br> thyr <br> -oid <br> -ism | P <br> R <br> S <br> S | excessive <br> thyroid, shield <br> resemble <br> condition | Excessive secretion of thyroid hormone, a condition that can affect many body systems. See Figure 13–14 ▶. ✶ See Pathology Spotlight: Hyperthyroidism on page 436. |
| **hypogonadism** <br> (hī″ pō-gō′ năd-ĭzm) | hypo- <br> gonad <br> -ism | P <br> R <br> S | deficient <br> seed <br> condition | Condition caused by deficient internal secretion of the gonads |
| **hypopara-thyroidism** <br> (hī″ pō-păr″ ă-thī′ royd-ĭzm) | hypo- <br> para- <br> thyr <br> -oid <br> -ism | P <br> P <br> R <br> S <br> S | deficient <br> beside <br> thyroid, shield <br> resemble <br> condition | Deficient internal secretion of the parathyroid glands |
| **hypophysis** <br> (hī-pŏf′ ĭ-sĭs) | hypo- <br> -physis | P <br> S | deficient, under <br> growth | Any undergrowth; the pituitary body |
| **hypothyroidism** <br> (hī″ pō-thī′ royd-ĭzm) | hypo- <br> thyr <br> -oid <br> -ism | P <br> R <br> S <br> S | deficient <br> thyroid, shield <br> resemble <br> condition | Deficient secretion of thyroid hormone, a condition that can affect many body systems. See Figure 13–15 ▶. ✶ See Pathology Spotlight: Hypothyroidism on page 433. |
| **insulin** <br> (in′ sū-lĭn) | insul <br> -in | R <br> S | insulin, island <br> chemical | Hormone produced by the beta cells of the islets of Langerhans of the pancreas; acts to regulate the metabolism of glucose and the process necessary for the intermediary metabolism of carbohydrates, fats, and proteins; used in the management of diabetes mellitus |
| **insulinogenic** <br> (ĭn″ sū-lĭn″ ō-jĕn′ ĭk) | insulin/o <br> -genic | CF <br> S | insulin, island <br> formation, produce | Formation or production of insulin |
| **iodine** <br> (ī′ ō-dīn) | | | | Trace mineral that aids in the development and functioning of the thyroid gland |
| **lethargic** <br> (lĕ-thar′ jĭk) | letharg <br> -ic | R <br> S | drowsiness <br> pertaining to | Pertaining to drowsiness, sluggish |
| **myxedema** <br> (mĭks″ ĕ-dē′ mă) | myx <br> -edema | R <br> S | mucus <br> swelling | Literally means *condition of mucus swelling*; it is the most severe form of hypothyroidism, characterized by marked edema of the face, a somnolent look, and hair that is stiff and without luster. ✶ See Pathology Spotlight: Hypothyroidism on page 433 and Figure 13–19. |

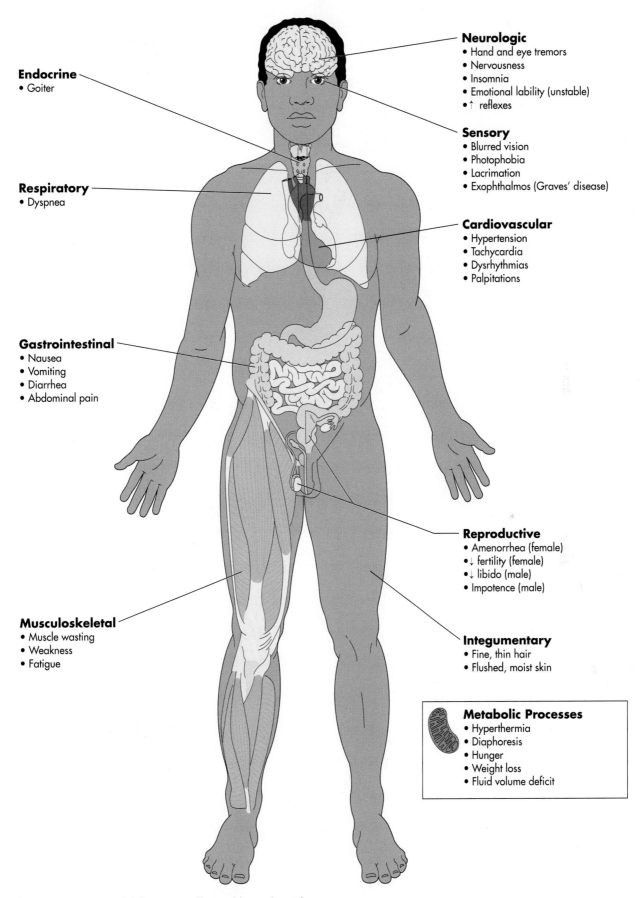

**Endocrine**
• Goiter

**Respiratory**
• Dyspnea

**Gastrointestinal**
• Nausea
• Vomiting
• Diarrhea
• Abdominal pain

**Musculoskeletal**
• Muscle wasting
• Weakness
• Fatigue

**Neurologic**
• Hand and eye tremors
• Nervousness
• Insomnia
• Emotional lability (unstable)
• ↑ reflexes

**Sensory**
• Blurred vision
• Photophobia
• Lacrimation
• Exophthalmos (Graves' disease)

**Cardiovascular**
• Hypertension
• Tachycardia
• Dysrhythmias
• Palpitations

**Reproductive**
• Amenorrhea (female)
• ↓ fertility (female)
• ↓ libido (male)
• Impotence (male)

**Integumentary**
• Fine, thin hair
• Flushed, moist skin

**Metabolic Processes**
• Hyperthermia
• Diaphoresis
• Hunger
• Weight loss
• Fluid volume deficit

▶ FIGURE 13–14  Multisystem effects of hyperthyroidism.

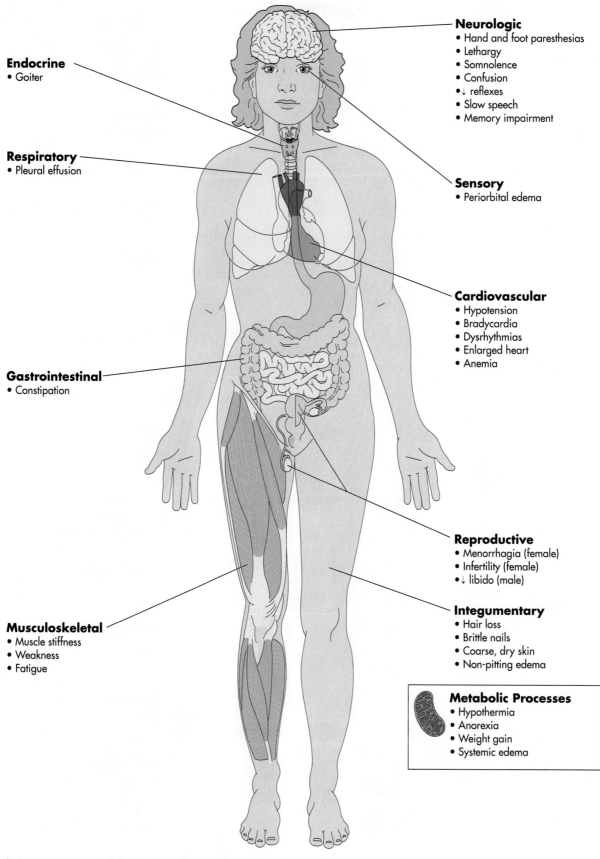

**Neurologic**
- Hand and foot paresthesias
- Lethargy
- Somnolence
- Confusion
- ↓ reflexes
- Slow speech
- Memory impairment

**Endocrine**
- Goiter

**Respiratory**
- Pleural effusion

**Sensory**
- Periorbital edema

**Cardiovascular**
- Hypotension
- Bradycardia
- Dysrhythmias
- Enlarged heart
- Anemia

**Gastrointestinal**
- Constipation

**Reproductive**
- Menorrhagia (female)
- Infertility (female)
- ↓ libido (male)

**Musculoskeletal**
- Muscle stiffness
- Weakness
- Fatigue

**Integumentary**
- Hair loss
- Brittle nails
- Coarse, dry skin
- Non-pitting edema

**Metabolic Processes**
- Hypothermia
- Anorexia
- Weight gain
- Systemic edema

▶ **FIGURE 13–15**    Multisystem effects of hypothyroidism.

| MEDICAL WORD | WORD PARTS (WHEN APPLICABLE) | | | DEFINITION |
|---|---|---|---|---|
| | Part | Type | Meaning | |
| **norepinephrine**<br>(nŏr-ĕp″ĭ-nĕf′rĭn) | nor-<br>epi-<br>nephr<br>-ine | P<br>P<br>R<br>S | not<br>upon<br>kidney<br>substance | Hormone produced by the adrenal medulla; used as a vasoconstrictor of peripheral blood vessels in acute hypotensive states |
| **oxytocin**<br>(ŏk″sĭ-tō′sĭn) | | | | Hormone that stimulates uterine contraction during childbirth and stimulates the release of milk during suckling |
| **pancreatic**<br>(păn″krē-ăt′ĭk) | pancreat<br>-ic | R<br>S | pancreas<br>pertaining to | Pertaining to the pancreas |
| **parathyroid glands**<br>(păr″ă-thī′royd glă′nds) | para-<br>thyr<br>-oid | P<br>R<br>S | beside<br>thyroid, shield<br>resemble | Endocrine glands located beside the thyroid gland |
| **pineal**<br>(pĭn′ē-ăl) | pine<br>-al | R<br>S | pine cone<br>pertaining to | Endocrine gland shaped like a small pine cone |
| **pituitarism**<br>(pĭt-ū′ĭ-tă-rĭzm) | pituitar<br>-ism | R<br>S | pituitary gland<br>condition | Any condition of the pituitary gland |
| **pituitary**<br>(pĭ-tū′ĭ-tăr″ē) | pituitar<br>-y | R<br>S | pituitary gland<br>pertaining to | Pertaining to the pituitary gland, the hypophysis |
| **progeria**<br>(prō-jē′rĭ-ă) | pro-<br>ger<br>-ia | P<br>R<br>S | before<br>old age<br>condition | Condition of premature old age occurring in childhood |
| **progesterone**<br>(prō-jĕs′tĕr-ōn) | pro-<br>gester<br>-one | P<br>R<br>S | before<br>to bear<br>hormone | Hormone produced by the corpus luteum of the ovary, the adrenal cortex, or the placenta; released during the second half of the menstrual cycle |
| **Simmonds' disease**<br>(sĭm′mŏnds dĭ-zēz′) | | | | Condition in which complete atrophy of the pituitary gland causes loss of function of the thyroid, adrenals, and gonads; symptoms include premature senility, psychic symptoms, and cachexia; also called *panhypopituitarism*. Treatment involves regular administration of the various hormones whose release is normally dependent on pituitary function. |
| **somatotropin**<br>(sō-măt′ō-trō″pĭn) | somat/o<br>trop<br>-in | CF<br>R<br>S | body<br>turn<br>chemical | Growth-stimulating hormone produced by the anterior lobe of the pituitary gland |
| **steroids**<br>(stĕr′oydz) | ster<br>-oid | R<br>S | solid<br>resemble | Group of chemical substances that includes hormones, vitamins, sterols, cardiac glycosides, and certain drugs |
| **testosterone**<br>(tĕs-tŏs′tĕr-ōn) | test/o<br>ster<br>-one | CF<br>R<br>S | testicle<br>solid<br>hormone | Hormone produced by the testes; male sex hormone important in the development of secondary sex characteristics and masculinization |

| MEDICAL WORD | WORD PARTS (WHEN APPLICABLE) | | | DEFINITION |
|---|---|---|---|---|
| | Part | Type | Meaning | |
| **thymectomy**<br>(thī-měk′ tō-mē) | thym<br>-ectomy | R<br>S | thymus<br>surgical excision | Surgical excision of the thymus gland |
| **thymitis**<br>(thī-mī′ tǐs) | thym<br>-it is | R<br>S | thymus<br>inflammation | Inflammation of the thymus gland |
| **thyroid**<br>(thī′ royd) | thyr<br>-oid | R<br>S | thyroid, shield<br>resemble | Resembling a shield; one of the endocrine glands. See Figure 13–16 ▼. |
| **thyroidectomy**<br>(thī″ royd-ěk′ tō-mē) | thyr<br>-oid<br>-ectomy | R<br>S<br>S | thyroid, shield<br>resemble<br>surgical excision | Surgical excision of the thyroid gland |
| **thyroiditis**<br>(thī″ royd′ ǐ′ tǐs) | thyr<br>-oid<br>-itis | R<br>S<br>S | thyroid, shield<br>resemble<br>inflammation | Inflammation of the thyroid gland |
| **thyrotoxicosis**<br>(thī″ rō-tŏks″ ǐ-kō′ sǐs) | thyr/o<br>toxic<br>-osis | CF<br>R<br>S | thyroid, shield<br>poison<br>condition (usually abnormal) | Poisonous condition of the thyroid gland caused by hyperactivity |
| **thyroxine (T4)**<br>(thī-rŏks′ ēn) | thyro<br>-ine | R<br>S | thyroid, shield<br>substance | Hormone produced by the thyroid gland; important in growth and development and regulation of the body's metabolic rate and metabolism of carbohydrates, fats, and proteins |
| **vasopressin (VP)**<br>(văs″ ō-prěs′ ǐn) | vas/o<br>press<br>-in | CF<br>R<br>S | vessel<br>to press<br>chemical | Hormone produced by the hypothalamus and stored in the posterior lobe of the pituitary gland; also called *antidiuretic hormone (ADH)* |
| **virilism**<br>(vǐr′ ǐl-ǐzm) | viril<br>-ism | R<br>S | masculine<br>condition | Condition of masculinity developed in a woman |

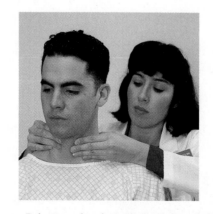

▶ FIGURE 13–16  Palpating the thyroid gland from behind the patient.

# DRUG HIGHLIGHTS

| | |
|---|---|
| **Thyroid hormones** | Increase metabolic rate, cardiac output, oxygen consumption, body temperature, respiratory rate, blood volume, and carbohydrate, fat, and protein metabolism; influence growth and development at cellular level. Thyroid hormones are used as supplements or replacement therapy in hypothyroidism, myxedema, and cretinism.<br><br>*Examples: Levothroid and Synthroid (levothyroxine sodium), Cytomel (liothyronine sodium), Thyrolar (liotrix), and thyroid, USP* |
| **Antithyroid hormones** | Inhibit the synthesis of thyroid hormones by decreasing iodine use in manufacture of thyroglobin and iodothyronine; do not inactivate or inhibit thyroxine or triiodothyronine. They are used in the treatment of hyperthyroidism.<br><br>*Example: Tapazole (methimazole), potassium iodide solution, Lugol's solution (strong iodine solution), and PTU (propylthiouracil)* |
| **Insulin** | Stimulates carbohydrate metabolism by increasing the movement of glucose and other monosaccharides into cells. It also influences fat and carbohydrate metabolism in the liver and adipose cells. It decreases blood sugar, phosphate, and potassium, and increases blood pyruvate and lactate. Insulin is used to treat insulin-dependent diabetes mellitus (Type 1), noninsulin-dependent diabetes mellitus (Type 2) when other regimens are not effective, and to treat ketoacidosis. |
| **Insulin preparations** | Insulin is given by subcutaneous injection and is available in rapid-acting, intermediate-acting, and long-acting preparations. In 2006, the FDA approved the first inhaled insulin combination product for treatment of diabetes. It is an inhaled, rapid-acting, dry-powder formulation of recombinant human insulin (rDNA) that is inhaled into the lungs via the mouth before meals using a handheld device. |
| Rapid acting | *Examples: Regular, Novolin R, Velosulin, and Humalog.*<br><br>Onset of Action ½ hour        Appearance—clear |
| Intermediate acting | *Examples: NPH, Novolin N, Humulin N, Lente Insulin, and Novolin L*<br><br>Onset of action—1–1½ hours        Appearance—cloudy |
| Long acting | *Examples: Ultralente and Humulin U*<br><br>Onset of action—3–5 hours     Appearance—cloudy |
| Inhaled insulin | *Example: Exubera        Delivered by handheld device*<br><br>Onset of action—rapid |
| **Oral hypoglycemic agents** | Stimulate insulin secretion from pancreatic cells in noninsulin-dependent diabetics with some pancreatic function. They are agents of the sulfonylurea class.<br><br>*Examples: Diabinese (chlorpropamide), Glucotrol (glipizide), DiaBeta and Micronase (glyburide), Tolinase (tolazamide), Orinase (tolbutamide), and Avandia (rosiglitazone maleate)* |
| **Hyperglycemic agents** | Cause an increase in blood glucose of diabetic patients with severe hypoglycemia (insulin shock). In patients with mild hypoglycemia, the administration of an oral carbohydrate such as orange juice, candy, or a lump of sugar generally corrects the condition. If comatose, the patient is given dextrose solution IV. For management of severe hypoglycemia, the following agents may be used.<br><br>*Examples: Glucagon (an insulin antagonist), Proglycem (diazoxide), and Glutose, Insta-Glucose (glucose)* |

# DIAGNOSTIC AND LAB TESTS

| TEST | DESCRIPTION |
|------|-------------|
| Catecholamines (kăt″ ĕ-kōl′ ă-mēns) | Test performed on urine to determine the amount of epinephrine and norepinephrine present. These adrenal hormones increase in times of stress. |
| Corticotropin, corticotropin-releasing factor (CRF) (kor″ tĭ-kō-trō′ pin) | Test performed on blood plasma to determine the amount of corticotropin present. Increased levels can indicate stress, adrenal cortical hypofunction, and/or pituitary tumors. Decreased levels can indicate adrenal neoplasms and/or Cushing's syndrome. |
| Fasting blood sugar (FBS) | Test performed on blood to determine the level of sugar in the bloodstream. Increased levels can indicate diabetes mellitus, diabetic acidosis, and many other conditions. Decreased levels can indicate hypoglycemia, hyperinsulinism, and many other conditions. Also referred to as fasting blood glucose (FBG). |
| Glucose tolerance test (GTT) (gloo′ kōs) | Blood sugar test performed at specified intervals after the patient has been given a certain amount of glucose. Blood samples are drawn, and the glucose level of each sample is measured. It is more accurate than other blood sugar tests and is used to diagnose diabetes mellitus. |
| 17-hydroxycortico-steroids (17-OHCS) (hī-drŏk″ sē-kor tĭ-kō-) | Test performed on urine to identify adrenocorticosteroid hormones and to determine adrenal cortical function. |
| 17-ketosteroids (17-KS) (kē″ tō-stĕr′ oyds) | Test performed on urine to determine the amount of 17-KS present, the end product of androgens that is secreted from the adrenal glands and testes. It is used to diagnose adrenal tumors. |
| Protein-bound iodine (PBI) (prō′ tēn bound ī′ ō-dīn) | Test performed on serum to indicate the amount of iodine that is attached to serum protein. It can be used to indicate thyroid function. |
| Radioactive iodine uptake (RAIU) (rā″ dē-ō-ăk′ tīv ī′ ō-dīn) | Test to measure the ability of the thyroid gland to concentrate ingested iodine. Increased level can indicate hyperthyroidism, cirrhosis, and/or thyroiditis. Decreased level can indicate hypothyroidism. |
| Radioimmunoassay (RIA) (rā″ dē-ō-ĭmŭ″ -nō-ăs′ ā) | Standard assay method used to measure minute quantities of specific antibodies and/or antigens. It can be used for clinical laboratory measurements of hormones, therapeutic drug monitoring, and substance abuse screening. |
| Thyroid scan (thī′ royd skăn) | Test to detect tumors of the thyroid gland. The patient is given radioactive iodine 131, which localizes in the thyroid gland, which is then visualized with a scanner device. |
| Thyroxine (T4) (thī-rŏks′ ĭn) | Test performed on blood serum to determine the amount of thyroxine present. Increased levels can indicate hyperthyroidism; decreased levels can indicate hypothyroidism. |
| Triiodothyronine uptake (T3U) (trī″ ī-ō″ dō-thī′ rō-nĭn) | Test performed on blood serum to determine the amount of triiodothyronine present. Increased levels can indicate thyrotoxicosis, toxic adenoma, and/or Hashimoto's struma. Decreased levels can indicate starvation, severe infection, and severe trauma. |
| Total calcium (tōt′ l kăl′ sē-ŭm) | Test performed on blood serum to determine the amount of calcium present. Increased levels can indicate hyperparathyroidism; decreased levels can indicate hypoparathyroidism. |
| Ultrasonography (ŭl-tră-sŏn-ŏg′ ră-fē) | Use of high-frequency sound waves as a screening test or as a diagnostic tool to visualize the structure being studied; can be used to visualize the pancreas, thyroid, and any other gland. |

# ABBREVIATIONS

| ABBREVIATION | MEANING |
|---|---|
| 17-KS | 17-ketosteroids |
| 17-OHCS | 17-hydroxycorticosteroids |
| ACTH | adrenocorticotropic hormone |
| ADA | American Diabetes Association |
| ADH | antidiuretic hormone |
| BG | blood glucose |
| BMR | basal metabolic rate |
| CHT | congenital hypothyroidism |
| cm | centimeter |
| CRF | corticotropin-releasing factor |
| DI | diabetes insipidus |
| DM | diabetes mellitus |
| FBG | fasting blood glucose |
| FBS | fasting blood sugar |
| FSH | follicle-stimulating hormone |
| g | gram |
| GH | growth hormone |
| GHRF | growth hormone-releasing factor |
| GnRF | gonadotropin-releasing factor |
| GTT | glucose tolerance test |
| IDDM | insulin-dependent diabetes mellitus |
| K | potassium |
| LH | luteinizing hormone |
| LTH | lactogenic hormone |
| MIF | melanocyte-stimulating hormone release-inhibiting factor |

| ABBREVIATION | MEANING |
|---|---|
| MRF | melanocyte-stimulating hormone-releasing factor |
| MSH | melanocyte-stimulating hormone |
| Na | sodium |
| NIDDM | non-insulin-dependent diabetes mellitus |
| PBI | protein-bound iodine |
| PIF | prolactin release-inhibiting factor |
| PRF | prolactin-releasing factor |
| PRL | prolactin hormone |
| PTH | parathyroid (parathormone hormone) |
| RAIU | radioactive iodine uptake |
| rDNA | recombinant deoxyribonucleic acid |
| RIA | radioimmunoassay |
| STH | somatotropin hormone |
| T3 | triiodothyronine |
| T3U | triiodothyronine uptake |
| T4 | thyroxine |
| TFS | thyroid function studies |
| TH | thyroid hormone |
| TRH | thyrotropin-releasing hormone |
| TSH | thyroid-stimulating hormone |
| VP | vasopressin |

# PATHOLOGY SPOTLIGHTS

## ＊ Addison's Disease

**Addison's disease** occurs when the cortex of the adrenal gland is damaged and there is a deficiency in the production of the adrenocortical hormones. The most common cause of this condition is the result of the body attacking itself (autoimmune disease). For unknown reasons, the immune system views the adrenal cortex as a foreign body, something to attack and destroy. Other causes of Addison's disease include infections of the adrenal glands, spread of cancer to the glands, and hemorrhage into the glands.

Named for the 19th century English physician, Thomas Addison, who identified and described the condition, Addison's disease can occur at any age, including infancy, and is equally prevalent among males and females. The signs and symptoms of Addison's disease can include the following:

- Weight loss.
- Anorexia.
- Weakness and lethargy.
- Increased pigmentation of the skin and mucous membranes.
- Low blood sugar (hypoglycemia).
- Joint and muscle aches.
- Persistent fever.
- Nausea, vomiting, diarrhea, and abdominal discomfort.

The diagnosis of Addison's disease is determined by blood and urine tests that measure the amount of corticosteroid hormones present. With Addison's, the level of the hormones is very low. When Addison's disease is diagnosed early, treatment generally consists of replacement of the adrenocortical hormones and supplemental sodium.

## ✱ Diabetes Mellitus

**Diabetes mellitus** is a complex disorder of metabolism in which the body does not produce or properly use insulin, a hormone needed to convert sugar, starches, and other food into energy needed for daily life.

According to the American Diabetes Association (ADA), approximately 18.2 million people in the United States, or 6.3% of the population, have diabetes. While an estimated 13 million have been diagnosed, 5.2 million people unfortunately are unaware that they have the disease. Each year about 1.5 million people age 20 or older are diagnosed with diabetes.

There are three major types of diabetes: Type 1, Type 2, and gestational diabetes. Type 1 is an autoimmune disease and results from the body's failure to produce insulin. An individual with this type of diabetes needs to take insulin each day for the rest of his or her life. It is estimated that 5% to 10% of Americans who are diagnosed with diabetes have Type 1 diabetes. It develops most often in children and young adults but can appear at any age. If not diagnosed and treated with insulin, a person with Type 1 diabetes can lapse into a life-threatening diabetic coma or diabetic ketoacidosis.

Type 2 diabetes is the most common type of diabetes. Approximately 90% to 95% of Americans who have diabetes have Type 2 diabetes. It results from a combination of defective insulin secretion and defective responsiveness to insulin (reduced insulin sensitivity) and is associated with obesity and aging. It used to be known as noninsulin-dependent diabetes mellitus, NIDDM, or adult-onset diabetes. Factors contributing to developing this form of diabetes include heredity, obesity, sedentary lifestyle, high-fat low-fiber diet, hypertension, and aging.

Type 2 diabetes used to be rare in children. But with the increase in obesity in children, doctors are now finding that as many as 1 out of 20 children who have diabetes has Type 2 diabetes. It may be possible to prevent the onset of Type 2 diabetes by making even modest lifestyle changes. The key is to eat a healthy diet, exercise 30 minutes a day at least 5 days a week, and maintain a proper body weight for age and body type. See Table 13–2 for the warning signs and symptoms of diabetes mellitus.

Untreated diabetes mellitus or complications of diabetes can result in various multi-system effects. Progressive complications include hyperglycemia (excessive amount of sugar in the blood) and hypoglycemia (deficient amount of sugar in the blood). **Hyperglycemia** can lead to diabetic **ketoacidosis** (accumulation of ketones and acids in the body due to faulty metabolism of carbohydrates and the improper burning of fats) and the development

TABLE 13–2  **Warning Signs and Symptoms of Diabetes Mellitus**

| Type 1 | Type 2 |
|---|---|
| Frequent urination (polyuria) | Any Type 1 symptom |
| Excessive thirst (polydipsia) | Tingling or numbness in the feet |
| Extreme hunger (polyphagia) | Frequent vaginal or skin infection |
| Unusual weight loss | |
| Increased fatigue | |
| Blurred vision | |
| Irritability | |

of a coma when the blood sugar is too high or an insufficient amount of insulin has been received. **Hypoglycemia** occurs when too much insulin has been taken. Insulin shock is a severe form of hypoglycemia and requires an immediate dose of glucose. Convulsions, coma, and death can occur if the patient is not treated. See Figure 13–17 ▶ for other complications of diabetes.

**Gestational diabetes** or pregnancy-induced diabetes develops in about 4% of all pregnant women (about 135,000 cases in the United States each year). In most cases, this type of diabetes goes away after the pregnancy.

**Prediabetes** is a condition that occurs when a person's blood glucose levels are higher than normal but not high enough for a diagnosis of Type 2 diabetes. It is estimated that at least 16 million Americans have prediabetes in addition to the 18.2 million with diabetes. Without lifestyle changes, most people who have prediabetes progress to Type 2 diabetes within 10 years.

## ✴ Hypothyroidism

**Hypothyroidism** is a condition in which the thyroid gland does not produce adequate amounts of thyroid hormone. Approximately 6 to 7 million Americans, mainly women older than age 40, have an underactive thyroid. Symptoms include fatigue, decreased concentration, intolerance to cold environments, constipation, loss of appetite, muscle cramping and stiffness, and weight gain. Some individuals notice hair loss, dry skin, or nail changes.

Untreated hypothyroidism can lead to a number of health problems. Constant stimulation of the thyroid to release more hormones can cause the gland to become larger, a condition known as a **goiter.** Hashimoto's thyroiditis, an autoimmune inflammation of the thyroid, is one of the most common causes of a goiter. Another type of goiter is an *endemic goiter* that develops in certain geographic regions where the iodine content in food and water is deficient (see Figure 13–18 ▶).

Complications of hypothyrodism include an increased risk of heart disease, depression, decreased sexual desire, and slowed mental functioning. **Myxedema** is the most severe form of hypothyrodism. It is characterized by pronounced edema of the face and a somnolent look. The hair is stiff and dull. Without treatment, coma and death can occur. See Figure 13–19 ▶.

Treatment of hypothyroidism involves the replacement of thyroxine with daily regulated doses of levothyroxine sodium (Levothroid, Synthroid). The medication should be taken before breakfast, and the patient is advised to avoid foods and over-the-counter medications that contain iodine.

**Congenital hypothyroidism** (CHT) is a condition that affects infants from birth (congenital) and results from a partial or complete loss of thyroid function (hypothyroidism). Congenital hypothyroidism occurs when the thyroid gland fails to develop or

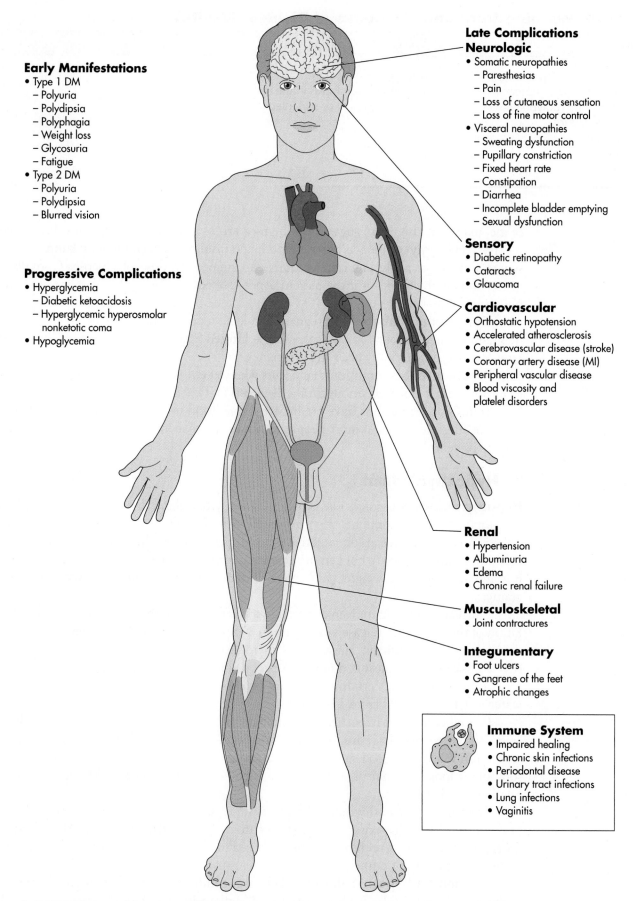

**Early Manifestations**
- Type 1 DM
  - Polyuria
  - Polydipsia
  - Polyphagia
  - Weight loss
  - Glycosuria
  - Fatigue
- Type 2 DM
  - Polyuria
  - Polydipsia
  - Blurred vision

**Progressive Complications**
- Hyperglycemia
  - Diabetic ketoacidosis
  - Hyperglycemic hyperosmolar nonketotic coma
- Hypoglycemia

**Late Complications**
**Neurologic**
- Somatic neuropathies
  - Paresthesias
  - Pain
  - Loss of cutaneous sensation
  - Loss of fine motor control
- Visceral neuropathies
  - Sweating dysfunction
  - Pupillary constriction
  - Fixed heart rate
  - Constipation
  - Diarrhea
  - Incomplete bladder emptying
  - Sexual dysfunction

**Sensory**
- Diabetic retinopathy
- Cataracts
- Glaucoma

**Cardiovascular**
- Orthostatic hypotension
- Accelerated atherosclerosis
- Cerebrovascular disease (stroke)
- Coronary artery disease (MI)
- Peripheral vascular disease
- Blood viscosity and platelet disorders

**Renal**
- Hypertension
- Albuminuria
- Edema
- Chronic renal failure

**Musculoskeletal**
- Joint contractures

**Integumentary**
- Foot ulcers
- Gangrene of the feet
- Atrophic changes

**Immune System**
- Impaired healing
- Chronic skin infections
- Periodontal disease
- Urinary tract infections
- Lung infections
- Vaginitis

▶ **FIGURE 13–17**   Multisystem effects of diabetes mellitus.

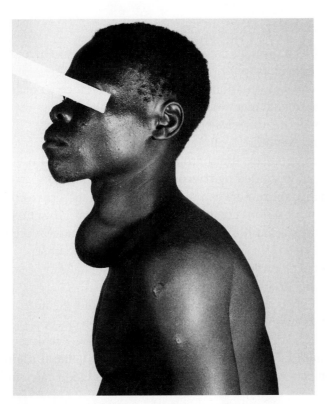

▶ **FIGURE 13–18** Endemic goiter.

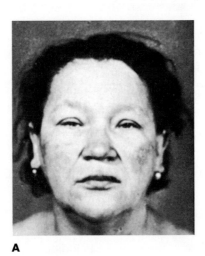

**A**

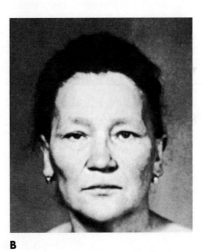

**B**

▶ **FIGURE 13–19** (A) A 62-year-old patient with myxedema exhibiting marked edema of the face and a somnolent look. The hair is stiff and without luster. (B) The same patient after 3 months of treatment with thyroxine.

function properly. In 80% to 85% of cases, the thyroid gland is absent, abnormally located, or severely reduced in size. In the remaining cases, a normal-size or enlarged thyroid gland is present, but production of thyroid hormones is decreased or absent. If untreated, congenital hypothyroidism can lead to mental retardation and abnormal growth. In the United States and many other countries, all newborns are tested for congenital hypothyroidism. If treatment begins in the first month after birth, infants usually develop normally.

### ✳ Hyperthyroidism

**Hyperthyroidism** is a disorder caused by elevated levels of thyroid hormone. Symptoms can include nervousness, palpitations, tremors, sweating, increased activity in the intestinal tract, changes in menstruation, weight loss, intolerance to heat, anxiety, restlessness, irregular heartbeat, and changes in fingernails and hair.

The most common etiologies of hyperthyroidism are Graves' disease and toxic multinodular goiter. *Graves' disease* is an autoimmnue disease in which antibodies produced by the immune system stimulate the thyroid to produce too much thyroxine. Other forms of hyperthyroidism can be caused by **thyroiditis,** or inflammation of the thyroid gland. Certain benign or malignant tumors can also produce too much thyroid hormone.

Some of the most serious complications of hyperthyroidism involve the heart, including a rapid heart rate, atrial fibrillation, and congestive heart failure. Untreated hyperthyroidism can also lead to weak, brittle bones (osteoporosis). People with Graves' ophthalmopathy develop eye problems, including bulging, red or swollen eyes, sensitivity to light, and blurring or double vision.

Hyperthyroidism is usually treated with antithyroid medications, radioactive iodine (which destroys the thyroid and thus stops the excess production of hormones), or surgery (thyroidectomy). If the thyroid must be removed or destroyed, replacement thyroid hormones (levothyroxine) must be taken for the rest of the person's life. If the parathyroid glands are also removed, the patient needs medication to keep the blood calcium levels normal.

# ✓PATHOLOGY CHECKPOINT

*Following is a concise list of the pathology-related terms that you have seen in the chapter. Review this checklist to make sure that you are familiar with the meaning of each term before moving to the next section.*

### Conditions and Symptoms ✳

- ❑ acidosis
- ❑ acromegaly
- ❑ Addison's disease
- ❑ adenoma
- ❑ adenosis
- ❑ adrenopathy
- ❑ congenital hypothyroidism
- ❑ cretinism
- ❑ Cushing's disease
- ❑ diabetes
- ❑ dwarfism
- ❑ exophthalmic
- ❑ galactorrhea
- ❑ gigantism
- ❑ hirsutism
- ❑ hypergonadism
- ❑ hyperinsulinism
- ❑ hyperkalemia
- ❑ hyperthyroidism

- ❑ hypogonadism
- ❑ hypoparathyroidism
- ❑ hypothyroidism
- ❑ lethargic
- ❑ myxedema
- ❑ pituitarism
- ❑ progeria
- ❑ Simmonds' disease
- ❑ thymitis
- ❑ thyroiditis
- ❑ thyrotoxicosis
- ❑ virilism

### Diagnosis and Treatment ✳

- ❑ adenectomy
- ❑ adrenalectomy
- ❑ aldosterone
- ❑ androgen
- ❑ catecholamines
- ❑ cortisone

- ❑ dopamine
- ❑ epinephrine
- ❑ estrogen
- ❑ glucocorticoid
- ❑ hormone
- ❑ hydrocortisone
- ❑ insulin
- ❑ iodine
- ❑ norepinephrine
- ❑ oxytocin
- ❑ progesterone
- ❑ somatotropin
- ❑ steroids
- ❑ testosterone
- ❑ thymectomy
- ❑ thyroidectomy
- ❑ thyroxine
- ❑ vasopressin

# STUDY AND REVIEW

## Anatomy and Physiology

*Write your answers to the following questions. Do not refer to the text.*

1. Name the primary glands of the endocrine system.

   a. _____     b. _____

   c. _____     d. _____

   e. _____     f. _____

   g. _____     h. _____

2. Name the secondary glands of the endocrine system.

   a. _____     b. _____

   c. _____

3. State the vital function of the endocrine system. _____

   _____

4. Define *hormone.* _____

5. State the vital role of the hypothalamus in regulating endocrine functions.

   _____

   _____

   _____

6. Why is the pituitary gland known as the master gland of the body?

   _____

7. Name the hormones secreted by the adenohypophysis.

   a. _____     b. _____

   c. _____     d. _____

   e. _____     f. _____

   g. _____

8. Name the hormones secreted by the neurohypophysis.

   a. _____     b. _____

9. The pineal gland secretes the hormones _____ and _____.

10. State the vital role of the thyroid gland.

   _____

11. Name the hormones stored and secreted by the thyroid gland.

   a. _____     b. _____

   c. _____

12. Parathyroid (parathormone hormone) is essential for the maintenance of a

   normal level of _____ and also plays a role in the metabolism of

   _____.

13. Insulin is essential for the maintenance of a normal level of _____.

14. The adrenal cortex secretes a group of hormones known as the _____,

   the _____, and the _____.

15. Name four functions of cortisol.

   a. _____     b. _____

   c. _____     d. _____

16. Name four functions of corticosterone.

   a. _____     b. _____

   c. _____     d. _____

17. _____ is the principal mineralocorticoid secreted by the adrenal cortex.

18. Define *androgen.* _____

19. Name the three main catecholamines synthesized, secreted, and stored by the
   adrenal medulla.

   a. _____     b. _____

   c. _____

20. Name three functions of the hormone epinephrine.

   a. _____

   b. _____

   c. _____

21. The ovaries produce the hormones _____ and _____.

22. The testes produce the hormone _____.

23. Name the two hormones secreted by the thymus.

a. _____     b. _____

24. Name the four hormones secreted by the gastrointestinal mucosa.

a. _____     b. _____

c. _____     d. _____

## Word Parts

1. In the spaces provided, write the definitions of these prefixes, roots, combining forms, and suffixes. Do not refer to the listings of medical words. Leave blank those words you cannot define.

2. After completing as many as you can, refer to the medical word listings to check your work. For each word missed or left blank, write the word and its definition several times on the margins of these pages or on a separate sheet of paper.

3. To maximize the learning process, it is to your advantage to do the following exercises as directed. To refer to the word-building section before completing these exercises invalidates the learning process.

## PREFIXES

*Give the definitions of the following prefixes.*

1. dia- _____     2. endo- _____

3. eu- _____     4. ex- _____

5. exo- _____     6. hyper- _____

7. hypo- _____     8. para- _____

9. pro- _____    10. epi- _____

11. hydro- _____

## ROOTS AND COMBINING FORMS

*Give the definitions of the following roots and combining forms.*

1. acid _____     2. acr/o _____

3. aden _____     4. aden/o _____

5. cortic _____     6. creat _____

7. cretin _____     8. andr/o _____

9. crine _____    10. crin/o _____

11. dwarf _____    12. galact/o _____

13. ger _____

14. gigant _____

15. glandul _____

16. gluc/o _____

17. gonad _____

18. hirsut _____

19. insul _____

20. cortis _____

21. insulin/o _____

22. kal _____

23. letharg _____

24. log _____

25. myx _____

26. ophthalm _____

27. pine _____

28. nephr _____

29. pituitar _____

30. ren _____

31. ren/o _____

32. estr/o _____

33. thym _____

34. gester _____

35. thyr _____

36. thyr/o _____

37. toxic _____

38. trop _____

39. viril _____

40. somat/o _____

41. test/o _____

42. ster _____

43. thyrox _____

44. vas/o _____

45. press _____

46. adren _____

47. adren/o _____

48. pancreat _____

## SUFFIXES

*Give the definitions of the following suffixes.*

1. -al _____

2. -gen _____

3. -ar _____

4. -betes _____

5. -ectomy _____

6. -edema _____

7. -emia _____

8. -genic _____

9. -ia _____

10. -ic _____

11. -ism _____

12. -ist _____

13. -itis _____

14. -logy _____

15. -one _____

16. -megaly _____

17. -oid _____

18. -oma _____

19. -osis _____

20. -pathy _____

21. -ine _____

22. -physis _____

23. -in _____

24. -rrhea _____

25. -y _____

## Identifying Medical Terms

*In the spaces provided, write the medical terms for the following meanings.*

1. _____ Any disease condition of a gland

2. _____ Congenital deficiency in secretion of the thyroid hormones

3. _____ Disease characterized by excessive discharge of urine

4. _____ Study of the endocrine system

5. _____ Normal activity of the thyroid gland

6. _____ External secretion of a gland

7. _____ Condition of being abnormally large

8. _____ General classification of the adrenal cortex hormones

9. _____ Excessive amount of potassium in the blood

10. _____ Deficient internal secretion of the gonads

11. _____ Pertaining to drowsiness; sluggishness

12. _____ Inflammation of the thymus

## Spelling

*In the spaces provided, write the correct spelling of these misspelled words.*

1. catcholamines _____

2. crtinism _____

3. exopthalmic _____

4. hypthyoidism _____

5. myexdema _____

6. pinael _____

7. pitutary _____

8. thyoid _____

9. oxytoin _____

10. virlism _____

## Matching

*Select the appropriate lettered meaning for each of the following words.*

_____ 1. aldosterone

_____ 2. androgen

_____ 3. catecholamines

_____ 4. cortisone

_____ 5. dopamine

_____ 6. epinephrine

_____ 7. insulin

_____ 8. iodine

_____ 9. thyroxine

_____ 10. vasopressin

a. Also called *antidiuretic hormone, ADH*

b. Biochemical substances, epinephrine, norepinephrine, and dopamine

c. Hormone essential for the metabolism of carbohydrates and fats

d. Hormone produced by the thyroid gland

e. Principal mineralocorticoid secreted by the adrenal cortex

f. Hormones that produce or stimulate the development of male characteristics

g. Glucocorticoid hormone used as an antiinflammatory agent

h. Intermediate substance in the synthesis of norepinephrine

i. Also called *adrenaline, Adrenalin*

j. Trace mineral that aids in the development and functioning of the thyroid gland

k. Hormone produced by the testes

## Abbreviations

*Place the correct word, phrase, or abbreviation in the space provided.*

1. basal metabolic rate _____

2. diabetes mellitus _____

3. FBS _____

4. GTT _____

5. protein bound iodine _____

6. PTH _____

7. RIA _____

8. somatotropin hormone _____

9. TFS _____

10. VP _____

## Diagnostic and Laboratory Tests

*Select the best answer to each multiple choice question. Circle the letter of your choice.*

1. A test performed on urine to determine the amount of epinephrine and norepinephrine present.
   a. catecholamines
   b. corticotropin
   c. protein bound iodine
   d. total calcium

2. Increased levels can indicate diabetes mellitus, diabetes acidosis, and many other conditions.
   a. protein-bound iodine
   b. total calcium
   c. fasting blood sugar
   d. thyroid scan

3. Test used to detect tumors of the thyroid gland.
   a. thyroxine
   b. total calcium
   c. thyroid scan
   d. protein-bound iodine

4. Blood sugar test performed at specific intervals after the patient has been given a certain amount of glucose.
   a. fasting blood sugar
   b. glucose tolerance test
   c. protein bound iodine
   d. corticotropin

5. A test used in the diagnosing of adrenal tumors.
   a. 17-HCS
   b. 17-OHCS
   c. 17-KS
   d. 17-HDL

# PRACTICAL APPLICATION

## S O A P : Chart Note Analysis

*This exercise will make you aware of information, abbreviations, and medical terminology typically found in a family practice patient's chart.*

---

**Abbreviations Key**

| | | | | |
|---|---|---|---|---|
| **Abd** | abdominal | | **MS** | musculoskeletal |
| **ADA** | American Diabetes Association | | **Neuro** | neurology |
| **BMI** | body mass index | | **NKDA** | no known drug allergies |
| **BP** | blood pressure | | **P** | pulse |
| **BG** | blood glucose | | **PERRLA** | pupils equal, round, react to light |
| **c/o** | complains of | | | and accomodation |
| **CTA** | clear to auscultation | | **R** | respiration |
| **DM** | diabetes mellitus | | **ROM** | range of motion |
| **DOB** | date of birth | | **SOAP** | subjective, objective, assessment, plan |
| **F** | Fahrenheit | | **T** | temperature |
| **GTT** | glucose tolerance test | | **TM** | tympanic membrane |
| **HEENT** | head, eyes, ears, nose, throat | | **WNL** | within normal limits |
| **Ht** | height | | **Wt** | weight |
| **lb** | pound | | **y/o** | year(s) old |

---

*Read the following chart note and then answer the questions that follow.*

---

**PATIENT:** Marshall, Matthew J.   **DATE:** 03/23/2007
**DOB:** 06/01/91   **AGE:** 15   **SEX:** Male
**INSURANCE:** Millennia Health Insurance

**Vital Signs:**
  T: 98.4 F
  P: 78
  R: 18
  BP: 132/70
  Ht: 5' 5"
  Wt: 160 lb

**Allergies:** NKDA

**Chief Complaint:** Polydipsia, polyphagia, polyuria, fatigue

**S** **Subjective:** 15 y/o white male c/o of being "thirsty, hungry, and urinating a lot." He states, "I am tired and just don't have any energy. I eat like a horse, but I stay hungry. I am afraid that I have 'sugar.' My dad and my grandfather both take insulin."

**O** **Objective:**
**General Appearance:** Appeared concerned about his condition with troubled expression and slightly flushed complexion. Overweight for age.
**BMI:** 26.6

**Heent:** PERRLA. TM pearly gray in color, landmarks intact. Nasal mucosa pink, no discharge.

**Heart:** Regular rate and rhythm. No murmurs.

**Lungs:** CTA

**Abd:** Noted excessive adipose tissue. Soft, nontender, no masses, no liver enlargement.

**MS:** Muscles and joints symmetric. Mobility of hands, fingers and wrists WNL. No tenderness or swelling noted. Full ROM.

**Neuro:** Reflexes WNL, no decrease sensation of feet bilaterally as noted with monofilament, tuning fork and palpation.

**Skin:** Warm and dry, no lesions, no discoloration of lower extremities

---

**A**    **Assessment:** Diabetes mellitus Type 1

---

**P**    **Plan:**

1. Because of the characteristic symptoms, family history, and the results of the BG test and GTT, this patient is scheduled to attend the next health education seminar on Thursday of next week. Explained that this seminar will involve the treatment regimen for diabetes, including insulin therapy, diet therapy, and glucose monitoring, plus the importance of exercise and weight control, healthy lifestyle choices, and prevention of possible future complications. One or both parents are to attend the seminar with Matthew.

2. Patient is to return in two weeks for a follow-up visit and then every four weeks until blood sugar level is stabilized and patient and his family are comfortable with the treatment program.

3. Inform the patient about MedicAlert identification bracelet and medical ID necklace and their importance. Give the patient the following telephone number 1-888-633-4298 and website address: www.medicalert.org.

4. Provide the patient with resource material, such as the Novo Nordisk *Keeping Well with Diabetes* series, and how to obtain more information on diabetes.

---

**FYI:** Individuals who are overweight, have a BMI greater than or equal to 25, and who have immediate family members with diabetes are at a higher risk of developing diabetes. For more information on diabetes, call 1-800-DIABETES or visit the following Web sites:

American Diabetes Association (ADA)    www.diabetes.org

National Diabetes Education Program    www.ndep.nih.gov

To receive information on *Keeping Well with Diabetes,* call 1-800-727-6500 or go to www.kwwd.com.

## Chart Note Questions
*Place the correct answer in the space provided.*

1. Signs and symptoms of diabetes mellitus Type 1 include _____, polyphagia, and polyuria.

2. The diagnosis was determined by the characteristic symptoms, family history, a blood glucose test, and a _____ tolerance test.

3. Treatment for diabetes mellitus Type 1 includes insulin therapy, _____ therapy, an exercise program, and lifestyle changes.

4. The medical word for excessive thirst is _____.

5. The medical word for frequent urination is _____.

6. The medical word for extreme hunger is _____.

7. What is the medical word for lack of energy? _____

8. During the abdominal exam, the physician noted _____.

9. What does the abbreviation GTT mean? _____

10. A BMI over _____ may indicate a higher risk of developing diabetes.

# MULTIMEDIA PREVIEW

*Additional interactive resources and activities for this chapter can be found on the Companion Website. For videos, audio glossary, and review, access the accompanying CD-ROM in this book.*

 **CD-ROM HIGHLIGHTS**

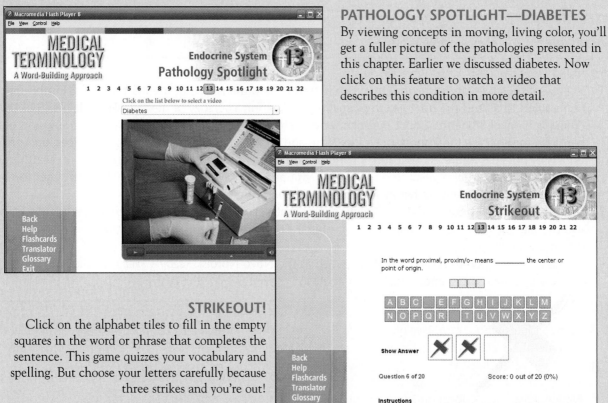

## PATHOLOGY SPOTLIGHT—DIABETES

By viewing concepts in moving, living color, you'll get a fuller picture of the pathologies presented in this chapter. Earlier we discussed diabetes. Now click on this feature to watch a video that describes this condition in more detail.

## STRIKEOUT!

Click on the alphabet tiles to fill in the empty squares in the word or phrase that completes the sentence. This game quizzes your vocabulary and spelling. But choose your letters carefully because three strikes and you're out!

 **WEBSITE HIGHLIGHTS—www.prenhall.com/rice**

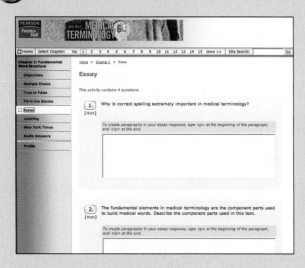

## ESSAY QUESTIONS

Click here and take advantage of the free-access on-line study guide that accompanies your textbook. You'll find a series of short answer essay questions that correspond to the concepts in this chapter. By clicking on this URL you'll also access links to download mp3 audio reviews, current news articles, and an audio glossary.

# Nervous System

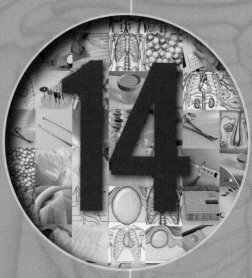

**14**

## ■ OBJECTIVES

*On completion of this chapter, you will be able to:*

- Describe the tissues of the nervous system.
- Describe nerve fibers, nerves, and tracts.
- Describe the transmission of nerve impulses.
- Describe the central nervous system.
- Describe the peripheral nervous system.
- Describe the autonomic nervous system.
- Analyze, build, spell, and pronounce medical words.
- Comprehend the drugs highlighted in this chapter.
- Describe diagnostic and laboratory tests related to the nervous system.
- Identify and define selected abbreviations.
- Describe each of the conditions presented in the Pathology Spotlights.
- Review the Pathology Checkpoint.
- Complete the Study and Review section and the Chart Note Analysis.

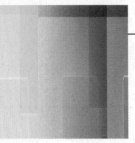

# Anatomy and Physiology Overview

The nervous system is usually described as having two interconnected divisions: the central nervous system (CNS) and the peripheral nervous system (PNS). The CNS includes the brain and spinal cord. It is enclosed by the bones of the skull and spinal column. The PNS consists of the network of nerves and neural tissues branching throughout the body from 12 pairs of cranial nerves and 31 pairs of spinal nerves. See Figure 14–1 ▼. A general description of the nervous system and its functions is provided in this overview.

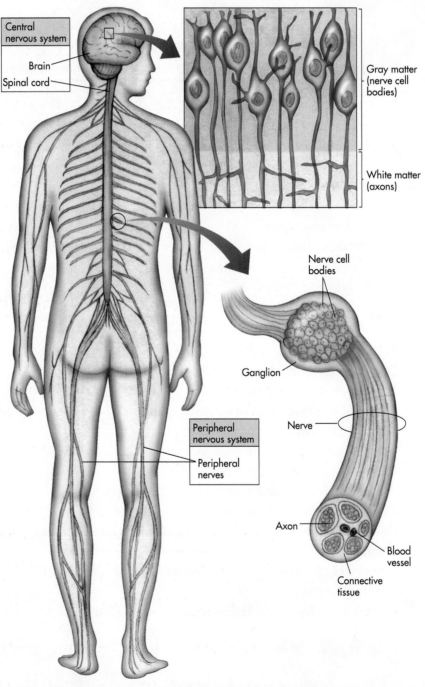

▶ **FIGURE 14–1**   The nervous system is described as having two interconnected divisions: the central nervous system (CNS) consisting of the brain and spinal cord and the peripheral nervous system (PNS) consisting of peripheral nerves.

## Nervous System

| Organ/Structure | Primary Functions |
| --- | --- |
| Neurons (nerve cells) | Structural and functional units of the nervous system act as specialized conductors of impulses that enable the body to interact with its internal and external environments |
| Neuroglia | Act as supporting tissue |
| Nerve fibers and tracts | Conduct impulses from one location to another |
| Central nervous system | Receives impulses from throughout the body, processes the information, and responds with an appropriate action |
| *Brain* | Governs sensory perception, emotions, consciousness, memory, and voluntary movements |
| *Spinal cord* | Conducts sensory impulses to the brain and motor impulses from the brain to body parts, also serves as a reflex center for impulses entering and leaving the spinal cord without involvement of the brain |
| Peripheral Nervous System | Links the central nervous system with other parts of the body |
| *Cranial nerves (12 pairs)* | Provide sensory input and motor control, or a combination of these |
| *Spinal nerves (31 pairs)* | Carry impulses to the spinal cord and to muscles, organs, and glands |
| Autonomic nervous system | Controls involuntary bodily functions such as sweating and arterial blood pressure |

# TISSUES OF THE NERVOUS SYSTEM

The nervous system has two principal tissue types. These tissues are made up of **neurons** or nerve cells and their supporting tissues, collectively called **neuroglia.** See Figure 14–2 ▶. Neurons are the structural and functional units of the nervous system. These cells are specialized conductors of impulses that enable the body to interact with its internal and external environments. There are several types of neurons, three of which are described in the following sections.

## Motor Neurons

**Motor neurons** cause contractions in muscles and secretions from glands and organs. They also act to inhibit the actions of glands and organs, thereby controlling most of the body's functions. Motor neurons can be described as being *efferent processes* because they transmit impulses away from the neural cell body to the muscles or organs to be innervated. Motor neurons consist of a nucleated cell body with protoplasmic processes extending away from it in several directions. These processes are known as the **axon** and **dendrites.** Most axons are long and are covered with a fatty substance, the myelin sheath, which acts as an insulator and increases the transmission velocity of the nerve fiber it surrounds. Axons may be as long as several feet and reach from the cell body to the area to be activated. Dendrites resemble the branches of a tree, are short, or unsheathed, and transmit impulses to the cell body. Neurons usually have several dendrites and only one axon.

## Sensory Neurons

**Sensory neurons** differ in structure from motor neurons because they do not have true dendrites. The processes transmitting sensory information to the cell bodies of these neurons are called *peripheral processes*, are sheathed, and resemble axons. They are attached to sensory receptors and transmit impulses to the central nervous system (CNS). In turn, the CNS can stimulate motor neurons in response to this sensory information. Sensory neurons

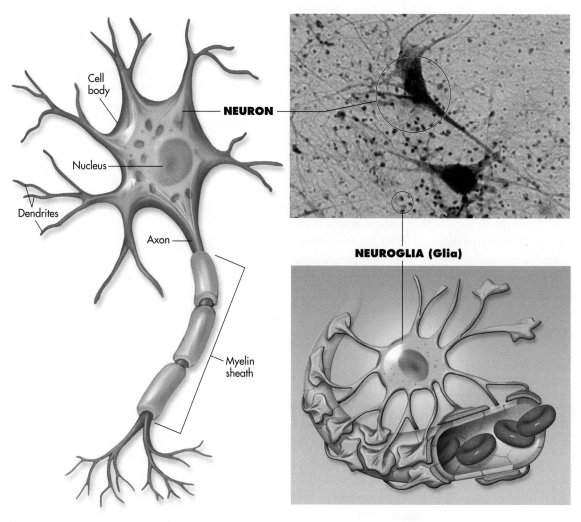

Cell body

Nucleus

Dendrites

Axon

Myelin sheath

**NEURON**

**NEUROGLIA (Glia)**

▶ **FIGURE 14–2** Two main types of nerve cells.

are sometimes referred to as *afferent nerves* because they carry impulses from the sensory receptors to the synaptic endings in the central nervous system.

### Interneurons

**Interneurons** are sometimes called *central* or *associative neurons* and are located entirely within the central nervous system. They function to mediate impulses between sensory and motor neurons.

## NERVE FIBERS, NERVES, AND TRACTS

The terms *nerve fiber*, *nerve*, and *tract* are used to describe neuronal processes conducting impulses from one location to another.

### Nerve Fibers

A single elongated process, usually a long axon or a peripheral process from a sensory neuron, is called a **nerve fiber.** Nerve fibers of the peripheral nervous system are wrapped by protective membranes called **sheaths.** The PNS has two types of sheaths: *myelinated* and *unmyelinated*, which are formed by accessory cells. Myelinated fibers have an inner sheath of myelin, a thick fatty substance, and an outer sheath or **neurilemma** composed of

*Schwann cells.* Unmyelinated fibers lack myelin and are sheathed only by the neurilemma. Nerve fibers of the central nervous system do not contain Schwann cells, which are necessary for the regeneration of a damaged nerve fiber. Therefore, damage to fibers of the CNS is permanent, whereas damage to a peripheral nerve can be reversible.

### Nerves

A **nerve** is a bundle of nerve fibers, located outside the brain and spinal cord, that connects to various parts of the body. Nerves are usually described as being **afferent** (*conducting to the CNS*) or **efferent** (*conducting to muscles, organs, and glands*). Some nerves called **mixed nerves** contain a mixture of afferent and efferent fibers. Nerves are also referred to as *sensory* (afferent) and *motor* (efferent).

### Tracts

Groups of nerve fibers within the central nervous system are sometimes referred to as **tracts** when they have the same origin, function, and termination. The spinal cord contains afferent sensory tracts ascending to the brain and efferent motor tracts descending from the brain. The brain itself contains numerous tracts, the largest of which is the *corpus callosum* joining the left and right hemispheres.

## TRANSMISSION OF NERVE IMPULSES

Stimulation of a nerve occurs at a *receptor.* Sensory receptors are of different types, ranging from the simplest, which are free nerve endings for pain, to the most complex, as in the retina of the eye for vision. Receptors are generally specialized to specific types of stimulation such as heat, cold, light, pressure, or pain and react by initiating a chemical change or impulse. The transmission of an impulse by a nerve fiber is based on the **all-or-none principle.** This means that no transmission occurs until the stimulus reaches a set minimum strength, which can vary for different receptors. Once the minimum stimulus or threshold is reached, a maximum impulse is produced. The impulse is then transmitted via a **synapse,** a specialized knoblike branch ending, with the help of certain chemical agents, across a space separating the axon's end knobs from the dendrites of the next neuron or from a motor end plate attached to a muscle. This space is called a **synaptic cleft,** and the chemical agents released are called **neurotransmitters.**

## CENTRAL NERVOUS SYSTEM

Consisting of the brain and spinal cord, the **central nervous system** (CNS) receives impulses from throughout the body, processes the information, and responds with an appropriate action. This activity can be at the conscious or unconscious level, depending on the source of the sensory stimulus. Both the brain and spinal cord can be divided into **gray matter** and **white matter.** The gray matter consists of unsheathed cell bodies and true dendrites. The white matter is composed of myelinated nerve fibers. In the spinal cord, the arrangement of white and gray matter results in an H-shaped core of gray cell bodies surrounded by tracts of nerve fibers interconnected to the brain. The reverse is generally true of the brain where the surface layer or cortex is gray matter and most of the internal structures are white matter.

## Brain

The nervous tissue of the **brain** consists of millions of nerve cells and fibers. It is the largest mass of nervous tissue in the body, weighing about 1380 g in the male and 1250 g in the female. When fully developed, the brain fills the cranial cavity and is enclosed by three membranes known collectively as the **meninges.** From the outside in, these are the *dura mater, arachnoid,* and *pia mater.* The major structures of the brain are the *cerebrum, cerebellum, diencephalon,* and the *brainstem,* which is composed of the *midbrain, pons,* and *medulla oblongata.* See Figure 14–3 ▼.

## Cerebrum

Representing seven-eighths of the brain's total weight, the **cerebrum** contains nerve centers that govern all sensory and motor activity, including sensory perception, emotions, consciousness, memory, and voluntary movements. See Table 14–1.

The cerebrum is divided by the longitudinal fissure into two cerebral hemispheres, the right and left, that are joined by large fiber tracts (*corpus callosum*) that allow information to pass from one hemisphere to the other. The surface or *cortex* of each hemisphere is arranged in folds creating bulges and shallow furrows. Each bulge is called a **gyrus** or **convolution.** A furrow is known as a **sulcus.** This surface is composed of gray, unmyelinated cell bodies and is known as the **cerebral cortex.** The cortex has been divided into lobes as a means of identifying certain locations. These lobes correspond to the overlying bones of the skull and are the *frontal, parietal, temporal,* and *occipital lobes.*

Electrical stimulation of the various areas of the cortex during neurosurgery has identified specialized cell activity within the different lobes. The **frontal lobe** has been identified as the brain's major motor area and the site for personality and speech. The **parietal**

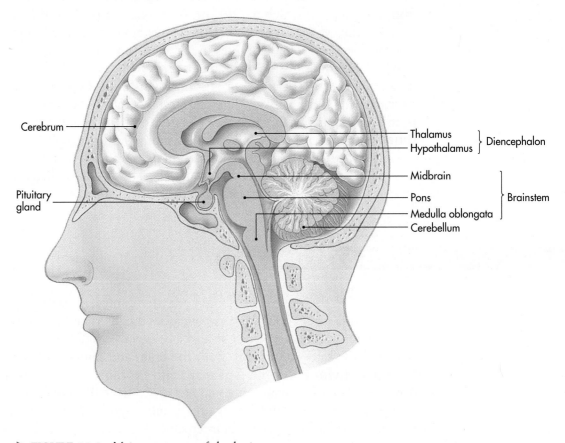

▶ **FIGURE 14–3**  Major structures of the brain.

TABLE 14–1 **Major Divisions of the Brain and Their Functions**

| Brain Area | Functions |
| --- | --- |
| Cerebrum | Governs all sensory and motor activity; sensory perception, emotions, consciousness, memory, and voluntary movements |
| Cerebellum | Plays an important role in the integration of sensory perception and motor output. Its neural pathways link with the motor cortex, which sends information to the muscles causing them to move, and the spinocerebellar tract, which provides feedback on the position of the body in space (proprioception). The cerebellum integrates these pathways using the constant feedback on body position to fine tune motor movements. Modern research shows that the cerebellum also has a broader role in a number of key cognitive functions, including attention and the processing of language, music, and other sensory temporal stimuli. |
| Diencephalon | |
| *Thalamus* | Is the relay center for all sensory impulses (except olfactory) being transmitted to the sensory areas of the cortex, and relays motor impulses from the cerebellum and the basal ganglia to motor areas of the cortex, thought to be involved with emotions and arousal mechanisms |
| *Hypothalamus* | Serves as the principal regulator of autonomic nervous activity that is associated with behavior and expression, also contains neurosecretions that are important for the control of certain metabolic activities such as maintenance of water balance, sugar and fat metabolism, regulation of body temperature, sleep-cycle control, appetite, and sexual arousal. |
| Brainstem | |
| *Midbrain* | Is a two-way conduction pathway and acts as a relay center for visual and auditory impulses; found in the midbrain are four small masses of gray cells known collectively as the *corpora quadrigemina*. The upper two, called the *superior colliculi*, are associated with visual reflexes. The lower two, or *inferior colliculi*, are involved with the sense of hearing. |
| *Pons* | Links the cerebellum and medulla to higher cortical areas; plays a role in somatic and visceral motor control |
| *Medulla oblongata* | Acts as the cardiac, respiratory, and vasomotor control center; regulates and controls breathing, swallowing, coughing, sneezing, and vomiting as well as heartbeat and arterial blood pressure, thereby exerting control over the circulation of blood |

**lobe** contains centers for sensory input from all parts of the body and is known as the *somesthetic area* and the site for the interpretation of language. Temperature, pressure, touch, and an awareness of muscle control are some of the sensory activities centered in this area. The **temporal lobe** contains centers for hearing, smell, and language input, and the **occipital lobe** is considered to be the primary sensory area for vision. The occipital lobe is the lower rear part of the cerebrum beneath the parietal lobe and posterior to the temporal lobe (see Figure 14–4 ▶).

### Cerebellum

The **cerebellum** is the second largest part of the brain. It occupies a space in the back of the skull, inferior to the cerebrum and dorsal to the pons and medulla oblongata. The cerebellum is oval in shape and divided into lobes by deep fissures. Its has a cortex of gray cell bodies, and its interior contains nerve fibers and white matter connecting it to every part of the central nervous system. The cerebellum plays an important part in the coordination of voluntary and involuntary complex patterns of movement and adjusts muscles to automatically maintain posture. See Table 14–1.

### Diencephalon

The word **diencephalon** means *second portion of the brain* and refers to the thalamus and hypothalamus.

Thalamus.    The **thalamus** is the larger of the two divisions of the diencephalon and is actually two large masses of gray cell bodies joined by a third or intermediate mass. The

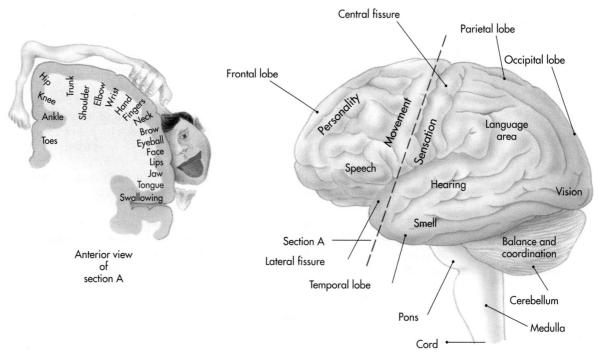

▶ FIGURE 14–4  Brain: lateral view showing the location of certain sensory and motor areas.

thalamus serves as a relay center for all sensory impulses (except olfactory) being transmitted to the sensory areas of the cortex. Besides its sensory function, the thalamus also relays motor impulses from the cerebellum and the basal ganglia to motor areas of the cortex. Some impulses related to emotional behavior are also passed from the hypothalamus, through the thalamus, to the cerebral cortex. See Table 14–1.

Hypothalamus.　The **hypothalamus** lies beneath the thalamus and is a principal regulator of autonomic nervous activity that is associated with behavior and emotional expression. It also produces neurosecretions for the control of water balance, sugar and fat metabolism, regulation of body temperature, and other metabolic activities. Additionally, the hypothalamus produces hormones for the posterior pituitary gland and exerts control over secretions from both the anterior and posterior pituitary. See Table 14–1. The pituitary gland is attached to the hypothalamus by a narrow stalk, the *infundibulum*.

### Brainstem

The **brainstem** consists of three structures: the mesencephalon or *midbrain*, the pons, and the medulla oblongata. These structures contain centers that, along with other important functions, process visual, auditory, and sensory data and relay information to and from the cerebrum.

Midbrain.　The **midbrain** is located below the cerebrum and above the pons. Found in the midbrain are four small masses of gray cells known collectively as the **corpora quadrigemina.** The upper two of these masses, called the **superior colliculi,** are associated with visual reflexes such as the tracking movements of the eyes. The lower two, or **inferior colliculi,** are involved with the sense of hearing. See Table 14–1.

Pons.　The **pons** is a broad band of white matter located anterior to the cerebellum and between the midbrain and the medulla oblongata. The pons contains fiber tracts linking the cerebellum and medulla to higher cortical areas. It also plays a role in somatic and visceral motor control. See Table 14–1.

Medulla Oblongata.    The **medulla oblongata** is that part of the brainstem that connects the pons and the rest of the brain to the spinal cord. All afferent and efferent tracts from the spinal cord either pass through or terminate in the medulla oblongata. It also contains nerve centers instrumental to the regulation and control of breathing, swallowing, coughing, sneezing, and vomiting. Other centers in the medulla regulate heartbeat and arterial blood pressure, thereby exerting control over the circulation of blood. See Table 14–1.

## Spinal Cord

As previously mentioned, the **spinal cord** has an H-shaped gray area of cell bodies encircled by an outer region of white matter. The white matter consists of nerve tracts and fibers providing sensory input to the brain and conducting motor impulses from the brain to spinal neurons. Other fibers connect nerve cells within the spinal cord with other areas of the cord. The adult spinal cord is about 44 centimeter (cm) long and extends down the vertebral canal from the medulla to terminate near the junction of the first ($L_1$) and second ($L_2$) lumbar vertebrae. Between the 12th thoracic ($T_{12}$) and $L_1$ is a region known as the **conus medullaris,** where the spinal cord becomes conically tapered. The **filum terminale** or terminal thread of fibrous tissue extends from the conus medullaris to the second sacral vertebra. The **cauda equina** (known as the horse's tail) is the terminal portion of the spinal cord that forms the nerve fibers that are the lumbar, sacral, and coccygeal spinal nerves. The functions of the spinal cord are to conduct sensory impulses to the brain, to conduct motor impulses from the brain, and to serve as a reflex center for impulses entering and leaving the spinal cord without involvement of the brain (see Figure 14–5 ▶).

## Cerebrospinal Fluid

The brain and spinal cord are surrounded by **cerebrospinal fluid** (CSF). This colorless fluid is produced by the *choroid plexuses* within the *ventricles* of the brain. Cerebrospinal fluid circulates through the ventricles, the central canal, and the subarachnoid space. Cerebrospinal fluid is removed from circulation by the **arachnoid villi,** which are small projections of the arachnoid membrane that penetrate the tough outer membrane, the dura mater. The arachnoid villi allow the fluid to drain into the superior sagittal sinus. The normal adult will have between 120 and 150 milliliter (mL) of cerebrospinal fluid in circulation. The fluid serves to cushion the brain and cord from shocks that could cause injury. It also helps to support the brain by allowing it to float within the supporting liquid. It also contains neurotransmitters such as monoamines, acetylcholine (ACh), and neuropeptides.

# PERIPHERAL NERVOUS SYSTEM

The network of nerves branching throughout the body from the brain and spinal cord is known as the **peripheral nervous system** (PNS). There are 12 pairs of cranial nerves that attach to the brain and 31 pairs of spinal nerves connected to the spinal cord.

## Cranial Nerves

The nerves described in the following sections attach to the brain and provide sensory input, motor control, or a combination of these functions. They are arranged symmetrically, 12 to each side of the brain, and generally are named for the area or function they serve (see Figure 14–6 ▶ and Table 14–2).

### Olfactory Nerve (I)

The **olfactory nerve** provides sensory input only and carries impulses for smell to the brain. The cell bodies of these nerve fibers are located in the nasal mucous membrane and serve as receptors for the sense of smell.

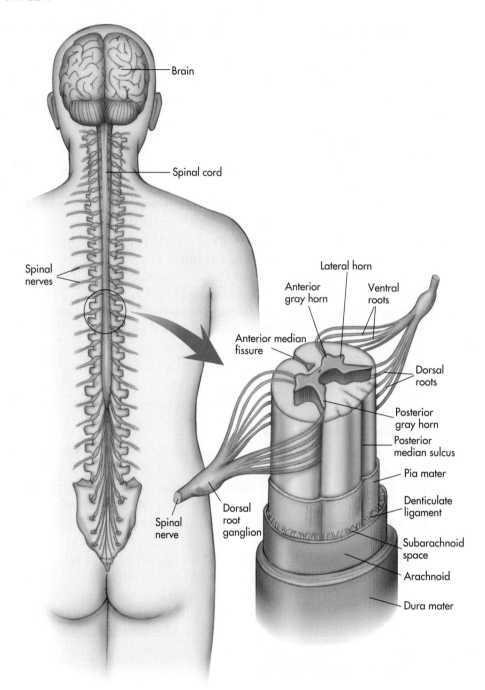

▶ **FIGURE 14–5** Brain, spinal cord, and spinal nerves with an expanded view of a spinal nerve.

## Optic Nerve (II)

The **optic nerve** provides sensory input only and carries impulses for vision to the brain. The rods and cones of the eyes are receptors and transmit images through the cells of the retina to processes that form the optic nerve. The optic nerves from each eye unite after they enter the cranial cavity to form the optic chiasm from which tracts carrying images from both eyes connect to the brain.

## Oculomotor Nerve (III)

The **oculomotor nerve** conducts motor impulses to four of the six external muscles of the eye and to the muscle that raises the eyelid. The cell bodies of motor nerves are located in the brain.

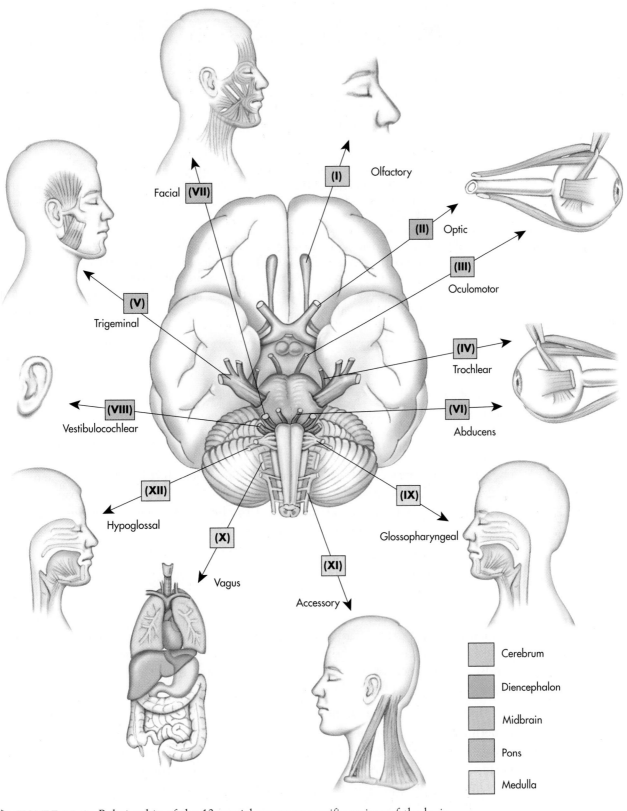

Olfactory (I)

Optic (II)

Oculomotor (III)

Trochlear (IV)

Abducens (VI)

Facial (VII)

Trigeminal (V)

Vestibulocochlear (VIII)

Hypoglossal (XII)

Vagus (X)

Accessory (XI)

Glossopharyngeal (IX)

Cerebrum

Diencephalon

Midbrain

Pons

Medulla

▶ FIGURE 14–6  Relationship of the 12 cranial nerves to specific regions of the brain.

## TABLE 14–2  Cranial Nerves and Functions

| Nerve/Number | Function |
| --- | --- |
| Olfactory (I) | Provides sense of smell |
| Optic (II) | Provides vision |
| Oculomotor (III) | Conducts motor impulses to four of the six external muscles of the eye and to the muscle that raises the eyelid |
| Trochlear (IV) | Conducts motor impulses to control the superior oblique muscle of the eyeball |
| Trigeminal (V) | Provides sensory input from the face, nose, mouth, forehead, and top of the head; motor fibers to the muscles of the jaw (chewing) |
| Abducens (VI) | Conducts motor impulses to the lateral rectus muscle of the eyeball |
| Facial (VII) | Controls the muscles of the face and scalp; the lacrimal glands of the eye and the submandibular and sublingual salivary glands; input from the tongue for the sense of taste |
| Vestibulocochlear (Acoustic) (VIII) | Provides input for hearing and equilibrium |
| Glossopharyngeal (IX) | Provides general sense of taste; regulates swallowing; controls secretion of saliva |
| Vagus (X) | Controls muscles of the pharynx, larynx, thoracic, and abdominal organs; swallowing, voice production, slowing of heartbeat, acceleration of peristalsis |
| Accessory (XI) | Controls the trapezius and sternocleidomastoid muscles, permitting movement of the head and shoulders |
| Hypoglossal (XII) | Controls the tongue; tongue movements |

### Trochlear Nerve (IV)

The **trochlear nerve** conducts motor impulses to control the superior oblique muscle of the eyeball.

### Trigeminal Nerve (V)

The **trigeminal nerve** has both sensory and motor fibers. Its fibers form three sensory divisions, the ophthalmic, maxillary, and mandibular. These fibers provide sensory input from the face, nose, mouth, forehead, and top of the head. The mandibular division also contains motor fibers to the muscles of the jaw.

### Abducens Nerve (VI)

The **abducens nerve** conducts motor impulses to the lateral rectus muscle of the eyeball.

### Facial Nerve (VII)

The **facial nerve** has both sensory and motor fibers. Its motor fibers control the muscles of the face and scalp, thereby providing for facial expression. It also provides efferent fibers to control the lacrimal glands of the eyes as well as the submandibular and sublingual salivary glands. Sensory fibers of the facial nerve provide input from the forward two-thirds of the tongue for the sense of taste.

### Vestibulocochlear Nerve (Acoustic) (VIII)

Sometimes called the *acoustic* or *auditory* nerve, the **vestibulocochlear nerve** provides sensory input for hearing and equilibrium. Fibers of the cochlear division connect with receptors in the cochlea of the ear for hearing. Fibers of the vestibular division connect to receptors in the semicircular canals and vestibule located in the ear for the sense of equilibrium.

### Glossopharyngeal Nerve (IX)

The **glossopharyngeal nerve** has both sensory and motor fibers. The sensory fibers provide for the general sense of taste and attach to the back of the tongue and pharynx. Motor fibers innervate the stylopharyngeus muscle and are important to the act of the swallowing. Other efferent fibers control the secretion of saliva from the parotid gland.

### Vagus Nerve (X)

The **vagus nerve** contains both sensory and motor fibers and is the longest of the cranial nerves. The motor fibers innervate palatal and pharyngeal muscles and branch to the heart, lungs, stomach, and intestines. The sensory fibers provide input from the pharynx, the external ear, the diaphragm, and the organs of the thoracic and abdominal cavities.

### Accessory Nerve (XI)

The **accessory nerve** conducts motor impulses for the control of the trapezius and sternocleidomastoid muscles, permitting movement of the head and shoulders.

### Hypoglossal Nerve (XII)

The **hypoglossal nerve** conducts motor impulses for control of the muscles of the tongue.

## Spinal Nerves

There are 31 pairs of **spinal nerves** distributed along the length of the spinal cord and emerging from the vertebral canal on either side through the intervertebral foramina. At the point of attachment, each nerve is divided into *two roots* (see Figure 14–5). The **dorsal** or **sensory root** is composed of afferent fibers carrying impulses to the cord, and the **ventral root** contains motor fibers carrying efferent impulses to muscles and organs. Named for the region of the vertebral column from which they exit, there are 8 pairs of **cervical spinal nerves**, 12 pairs of **thoracic spinal nerves**, 5 pairs of **lumbar spinal nerves**, 5 pairs of **sacral spinal nerves**, and 1 pair of **coccygeal spinal nerves**. See Figure 14–7 ▼.

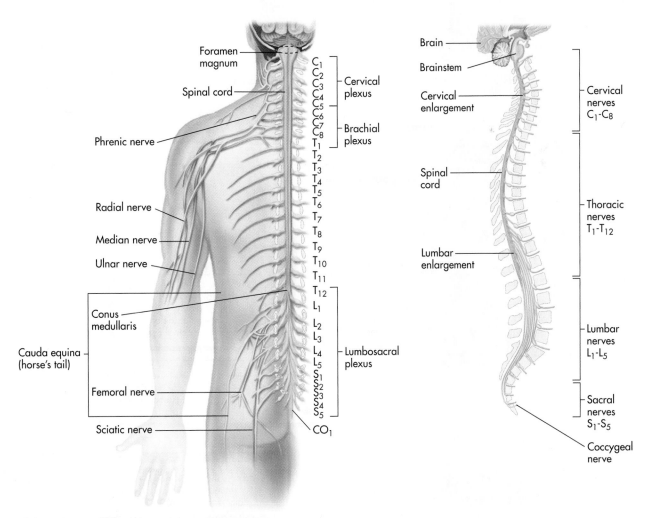

▶ **FIGURE 14–7**   The 31 pairs of spinal nerves.

A short distance from the cord, the fibers of the two roots unite to form a spinal nerve. Having formed a single nerve composed of afferent and efferent fibers, each spinal nerve then branches into several smaller nerves. The two primary branches from each spinal nerve are the **dorsal** and **ventral rami.** The dorsal rami (*branches*) carry motor and sensory fibers to the muscles and skin of the back and serve an area from the back of the head to the coccyx. The ventral rami, serving a much larger area, carry both motor and sensory fibers to the muscles and organs of the body, including the arms, legs, hands, and feet.

# AUTONOMIC NERVOUS SYSTEM

Actually a part of the peripheral nervous system, the **autonomic nervous system** (ANS) controls involuntary bodily functions such as sweating, secretions of glands, arterial blood pressure, smooth muscle tissue, and the heart. The autonomic nervous system is primarily composed of efferent fibers from certain cranial and spinal nerves and can be functionally divided into two divisions, the **sympathetic** and **parasympathetic.** These two divisions counteract each other's activity to keep the body in a state of homeostasis. See Figure 14–8 ▼.

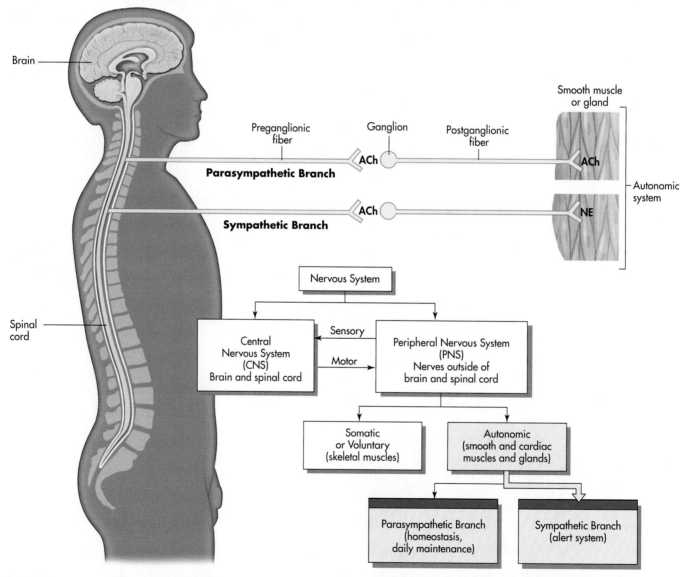

▶ **FIGURE 14–8**  General representation of the autonomic nervous system.

## Sympathetic Division

Branches from the ventral roots of the 12 thoracic and the first 3 lumbar spinal nerves form the first part of the **sympathetic division.** The cell bodies of these nerve fibers are located in the *gray matter* of the spinal cord. Just outside the spinal cord, axons of these nerve cells leave the spinal nerves and enter almost immediately into masses of nerve cell bodies, the **sympathetic ganglia,** which form a chain that runs next to the vertebral column. This chain of about 23 ganglia runs from the base of the head to the coccyx and is known as the **sympathetic trunk.** Within the ganglia of the sympathetic trunk, fibers from the spinal nerves synapse with ganglionic nerve cell bodies. These ganglionic neurons produce long axons that reach to the parts of the body to be innervated. This arrangement, characteristic of autonomic nerves, creates a two-neuron chain as opposed to single-neuron control of regular motor nerves (see Figure 14–9 ▼).

Because of the arrangement in which *sympathetic fibers* from spinal nerves synapse with many cell bodies in the sympathetic ganglia, they tend to produce widespread innervation when activated. This condition has been described as preparing the individual for *fight or flight.* During the *fight-or-flight response,* a person experiences increased alertness, increased metabolic rate, decreased digestive and urinary function, an increase in respiration, blood pressure, and heart rate and a corresponding warming of the body that can activate the sweat glands. The sympathetic system stimulates the adrenal gland to release epinephrine (adrenaline), the hormone that causes the familiar adrenaline rush.

## Parasympathetic Division

Very long fibers branching from cranial nerves III, VII, IX, and X along with long fibers of sacral nerves II, III, and IV form the first stage of the **parasympathetic division.** Cell bodies for these long fibers are located in the brain and spinal cord. These long fibers extend to ganglia located near the organs to be innervated. Fibers of **cranial** and **sacral nerves** synapse with ganglionic cell bodies, which then conduct impulses over short axons to the gland, smooth muscle tissue, or organ to be innervated. Fibers from the cranial nerves serve

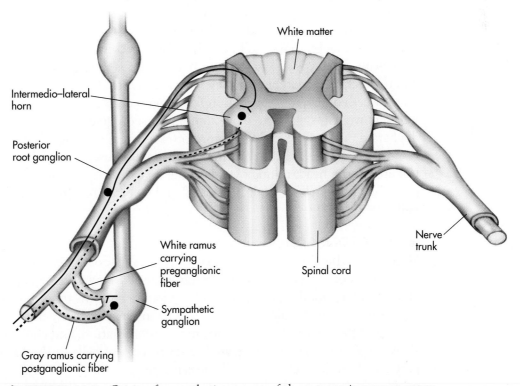

▶ **FIGURE 14–9** Origin of sympathetic neurons of the autonomic nervous system.

the iris and ciliary muscles of the eye, lacrimal glands, and salivary glands through four ganglia located in the head. Cranial nerve fibers extend via the vagus nerve to ganglia serving the thoracic, abdominal, and pelvic viscera. The fibers of the sacral spinal nerves form the pelvic nerve, which branches to synapse with small ganglia near or within the organs to be innervated. The cell bodies of these ganglia serve the lower colon, rectum, bladder, and reproductive organs.

The parasympathetic division works to conserve energy and innervate the digestive system. When activated, it stimulates the salivary and digestive glands, decreases the metabolic rate, slows the heart rate, reduces blood pressure, and promotes the passage of material through the intestines along with absorption of nutrients by the blood.

# LIFE SPAN CONSIDERATIONS

## ■ THE CHILD

Neural tube development occurs about the third to fourth week of embryonic life. This development becomes the **central nervous system.** At 6 weeks, a developing baby's brain waves are measurable. At 28 weeks, the fetal nervous system begins some regulatory functions. At 32 weeks, the fetal nervous system is continuing to mature so that rhythmic respirations and regulation of body temperature are possible if delivery of the fetus occurs at this time. Brain and nerve cell growth are most rapid from birth until about 4 years of age.

A baby's **brain** has three main structural parts: the **cerebrum,** the **cerebellum,** and the **brainstem.** The cerebrum serves as a control center as it receives, processes, and acts on information. The cerebellum helps coordinate muscle activities and maintains posture and balance. The brainstem maintains vital body functions, such as breathing, heartbeat, blood pressure, digestion, and swallowing. While the brain of an infant resembles that of an adult, one area is relatively unrefined. In an infant, the right and left hemispheres of the brain have not yet developed their own specific tasks. By the time a child is 3 years old, the two sides of the brain are well on their way to becoming specialized in different tasks.

While a baby is still in the womb, the brain is forging connections in the cerebellum, and the kicks and twitches that the fetus delivers to the mother are proof of this. At about 4 to 6 weeks of life, motor function is the main connection taking place in the brain. The initial movements characteristic of an infant soon give way to the repetition of smoother, deliberate ones as the brain's motor cortex process new signals and strengthens connections. Over the next 12 months, a baby's brain focuses first on gross motor skills, such as holding up the head, rolling over, pushing up to a seated position, crawling, and using the pincer grasp to pick up food. Between 2 and 4 years, the child will learn to run and kick a ball.

## ■ THE OLDER ADULT

With aging, the number of nerve cells decreases, as does brain mass. Loss can occur in different areas of the brain and to varying degrees. Many older adults experience very little change in function because a person has more nerve cells than needed. The levels of **neurotransmitters** or chemicals communicating in synapses between nerve cells decrease. This generally affects short-term memory, motor coordination, and control. The older adult has slower response time and decreased reflexes. Loss of cells in the brainstem changes sleep patterns. The older adult generally does not sleep as long or as well as a younger person. As people age, however, the learning of new information and skills continues.

# BUILDING YOUR MEDICAL VOCABULARY

This section provides the foundation for learning medical terminology. Review the following alphabetized word list. Note how common prefixes and suffixes are repeatedly applied to word roots and combining forms to create different meanings.

| | |
|---|---|
| **P** | Prefix |
| **R** | Root |
| **CF** | Combining form |
| **S** | Suffix |

| | |
|---|---|
| **Pink words** | Terms not built from word parts. |
| **\*** | Indicates words covered in the Pathology Spotlights section. |
| (CD-ROM) | Check the CD-ROM for more information. |

| MEDICAL WORD | WORD PARTS (WHEN APPLICABLE) | | | DEFINITION |
|---|---|---|---|---|
| | **Part** | **Type** | **Meaning** | |
| **acetylcholine (ACh)** (ăs″ ĕ-tĭl-kō′ lēn) | | | | Cholinergic neurotransmitter in various tissues and organs of the body; plays an important role in the transmission of nerve impulses at synapses and myoneural junctions |
| **akathesia** (ăk″ ă-thē′ zĭ ă) | | | | Inability to remain still; motor restlessness and anxiety |
| **akinesia** (ă″ kĭ-nē′ zĭ-ă) | a- -kinesia | P S | lack of motion, movement | Loss or lack of the power of voluntary motion |
| **Alzheimer's disease (AD)** (ahlts′ hĭ-merz dĭ-zēz′) (CD-ROM) | | | | Severe form of senile dementia; perhaps due to some defect in the neurotransmitter system. Cortical destruction causes variable degrees of confusion, memory loss, and other cognitive defects. \* See Pathology Spotlight: Alzheimer's Disease on page 478. |
| **amnesia** (ăm-nē′ zĭ-ă) | a- mnes -ia | P R S | lack of memory condition | Condition in which there is a loss or lack of memory |
| **amyotrophic lateral sclerosis (ALS)** (ă-mī″ ō-trŏf′ ĭk lăt′ ĕr-ăl sklĕ-rō′ sĭs) | a- my/o -troph (y) -ic later -al scler -osis | P CF S S R S R S | lack of muscle nourishment pertaining to side pertaining to hardening condition (usually abnormal) | Muscular weakness, atrophy, with spasticity caused by degeneration of motor neurons of the spinal cord, medulla, and cortex; also called *Lou Gehrig's disease* |
| **analgesia** (ăn″ ăl-jē′ zĭ-ă) | an- -algesia | P S | lack of condition of pain | Condition in which there is a lack of the sense of pain |

| MEDICAL WORD | WORD PARTS (WHEN APPLICABLE) | | | DEFINITION |
|---|---|---|---|---|
| | Part | Type | Meaning | |
| **anencephaly**<br>(ăn″ ĕn-sĕf′ ăl-ē) | an-<br>encephal<br>-y | P<br>R<br>S | lack of<br>brain<br>condition | Congenital condition in which there is a lack of development of the brain |
| **anesthesia**<br>(ăn″ ĕs-thē′ zĭ-ă) | an-<br>-esthesia | P<br>S | lack of<br>feeling | Loss or lack of the sense of feeling |
| **anesthesiologist**<br>(ăn″ ĕs-thē′ zĭ-ŏl′ ō-jĭst) | an-<br>esthesi/o<br>log<br>-ist | P<br>CF<br>R<br>S | lack of<br>feeling<br>study of<br>one who specializes | Physician who specializes in the science of anesthesia |
| **aphagia**<br>(ă-fā′ jĭ-ă) | a-<br>-phagia | P<br>S | lack of<br>to eat, swallow | Loss or lack of the ability to eat or swallow |
| **aphasia**<br>(ă-fā′ zĭ-ă) | a-<br>-phasia | P<br>S | lack of<br>to speak, speech | Loss or lack of the ability to speak due to neurological impairment. A person may also have difficulty understanding others and/or expressing him- or herself verbally. |
| **apraxia**<br>(ă-prăks′ ĭ-ă) | a-<br>-praxia | P<br>S | lack of<br>action | Loss or lack of the ability to use objects properly; inability to perform motor tasks or activities of daily living, such as dressing and bathing |
| **asthenia**<br>(ăs-thē′ nĭ-ă) | a-<br>-sthenia | P<br>S | lack of<br>strength | Loss or lack of strength |
| **astrocytoma**<br>(ăs″ trō-sī-tō′ mă) | astro-<br>cyt<br>-oma | P<br>R<br>S | star-shaped<br>cell<br>tumor | A primary tumor of the brain composed of astrocytes (star shaped neuroglial cells) characterized by slow growth, cyst formation, metastasis, and malignant glioblastoma within the tumor mass. Surgical intervention is possible in the early developmental stage of the tumor; also called *astrocytic glioma*. |
| **ataxia**<br>(ă-tăks′ ĭ-ă) | a-<br>-taxia | P<br>S | lack of<br>order, coordination | Loss or lack of muscular coordination |
| **bradykinesia**<br>(brăd″ ĭ-kĭ-nē′ sĭ-ă) | brady-<br>-kinesia | P<br>S | slow<br>motion, movement | Abnormal slowness of motion |
| **cephalalgia**<br>(sĕf″ ă-lăl′ jĭ-ă) | cephal<br>-algia | R<br>S | head<br>pain | Head pain; *headache* |
| **cerebellar**<br>(sĕr″ ĕ-bĕl′ ăr) | cerebell<br>-ar | R<br>S | little brain<br>pertaining to | Pertaining to the cerebellum |
| **cerebral palsy (CP)**<br>(sĕr″ ĕ-br′ăl pawl′ zē) | | | | Disorder of movement and posture secondary to lesions or anomalies of the brain, arising in the early stages of its development. Most common chronic disorder of childhood involving four motor dysfunctions: spastic, dyskinetic, ataxic, and mixed. See Figure 14–10 ▶. |

| MEDICAL WORD | WORD PARTS (WHEN APPLICABLE) | | | DEFINITION |
|---|---|---|---|---|
| | **Part** | **Type** | **Meaning** | |
| **cerebrospinal** (sĕr″ ĕ-brō-spī′ năl) | cerebr/o spin -al | CF R S | cerebrum a thorn, spine pertaining to | Pertaining to the cerebrum and the spinal cord |
| **chorea** (kō-rē′ ă) | | | | Condition of rapid, jerky involuntary muscular movements of the limbs or face |
| **coma** (kō′ ma) | | | | Unconscious state or stupor from which the patient cannot be aroused |
| **concussion (brain)** (kŏn-kŭsh′ ŭn) | concuss -ion | R S | shaken violently process | Loss of consciousness, temporary or prolonged, caused by a blow to the head |
| **craniectomy** (krā″ nĭ-ĕk′ tō-mē) | cran/i -ectomy | CF S | skull surgical excision | Surgical excision of a portion of the skull |
| **craniotomy** (krā″ nĭ-ŏt′ ō-mē) | crani/o -tomy | CF S | skull incision | Surgical opening into the skull. A series of burr holes is made and then the bone between the holes is cut and the scalp is pulled back to allow access to the brain. Used to repair defects associated with traumatic head injuries or to repair a cerebral aneurysm. See Figure 14–11 ▼. |

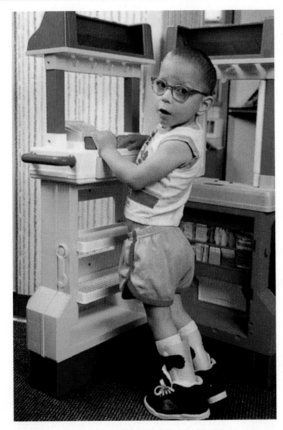

▶ **FIGURE 14–10** Child with cerebral palsy has abnormal muscle tone and lack of physical coordination.

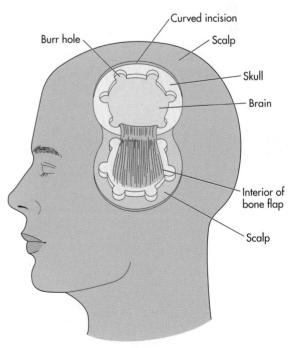

▶ **FIGURE 14–11** In a craniotomy, a portion of the skull and overlying scalp is pulled back to allow access to the brain.

| MEDICAL WORD | WORD PARTS (WHEN APPLICABLE) | | | DEFINITION |
|---|---|---|---|---|
| | Part | Type | Meaning | |
| **deep brain stimulation (DBS)** (dēp brān stĭm' ū- lā' shŭn) | | | | Technique used to stop uncontrollable movements in Parkinson's disease. Electrodes are implanted in the thalamus or globus pallidus of the brain and connected to a pacemakerlike device, which the patient can switch on or off as symptoms dictate. |
| **dementia** (dē-mĕn' shē-ă) | de- ment -ia | P R S | down mind condition | Refers to a group of symptoms marked by memory loss and other cognitive functions such as perception, thinking, reasoning, and remembering. Alzheimer's is the most common form of dementia. |
| **diskectomy** (dĭs-kĕk' tō-mē) | disk -ectomy | R S | a disk surgical excision | Surgical excision of an intervertebral disk |
| **dyslexia** (dĭs-lĕks' ĭ-ă) | dys- -lexia | P S | difficult diction, word, phrase | Condition in which an individual has difficulty in using and comprehending written language |
| **dysphasia** (dĭs-fā' zĭ-ă) | dys- -phasia | P S | difficult speak, speech | Impairment of speech caused by a brain lesion |
| **electroencephalograph** (ē-lĕk" trō-ĕn-sĕf' ă-lō-grăf) | electr/o encephal/o -graph | CF CF S | electricity brain instrument for recording | Instrument used to record the electrical activity of the brain |
| **electromyography** (ē-lĕk" trō-mī-ŏg' ră-fē) | electr/o my/o -graphy | CF CF S | electricity muscle recording | Process of recording the contraction of a skeletal muscle as a result of electrical stimulation; used in diagnosing disorders of nerves supplying muscles |
| **encephalitis** (ĕn-sĕf" ă-lī' tĭs) | encephal -itis | R S | brain inflammation | Inflammation of the brain. ✱ See Pathology Spotlight: Encephalitis on page 479. |
| **encephalopathy** (ĕn-sĕf" ă-lōp'ă-thē) | encephal/o -pathy | CF S | brain disease | Any dysfunction of the brain. HIV encephalopathy is called *AIDS-dementia complex.* |
| **endorphins** (ĕn-dor' fĭns) | | | | Chemical substances produced in the brain that act as natural analgesics (*opiates*) |
| **epidural** (ĕp" ĭ-dū' răl) | epi- dur -al | P R S | upon dura, hard pertaining to | Pertaining to situated on the dura mater |
| **epiduroscopy** (ep" ĭ-du-ros' kō-pē) | epi- dur/o -scopy | P CF S | upon dura, hard visual examination, to view, examine | Minimally invasive form of surgery that introduces medication via an endoscope into the epidural space; used for back pain relief when all other conservative treatments have failed |

| MEDICAL WORD | WORD PARTS (WHEN APPLICABLE) | | | DEFINITION |
|---|---|---|---|---|
| | **Part** | **Type** | **Meaning** | |
| **epilepsy**<br>(ĕp′ ĭ-lĕp″ sē) | epi-<br>-lepsy | P<br>S | upon<br>seizure | Disorder of cerebral function resulting from abnormal electrical activity or malfunctioning of the chemical substances of the brain. ✱ See Pathology Spotlight: Epilepsy on page 480. |
| **ganglionectomy**<br>(gang″ lĭ-ō-nĕk′ tō-mē) | ganglion<br>-ectomy | R<br>S | knot<br>surgical excision | Surgical excision of a ganglion (a mass of nerve tissue outside the brain and spinal cord) |
| **glioma**<br>(glī-ō′ mă) | gli<br>-oma | R<br>S | glue<br>tumor | Tumor composed of neuroglial tissue |
| **Guillain-Barré syndrome**<br>(gē-yă′băr-rā sĭn′drōm) | | | | Condition in which the myelin sheaths covering peripheral nerves are destroyed, resulting in decreased nerve impulses, loss of reflex response, and sudden muscle weakness. Generally an acute viral infection occurs 1 to 3 weeks before the onset of the syndrome; also called *infectious polyneuritis, acute febrile polyneuritis, acute idiopathic polyneuritis.* |
| **hemiparesis**<br>(hĕm″ ĭ-păr′ ĕ-sĭs) | hemi-<br>-paresis | P<br>S | half<br>weakness | Slight paralysis that affects one side of the body |
| **hemiplegia**<br>(hĕm″ ĭ-plē′ jĭ-ă) | hemi-<br>-plegia | P<br>S | half<br>stroke, paralysis | Paralysis of one half of the body when it is divided along the median sagittal plane. See Figure 14–12 ▼. |

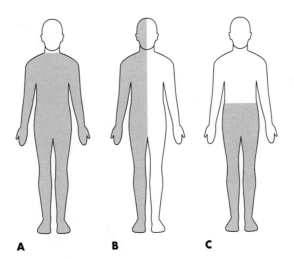

A  B  C

▶ **FIGURE 14–12** Types of paralysis: (A) Quadriplegia is complete or partial paralysis of the upper extremities and complete paralysis of the lower part of the body. (B) Hemiplegia is paralysis of one half of the body when it is divided along the median sagittal plane. (C) Paraplegia is a paralysis of the lower part of the body.

| MEDICAL WORD | WORD PARTS (WHEN APPLICABLE) | | | DEFINITION |
|---|---|---|---|---|
| | Part | Type | Meaning | |
| **herniated disk syndrome (HDS)** (hĕr-nē-ā'tĕd dĭs-kĕk' sĭn'drōm) | | | | Condition in which part or all of the soft, gelatinous central portion of an intervertebral disk (the nucleus pulposus) is forced through a weakened part of the disk. Compression on the nerves can cause *sciatica* or lumbar back pain that radiates down one or both legs; also called *herniated intervertebral disk, ruptured disk, herniated nucleus pulposus (HNP),* or *slipped disk.* See Figure 14–13 ▼. |
| **herpes zoster** (hĕr' pēz zŏs' tĕr) | | | | Acute viral disease characterized by painful vesicular eruptions along the segment of the spinal or cranial nerves; also called *shingles.* See Figures 14–14 ▼ and 14–15 ▼. |

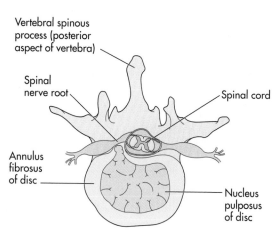

▶ **FIGURE 14–13**   Herniated intervertebral disk: the herniated nucleus pulposus is applying pressure against the nerve root.

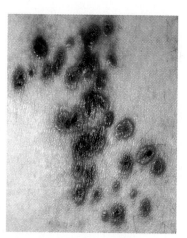

▶ **FIGURE 14–14**   Herpes zoster.
(Courtesy of Jason L. Smith, MD)

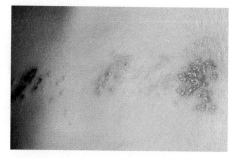

▶ **FIGURE 14–15**   Herpes zoster.
(Courtesy Jason L. Smith, MD)

| MEDICAL WORD | WORD PARTS (WHEN APPLICABLE) | | | DEFINITION |
|---|---|---|---|---|
| | Part | Type | Meaning | |
| **hydrocephalus** (hī″ drō-sĕf′ ă-lŭs) | hydro- cephal -us | P R S | water head pertaining to | Pertaining to an increased amount of cerebrospinal fluid within the brain. See Figure 14–16 ▼. |
| **hyperesthesia** (hī″ pĕr-ĕs-thē′ zĭ-ă) | hyper- -esthesia | P S | excessive feeling | Excessive feelings of sensory stimuli, such as pain, touch, or sound |
| **hyperkinesis** (hī″ pĕr-kĭn-ē′ sĭs) | hyper- -kinesis | P S | excessive motion | Excessive muscular movement and motion; inability to be still; also known as *hyperactivity* |
| **hypnosis** (hĭp-nō′ sĭs) | hypn -osis | R S | sleep condition (usually abnormal) | Artificially induced trancelike state resembling somnambulism (sleepwalking) |
| **intracranial** (ĭn″ trăh-krā′ nĕ-ăl) | intra- crani -al | P R S | within skull pertaining to | Pertaining to within the skull |
| **laminectomy** (lăm″ ĭ-nĕk′ tō-mē) | lamin -ectomy | R S | thin plate surgical excision | Surgical excision of a vertebral posterior arch |
| **lobotomy** (lō-bŏt′ ō-mē) | lob/o -tomy | CF S | lobe incision | Surgical incision into the prefrontal or frontal lobe of the brain |
| **meningioma** (mĕn-ĭn″ jĭ-ō′ mă) | mening/i -oma | CF S | membrane, meninges tumor | Tumor of the meninges that originates in the arachnoidal tissue |
| **meningitis** (mĕn″ ĭn-jī′ tĭs) | mening -itis | R S | membrane, meninges inflammation | Inflammation of the meninges of the spinal cord or brain. ✷ See Pathology Spotlight: Meningitis on page 479. |
| **meningocele** (mĕn-ĭn-gō-sēl) | mening/o -cele | CF S | membrane, meninges hernia | Congenital hernia (saclike protrusion) in which the meninges protrude through a defect in the skull or spinal column. See Figure 14–17 ▶. |

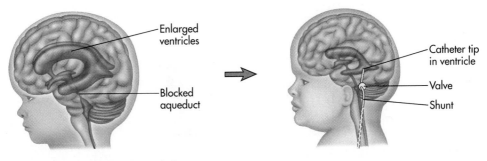

▶ FIGURE 14–16  Hydrocephalus.

| MEDICAL WORD | WORD PARTS (WHEN APPLICABLE) | | | DEFINITION |
|---|---|---|---|---|
| | **Part** | **Type** | **Meaning** | |
| **meningomyelocele**<br>(měn-ĭn″ gō-mī-ěl′ ō-sēl) | mening/o<br><br>myel/o<br>-cele | CF<br><br>CF<br>S | membrane,<br>meninges<br>spinal cord<br>hernia | Congenital herniation of the spinal cord and meninges through a defect in the vertebral column. See Figure 14–17 ▼. |
| **microcephalus**<br>(mī″ krō-sěf′ ă-lŭs) | micro-<br>cephal<br>-us | P<br>R<br>S | small<br>head<br>pertaining to | Abnormally small head; congenital anomaly characterized by an abnormal smallness of the head in relation to the rest of the body |
| **multiple sclerosis (MS)**<br>(mŭl′ tĭ-pl sklē′ -rō′ sĭs) | scler<br>-osis | R<br>S | hardening<br>condition (usu-<br>ally abnormal) | Chronic disease of the central nervous system marked by damage to the myelin sheath. Plaques occur in the brain and spinal cord causing tremor, weakness, incoordination, paresthesia, and disturbances in vision and speech. ✳ See Pathology Spotlight: Multiple Sclerosis on page 481. |
| **myelitis**<br>(mī″ ě-lī′ tĭs) | myel<br>-itis | R<br>S | spinal cord<br>inflammation | Inflammation of the spinal cord |
| **myelography**<br>(mī″ ě-lŏg′ ră-fē) | myel/o<br>-graphy | CF<br>S | spinal cord<br>recording | X-ray recording of the spinal cord after injection of a radiopaque medium into the spinal canal |
| **narcolepsy**<br>(nar′ kō-lěp″ sē) | narc/o<br><br>-lepsy | CF<br><br>S | numbness, sleep,<br>stupor<br>seizure | Chronic condition with recurrent attacks of uncontrollable drowsiness and sleep |

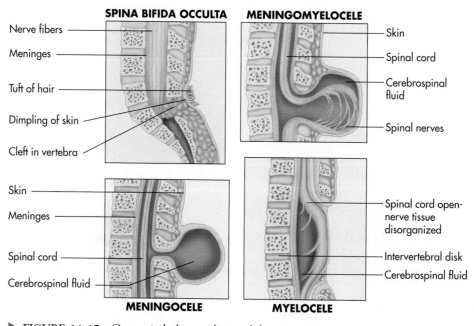

▶ FIGURE 14–17  Congenital abnormalities of the spine.

| MEDICAL WORD | WORD PARTS (WHEN APPLICABLE) | | | DEFINITION |
|---|---|---|---|---|
| | **Part** | **Type** | **Meaning** | |
| **neuralgia**<br>(nū-răl′ jĭ-ă) | neur<br>-algia | R<br>S | nerve<br>pain | Pain in a nerve or nerves |
| **neurasthenia**<br>(nū″ răs-thē′ nĭ-ă) | neur<br>-asthenia | R<br>S | nerve<br>weakness | Abnormal condition characterized by nervous weakness, exhaustion, and prostration that often follows depression |
| **neurectomy**<br>(nū-rĕk′ tō-mē) | neur<br>-ectomy | R<br>S | nerve<br>surgical excision | Surgical excision of a nerve |
| **neurilemma**<br>(nū′ rĭ-lĕm″ mă) | neur/i<br>-lemma | CF<br>S | nerve<br>a sheath, husk, rind | Thin membranous sheath that envelops a nerve fiber; also called *sheath of Schwann* or *neurolemma* |
| **neuritis**<br>(nū-rī′ tĭs) | neur<br>-itis | R<br>S | nerve<br>inflammation | Inflammation of a nerve |
| **neuroblast**<br>(nū′ rō-blăst) | neur/o<br>-blast | CF<br>S | nerve<br>germ cell | Germ cell from which nervous tissue is formed |
| **neuroblastoma**<br>(nū″ rō-blăs-tō′ mă) | neur/o<br>-blast<br>-oma | CF<br>S<br>S | nerve<br>germ cell<br>tumor | Malignant tumor composed of cells resembling neuroblasts; occurs mostly in infants and children |
| **neurocyte**<br>(nū′ rō-sīt) | neur/o<br>-cyte | CF<br>S | nerve<br>cell | Nerve cell, neuron |
| **neurofibroma**<br>(nū″ rō-fī-brō′ mă) | neur/o<br>fibr<br>-oma | CF<br>R<br>S | nerve<br>fiber<br>tumor | Fibrous connective tissue tumor, especially involving the Schwann cells of a nerve. See Figure 14–18 ▼. |
| **neuroglia**<br>(nū-rŏg′ lĭ-ă) | neur/o<br>-glia | CF<br>S | nerve<br>glue | Supporting or connective tissue cells of the central nervous system (*astrocytes, oligodendroglia, microglia,* and *ependymal cells*) |
| **neurologist**<br>(nū-rŏl′ ō-jĭst) | neur/o<br>log<br>-ist | CF<br>R<br>S | nerve<br>study of<br>one who specializes | Physician who specializes in the study of the nervous system |

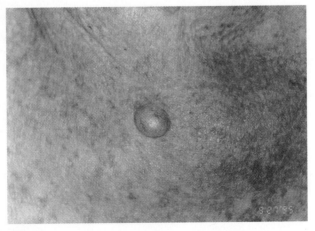

▶ **FIGURE 14–18**    Neurofibroma. (Courtesy of Jason L. Smith, MD)

| MEDICAL WORD | WORD PARTS (WHEN APPLICABLE) | | | DEFINITION |
|---|---|---|---|---|
| | Part | Type | Meaning | |
| **neurology (Neuro)** (nū-rŏl′ ō-jē) | neur/o -logy | CF S | nerve study of | Study of the nervous system |
| **neuroma** (nū-rō′ mă) | neur -oma | R S | nerve tumor | Tumor of nerve cells and nerve fibers |
| **neuropathy** (nū-rŏp′ ă-thē) | neur/o -pathy | CF S | nerve disease | Any nerve disease |
| **neurotransmitter** (nū″ rō-trăns′ mĭt-ĕr) | | | | Substances within neurons and the cerebrospinal fluid that allow nerve cells to communicate with one another |
| **oligodendro-glioma** (ŏl″ ĭ-gō-dĕn″ drō-glĭ-ō′ mă) | oligo- dendr/o gli -oma | P CF R S | little tree glue tumor | Malignant tumor derived and composed of oligodendroglia (a type of cell that makes up one component of the tissue of the CNS) |
| **pallidotomy** (păl″ ĭ-dŏt-ō-mē) | pallid/o -tomy | CF S | globus pallidus incision | Surgical destruction of the globus pallidus of the brain done to treat involuntary movements or muscular rigidity in Parkinson's disease |
| **palsy** (pawl′ zē) | | | | Loss of sensation or an impairment of motor function; also called *paralysis*. There are many types of palsy; one example is Bell's palsy, a unilateral paralysis of the facial (VII) nerve. The facial expression is distorted and the patient could be unable to close an eye or control salivation on the affected side. See Figure 14–19 ▼. |
| **papilledema** (păp″ ĭl-ĕ-dē′ mă) | papill -edema | R S | papilla swelling | Swelling of the optical disk, usually caused by increased intracranial pressure (ICP); also called *choked disk* |

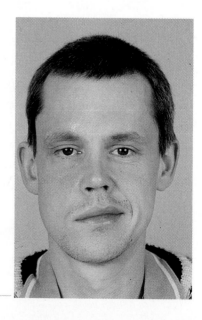

▶ **FIGURE 14–19**   Man with Bell's palsy shows typical drooping of the one side of the face. (Courtesy of Phototake, Inc.)

| MEDICAL WORD | WORD PARTS (WHEN APPLICABLE) | | | DEFINITION |
|---|---|---|---|---|
| | **Part** | **Type** | **Meaning** | |
| **paraplegia**<br>(păr″ ă-plē′ jĭ-ă) | para-<br>-plegia | P<br>S | beside<br>stroke, paralysis | Paralysis of the lower part of the body and of both legs. See Figure 14–12 on page 467. |
| **paresis**<br>(păr′ ē-sĭs) | | | | Slight, partial, or incomplete paralysis |
| **paresthesia**<br>(păr″ ĕs-thē′ zĭ-ă) | par-<br>-esthesia | P<br>S | beside<br>feeling | Abnormal sensation, feeling of numbness, prickling, or tingling |
| **Parkinson's disease**<br>(păr′ kĭn-sŭnz dĭ-zēz′) | | | | Chronic disease of the nervous system characterized by a loss of equilibrium and by salivation, frustration, nausea, dryness of the mouth, and muscular tremors; also called *paralysis agitans, shaking palsy.*<br>✱ See Pathology Spotlight: Parkinson's Disease on page 481. |
| **paroxysm**<br>(păr′ ok-sĭzm) | | | | Sudden recurrence of the symptoms of a disease, an exacerbation; also means a *spasm* or *seizure* |
| **pheochromocytoma**<br>(fē-ō-krō″ mō-sī-tō′ mă) | phe/o<br>chrom/o<br>cyt<br>-oma | CF<br>CF<br>R<br>S | dusky<br>color<br>cell<br>tumor | Chromaffin cell tumor of the adrenal medulla or of the sympathetic nervous system |
| **poliomyelitis**<br>(pōl″ ĭ-ō-mī″ ĕl-ī′ tĭs) | poli/o<br>myel<br>-itis | CF<br>R<br>S | gray<br>spinal cord<br>inflammation | Inflammation of the gray matter of the spinal cord |
| **polyneuritis**<br>(pŏl″ ē nū-rī′ tĭs) | poly-<br>neur<br>-itis | P<br>R<br>S | many<br>nerve<br>inflammation | Inflammation of many nerves |
| **quadriplegia**<br>(kwŏd″ rĭ plē′ jĭ-ă) | quadri-<br>-plegia | P<br>S | four<br>stroke, paralysis | Paralysis of all four extremities and usually the trunk due to injury to the spinal cord in the cervical spine; also called *tetraplegia.* See Figure 14–12 on page 467. |
| **receptor**<br>(rē-sĕp′ tōr) | | | | Sensory nerve ending that receives and relays responses to stimuli |
| **Reye's syndrome**<br>(rīz sĭn′ drōm) | | | | Acute disease that causes edema of the brain and increased intracranial pressure, hypoglycemia, and fatty infiltration of the liver and other vital organs; occurs in children and has a relation to aspirin administration; can be viral in origin |
| **sciatica**<br>(sī-ăt′ ĭ-kă) | | | | Severe pain along the course of the sciatic nerve |
| **sleep**<br>(slēp) | | | | State of rest for the body and mind; has two distinct types: REM for rapid eye movement, sometimes called *dream sleep,* and NREM for no rapid eye movement |
| **somnambulism**<br>(sŏm-năm′ bū-lĭzm) | somn<br>ambul<br>-ism | R<br>R<br>S | sleep<br>to walk<br>condition | Condition of sleepwalking |

| MEDICAL WORD | WORD PARTS (WHEN APPLICABLE) | | | DEFINITION |
|---|---|---|---|---|
| | Part | Type | Meaning | |
| **spondylosyndesis**<br>(spŏn″ dĭ-lō-sĭn′ dĕ-sĭs) | spondyl/o<br>syn-<br>-desis | CF<br>P<br>S | vertebra<br>together<br>binding | Surgical procedure to bind vertebra after removal of a herniated disk; also called *spinal fusion* |
| **stroke**<br>(strōk) | | | | Death of brain tissue that occurs when the brain does not get enough blood and oxygen; also called cerebrovascular accident (CVA) or brain attack. ✱ See Pathology Spotlight: Stroke on page 483 and Figures 14–24 and 14–25. |
| **subdural**<br>(sŭb-dū′ răl) | sub-<br>dur<br>-al | P<br>R<br>S | below<br>dura, hard<br>pertaining to | Pertaining to below the dura mater |
| **sundowning**<br>(sŭn′ dōwnĭng) | | | | Increased agitation or restlessness that occurs in the late afternoon or early evening in patients with cognitive impairment; most common with Alzheimer's type dementia and Parkinson's disease |
| **sympathectomy**<br>(sĭm″ pă-thĕk′ tō-mē) | sympath<br>-ectomy | R<br>S | sympathy<br>surgical excision | Surgical excision of a portion of the sympathetic nervous system |
| **syncope**<br>(sĭn′ kŭ-pē) | | | | Temporary loss of consciousness caused by a lack of blood supply to the brain; also called *fainting* |
| **tactile**<br>(tăk′ tĭl) | | | | Pertaining to the sense of touch |
| **Tay-Sachs disease**<br>(tā săks′ dĭ-zēz′) | | | | Inherited, progressive disease marked by degeneration of brain tissue; predominantly affects Jewish children of Ashkenazi origin |
| **transcutaneous electrical nerve stimulations (TENS)**<br>(trăns-kū-tā′ nē-ŭs nerv stĭm′ ŭ-lā′ shŭn) | | | | Use of mild electrical stimulation to interfere with the transmission of painful stimuli; has proved useful in relieving pain in some patients |
| **vagotomy**<br>(vā-gŏt′ ō-mē) | vag/o<br>-tomy | CF<br>S | vagus, wandering<br>incision | Surgical incision of the vagus nerve |
| **ventriculometry**<br>(vĕn-trĭk″ ū-lōm′ ĕtrē) | ventricul/o<br>-metry | CF<br>S | little belly<br>measurement | Measurement of intracranial pressure |

# DRUG HIGHLIGHTS

| | |
|---|---|
| **Analgesics** | Inhibit ascending pain pathways in the central nervous system. They increase pain threshold and alter pain perception. |
| Narcotic | *Examples: codeine phosphate, codeine sulfate, Dilaudid (hydromorphone HCl), Demerol (meperidine HCl), Darvon-N (propoxyphene napsylate), morphine sulfate, and Talwin (pentazocine HCl)* |
| Non-narcotic | *Examples: Stadol (butorphanol tartrate) and Nubain (nalbuphine HCl)* |
| **Analgesics–Antipyretics** | Act to relieve pain (analgesic effect) and reduce fever (antipyretic effect). |
| | *Examples: Tylenol (acetaminophen); aspirin; Advil, Motrin, Nuprin (ibuprofen); and Naprosyn, Aleve (naproxen)* |
| **Sedatives and hypnotics** | Depress the central nervous system by interfering with the transmission of nerve impulses. Depending upon the dosage, barbiturates, benzodiazepines, and certain other drugs can produce either a sedative or a hypnotic effect. When used as a sedative, the dosage is designed to produce a calming effect without causing sleep. Used as a hypnotic, the dosage is sufficient to cause sleep. |
| Barbiturates | *Examples: Nembutal (pentobarbital), Seconal (secobarbital), and Luminal (phenobarbital)* |
| Non-barbiturates | *Examples: Aquachloral (chloral hydrate), Dalmane (flurazepam HCl), Restoril (temazepam), and Halcion (triazolam)* |
| **Antiparkinsonism drugs** | Used for palliative relief from such major symptoms as bradykinesia, rigidity, tremor, and disorder of equilibrium and posture. Therapy involves an attempt to replenish dopamine levels and/or inhibit the effects of the neurotransmitter acetylcholine. |
| | *Examples: Symmetrel (amantadine HCl), Dopar (levodopa), Artane (trihexyphenidyl HCl), Cogentin (benztropine mesylate), Requip (ropinirole), Tasmar (tolcapone), and Stalevo (carbidopa, levodopa, and entacapone)* |
| **Anticonvulsants** | Inhibit the spread of seizure activity in the motor cortex. |
| | *Examples: Dilantin (phenytoin), Depakene (valproic acid), Tegretol (carbamazepine), Klonopin (clonazepam), and Mysoline (primidone)* |
| **Cholinesterase inhibitors** | Increase the brain's levels of acetylcholine, which helps to restore communication between brain cells. These medications can be used to improve global functioning (including activities of daily living, behavior, and cognition) in some patients with Alzheimer's disease. |
| | *Examples: Cognex (tacrine), Aricept (donepezil hydrochloride), and Exelon (rivastigmine tartrate)* |
| **Anesthetics** | Interfere with the conduction of nerve impulses and are used to produce loss of sensation, muscle relaxation, and/or complete loss of consciousness; block nerve transmission in the area to which they are applied. |
| Local | Block nerve transmission in the area to which they are applied. |
| | *Examples: Novocain (procaine HCl), Xylocaine (lidocaine HCl), Marcaine (bupivacaine HCl), Dyclone (dyclonine HCl), and Pontocaine (tetracaine HCl)* |
| General | Affect the central nervous system and produce either partial or complete loss of consciousness. They also produce analgesia, skeletal muscle relaxation, and reduction of reflex activity. |
| | *Examples: Pentothal (thiopental sodium), Fluothane (halothane), Penthrane (methoxyflurane), and nitrous oxide* |

# DIAGNOSTIC AND LAB TESTS

| TEST | DESCRIPTION |
|------|-------------|
| **Cerebral angiography** (sĕr′ ĕ-brăl ăn jĭ-ŏg′ ră-fē) | Process of making an x-ray record of the cerebral arterial system. A radiopaque substance is injected into an artery of the arm or neck, and x-ray films of the head are taken to visualize cerebral aneurysms, tumors, or ruptured blood vessels. |
| **Cerebrospinal fluid (CSF) analysis** (sĕr ĕ-brŏ-spī′ năl floo′ ĭd) | Examination of spinal fluid for color, pressure, pH, and the levels of protein, glucose, and leukocytes. Abnormal results can indicate hemorrhage, tumor, and various disease processes. |
| **Computed tomography (CT)** (kŏm-pū′ tĕd tō-mŏg″ ră-fe) | Diagnostic procedure used to study the structure of the brain. Computerized three-dimensional x-ray images allow the radiologist to differentiate among intracranial tumors, cysts, edema, and hemorrhage. |
| **Echoencephalography** (ĕk ō-ĕn-sĕf′ ă-lŏg′ ră-fē) | Process of using ultrasound to determine the presence of a centrally located mass in the brain. |
| **Electroencephalography (EEG)** (ē-lĕk-trō-ĕn-sĕf′ ă-lŏg′ ră-fē) | Process of measuring the electrical activity of the brain via an electroencephalograph. Abnormal results can indicate epilepsy, brain tumor, infection, abscess, hemorrhage, and/or coma. Also, brain "death" can be determined by an EEG. |
| **Lumbar puncture (LP)** (lŭm′ băr pŭnk′ chūr) | Insertion of a needle into the lumbar subarachnoid space for removal of spinal fluid. The fluid is examined for color, pressure, and the level of protein, chloride, glucose, and leukocytes. See Figure 14–20 ▶. |
| **Myelogram** (mī′ ĕ-lō-grăm) | X-ray of the spinal canal after the injection of a radiopaque dye. Useful in diagnosing spinal lesions, cysts, herniated disks, tumors, and nerve root damage. |
| **Neurologic examination** (nū″ -rō-lōj′ ĭk ĕks-ăm ĭ-nā′ shŭn) | Assessment of a patient's vision, hearing, sense of taste, smell, touch and pain, position, temperature, gait, muscle strength, coordination, and reflex action to determine neurologic status. |
| **Positron emission tomography (PET)** (pŏz′ ĭ-trŏn ē-mĭsh′ ŭn tō-mŏg′ ră-fē) | Computer-based nuclear imaging procedure that can produce three-dimensional pictures of actual organ functioning. Useful in locating brain lesion, identifying blood flow and oxygen metabolism in stroke patients, showing metabolic changes in Alzheimer's disease, and studying biochemical changes associated with mental illness. |
| **Ultrasonography, brain** (ŭl-tră-sŏn-ŏg′ ră-fē) | Use of high-frequency sound waves to record echoes on an oscilloscope and film. Used as screening test or diagnostic tool. |

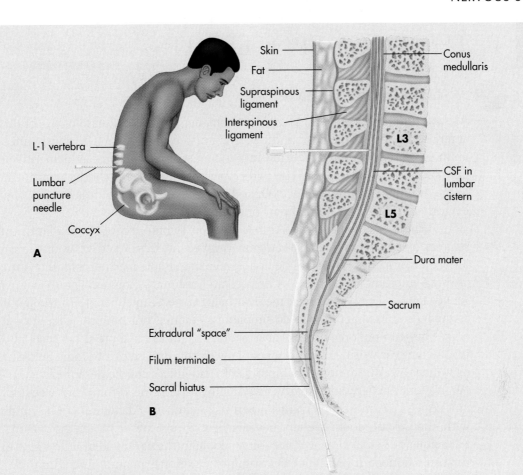

**FIGURE 14–20** (A) Lumbar puncture, also known as *spinal tap*, (B) section of the vertebral column showing the spinal cord and membranes with a lumbar puncture needle at L3–4 and in the sacral hiatus.

# ABBREVIATIONS

| ABBREVIATION | MEANING | ABBREVIATION | MEANING |
|---|---|---|---|
| ACh | acetylcholine | ICP | intracranial pressure |
| AD | Alzheimer's disease | LP | lumbar puncture |
| ALS | amyotrophic lateral sclerosis | mL | milliliter |
| | | MS | multiple sclerosis |
| ANS | autonomic nervous system | Neuro | neurology |
| cm | centimeter | NREM | no rapid eye movement (sleep) |
| CNS | central nervous system | | |
| CP | cerebral palsy | PET | positron emission tomography |
| CSF | cerebrospinal fluid | | |
| CT | computerized tomography | PNS | peripheral nervous system |
| | | REM | rapid eye movement (sleep) |
| CVA | cerebrovascular accident | | |
| DBS | deep brain stimulation | TENS | transcutaneous electrical nerve stimulation |
| EEG | electroencephalogram | | |
| HDS | herniated disk syndrome | TIA | transient ischemic attack |
| HNP | herniated nucleus pulposus | | |

# PATHOLOGY SPOTLIGHTS

 **✻ Alzheimer's Disease**

**Alzheimer's disease** (AD) is a progressive, degenerative disease of the brain that is characterized by loss of memory and other cognitive functions. It seriously affects a person's ability to carry out daily activities. It is the most common cause of dementia among people age 65 or older. AD involves the parts of the brain that control thought, memory, and language. It usually begins after age 60, and risk goes up with age. It is important to note, however, that AD is not a normal part of aging.

Alzheimer's begins slowly. At first, the only symptom could be mild forgetfulness. In this stage, people may have trouble remembering recent events, activities, or the names of familiar people or things. They can be unable to solve simple math problems. As the disease progresses, symptoms are more easily noticed and become serious enough to cause a person with AD or family members to seek medical help. For example, people in the moderate stage of Alzheimer's can forget how to do simple tasks such as brushing their teeth or combing their hair. They can no longer think clearly. They begin to have problems speaking, understanding, reading, or writing. Later on, people with this disease can become anxious or aggressive or wander away from home. Symptoms of Alzhemier's can be described as the 4 A's: Anger, Aggression, Anxiety, and Apathy. Eventually, patients need total care. See Table 14–3.

Age is the most important known risk factor for Alzheimer's. The number of people with the disease doubles every 5 years beyond age 65. To date, no treatment can stop Alzheimer's disease. However, for some people in the early and middle stages of the disease, the drugs donepezil (Aricept), rivastigmine (Exelon), galantamine (Razalyne), or memantine (Namenda) can help prevent some symptoms from becoming worse for a limited time.

**TABLE 14–3  Signs and Symptoms in the Progression of Alzheimer's Disease**

| Mild Alzheimer's | Moderate Alzheimer's | Severe Alzheimer's |
|---|---|---|
| Loses recent memory | Mixes identity of people, such as thinking a son is a brother | Does not recognize self or close family |
| Loses judgment about money | Cannot organize thoughts or follow logical explanations | Speaks in gibberish, is mute or difficult to understand |
| Requires more time to complete routine tasks | Can accuse, curse, fidget, or behave inappropriately—hitting, screaming, biting, or grabbing | Can groan, scream, or mumble loudly |
| Has difficulty with new learning and making new memories | Can be able to read but not to respond to a written request | Can refuse to eat, chokes, or forgets to swallow |
| Has trouble organizing and thinking logically | Loses spark or zest for life; does not initiate new projects | Sleeps more |
| Is occasionally confused about the location of familiar places | Exhibits restlessness, agitation, anxiety, tearfulness, and wandering in the late afternoon or evening (**sundowning**) | Has lack of bladder and bowel control |
| Has decreased attention span | Makes repetitive statements or movements | Has loss of physical coordination |
| Withdraws, loses interest, is irritable, angry when frustrated | Continuously repeats stories, favorite words, statements, or motions (tearing tissues) | Loses weight; skin becomes thin and tears easily |
| Has trouble finding words; substitutes words that sound alike or have a similar meaning | Has loss of impulse control resulting in behavior inappropriate for the situation, inappropriate vulgarity | Needs total assistance for all activities of daily living |

Also, some medicines can help control behavioral symptoms of AD such as sleeplessness, agitation, wandering, anxiety, and depression. Treating these symptoms often makes patients more comfortable and makes their care easier for caregivers.

## ✳ Encephalitis and Meningitis

**Encephalitis** is an inflammation of the brain. There are numerous types of encephalitis, many of which are caused by viral infection. Symptoms include sudden fever, headache, vomiting, photophobia (abnormal visual sensitivity to light), stiff neck and back, confusion, drowsiness, clumsiness, unsteady gait, and irritability. Symptoms that require emergency treatment include loss of consciousness, poor responsiveness, seizures, muscle weakness, sudden severe dementia, memory loss, withdrawal from social interaction, and impaired judgement.

Antiviral medications can be prescribed for herpes encephalitis or other severe viral infections. Antibiotics can be prescribed for bacterial infections. Anticonvulsants are used to prevent or treat seizures. Corticosteroids are used to reduce brain swelling and inflammation. The prognosis for encephalitis varies. Some cases are mild, short, and relatively benign, and patients have full recovery. Other cases are severe, and permanent impairment or death is possible. The acute phase of encephalitis may last for 1 to 2 weeks with gradual or sudden resolution of fever and neurological symptoms. Neurological symptoms can require many months before full recovery.

**Meningitis** is an infection of the membranes (called *meninges*) that surround the brain and spinal cord. Symptoms, which can appear suddenly, often include high fever, severe and persistent headache, stiff neck, nausea, and vomiting. Changes in behavior such as confusion, sleepiness, and difficulty waking up are extremely important symptoms and can require emergency treatment. In infants, symptoms of meningitis can include irritability or tiredness, poor feeding, and fever. Meningitis can be caused by many different viruses and bacteria. Viral meningitis cases are usually self-limited to 10 days or less. Some types of meningitis can be deadly if not treated promptly. Anyone experiencing symptoms of meningitis should see a doctor immediately.

With early diagnosis and prompt treatment, most patients recover from meningitis. Individuals with bacterial meningitis are usually hospitalized for treatment. The child with bacterial meningitis assumes an **opisthotonic** (opisth/o **CF** backward; ton **R** tone/tension; –ic **S** pertaining to) **position,** with the neck and head hyperextended to relieve discomfort. See Figure 14–21 ▼.

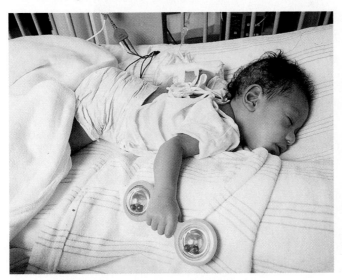

▶ **FIGURE 14–21**   Child with bacterial meningitis assumes an opisthotonic position, with the neck and head hyperextended to relieve discomfort.

## ✳ Epilepsy

**Epilepsy** is a brain disorder involving repeated seizures of any type. Seizures are episodes of disturbed brain function that cause changes in attention and/or behavior. They are caused by abnormal electrical excitation in the brain.

In epilepsy, clusters of nerve cells, or neurons, in the brain sometimes signal abnormally. The normal pattern of neuronal activity becomes disturbed, causing strange sensations, emotions, and behavior or sometimes convulsions, muscle spasms, and loss of consciousness.

Epilepsy is classified as idiopathic or symptomatic in origin, depending upon whether or not the cause of the condition is known. The majority of cases are idiopathic (cause not identified) and symptoms begin during childhood or early adolescence.

The types of seizures experienced by those with epilepsy are classified into four main categories.

1. **Partial seizures** (focal seizures) are those in which electrical disturbances are localized to areas of the brain near the source or focal point of the seizure.

2. **Generalized seizures** (bilateral, symmetrical) are those without local onset that involve both the right and left hemispheres of the brain.

3. **Unilateral seizures** are those in which the electrical discharge is predominately confined to one of the two hemispheres of the brain.

4. **Unclassified seizures** are those that cannot be placed into one of the other three categories because of incomplete data.

With all types of epilepsy, the objective is to obtain the greatest degree of control over the seizures without the patient experiencing intolerable side effects from the prescribed medication. The care of a patient during a seizure is important:

- Protect the patient from nearby hazards by moving hazards away.
- A child who has a seizure while standing should be gently assisted to the floor and placed in a side lying position. See Figure 14–22 ▼.

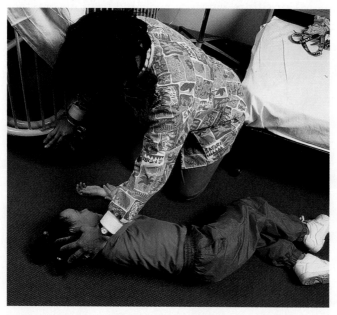

▶ **FIGURE 14–22** Child who has a seizure when standing should be gently assisted to the floor and placed in a side-lying position.

- Do not move the patient or restrain the patient.
- Do not put anything in the patient's mouth.
- Do not try to hold the patient's tongue; it cannot be swallowed.

## ✳ Multiple Sclerosis

**Multiple sclerosis** (MS) is a chronic, potentially debilitating disease that affects the brain and spinal cord (central nervous system). The illness is probably an autoimmune disease, which means that the immune system responds as if part of the body is a foreign substance.

MS causes the body to direct antibodies and white blood cells against proteins in the myelin sheath surrounding nerves in the brain and spinal cord. This causes inflammation and injury to the sheath and ultimately to the nerves. The damage slows or blocks muscle coordination, visual sensation, and other nerve signals.

The disease varies in severity, ranging from a mild illness to one that results in permanent disability. The manifestations of multiple sclerosis vary according to the areas destroyed by demyelination and the affected body system. Symptoms include weakness, paralysis, and/or tremor of one or more extremities; muscle spasticity (uncontrollable spasm of muscle groups); numbness, decreased, or abnormal sensation (in any area); tingling; urinary hesitancy, urgency, and/or frequency. Symptoms vary with each attack. The multisystem effects of MS are shown in Figure 14–23 ▶.

The exact cause of the inflammation associated with MS is unknown. There seems to be a genetic link to the disease; some families are more likely to be affected than others. Certain genetic markers are more common in people with MS than in the general population. An estimated 400,000 Americans have MS. It generally first occurs in people between the ages of 20 and 50. The disease is twice as common in women as in men.

There is no known cure for multiple sclerosis at this time. However, promising therapies could decrease exacerbations and delay progression of the disease. Treatment is aimed at controlling symptoms and maintaining function to give the maximum quality of life.

## ✳ Parkinson's Disease

**Parkinson's disease** is a progressive disorder caused by degeneration of nerve cells in the part of the brain that controls movement. This degeneration creates a shortage of the brain signaling chemical (neurotransmitter) known as *dopamine*, causing the movement impairments that characterize the disease.

Often the first symptom of Parkinson's disease is tremor (trembling or shaking) of a limb, especially when the body is at rest. The tremor often begins on one side of the body, frequently in one hand. Other common symptoms include slow movement (**bradykinesia**), an inability to move (**akinesia**), rigid limbs, a shuffling gait, and a stooped posture. People with Parkinson's disease often show reduced facial expressions and speak in a soft voice. The disease can also cause depression, personality changes, dementia, sleep disturbances, speech impairments, or sexual difficulties. The severity of Parkinson's symptoms tends to worsen over time.

An estimated 500,000 Americans have Parkinson's disease, and 50,000 new cases are reported annually. The disorder appears to be slightly more common in men than women. The average age of onset is about 60. Both prevalence and incidence increase with advancing age; the rates are very low in people under 40 and rise among people in their 70s and 80s.

Parkinson's disease is usually diagnosed by a neurologist who can evaluate symptoms and their severity. Tests, such as a brain scan, can help a physician determine whether a patient has true Parkinson's disease or some other disorder that resembles it.

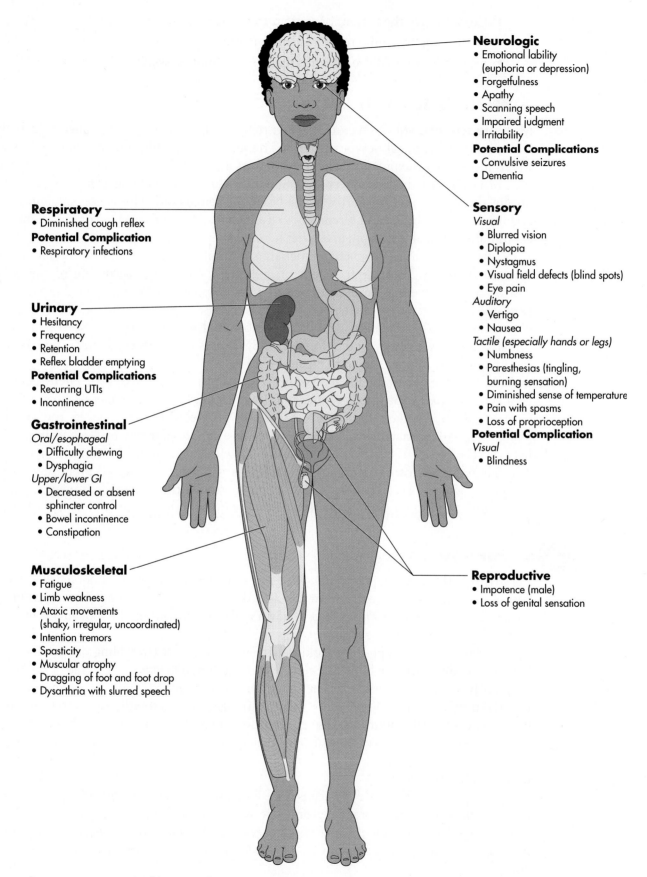

**Neurologic**
- Emotional lability (euphoria or depression)
- Forgetfulness
- Apathy
- Scanning speech
- Impaired judgment
- Irritability

**Potential Complications**
- Convulsive seizures
- Dementia

**Sensory**

*Visual*
- Blurred vision
- Diplopia
- Nystagmus
- Visual field defects (blind spots)
- Eye pain

*Auditory*
- Vertigo
- Nausea

*Tactile (especially hands or legs)*
- Numbness
- Paresthesias (tingling, burning sensation)
- Diminished sense of temperature
- Pain with spasms
- Loss of proprioception

**Potential Complication**
*Visual*
- Blindness

**Respiratory**
- Diminished cough reflex

**Potential Complication**
- Respiratory infections

**Urinary**
- Hesitancy
- Frequency
- Retention
- Reflex bladder emptying

**Potential Complications**
- Recurring UTIs
- Incontinence

**Gastrointestinal**
*Oral/esophageal*
- Difficulty chewing
- Dysphagia

*Upper/lower GI*
- Decreased or absent sphincter control
- Bowel incontinence
- Constipation

**Musculoskeletal**
- Fatigue
- Limb weakness
- Ataxic movements (shaky, irregular, uncoordinated)
- Intention tremors
- Spasticity
- Muscular atrophy
- Dragging of foot and foot drop
- Dysarthria with slurred speech

**Reproductive**
- Impotence (male)
- Loss of genital sensation

▶ **FIGURE 14–23** Multisystem effects of multiple sclerosis.

There is no cure for Parkinson's disease. Treatment involves drug therapy to replenish dopamine levels and/or inhibit the effects of the neurotransmitter acetylcholine. Surgical interventions that can be used to stop uncontrollable movements include **pallidotomy** and **deep brain stimulation** (brain implant).

## ✳ Stroke

A **stroke,** which is also called a *cerebrovascular accident (CVA)*, or *brain attack*, is the death of brain tissue that occurs when the brain does not get enough blood and oxygen. If the flow of blood in an artery supplying the brain is interrupted for longer than a few seconds, brain cells can die, causing permanent damage. The interruption can be caused either by bleeding or blood clots in the brain. See Figure 14–24 ▼.

Stroke is the third leading cause of death in the United States and many other countries and the leading cause of disability in adults. The risk doubles with each decade after age 35. Stroke occurs in men more often than women.

A very common cause of stroke is atherosclerosis. Fatty deposits and blood platelets collect on the wall of the arteries, forming plaques. Over time, the plaques slowly begin to block the flow of blood. The plaque itself can block the artery enough to cause a stroke.

In some cases, the plaque causes the blood to flow abnormally, which leads to a blood clot. A clot can stay at the site of narrowing and prevent blood flow to all of the smaller arteries it supplies. This type of clot, which does not travel, is called a **thrombus.** In other cases, the clot can travel and wedge into a smaller vessel. A clot that travels is called an **embolism** (see Figure 14–25 ▶). Strokes caused by embolisms are most commonly caused by heart disorders.

A second major cause of stroke is bleeding in the brain (hemorrhagic stroke). This can occur when small blood vessels in the brain become weak and burst. Some people have defects in the blood vessels of the brain that makes this more likely. The flow of blood after the break damages brain cells. This type of stroke can also occur if a clot caused by atherosclerosis or other conditions blocks a vessel, which then breaks and damages surrounding tissue.

The following sudden symptoms are the warning signs of stroke:

- Numbness or weakness of face, arm, or leg, especially on one side of the body.
- Confusion; trouble speaking or understanding.
- Trouble seeing in one or both eyes.
- Trouble walking, dizziness, loss of balance or coordination.
- Severe headache with no known cause.

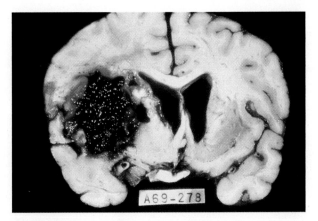

▶ **FIGURE 14–24** Cross-section of brain showing cerebrovascular accident.

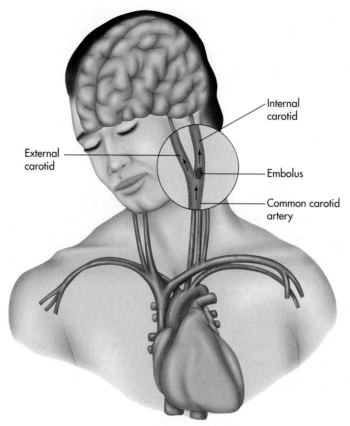

▶ **FIGURE 14–25** Embolus traveling to the brain.

A *transient ischemic attack* (TIA) is a temporary interference in the blood supply to the brain. It sometimes is referred to as a *ministroke,* and symptoms can last for a few minutes or several hours. After the attack, there is usually no evidence of residual brain damage or neurological damage. The specific signs and symptoms depend on the portion of the brain affected. Disturbance of normal vision in one or both eyes, dizziness, weakness, dysphasia, numbness, or unconsciousness can occur.

# ✔PATHOLOGY CHECKPOINT

*Following is a concise list of the pathology-related terms that you have seen in the chapter. Review this checklist to make sure that you are familiar with the meaning of each term before moving to the next section.*

## Conditions and Symptoms

- ❏ akathesia
- ❏ akinesia
- ❏ Alzheimer's disease
- ❏ amnesia
- ❏ amyotrophic lateral sclerosis
- ❏ anencephaly
- ❏ aphagia
- ❏ aphasia
- ❏ apraxia
- ❏ asthenia
- ❏ astrocytoma
- ❏ ataxia
- ❏ Bell's palsy
- ❏ bradykinesia
- ❏ brain attack
- ❏ cephalalgia
- ❏ cerebral palsy
- ❏ cerebrovascular accident
- ❏ chorea
- ❏ coma
- ❏ concussion (brain)
- ❏ dementia
- ❏ dyslexia
- ❏ dysphasia
- ❏ encephalitis
- ❏ encephalopathy
- ❏ epilepsy
- ❏ glioma
- ❏ hemiparesis
- ❏ hemiplegia
- ❏ herniated disk syndrome

- ❏ herpes zoster
- ❏ hydrocephalus
- ❏ hyperesthesia
- ❏ hyperkinesis
- ❏ meningioma
- ❏ meningitis
- ❏ meningocele
- ❏ meningomyelocele
- ❏ microcephalus
- ❏ multiple sclerosis
- ❏ myelitis
- ❏ narcolepsy
- ❏ neuralgia
- ❏ neurasthenia
- ❏ neuritis
- ❏ neuroblastoma
- ❏ neurofibroma
- ❏ neuroma
- ❏ neuropathy
- ❏ oligodendroglioma
- ❏ palsy
- ❏ papilledema
- ❏ paraplegia
- ❏ paresis
- ❏ paresthesia
- ❏ Parkinson's disease
- ❏ paroxysm
- ❏ pheochromocytoma
- ❏ poliomyelitis
- ❏ polyneuritis
- ❏ quadriplegia
- ❏ Reye's syndrome

- ❏ sciatica
- ❏ somnambulism
- ❏ spondylosyndesis
- ❏ stroke
- ❏ syncope
- ❏ Tay-Sachs disease
- ❏ transient ischemic attack

## Diagnosis and Treatment

- ❏ analgesia
- ❏ anesthesia
- ❏ craniectomy
- ❏ craniotomy
- ❏ deep brain stimulation
- ❏ diskectomy
- ❏ electroencephalograph
- ❏ electromyography
- ❏ epiduroscopy
- ❏ ganglionectomy
- ❏ hypnosis
- ❏ laminectomy
- ❏ lobotomy
- ❏ myelography
- ❏ neurectomy
- ❏ pallidotomy
- ❏ sympathectomy
- ❏ transcutaneous electrical nerve stimulations
- ❏ vagotomy
- ❏ ventriculometry

# STUDY AND REVIEW

## Anatomy and Physiology

*Write your answers to the following questions. Do not refer to the text.*

1. Name the two interconnected divisions of the nervous system.

   a. _____     b. _____

2. _____ are the structural and functional units of the nervous system.

3. State the three actions of motor neurons.

   a. _____     b. _____

   c. _____

4. Describe an axon. _____

5. Describe a dendrite. _____

6. State an action of sensory neurons. _____

7. _____ function to mediate impulses between sensory and motor neurons.

8. Define the following terms:

   a. *Nerve fiber* _____

   b. *Nerve* _____

   c. *Tracts* _____

9. The central nervous system consists of the _____ and the

   _____ _____.

10. State three functions of the central nervous system.

    a. _____     b. _____

    c. _____

11. Name the three meninges enclosing the brain.

    a. _____     b. _____

    c. _____

12. Name the seven major divisions of the brain.

    a. _____        b. _____

    c. _____        d. _____

    e. _____        f. _____

    g. _____

13. The _____ _____ has been identified as the brain's major motor area.

14. The parietal lobe is also known as the _____ _____

15. The temporal lobe contains centers for _____ and

    _____ input.

16. The occipital lobe is the primary area for _____.

17. State the functions of the thalamus.

    a. _____        b. _____

18. State three functions of the hypothalamus.

    a. _____        b. _____

    c. _____

19. The cerebellum plays an important role in the integration of _____

    and _____.

20. State five functions of the medulla oblongata.

    a. _____        b. _____

    c. _____        d. _____

    e. _____

21. State the three functions of the spinal cord.

    a. _____        b. _____

    c. _____

22. The normal adult has between _____ and _____
    mL of cerebrospinal fluid in circulation.

23. Name the 12 pairs of cranial nerves.

    a. _____        b. _____

    c. _____        d. _____

    e. _____        f. _____

    g. _____        h. _____

    i. _____        j. _____

    k. _____        l. _____

24. State four functions of the autonomic nervous system.

    a. _____    b. _____

    c. _____    d. _____

25. Name the two divisions of the autonomic nervous system.

    a. _____    b. _____

## Word Parts

1. In the spaces provided, write the definitions of these prefixes, roots, combining forms, and suffixes. Do not refer to the listings of medical words. Leave blank those words you cannot define.

2. After completing as many as you can, refer to the medical word listings to check your work. For each word missed or left blank, write the word and its definition several times on the margins of these pages or on a separate sheet of paper.

3. To maximize the learning process, it is to your advantage to do the following exercises as directed. To refer to the word-building section before completing these exercises invalidates the learning process.

## PREFIXES

*Give the definitions of the following prefixes.*

1. a- _____    2. an- _____

3. astro- _____    4. brady- _____

5. de- _____    6. dys- _____

7. epi- _____    8. hemi- _____

9. hydro- _____    10. hyper- _____

11. intra- _____    12. micro- _____

13. oligo- _____    14. par- _____

15. para- _____    16. poly- _____

17. quadri- _____    18. sub- _____

## ROOTS AND COMBINING FORMS

*Give the definitions of the following roots and combining forms.*

1. ambul _____

2. dur/o _____

3. cephal _____

4. later _____

5. cerebell _____

6. cerebr/o _____

7. chrom/o _____

8. concuss _____

9. cran/i _____

10. crani/o _____

11. cyt _____

12. dendr/o _____

13. disk _____

14. dur _____

15. electr/o _____

16. encephal _____

17. encephal/o _____

18. esthesi/o _____

19. narc/o _____

20. ganglion _____

21. gli _____

22. hypn _____

23. pallid/o _____

24. lamin _____

25. lob/o _____

26. log _____

27. mening _____

28. mening/i _____

29. mening/o _____

30. ment _____

31. mnes _____

32. myel _____

33. myel/o _____

34. my/o _____

35. neur _____

36. neur/i _____

37. neur/o _____

38. papill _____

39. phe/o _____

40. poli/o _____

41. scler _____

42. spin _____

43. spondyl/o _____

44. somn _____

45. sympath _____

46. vag/o _____

47. ventricul/o _____

## SUFFIXES

*Give the definitions of the following suffixes.*

1. -al _____

2. -algesia _____

3. -algia _____

4. -ar _____

5. -asthenia _____

6. -blast _____

7. -cele _____

8. -cyte _____

9. -desis _____

10. -ectomy _____

11. -edema _____

12. -esthesia _____

13. -glia _____

14. -gram _____

15. -graph _____

16. -graphy _____

17. -ia _____

18. -ic _____

19. -ion _____

20. -ism _____

21. -ist _____

22. -itis _____

23. -kinesia _____

24. -kinesis _____

25. -lepsy _____

26. -lemma _____

27. -lexia _____

28. -logy _____

29. -troph(y) _____

30. -metry _____

31. -scopy _____

32. -oma _____

33. -osis _____

34. -paresis _____

35. -pathy _____

36. -phagia _____

37. -phasia _____

38. -praxia _____

39. -sthenia _____

40. -taxia _____

41. -tomy _____

42. -us _____

43. -y _____

## Identifying Medical Terms

*In the spaces provided, write the medical terms for the following meanings.*

1. _____ Condition in which there is a loss or lack of memory

2. _____ Lack of the sense of pain

3. _____ Loss or lack of the ability to eat or swallow

4. _____ Loss or lack of muscular coordination

5. _____ Head pain; headache

6. _____ Pertaining to the cerebellum

7. _____ Surgical excision of a portion of the skull

8. _____ Condition in which an individual has difficulty in comprehending written language

9. _____ Inflammation of the brain

10. _____ Pertaining to, situated on the dura mater

11. _____ Paralysis that affects one side of the body

12. _____ Inflammation of the meninges of the spinal cord or brain

13. _____ Pain in a nerve or nerves

14. _____ Inflammation of a nerve

15. _____ Nerve cell, neuron

16. _____ Study of the nervous system

17. _____ Tumor of nerve cells and nerve fibers

18. _____ Loss of sensation or an impairment of motor function

19. _____ Inflammation of many nerves

20. _____ Condition of sleepwalking

21. _____ Surgical incision of the vagus nerve

22. _____ Measurement of intracranial pressure

## Spelling

*In the spaces provided, write the correct spelling of these misspelled words.*

1. anestesia _____

2. bradkinesia _____

3. cerebospinal _____

4. cranitomy _____

5. epilepisy _____

6. meningoma _____

7. meningmyelcele _____

8. neurpathy _____

9. polomyelitis _____

10. ventriulometry _____

## Matching

*Select the appropriate lettered meaning for each of the following words.*

_____ 1. acetylcholine

_____ 2. Alzheimer's disease

_____ 3. stroke

_____ 4. endorphins

_____ 5. epilepsy

_____ 6. palsy

_____ 7. percutaneous diskectomy

_____ 8. epiduroscopy

_____ 9. dementia

_____ 10. sciatica

a. Group of symptoms marked by memory loss and other cognitive functions

b. Chemical substances produced in the brain that act as natural analgesics

c. Cerebrovascular accident

d. Severe form of senile dementia

e. Disorder of cerebral function resulting from abnormal electrical activity or malfunctioning of the chemical substances of the brain

f. Used for back pain relief

g. Cholinergic neurotransmitter that occurs in various tissues and organs of the body

h. Loss of sensation or an impairment of motor function

i. Severe pain along the course of the sciatic nerve

j. Surgical procedure that can be done on an outpatient basis for slipped disk

k. Anxiety syndrome and panic disorder

## Abbreviations

*Place the correct word, phrase, or abbreviation in the space provided.*

1. Alzheimer's disease _____

2. amyotrophic lateral sclerosis _____

3. CNS _____

4. CP _____

5. computerized tomography _____

6. herniated disk syndrome _____

7. ICP _____

8. LP _____

9. MS _____

10. positron emission tomography _____

## Diagnostic and Laboratory Tests

*Select the best answer to each multiple choice question. Circle the letter of your choice.*

1. Diagnostic procedure used to study the structure of the brain.
   a. computed tomography
   b. echoencephalography
   c. electroencephalography
   d. myelogram

2. Process of using ultrasound to determine the presence of a centrally located mass in the brain.
   a. computed tomography
   b. echoencephalography
   c. electroencephalography
   d. myelogram

3. X-ray of the spinal canal after the injection of a radiopaque dye.
   a. cerebral angiography
   b. computed tomography
   c. myelogram
   d. ultrasonography

4. Computer-based nuclear imaging procedure that can produce three-dimensional pictures of actual organ functioning.
   a. electroencephalography
   b. myelogram
   c. ultrasonography
   d. positron emission tomography

5. Use of high-frequency sound waves to record echoes on an oscilloscope and film.
   a. electroencephalography
   b. myelogram
   c. ultrasonography
   d. positron emission tomography

# PRACTICAL APPLICATION

## S O A P : Chart Note Analysis

*This exercise will make you aware of information, abbreviations, and medical terminology typically found in a neurology practice patient's chart.*

### Abbreviations Key

| | | | | |
|---|---|---|---|---|
| **Abd** | abdomen | | **NKDA** | no known drug allergies |
| **BP** | blood pressure | | **P** | pulse |
| **CT** | computed tomography | | **PERRLA** | pupils equal, round, react to light and accommodation |
| **CTA** | clear to auscultation | | | |
| **DOB** | date of birth | | **PIP** | proximal interphalangeal |
| **EEG** | electroencephalogram | | **R** | respiration |
| **EOM** | extraocular movement | | **ROM** | range of motion |
| **F** | Fahrenheit | | **SOAP** | subjective, objective, assessment, plan |
| **HEENT** | head, eyes, ears, nose, throat | | | |
| **Ht** | height | | **T** | temperature |
| **lb** | pound | | **TM** | tympanic membrane |
| **MMSE** | Mini Mental State Examination | | **Wt** | weight |
| **MS** | musculoskeletal | | **y/o** | year(s) old |
| **Neuro** | neurology | | | |

*Read the following chart note and then answer the questions that follow.*

**PATIENT:** Brown, Sadie E.                                                  **DATE:** 9/17/07

**DOB:** 8/09/29    **AGE:** 78    **SEX:** Female

**INSURANCE:** Reliant Healthcare

**Vital Signs:**
   T: 98.4F
   P: 72
   R: 20
   BP: 136/86
   Ht: 5′ 5″
   Wt: 154 lb

**Allergies:** NKDA

**Chief Complaint:** Confusion, memory loss, and inappropriate actions

**S**  **Subjective:** Husband of 78 y/o white female explains that he is very concerned about his wife. He states that he has noticed "she is becoming confused and forgets where she puts things. Last Monday, she put the iron in the freezer." The patient had very little to say about herself during this appointment.

**O**  **Objective:**

**General Appearance:** Anxious and somewhat distracted. No apparent physical distress.

**HEENT:** Normocephalic. TM pearly gray, landmarks intact. Nasal mucosa pink, no exudate. Uvula midline, gag reflex intact.

**Heart:** Regular rate and rhythm. No murmurs or rubs.

**Lungs:** CTA

**Abd:** Bowel sounds all 4 quadrants. No tenderness or masses noted.

**MS:** Bouchard's nodes bilaterally involving the PIP joints of first and second fingers of right hand. No heat or swelling. Full ROM without tenderness. Muscle strength—able to maintain flexion against resistance and without tenderness.

**Neuro: Cranial Nerves**

| | |
|---|---|
| I | Identifies an orange and coffee. |
| II | Vision corrected to 20/20 with glasses, peripheral fields intact, fundi normal. |
| III, IV, VI | EOM intact, no ptosis or nystagmus, PERRLA. |
| V | Sensation intact and equal bilaterally, jaw strength equal bilaterally. |
| VII | Facial symmetry, muscles intact. |
| VIII | Hearing intact. |
| IX, X | Swallowing intact, gag reflex present, uvula rises midline on phonation. |
| XI | Shoulder shrug, head movement equal bilaterally |
| XII | Tongue protrudes midline, no tremors |

**Sensory:** Slightly diminished vibratory sensation at the ankle, bilaterally.

**MMSE score:** 19 (missing at least 1 in each category). Noted difficulty with orientation to place and time, recent memory, word recall, and attention span.

**Skin:** Cool to touch and dry. Small, flat, brown macules noted on forearms and dorsa of the hands.

**A** **Assessment:** Dementia of the Alzheimer's type

**P** **Plan:** After completing a physical examination, a medical history, neurology test, EEG, mental status and cognitive function examination, and receiving the results from a CT scan, the diagnosis was confirmed.

1. The patient was placed on Aricept 5 mg at bedtime for 4 to 6 weeks, then to increase to 10 mg per day at bedtime.
2. Explain that Aricept is a cholinesterase inhibitor and that about 50% of patients who take the medication as prescribed should experience modest improvement in cognitive symptoms.
3. Advise the husband that it is very important to obtain information about Alzheimer's and support that is available for patients and caregivers. Provide the time and location of the Alzheimer's support group's next meeting. For more information on Alzheimer's, he can contact the Alzheimer's Association at 1-800-272-3900 or access www.alz.com.
4. Patient is to return in four weeks for a follow-up visit.

**FYI:** The MMSE is a test that consists of 11 questions that cover five cognitive areas: orientation, registration (ability to recognize and name specific items), attention, recall, and language. It is relatively easy to administer and takes only 5 to 10 minutes. It is a good screening tool used for diagnosis in the mild, moderate, and severe stages of Alzheimer's disease. Maximum score is 30, normal averages 27. Scores below 20 occur with dementia.

(*Note:* Bouchard's nodes are bony enlargements located at the proximal interphalangeal joints that result from osteoarthritis.)

## Chart Note Questions
*Place the correct answer in the space provided.*

1. Signs and symptoms of Alzheimer's disease include confusion, _____ loss, and apparent inappropriate behavior.

2. Bouchard's nodes indicate what condition? _____

3. Which cranial nerve is involved with the identification of an orange and coffee? _____

4. One test used to assist in diagnosing Alzheimer's disease is an EEG, which is the abbreviation for _____

5. Why was a CT scan performed? _____

6. Aricept is classified as a(n) _____

7. The MMSE concentrates on _____ functioning, not on mood.

8. What does the abbreviation NKDA mean? _____

9. Which cranial nerve is involved with being able to shrug the shoulder and move the head bilaterally? _____

10. Of the Alzheimer's patients who take a cholinesterase inhibitor, _____% experience a modest improvement in cognitive symptoms.

# MULTIMEDIA PREVIEW

*Additional interactive resources and activities for this chapter can be found on the Companion Website. For videos, audio glossary, and review, access the accompanying CD-ROM in this book.*

 **CD-ROM HIGHLIGHTS**

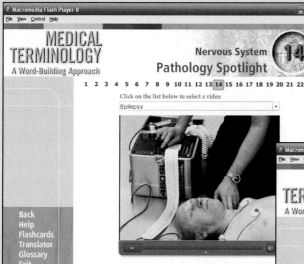

## PATHOLOGY SPOTLIGHT—EPILEPSY

By viewing concepts in moving, living color, you'll get a fuller picture of the pathologies presented in this chapter. Earlier we discussed epilepsy. Now click on this feature to watch a video that describes this condition in more detail.

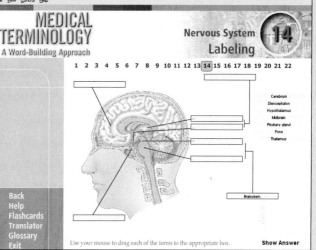

## LABELING EXERCISE

A picture is worth a thousand words . . . only if it's labeled correctly. To review anatomy, click and drag the terms that correlate to a figure from this chapter. All correct labels will lock into place beside the picture.

 **WEBSITE HIGHLIGHTS—www.prenhall.com/rice**

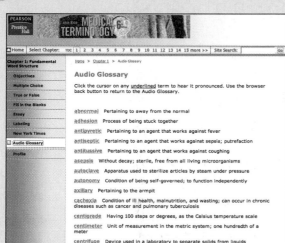

## AUDIO GLOSSARY

Click here and take advantage of the free-access on-line study guide that accompanies your textbook. You'll find an audio glossary with definitions and audio pronunciations for every term in the book. By clicking on this URL you'll also access a variety of quizzes with instant feedback, links to download mp3 audio reviews, and current news articles.

# Special Senses: The Ear

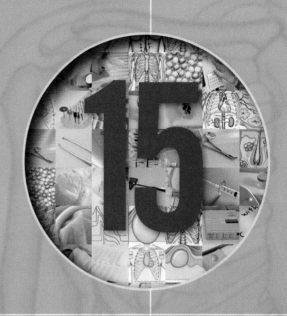

**15**

## ■ OUTLINE

## ■ OBJECTIVES

*On completion of this chapter, you will be able to:*

- Describe the anatomical structures of the ear.
- Describe the external ear.
- Describe the middle ear.
- Describe the inner ear.
- Analyze, build, spell, and pronounce medical words.
- Comprehend the drugs highlighted in this chapter.
- Describe diagnostic and laboratory tests related to the ear.
- Identify and define selected abbreviations.
- Describe each of the conditions presented in the Pathology Spotlights.
- Review the Pathology Checkpoint.
- Complete the Study and Review section and the Chart Note Analysis.

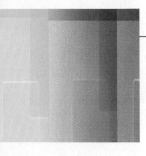

# Anatomy and Physiology Overview

The **ear** is the site of **hearing** and **equilibrium.** It contains specially designed anatomical structures that receive sound vibrations, are sensitive to the force of gravity, and react to the movements of the head. These anatomical structures are connected to sensory areas of the brain by specialized fibers from the eighth cranial nerve. The ear is generally described as having three distinct divisions: the external ear, the middle ear, and the inner ear. The following is a listing of the major components of the ear and some of their functions.

## Special Senses: The Ear

| Organ/Structure | Primary Functions |
|---|---|
| **External ear** | |
| *Auricle (pinna)* | Collects and directs sound waves into the auditory canal and then into the tympanic membrane |
| *External acoustic meatus (auditory canal)* | Numerous glands line the canal and secrete earwax to lubricate and protect the ear |
| *Tympanic membrane (eardrum)* | Separates the external ear from the middle ear |
| **Middle Ear** | |
| *Contains the ossicles: malleus, incus, and stapes; has several openings; is lined with mucous membrane* | Transmits sound vibrations |
| | Equalizes external/internal air pressure on the tympanic membrane |
| | Exerts control over potentially damaging or disruptive loud sounds |
| **Inner Ear** | |
| *Cochlea* | Contains the organ of Corti, the organ of hearing |
| *Vestibule* | Contains the utricle and saccule, membranous pouches containing perilymph. The utricle communicates with the semicircular canals and contains hair cell sensory receptors connected to fibers from the eighth cranial nerve. These hair cells react to the force of gravity and movement of **otoliths,** and are a part of the sense of equilibrium. |
| *Semicircular canals* | Contain nerve endings in the form of hair cells that note changes in the position of the head and reports such movement to the brain through fibers leading to the eighth cranial nerve |

## EXTERNAL EAR

The **external ear** is the appendage on the side of the head consisting of the *auricle* or *pinna,* the *external acoustic meatus* or *auditory canal,* and the *tympanic membrane* or *eardrum.* The auricle collects sound waves that then pass through the auditory canal to vibrate the tympanic membrane that separates the external ear from the middle ear. The auditory canal is an S-shaped tubular structure about 2.5 cm long. Numerous glands line the canal and secrete **cerumen** or **earwax** to lubricate and protect the ear (see Figure 15–1 ▶).

## MIDDLE EAR

Beyond the tympanic membrane is a tiny cavity in the temporal bone of the skull called the **middle ear.** This cavity contains three small bones or **ossicles** instrumental to the hearing process. These ossicles are the **malleus, incus,** and **stapes.** Sometimes referred to

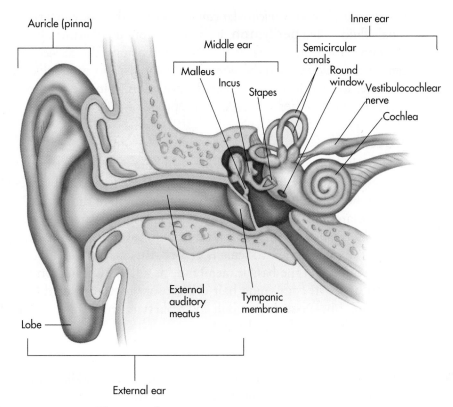

**Auricle (pinna)**

**Middle ear**

**Inner ear**

**Malleus**

**Incus**

**Stapes**

**Semicircular canals**

**Round window**

**Vestibulocochlear nerve**

**Cochlea**

**External auditory meatus**

**Tympanic membrane**

**Lobe**

**External ear**

▶ **FIGURE 15–1** The ear and its anatomic structures.

as the **hammer, anvil,** and **stirrup** because of their shapes, these bones mechanically transmit sound vibrations from the tympanic membrane, to which the malleus is attached, through the incus to the stapes, which attaches to a thin membrane covering a small opening, the oval window, that marks the beginning of the inner ear. During transmission, tympanic vibrations can be amplified as much as 22 times their original force.

The cavity of the middle ear has several openings, one that is covered by the tympanic membrane, another opening to the auditory or eustachian tube, a third opening to the mastoid cells, and two openings to the inner ear, the oval and round windows (see Figure 15–1). The cavity is lined by mucous membrane that is continuous with that found in the mastoid air cells, the eustachian tube, and the throat. The spread of infection from the throat along this membrane to the middle ear is called **otitis media** (OM). The continued spread of infection to one of the mastoid bones is called **mastoiditis.**

Three functions have been attributed to the middle ear:

- Transmits sound vibrations.
- Equalizes external/internal air pressure on the tympanic membrane.
- Exerts control over potentially damaging or disruptive loud sounds through reflex contractions of the stapedius and tensor tympani muscles, which are attached to the stapes and the malleus, respectively.

# INNER EAR

The **inner ear** consists of a membranous labyrinth or mazelike network of canals located within a bony labyrinth. These structures are called **labyrinths** because of their complicated shapes. The bony labyrinth, located in the temporal bone, consists of the *cochlea,* *vestibule,* and three *semicircular canals.* Within the bony labyrinth but separated from it by a pale fluid called **perilymph,** is the membranous labyrinth. It has much the same shape as the bony labyrinth and has three distinct divisions: the *cochlear duct* inside the cochlea, the *semicircular ducts* within the semicircular canals, and two saclike structures, the **utricle** and **saccule,** located in the vestibule. Nerve endings in the form of hair cells located in various parts of the inner ear serve as receptors for the senses of *hearing* and *equilibrium.*

## Cochlea

The **cochlea** is a spiral-shaped bony structure containing the cochlear duct; it is so named because it resembles a snail shell. The spiral cavity of the bony cochlea is partitioned into three tubelike channels that run the entire length of the spiral. Two membranes form these tubelike areas. The *basilar membrane* forms the lower channel or *scala tympani,* and the *vestibular membrane (Reissner's membrane)* forms the upper channel, which is called the *scala vestibuli.* Between the two scala is a space, the *cochlear duct,* formed by the vestibular membrane on top and the basilar membrane as a floor. Located on the basilar membrane is the **organ of Corti** containing hair cell sensory receptors for the sense of hearing. The fluid perilymph fills the scala vestibuli and scala tympani. A different fluid, **endolymph,** fills the cochlear duct (see Figure 15–2 ▼).

### Hearing Process in the Inner Ear

The scala vestibuli and scala tympani open to the middle ear through the oval and round windows, respectively. The stapes fits into the round window and causes vibration of the perilymph, which, in turn, vibrates the basilar membrane and endolymph of the cochlear duct, thereby exciting the nerve endings contained on the **organ of Corti.** These nerve endings transmit the sounds, via the *eighth cranial nerve,* to the auditory areas of the brain. The sound waves, having excited the fluid of the cochlear duct, then pass on to the perilymph of the scala tympani and are dissipated against the membrane covering the round window. The path of sound vibrations is shown in Figure 15–3 ▶. Sound travels in waves

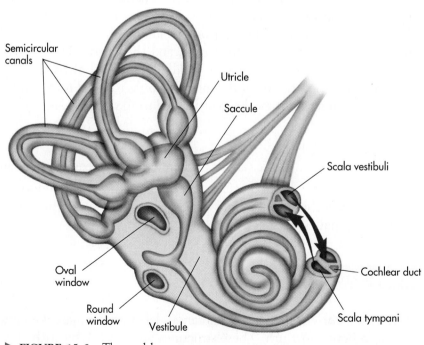

▶ **FIGURE 15–2** The cochlea.

Path of sound vibrations

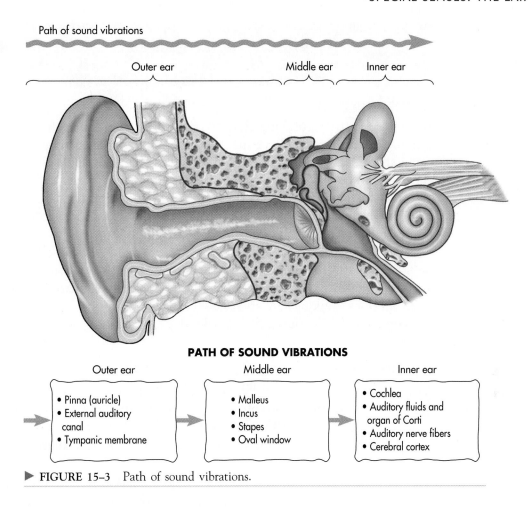

Outer ear          Middle ear    Inner ear

**PATH OF SOUND VIBRATIONS**

Outer ear

- Pinna (auricle)
- External auditory canal
- Tympanic membrane

Middle ear

- Malleus
- Incus
- Stapes
- Oval window

Inner ear

- Cochlea
- Auditory fluids and organ of Corti
- Auditory nerve fibers
- Cerebral cortex

▶ **FIGURE 15–3**   Path of sound vibrations.

from the outer ear, through the middle ear, and into the cochlea of the inner ear. These waves are transmitted by nerve fibers to the auditory region of the brain where sensations of sound are perceived within the cerebral cortex.

## Vestibule

The **vestibule** is a bony structure located between the cochlea and the three semicircular canals. The bony vestibule contains the **utricle** and **saccule,** membranous pouches containing perilymph. The utricle communicates with the semicircular canals and contains hair cell sensory receptors connected to fibers from the eighth cranial nerve. These hair cells react to the forces of gravity and movement of otoliths and are a part of the sense of *equilibrium*.

## Semicircular Canals

Located at right angles to each other are the superior, posterior, and inferior **semicircular canals.** Within the bony canals are the membranous semicircular ducts containing endolymph. At the base of each canal is an enlargement called an **ampulla** containing nerve endings in the form of hair cells. Changes in the position of the head cause the fluid in the canals to move against these sensory receptors, which, in turn, report such movement to the brain through fibers leading to the eighth cranial nerve. *Dizziness* and motion sickness are associated with rapid or erratic movement and the resulting sensory sensation in these areas.

# LIFE SPAN CONSIDERATIONS

## ■ THE CHILD

At 36 weeks, the identifying characteristics of the fetus are soft ear lobes, few creases on the soles of the foot, ample vernix caseosa, and diminishing lanugo. At 40 weeks, there are firm **ear lobes.** In newborns, the wall of the ear canal is pliable because of underdeveloped cartilage and bone. The **eustachian tube** in infants is shorter and straighter than in older children and adults. Because of this, an infant or young child is more predisposed to developing an ear infection. When this occurs, the child's ears should be examined very carefully. See Figure 15–4 ▼.

Babies respond to "mother-ese" and "parent-ese," whose melodic sounds actually provide a tutorial in the sounds that make up language. It is recommended that parents sing and talk to even the youngest infants because verbal stimulation is crucial to how well a child develops thinking and language skills later. According to Dr. William Staso, an expert in neurologic development, different kinds of stimulation should be emphasized at different ages.

| | |
|---|---|
| First Month | Low level of stimulation reduces stress and increases the infant's wakefulness and alertness. |
| 1 to 3 Months | Brain starts to discriminate among acoustic patterns of language such as intonation and pitch. |
| 3 to 5 Months | Infants rely primarily on vision to acquire information about the world. |
| 6 to 7 Months | Infants become alert to relationships such as cause and effect, the location of objects, and the function of objects. |
| 7 to 8 Months | Brain is oriented to make association between sound and some meaningful activity or object. |
| 9 to 12 Months | Learning adds up to a new level of awareness of the environment and increased interest in exploration; sensory and motor skills coordinate in a more mature fashion. |

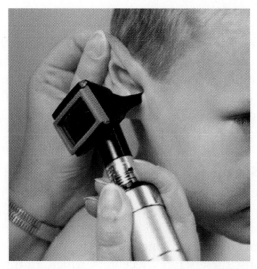

▶ **FIGURE 15–4**    To straighten the auditory canal, the pinna should be pulled back and up for children over 3 years; the pinna should be pulled down and back for children under 3 years of age.

## ■ THE OLDER ADULT

With aging, changes occur in the external, middle, and inner ear. The skin of the **auricle** can become dry and wrinkled. Production of cerumen declines and is drier. There is also dryness of the external canal, which causes itching. Hairs in the external canal become coarser and longer, especially in males. The eardrum thickens, and the bony joints in the middle ear degenerate.

Changes in the inner ear affect sensitivity to sound, understanding of speech, and balance. Degenerative changes include atrophy of the cochlea, the cochlear nerve cells, and the organ of Corti. These changes lead to the hearing loss, **presbycusis,** which is common in the older adult. Noisy surroundings make it difficult for older adults to discriminate between sounds, thereby impairing communication and socialization. The hearing distance (HD) of older adults can also be impaired.

# BUILDING YOUR MEDICAL VOCABULARY

This section provides the foundation for learning medical terminology. Review the following alphabetized word list. Note how common prefixes and suffixes are repeatedly applied to word roots and combining forms to create different meanings.

| | |
|---|---|
| P | Prefix |
| R | Root |
| CF | Combining form |
| S | Suffix |

| | |
|---|---|
| Pink words | Terms not built from word parts. |
| * | Indicates words covered in the Pathology Spotlights section. |
| 💿 | Check the CD-ROM for more information. |

| MEDICAL WORD | WORD PARTS (WHEN APPLICABLE) | | | DEFINITION |
|---|---|---|---|---|
| | **Part** | **Type** | **Meaning** | |
| **acoustic** (ă-koos′ tĭk) | acoust -ic | R S | hearing pertaining to | Pertaining to the sense of hearing |
| **audiogram** (ŏ′ dĭ-ō-grăm″) | audi/o -gram | CF S | to hear a mark, record | Record of hearing by audiometry |
| **audiologist** (ŏ″ dĭ-ŏl′ ō-jĭst) | audi/o log -ist | CF R S | to hear study of one who specializes | One who specializes in disorders of hearing |
| **audiology** (ŏ″ dĭ-ŏl′ ō-jĭ) | audi/o -logy | CF S | to hear study of | Study of hearing disorders |
| **audiometer** (ŏ dĭ-ŏm′ ĕ-tĕr) | audi/o -meter | CF S | to hear instrument to measure | Instrument used to measure hearing |

| MEDICAL WORD | WORD PARTS (WHEN APPLICABLE) | | | DEFINITION |
|---|---|---|---|---|
| | **Part** | **Type** | **Meaning** | |
| **audiometry**<br>(ŏ″ dĭ-ŏm′ ĕ-trē) | audi/o<br>-metry | CF<br>S | to hear<br>measurement | Measurement of the hearing sense |
| **audiphone**<br>(ŏ′ dĭ-fōn) | aud/i<br>phone | CF<br>R | to hear<br>voice | Instrument that conveys sound to the auditory nerve through teeth or bone |
| **auditory**<br>(ŏ′ dĭ-tō″ rē) | auditor<br>-y | R<br>S | hearing<br>pertaining to | Pertaining to the sense of hearing |
| **aural**<br>(ŏ′ răl) | aur<br>-al | R<br>S | the ear<br>pertaining to | Pertaining to the ear |
| **auricle**<br>(ŏ′ rĭ-kl) | aur/i<br>-cle | CF<br>S | ear<br>small | External portion of the ear, known as the *flap of the ear;* the *pinna* (pin′ na) |
| **binaural**<br>(bīn-aw′ răl) | bin<br>aur<br>-al | P<br>R<br>S | twice<br>ear<br>pertaining to | Pertaining to both ears |
| **cerumen**<br>(sē-roo′ měn) | | | | Earwax, the yellowish substance secreted by the glands in the canal of the external ear |
| **cholesteatoma**<br>(kō″ lē-stē″ ă-tō′ mă) | chol/e<br>steat<br>-oma | CF<br>R<br>S | gall or bile<br>fat<br>tumor | Tumorlike mass filled with epithelial cells and cholesterol |
| **cochlea**<br>(kŏk′ lē-ă) | | | | Portion of the inner ear shaped like a snail shell; contains the organ of hearing referred to as *the organ of Corti* |
| **deafness** | | | | Complete or partial loss of the ability to hear. *Hearing impairment* is often used to describe a minimal loss of hearing as compared to the use of the word *deafness* when there is complete or extensive loss of hearing. See Figure 15–5 ▶. ✱ See Pathology Spotlight: Hearing Loss on page 514. |
| **ear** | | | | Organ of hearing and equilibrium |
| **electrocochleography**<br>(ē-lěk″ trō-kŏk″ lē-ŏg′ ră-fē) | electr/o<br>cochle/o<br>-graphy | CF<br>CF<br>S | electricity<br>land snail<br>recording | Recording of the electrical activity produced when the cochlea is stimulated |
| **endaural**<br>(ěn′ dŏ″ răl) | end-<br>aur<br>-al | P<br>R<br>S | within<br>ear<br>pertaining to | Pertaining to within the ear |
| **endolymph**<br>(ěn′ dō-lǐmf) | endo-<br>-lymph | P<br>S | within<br>serum, clear fluid | Clear fluid contained within the labyrinth of the ear |
| **equilibrium**<br>(ē″ kwǐ-lǐb′ rē-ŭm) | | | | State of balance. In the inner ear, the semicircular canals are the sites of the organs of balance. |
| **eustachian tube**<br>(ū-stā′kē-ăn tūb) | | | | Narrow tube between the middle ear and the throat that serves to equalize pressure on both sides of the eardrum |

| MEDICAL WORD | WORD PARTS (WHEN APPLICABLE) | | | DEFINITION |
|---|---|---|---|---|
| | **Part** | **Type** | **Meaning** | |
| **fenestration**<br>(fĕn″ ĕs-trā′ shŭn) | fenestrat<br>-ion | R<br>S | window<br>process | Surgical operation in which a new opening is made in the labyrinth of the inner ear to restore hearing |
| **incus**<br>(ing′ kŭs) | | | | Middle of the three ossicles; also called the *anvil* |
| **labyrinth**<br>(lăb′ ĭ-rĭnth) | | | | The inner ear; made up of the *vestibule, cochlea,* and *semicircular canals* |
| **labyrinthectomy**<br>(lăb″ ĭ-rĭn-thĕk′ tō-mē) | labyrinth<br>-ectomy | R<br>S | maze, inner ear<br>surgical excision | Surgical excision of the labyrinth |
| **labyrinthitis**<br>(lăb″ ĭ-rĭn-thī′ tĭs) | labyrinth<br>-itis | R<br>S | maze, inner ear<br>inflammation | Inflammation of the labyrinth |
| **labyrinthotomy**<br>(lăb″ ĭ-rĭn-thŏt′ ō-mē) | labyrinth/o<br>-tomy | CF<br>S | maze, inner ear<br>incision | Incision of the labyrinth |
| **malleus**<br>(măl′ ē-ŭs) | | | | Largest of the three ossicles; also called the *hammer* |
| **mastoidalgia**<br>(măs″ toyd-ăl′ jĭ-ă) | mast<br><br>-oid<br>-algia | R<br><br>S<br>S | mastoid process, breast-shaped<br>resemble<br>pain | Pain in the mastoid process |
| **mastoiditis**<br>(măs″ toyd-ī′ tĭs) | mast<br><br>-oid<br>-itis | R<br><br>S<br>S | mastoid process, breast-shaped<br>resemble<br>inflammation | Inflammation of one of the mastoid bones; usually an extension of otitis media characterized by earache, fever, headache, and malaise |

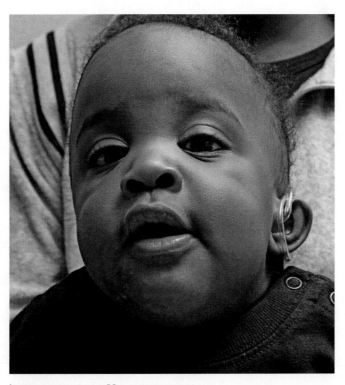

▶ FIGURE 15–5   Hearing impairment.

| MEDICAL WORD | WORD PARTS (WHEN APPLICABLE) | | | DEFINITION |
|---|---|---|---|---|
| | Part | Type | Meaning | |
| **Ménière's disease** (mān" ē-ārz) | | | | Disease of the inner ear *(labyrinth)* that presents a group of symptoms that recur. In acute attacks, bedrest is recommended. Vertigo and dizziness are the classic symptoms, and the patient experiences nausea, tinnitus, and a sensation of fullness or pressure in the ears. Deafness can occur. ✳ See Pathology Spotlight: Ménière's Disease on page 515. |
| **monaural** (mŏn-aw' răl) | mon(o)- aur -al | P R S | one ear pertaining to | Pertaining to one ear |
| **myringectomy** (mĭr-ĭn-jĕk' tō-mē) | myring -ectomy | R S | eardrum, tympanic membrane surgical excision | Surgical excision of the tympanic membrane |
| **myringoplasty** (mĭr-ĭn' gō-plăst" ē) | myring/o -plasty | CF S | eardrum, tympanic membrane surgical repair | Surgical repair of the tympanic membrane |
| **myringoscope** (mĭr-ĭn' gō-skōp) | myring/o -scope | CF S | eardrum, tympanic membrane instrument for examining | Instrument used to examine the eardrum |
| **myringotome** (mĭ-rĭn' gō-tōm) | myring/o -tome | CF S | eardrum, tympanic membrane instrument to cut | Instrument used for cutting the eardrum |
| **myringotomy** (mĭr-ĭn-gŏt' ō-mē) | myring/o -tomy | CF S | eardrum, tympanic membrane incision | Surgical incision of the tympanic membrane to remove unwanted fluids from the ear |
| **ossicle** (ŏs' ĭ-kl) | | | | Small bone; any one of the three bones of the middle ear: *the malleus, the incus,* or *the stapes* |
| **otic** (ō' tĭk) | ot -ic | R S | ear pertaining to | Pertaining to the ear |
| **otitis** (ō-tī' tĭs) | ot -itis | R S | ear inflammation | Inflammation of the ear. ✳ See Pathology Spotlight: Otitis Media on page 515. |
| **otitis media** (ō-tī' tĭs mē' dē-ă) | ot -itis med -ia | R S R S | ear inflammation middle condition | Inflammation of the middle ear. ✳ See Pathology Spotlight: Otitis Media on page 515. |
| **otodynia** (ō" tō-dĭn' ĭ-ă) | ot/o -dynia | CF S | ear pain | Pain in the ear, earache; also referred to as *otalgia* |

| MEDICAL WORD | WORD PARTS (WHEN APPLICABLE) | | | DEFINITION |
|---|---|---|---|---|
| | **Part** | **Type** | **Meaning** | |
| **otolaryngologist**<br>(ō″ tō-lar″ ĭn-gŏl″ ō-jĭst) | ot/o<br>laryng/o<br>log<br>-ist | CF<br>CF<br>R<br>S | ear<br>larynx, voice box<br>study of<br>one who specializes | Physician who specializes in the study of the ear and larynx (*voice box*) |
| **otolaryngology**<br>(ō″ tō-lar″ ĭn-gŏl′ ō-jē) | ot/o<br>laryng/o<br>-logy | CF<br>CF<br>S | ear<br>larynx, voice box<br>study of | Study of the ear and larynx (*voice box*) |
| **otolith**<br>(ō′ tō-lĭth) | ot/o<br>-lith | CF<br>S | ear<br>stone | Ear stone |
| **otomycosis**<br>(ō″ tō-mī-kō′ sĭs) | ot/o<br>myc<br>-osis | CF<br>R<br>S | ear<br>fungus<br>condition (usually abnormal) | Fungus condition of the ear |
| **otoneurology**<br>(ō″ tō-nū-rŏl′ ō-jē) | ot/o<br>neur/o<br>-logy | CF<br>CF<br>S | ear<br>nerve<br>study of | Study of ear conditions with nerve complications |
| **otopharyngeal**<br>(ō″ tō-far-ĭn′ jē-āl) | ot/o<br>pharyng/e<br>-al | CF<br>CF<br>S | ear<br>pharynx<br>pertaining to | Pertaining to the ear and pharynx |
| **otoplasty**<br>(ō′ tō-plăs″ tē) | ot/o<br>-plasty | CF<br>S | ear<br>surgical repair | Surgical repair of the ear |
| **otopyorrhea**<br>(ō″ tō-pī″ ō-rē′ ă) | ot/o<br>py/o<br>-rrhea | CF<br>CF<br>S | ear<br>pus<br>flow | Flow of pus from the ear |
| **otorhinolaryngology (ENT)**<br>(ō″ tō-rī″ nō-lăr″ ĭn-gŏl′ ō-jē) | ot/o<br>rhin/o<br>laryng/o<br>-logy | CF<br>CF<br>CF<br>S | ear<br>nose<br>larynx<br>study of | Study of the ear, nose, and larynx (*voice box*). The medical speciality is often referred to as *ENT* (*ear, nose, throat*); in this case, *throat* is used in a broad sense instead of *larynx*. |
| **otosclerosis**<br>(ō″ tō-sklē-rō′ sĭs) | ot/o<br>scler<br>-osis | CF<br>R<br>S | ear<br>hardening<br>condition (usually abnormal) | Hardening condition of the ear characterized by progressive deafness |
| **otoscope**<br>(ō′ tō-skōp) | ot/o<br>-scope | CF<br>S | ear<br>instrument for examining | Instrument used to examine the ear. See Figure 15–6 ▶. An inspection of the walls of the auditory canal should find no sign of irritation, discharge, or a foreign object. The walls are normally pink and some cerumen is present. The tympanic membrane is usually pearly gray and translucent. It reflects light and the ossicles are visible. |
| **oval window** | | | | Membrane in the middle ear into which the footplate of the stapes fits |

| MEDICAL WORD | WORD PARTS (WHEN APPLICABLE) | | | DEFINITION |
|---|---|---|---|---|
| | **Part** | **Type** | **Meaning** | |
| **perilymph**<br>(pĕr′ ĭ-lĭmf) | peri-<br>-lymph | P<br>S | around<br>serum, pale fluid | Serum fluid of the inner ear |
| **presbycusis**<br>(prĕz″ bĭ-kū′ sĭs) | presby<br>-cusis | R<br>S | old<br>hearing | Impairment of hearing that occurs with aging |
| **Rinne test**<br>(rĭn′ nē test) | | | | Hearing test utilizing a tuning fork to compare bone conduction (BC) hearing with air conduction (AC). After being struck, the vibrating tuning fork is held on the mastoid process until the patient no longer hears the sound.<br>See Figure 15–7 ▼. |
| **stapedectomy**<br>(stā″ pē-dĕk′ tō-mē) | staped<br>-ectomy | R<br>S | stapes, stirrup<br>surgical excision | Surgical excision of the stapes in the middle ear to improve hearing, especially in cases of otosclerosis. The stapes is replaced by a prosthesis. |
| **stapes**<br>(stā′ pēz) | | | | Innermost of the ossicles in the middle ear; also called the *stirrup* |
| **tinnitus**<br>(tĭn-ī′ tŭs) | | | | Ringing or jingling sound in the ear.<br>✱ See Pathology Spotlight: Tinnitus on page 517. |

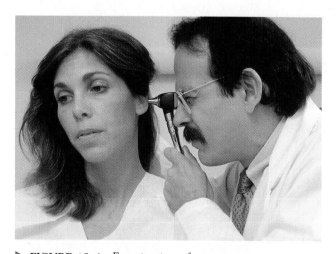

▶ **FIGURE 15–6**   Examination of ear using otoscope.

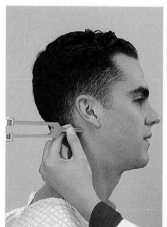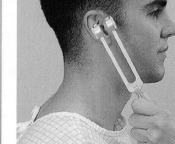

▶ **FIGURE 15–7**   Administration of the Rinne test.

| MEDICAL WORD | WORD PARTS (WHEN APPLICABLE) | | | DEFINITION |
|---|---|---|---|---|
| | Part | Type | Meaning | |
| **tuning fork** | | | | Instrument used in a hearing test, which, when struck at the forked end, vibrates and thus can be heard and felt |
| **tympanectomy** (tĭm″ păn-ĕk tō-mē) | tympan | R | eardrum, tympanic membrane | Surgical excision of the tympanic membrane (eardrum) |
| | -ectomy | S | surgical excision | |
| **tympanic** (tĭm-păn′ ĭk) | tympan | R | eardrum, tympanic membrane | Pertaining to the eardrum (tympanic membrane) |
| | -ic | S | pertaining to | |
| **tympanic thermometer** (tĭm-păn′ ĭk thĕr-mŏm′ ĕ-tĕr) | | | | Electronic thermometer used to determine core body temperature by measuring it from the tympanic membrane and its surrounding tissues. See Figure 15–8 ▼ and Figure 15–9 ▼. |
| **tympanitis** (tĭm-păn-ī′ tĭs) | tympan | R | eardrum, tympanic membrane | Inflammation of the eardrum (tympanic membrane) |
| | -itis | S | inflammation | |
| **tympanoplasty** (tĭm″ păn-ō-plăs′ tē) | tympan/o -plasty | CF S | eardrum, tympanic membrane surgical repair | Surgical repair of the tympanic membrane (eardrum) |
| **utricle** (ū′ trĭk-l) | | | | Small, saclike structure of the labyrinth of the inner ear |
| **vertigo** (ver′ tĭ-gō) | | | | Sensation of instability and loss of equilibrium; patients feel like they are spinning in space or objects around them are spinning. Caused by a disturbance in the semicircular canal of the inner ear or the vestibular nuclei of the brainstem. |

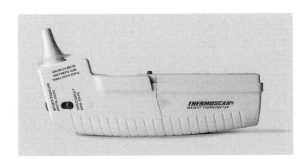

▶ **FIGURE 15–8**   Thermoscan instant thermometer (Courtesy of Thermoscan, Inc., San Diego, CA)

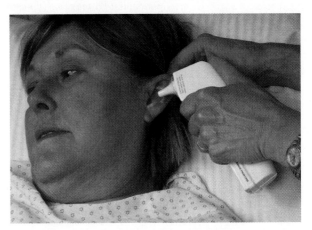

▶ **FIGURE 15–9**   Use of the tympanic thermometer to measure body temperature.

# DRUG HIGHLIGHTS

| | |
|---|---|
| **Analgesic** | Used to relieve pain without causing loss of consciousness. |
| | *Examples: Tylenol (acetaminophen), Advil, Motrin (ibuprofen), aspirin* |
| **Antipyretic** | Agent that reduces fever. |
| | *Examples: Tylenol (acetaminophen), aspirin* |
| | **Note:** *In children, aspirin should not be used as an analgesic or antipyretic because of the risk of Reye's syndrome.* |
| **Antibiotics** | Used to treat infectious diseases; can be natural or synthetic substances that inhibit the growth of or destroy microorganisms, especially bacteria. |
| Penicillins | Act by interfering with bacterial cell wall synthesis among newly formed bacterial cells. Penicillins are contraindicated in patients who are known to be allergic or hypersensitive to any of its varieties or to any of the cephalosporins. |
| | *Examples: penicillin G, ampicillin, penicillin V, piperacillin, amoxicillin, and ticarcillin* |
| Cephalosporins | Chemically and pharmacologically related to the penicillins, they act by inhibiting bacterial cell wall synthesis, thereby promoting the death of the developing microorganisms. Hypersensitivity to cephalosporins and/or penicillins can result in an allergic reaction. |
| | *Examples: Ancef (cefazolin sodium), Mandol (cefamandole nafate), Ceclor (cefaclor), Keflex (cephalexin), Suprax (cefixime), and Monocid (cefonicid)* |
| Tetracyclines | Primarily bacteriostatic and active against a wide range of gram-negative and gram-positive microorganisms, they inhibit protein synthesis in the bacterial cell. **Note:** Contraindicated in children 8 years of age and younger; they cause permanent discoloration of tooth enamel. |
| | *Examples: Achromycin, Sumycin, Panmycin (tetracycline hydrochloride); Declomycin DMCT (demeclocycline HCl), and Doryx, Vibramycin (doxycycline)* |
| Erythromycin | Works by inhibiting protein synthesis in susceptible bacteria. These drugs can be used for patients who are allergic to penicillin. |
| | *Examples: E-Mycin, Ilotycin, Ilosone, EES, EryPed, and Erythrocin* |
| **Drugs used to treat vertigo** | Vertigo is an illusion of movement that can be caused by a lesion or other process affecting the brain, the eighth cranial nerve, or the labyrinthine system of the ear. Drugs used for vertigo include anticholinergics, antihistamines, and antidopamines. |
| | *Examples: Dramamine (dimenhydrinate), Benadryl (diphenhydramine HCl), Antivert (meclizine HCl), Torecan (thiethylperazine maleate), Phenergan (promethazine HCl), Transderm-scop (scopolamine), and Torecan (thiethylperazine maleate)* |

# DIAGNOSTIC AND LAB TESTS

| TEST | DESCRIPTION |
|------|-------------|
| **Auditory-evoked response** (aw′ dǐ-tō rē ě-vōkd′) | Response to auditory stimuli (sound) that can be measured independently of the patient's subjective response. Use of an electroencephalograph can determine the intensity of sound and presence of response. This test is useful to test the hearing of children who are too young for standard tests, autistic, hyperkinetic, and/or retarded. |
| **Electronystagmography (ENG)** (ē-lěk″ trō-nǐs tăg-mǒg′ rǎ-fē) | Recording eye movement in response to specific stimuli, such as sound; used to determine the presence and location of a lesion in the vestibule of the ear, to help diagnose unilateral hearing loss of unknown origin, and to help identify the cause of vertigo, tinnitus, and dizziness. |
| **Falling test** | Test to observe the patient for marked swaying or falling. With eyes open, the patient is asked to stand on one foot, stand heel to toe, and then to walk forward. The patient is asked to repeat each of these with the eyes closed. Marked swaying or falling can indicate vestibular and cerebellar dysfunction. |
| **Past-pointing test** | Test that instructs the patient to reach out and touch the examiner's index finger, which is held at shoulder level, then to lower the arm, close the eyes, and to touch the finger again. The test is repeated using the finger of the examiner's opposite hand. The degree and direction of past-pointing is observed. |
| **Otoscopy** (ō-tǒs′ kō-pē) | Visual examination of the external auditory canal and the tympanic membrane via an otoscope. Pneumatic otoscopy uses a special attachment on the otoscope. This allows the examiner to direct a light stream of air toward the eardrum. The directed air current should then cause the tympanic membrane to vibrate. With dysfunction there is little or no vibration noted. |
| **Tuning fork test** | Method of testing hearing by the use of a tuning fork. Two types of hearing loss (conductive and perceptive) can be distinguished through the use of this test. Tuning forks are used in several types of test: the Weber, Bing, and Schwabach tests but the most commonly used test is the Rinne test. |
| **Tympanometry** (tīm″ păn-nǒm′ ě-trē) | Measurement of the movement of the tympanic membrane and pressure in the middle ear. It is used for detecting middle ear disorders. |

# ABBREVIATIONS

| ABBREVIATION | MEANING | ABBREVIATION | MEANING |
|--------------|---------|--------------|---------|
| AC | air conduction | ENT | ear, nose, throat (otorhinolaryngology) |
| BC | bone conduction | | |
| db, dB | decibel | HD | hearing distance |
| ENG | electronystagmography | OM | otitis media |

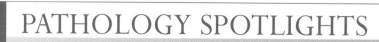

# PATHOLOGY SPOTLIGHTS

## ✳ Hearing Loss

Sustained noise over 85 decibels (db, dB) can cause permanent **hearing loss.** Risk doubles with each 5-decibel increase. About 2 in every 10 teens have lost some of their hearing ability from exposure to noise and are not aware of it, according to a study conducted at the University of Florida. Standard hearing tests given to middle and high school students identified some hearing loss in 17% of the students. High-pitched sounds are the first to be affected by noise exposure. As hearing loss progresses, a person can start to have difficulty hearing, particularly when there is noise in the background. Excessive noise can permanently damage the hair cell sensory receptors of the organ of Corti. These receptors are instrumental in transmitting sound to the brain. See Figure 15–10 ▼.

| Are You Harming Your Hearing? | Above 85 Decibels |
|---|---|
| Firecracker at 10 feet | 160 decibels |
| Rock concert | 125 decibels |
| Jet taking off at close range | 120 decibels |
| Stereo headset, volume at six | 115 decibels |
| Subway | 100 decibels |
| Car horn | 100 decibels |
| Garbage disposal | 95 decibels |
| City traffic | 90 decibels |

Noise can get in the way of learning and cause stress. Research shows that noise can cause anger, aggression, poor performance, and insomnia. It can also be a factor in hypertension and cardiovascular and digestive problems. If a noise is so loud that a person has to raise his or her voice to be heard, it is loud enough to hurt the person's hearing.

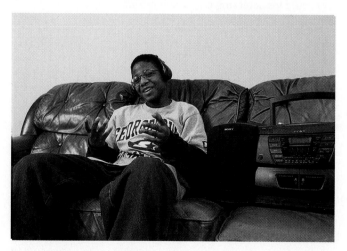

▶ **FIGURE 15–10**  Listening to loud music with headphones or at rock concerts is a frequent cause of hearing loss among teenagers and young adults.

According to Tedd Mitchell, "MD HealthSmart: Here's to Ears," *USA Weekend*, people can use the word *sound* to remember things that can cause ear problems.

- **Sensory overload.** If you need to raise your voice above the background noise for others to hear you, you need either to get away from the sound source or protect your ears.
- **Old age.** By age 55, 20% of people have hearing loss. By age 65, 33% are affected. Age-related hearing loss typically does not lead to complete deafness but can lead to auditory isolation.
- **Undiagnosed tumors or undertreated infections.** These condition can cause hearing loss and should be addressed by a physician.
- **Non-functioning ear canal or bones.** Anything that blocks the ear canal impedes sound flow.
- **Damage from drugs, trauma, or pressure.** Certain antibiotics, drugs for malaria, antiarrhythmics, and even aspirin can have toxic effects on hearing. Also, trauma such as a hole in the eardrum, fracture to the skull, noise trauma (gunfire, fireworks), and pressure trauma (underwater diving or pressurized airplane cabins) can damage the ear and cause hearing loss.

## ✱ Ménière's Disease

**Ménière's disease** is an abnormality of the inner ear causing a host of symptoms, including vertigo (severe dizziness), tinnitus (a roaring sound in the ears), fluctuating hearing loss, and the sensation of pressure or pain in the affected ear. The disorder usually affects only one ear and is a common cause of hearing loss. The disease is named after French physician Prosper Ménière who first described the syndrome in 1861.

The symptoms of Ménière's disease are associated with a change in fluid volume within the labyrinth and can occur suddenly and arise daily or as infrequently as once a year. **Vertigo,** often the most debilitating symptom of Ménière's disease, typically involves a whirling dizziness that forces the sufferer to lie down. Vertigo attacks can lead to severe nausea, vomiting, and sweating and often come with little or no warning.

Some individuals with Ménière's disease have attacks that start with **tinnitus,** then a loss of hearing, and/or a full feeling or pressure in the affected ear. All of these symptoms are unpredictable. Typically, the attack is characterized by a combination of vertigo, tinnitus, and hearing loss lasting several hours. People experience these discomforts at varying frequencies, durations, and intensities. Other occasional symptoms of Ménière's disease include headaches, abdominal discomfort, and diarrhea. A person's hearing tends to recover between attacks but over time becomes worse.

There is no cure for Ménière's disease. However, the symptoms of the disease are often controlled successfully by reducing the body's retention of fluids through dietary changes (such as a low-salt or salt-free diet and no caffeine or alcohol) or medication.

 ## ✱ Otitis Media

**Otitis** is an inflammation or infection of any part of the outer, middle, or inner ear. **Otitis media** (OM) is the most common type of otitis. This inflammation often begins when viral or bacterial infections that cause sore throats, colds, or other respiratory or breathing problems spread to the middle ear.

Children are more likely to suffer from otitis media than adults. Seventy-five percent of children experience at least one episode of otitis media by their third birthday. Almost half of these children will have three or more ear infections during their first three years.

Children are more likely to suffer from otitis media than adults for many reasons. First, children have more trouble fighting infections because their immune systems are still developing. Another reason has to do with the child's eustachian tube. It is shorter and straighter in the child than in the adult. It can contribute to otitis media in several ways. The eustachian tube is usually closed but opens regularly to ventilate or replenish the air in the middle ear. This tube also equalizes middle ear air pressure in response to air pressure changes in the environment. However, a eustachian tube that is blocked by swelling of its lining or plugged with mucus from a cold or for some other reason cannot open to ventilate the middle ear. The lack of ventilation can allow fluid from the tissue that lines the middle ear to accumulate. If the eustachian tube remains plugged, the fluid cannot drain and begins to collect in the normally air-filled middle ear.

One more factor that makes children more susceptible to otitis media is that adenoids in children are larger than they are in adults. *Adenoids* are composed largely of cells (lymphocytes) that help fight infections. They are positioned in the back of the upper part of the throat near the eustachian tubes. Enlarged adenoids can, because of their size, interfere with the eustachian tube opening. In addition, adenoids can themselves become infected, and the infection can spread into the eustachian tubes.

Bacteria reach the middle ear through the lining or the passageway of the eustachian tube and can then produce infection, which causes the lining of the middle ear to swell, blocking the eustachian tube, and white cells to migrate from the bloodstream to help fight the infection. In this process, the white cells accumulate, often killing bacteria and dying themselves, leading to the formation of pus, a thick yellowish-white fluid in the middle ear. As the fluid increases, the child can have trouble hearing because the eardrum and middle ear bones are unable to move as freely as they should. As the infection worsens, some children experience severe ear pain while others do not.

Otitis media is often difficult to detect because most children affected by this disorder do not yet have sufficient speech and language skills to tell others what is bothering them. Common signs of otitis media are these:

- Unusual irritability; fussiness.
- Difficulty sleeping; night awakening.
- Tugging or pulling at one or both ears. See Figure 15–11 ▼.

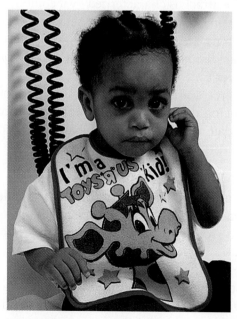

▶ **FIGURE 15–11**  This young child is pulling at the ear and acting fussy, two important signs of otitis media.

- Fever.
- Fluid draining from the ear.
- Loss of balance.
- Unresponsiveness to quiet sounds or other signs of hearing difficulty such as sitting too close to the television or being inattentive.

## ✳ Tinnitus

**Tinnitus,** the sensation of ringing or roaring sounds in one or both ears, is a symptom associated with damage to the auditory cells in the inner ear. It can also be a symptom of other health problems. According to estimates by the American Tinnitus Association, at least 12 million Americans have tinnitus. Of these, at least 1 million experience it so severely that it interferes with their daily activities, such as hearing, working, and sleeping.

There are several possible causes of tinnitus:

- **Hearing loss.** Doctors and scientists have discovered that people with different kinds of hearing loss, primarily from presbycusis or trauma-related damage to the inner ear, also have tinnitus.
- **Loud noise.** Too much exposure to loud noise can cause noise-induced hearing loss and tinnitus.
- **Medicine.** More than 200 medicines can cause tinnitus.
- **Other health problems.** Allergies, tumors, and problems in the heart and blood vessels, jaws, and neck can cause tinnitus.

A patient can be referred to an **otolaryngologist** for diagnosis, and/or an **audiologist,** who performs hearing tests. Although there is no cure for tinnitus, scientists and doctors have discovered several treatments that can provide some relief:

- **Hearing aids.** Many people with tinnitus also have a hearing loss. Wearing a hearing aid makes it easier for some people to hear the sounds they need to hear by making them louder.
- **Maskers.** Maskers are small electronic devices that use sound to make tinnitus less noticeable. Maskers do not make tinnitus go away, but they make the ringing or roaring seem softer. For some people, maskers hide their tinnitus so well that they can barely hear it.
- **Medicine or drug therapy.** Medications such as antiarrhythmics and antidepressants can help suppress tinnitus.

# ✔ PATHOLOGY CHECKPOINT

*Following is a concise list of the pathology-related terms that you have seen in the chapter. Review this checklist to make sure that you are familiar with the meaning of each term before moving to the next section.*

## Conditions and Symptoms

- ❏ cholesteatoma
- ❏ deafness
- ❏ labyrinthitis
- ❏ mastoidalgia
- ❏ mastoiditis
- ❏ Ménière's disease
- ❏ otalgia
- ❏ otitis
- ❏ otitis media
- ❏ otodynia
- ❏ otolith
- ❏ otomycosis
- ❏ otopyorrhea
- ❏ otosclerosis
- ❏ presbycusis
- ❏ tinnitus
- ❏ tympanitis
- ❏ vertigo

## Diagnosis and Treatment

- ❏ audiogram
- ❏ audiometer
- ❏ audiometry
- ❏ audiphone
- ❏ electrocochleography
- ❏ fenestration
- ❏ labyrinthectomy
- ❏ labyrinthotomy
- ❏ myringectomy
- ❏ myringoplasty
- ❏ myringoscope
- ❏ myringotome
- ❏ myringotomy
- ❏ otoplasty
- ❏ otoscope
- ❏ Rinne test
- ❏ stapedectomy
- ❏ tympanectomy
- ❏ tympanic thermometer
- ❏ tympanoplasty

# STUDY AND REVIEW

*Write your answers to the following questions. Do not refer to the text.*

1. The ear is the site of the senses of _____ and _____.

2. Name the three divisions of the ear.

   a. _____   b. _____

   c. _____

3. The external ear consists of the _____, the _____, and the

   _____.

4. Which structure of the external ear collects sound waves?

5. State the two functions of cerumen.

   a. _____   b. _____

6. Name the three ossicles of the middle ear.

   a. _____   b. _____

   c. _____

7. State the function of the ossicles.

   _____

8. State the three functions of the middle ear.

   a. _____   b. _____

   c. _____

9. The bony labyrinth of the inner ear consists of the _____,

   _____, and the _____.

10. Name the three divisions of the membranous labyrinth.

    a. _____   b. _____

    c. _____

11. Located on the basilar membrane is the _____, containing hair cell
    sensory receptors for the sense of hearing.

12. The _____ is a bony structure located between the cochlea and the
    three semicircular canals.

13. The auditory nerve is also known as the _____.

14. The hair cells located in each ampulla of the semicircular canals sense changes in _____ and report this information to the brain.

15. Name the two types of fluid found in the ear.

a. _____    b. _____

## Word Parts

1. In the spaces provided, write the definitions of these prefixes, roots, combining forms, and suffixes. Do not refer to the listings of medical words. Leave blank those words you cannot define.

2. After completing as many as you can, refer to the medical word listings to check your work. For each word missed or left blank, write the word and its definition several times on the margins of these pages or on a separate sheet of paper.

3. To maximize the learning process, it is to your advantage to do the following exercises as directed. To refer to the word-building section before completing these exercises invalidates the learning process.

## PREFIXES

*Give the definitions of the following prefixes.*

1. end- _____    2. endo- _____

3. peri- _____    4. bin- _____

5. mon(o)- _____

## ROOTS AND COMBINING FORMS

*Give the definitions of the following roots and combining forms.*

1. acoust _____    2. aud/i _____

3. audi/o _____    4. auditor _____

5. aur _____    6. chol/e _____

7. cochle/o _____    8. electr/o _____

9. labyrinth _____    10. labyrinth/o _____

11. laryng/o _____    12. log _____

13. mast _____    14. myc _____

15. myring _____    16. myring/o _____

17. neur/o _____    18. ot _____

19. ot/o _____

20. pharyng/e _____

21. phone _____

22. presby _____

23. py/o _____

24. rhin/o _____

25. scler _____

26. staped _____

27. steat _____

28. tympan _____

29. aur/i _____

30. fenestrat _____

31. med _____

32. tympan/o _____

## SUFFIXES

*Give the definitions of the following suffixes.*

1. -al _____

2. -algia _____

3. -cusis _____

4. -dynia _____

5. -ectomy _____

6. -gram _____

7. -graphy _____

8. -ic _____

9. -ist _____

10. -itis _____

11. -lith _____

12. -logy _____

13. -lymph _____

14. -meter _____

15. -metry _____

16. -oid _____

17. -oma _____

18. -osis _____

19. -plasty _____

20. -rrhea _____

21. -scope _____

22. -tome _____

23. -tomy _____

24. -y _____

25. -cle _____

26. -ion _____

27. -ia _____

## Identifying Medical Terms

*In the spaces provided, write the medical terms for the following meanings.*

1. _____ One who specializes in disorders of hearing

2. _____ Measurement of the hearing sense

3. _____ Pertaining to the sense of hearing

4. _____ Pertaining to within the ear

5. _____ Inflammation of the labyrinth

6. _____ Surgical repair of the tympanic membrane

7. _____ Instrument used for cutting the eardrum

8. _____ Pain in the ear, earache

9. _____ Study of the ear and larynx

10. _____ Pertaining to the ear and pharynx

11. _____ Instrument used to examine the ear

12. _____ Serum fluid of the inner ear

13. _____ Surgical excision of the stapes of the ear

14. _____ Surgical excision of the tympanic membrane

15. _____ A ringing or jingling sound in the ear

## Spelling

*In the spaces provided, write the correct spelling of these misspelled words.*

1. acostic _____

2. audilogy _____

3. cholestoma _____

4. electrochleography _____

5. labrinthitis _____

6. myringplasty _____

7. otomcosis _____

8. otosterosis _____

9. typanic _____

10. typanitis _____

## Matching

*Select the appropriate lettered meaning for each of the following words.*

_____ 1. auricle

_____ 2. binaural

_____ 3. cerumen

_____ 4. equilibrium

_____ 5. fenestration

_____ 6. labyrinth

_____ 7. myringotomy

_____ 8. ossicle

_____ 9. tympanoplasty

_____ 10. vertigo

a. State of balance
b. Inner ear
c. Small bone
d. Surgical repair of the tympanic membrane
e. Pertaining to both ears
f. Sensation of instability, loss of equilibrium
g. Surgical operation in which a new opening is made in the labyrinth
h. External portion of the ear
i. Earwax
j. Surgical incision of the tympanic membrane
k. Organ of hearing

## Abbreviations

*Place the correct word, phrase, or abbreviation in the space provided.*

1. air conduction _____

2. bone conduction _____

3. db, dB _____

4. electronystagmography _____

5. ENT _____

6. hearing distance _____

7. otitis media _____

## Diagnostic and Laboratory Tests

*Select the best answer to each multiple choice question. Circle the letter of your choice.*

1. The response to auditory stimuli that can be measured independent of the patient's subjective response.
   a. auditory-evoked response
   b. electronystagmography
   c. falling test
   d. otoscopy

2. Recording of eye movement in response to specific stimuli.
   a. auditory-evoked response
   b. electronystagmography
   c. falling test
   d. otoscopy

3. Test to observe the patient for marked swaying.
   a. auditory-evoked response
   b. electronystagmography
   c. falling test
   d. past-pointing test

4. Visual examination of the external auditory canal and the tympanic membrane.
   a. tuning fork test
   b. tympanometry
   c. electronystagmography
   d. otoscopy

5. Measurement of the movement of the tympanic membrane.
   a. tuning fork tests
   b. tympanometry
   c. otoscopy
   d. past-pointing test

# PRACTICAL APPLICATION

## S O A P : Chart Note Analysis

*This exercise will make you aware of the information, abbreviations, and medical terminology typically found in a pediatric patient's chart.*

### Abbreviations Key

| | | | | |
|---|---|---|---|---|
| Abd | abdomen | | NKDA | no known drug allergies |
| AOM | acute otitis media | | P | pulse |
| BP | blood pressure | | PO | orally, by mouth |
| CTA | clear to auscultation | | prn | as necessary |
| DOB | date of birth | | R | respiration |
| F | Fahrenheit | | SOAP | subjective, objective, assessment, plan |
| HEENT | head, eyes, ears, nose, throat | | T | temperature |
| Ht | height | | TM | tympanic membrane |
| kg | kilogram | | URI | upper respiratory infection |
| lb | pound | | Wt | weight |
| mg | milligram | | y/o | year(s) old |
| mL | milliliter | | | |

*Read the following chart note and then answer the questions that follow.*

**PATIENT:** Chamberlain, Takeshia                                                    **DATE:** 9/29/07
**DOB:** 6/19/05      **AGE:** 2      **SEX:** Female
**Insurance: Physicare Health Insurance**

   **Vital Signs:**
      **T:** 102.2 F
      **P:** 92
      **R:** 24
      **BP:** 78/56
      **Ht:** 34″
      **Wt:** 26 lb (12 kg)

**S**   **Subjective:** Mother of a 2 y/o black girl states that her baby has been unusually fussy for two days, and she has had to keep her at home instead of taking her to day care. "My baby felt like she was burning up late yesterday afternoon. I put her in the tub, but it didn't do much good. I gave her some baby Tylenol and it helped a little, but she won't stop pulling at her ear. Last night she woke me up just screaming."
**Allergies:**   NKDA
**Chief Complaint:**   Otodynia (otalgia), fever, irritability, and night awakening.

**O**   **Objective:**

**General Appearance:** Noted dark circles under both eyes. Appears to be in moderate pain and not feeling well. Pulling on left ear.

**Abd:** Bowel sounds in all 4 quadrants, abdomen soft and nontender

**HEENT:**

    Eyes: No exudate, conjunctivae clear, sclera white, bilateral red reflex present.

    Ears: Left TM red, dull, and bulging, diffuse light reflex with loss of landmarks. Pneumatic oto-scopy reveals immobile left TM. Right TM pearly gray, landmarks intact.

    Nose: Nasal mucosa dark red and swollen with moderate amount of discharge.

    Throat: Oral mucosa erythematous with yellow-white exudate, no lesions. Uvula rises in midline with phonation. Gag reflex present. No lymphadenopathy. Neck supple.

**Lungs:** CTA

**Heart:** Normal rate and rhythm. No murmurs.

**Skin:** No rashes or lesions, warm to the touch.

**A**    **Assessment:** Acute otitis media (AOM) left ear

**P**    **Plan:** After a visual examination of the ears, physical examination of the child, and the signs and symptoms described by the mother, the diagnosis was confirmed.

1. Ordered was an analgesic/antipyretic, acetaminophen (Tylenol) liquid, 1.6 mL (1 teaspoon) PO every 4 hours prn for pain and to reduce fever. For infection Takeshia is to take an antibiotic, amox-icillin (Amoxil) suspension 40mg per kg per day, in 3 divided doses, every 8 hours for 10 days.
2. Teach the mother that the most common adverse reaction to penicillin is an allergic one. Explain that anaphylaxis is a severe allergic reaction and can occur at anytime and she should look for signs such as unusual facial swelling, difficulty in breathing, bluish or grayish discoloration around the mouth, circulatory collapse, and convulsions. If such symptoms occur she should call 911 immediately. Inform that other adverse reactions can include nausea, vomiting, diarrhea, fever, chills, rash, itching, and signs of superinfection, which are black tongue, sore mouth, perianal infection and itching, foul-smelling vaginal discharge, loose stools, sudden fever, and cough. She should notify the physician's office if any of these symptoms appear in her baby.
3. Inform the mother that she should use the measuring device that comes with each medicine to give the correct dose to her baby. Instruct her to give the baby at least 8 ounces of water to drink following the administration of the antibiotic.
4. Explain that she should not give the antibiotic with soft drinks or fruit juices because the acid in these products could destroy the effectiveness of the drug.
5. Stress the importance of the baby taking the antibiotic as ordered for the entire 10 days and around the clock, every 8 hours. Explain that to effectively kill the microorganisms causing the infection, the medicine has to be taken exactly as the doctor prescribed.
6. Instruct the mother to bring the baby back to the clinic if symptoms do not improve in 48–72 hours.
7. Schedule a follow-up visit for three weeks.

**FYI:** When examining the tympanic membrane, the position, mobility, color, and degree of translu-cency are evaluated and described. The normal tympanic membrane is in the neutral position (nei-ther retracted nor bulging), pearly gray, translucent, and responds briskly to positive and negative pressure, indicating an air-filled space. An abnormal tympanic membrane can be retracted or bulging and immobile or poorly mobile in pneumatic otoscopy. The position of the tympanic mem-brane is a key for differentiating acute otitis media and otitis media with effusion. In acute otitis media, the tympanic membrane is usually bulging.

**Note:** Children age 2 and younger who attend day care centers are 36 times more likely to contract ear infections, pneumonia, and meningitis than stay-at-home children. Most middle ear infections are a result of an upper respiratory infection (URI) that has spread through the eustachian tube.

## Chart Note Questions
*Place the correct answer in the space provided.*

1. The signs and symptoms of acute otitis media in Takeshia included otodynia, fever, irritability, and _____.

2. Otodynia (otalgia) is a medical term for _____.

3. The diagnosis was determined by a visual examination of the ear called pneumatic _____, a physical examination of the child, and the signs and symptoms described by the mother.

4. A bulging, red, immobile left tympanic membrane indicates _____.

5. Tylenol is classified as a(n) _____ and is given to relieve _____ and reduce _____.

6. Amoxil is classified as a(n) _____ and is given for _____.

7. The most common adverse reaction to penicillin is a(n) _____.

8. Signs of anaphylaxis include unusual facial swelling, difficulty in _____, circulatory collapse, and convulsions.

9. The _____ in soft drinks and fruit juices can destroy the effectiveness of the antibiotic drug.

10. Most middle ear infections are a result of an URI that has spread through the _____.

# MULTIMEDIA PREVIEW

*Additional interactive resources and activities for this chapter can be found on the Companion Website. For videos, audio glossary, and review, access the accompanying CD-ROM in this book.*

 **CD-ROM HIGHLIGHTS**

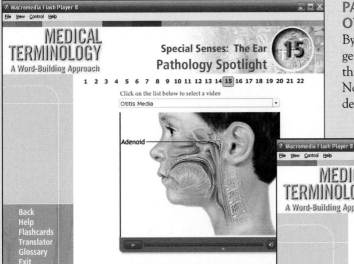

## PATHOLOGY SPOTLIGHT— OTITIS MEDIA

By viewing concepts in moving, living color, you'll get a fuller picture of the pathologies presented in this chapter. Earlier we discussed otitis media. Now click on this feature to watch a video that describes this condition in more detail.

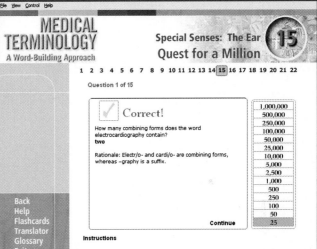

## QUEST FOR A MILLION

Who wants to win a million points? If it's you, then click on this game to begin your challenge. If you correctly answer 15 questions in a row, then you're a winner. But be very careful, because one wrong response will take you back down to zero.

 **WEBSITE HIGHLIGHTS—www.prenhall.com/rice**

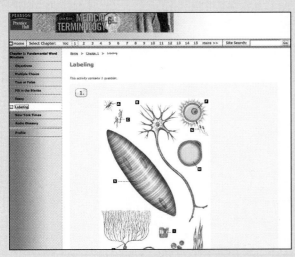

## LABELING EXERCISE

Click here and take advantage of the free-access on-line study guide that accompanies your textbook. You'll find an image labeling question that corresponds to the concepts in this chapter. By clicking on this URL you'll also access links to download mp3 audio reviews, current news articles, and an audio glossary.

# Special Senses:
# The Eye

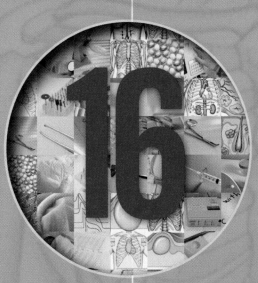

**16**

## ■ OUTLINE

## ■ OBJECTIVES

*On completion of this chapter, you will be able to:*

- Describe the anatomical structures of the eye.
- Describe the external structures of the eye.
- Describe the internal structures of the eye.
- Analyze, build, spell, and pronounce medical words.
- Comprehend the drugs highlighted in this chapter.
- Describe diagnostic and laboratory tests related to the eye.
- Identify and define selected abbreviations.
- Describe each of the conditions presented in the Pathology Spotlights.
- Review the Pathology Checkpoint.
- Complete the Study and Review section and the Chart Note Analysis.

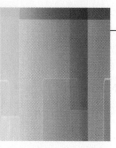

# Anatomy and Physiology Overview

The **eye** is composed of special anatomical structures that work together to facilitate sight. Light passes through the cornea, pupil, lens, and the vitreous body to stimulate sensory receptors (*rods* and *cones*) on the **retina** or innermost layer of the eye. **Vision** is made possible through the coordinated actions of nerves that control the movement of the eyeball, the amount of light admitted by the pupil, the focusing of that light on the retina by the lens, and the transmission of the resulting sensory impulses to the brain by the optic nerve.

## Special Senses: The Eye

| Organ/Structure | Primary Functions |
| --- | --- |
| Orbit | Contains the eyeball; cavity is lined with fatty tissue that cushions the eyeball and has several openings through which blood vessels and nerves pass |
| Muscles of the Eye | Six short muscles provide support and rotary movement of the eyeball |
| Eyelids | Protect the eyeballs from intense light, foreign particles, and impact |
| Conjunctiva | Acts as a protective covering for the exposed surface of the eyeball and helps keep the eyelid and eyeball moist |
| Lacrimal apparatus | Produces, stores, and removes tears that cleanse and lubricate the eye |
| Eyeball | Organ of vision |
| Sclera | Outer layer of the eyeball composed of fibrous connective tissue; at the front of the eye, it is visible as the white of the eye and ends at the cornea |
| Cornea | Transparent anterior portion of the eyeball which bends light rays and helps to focus them on the surface of the retina |
| Choroid | Pigmented vascular membrane that prevents internal reflection of light |
| Ciliary body | Smooth muscle that forms a part of the ciliary body that governs the convexity of the lens; secretes nutrient fluids that nourish the cornea, the lens, and surrounding tissues |
| Iris | Colored portion of the eyeball (can appear as blue, brown, green, hazel, or gray) attached to the ciliary body with a circular opening in its center, the pupil, and two muscles that contract; regulates the amount of light admitted by the pupil |
| Retina | Innermost layer with photoreceptive cells; translates light waves focused on its surface into nerve impulses |
| Lens | Sharpens the focus of light on the retina (accommodation [Acc]) |

# EXTERNAL STRUCTURES OF THE EYE

The orbit, the muscles of the eye, the eyelids, the conjunctiva, and the lacrimal apparatus make up the external structures of the eye.

## Orbit

The **orbit** is a cone-shaped cavity in the front of the skull that contains the *eyeball*. Formed by the combination of several bones, this cavity is lined with fatty tissue that cushions the eyeball and has several **foramina** (openings) through which blood vessels and nerves pass. The largest of these is the optic foramen for the optic nerve and ophthalmic artery.

## Muscles of the Eye

Six eye muscles control movement of the eye, allowing it to follow a moving object and move precisely. Of the six, four are rectus muscles and two are oblique muscles. *Rectus muscles* allow a person to see up, down, right, and left. *Oblique muscles* allow the eyes to turn to

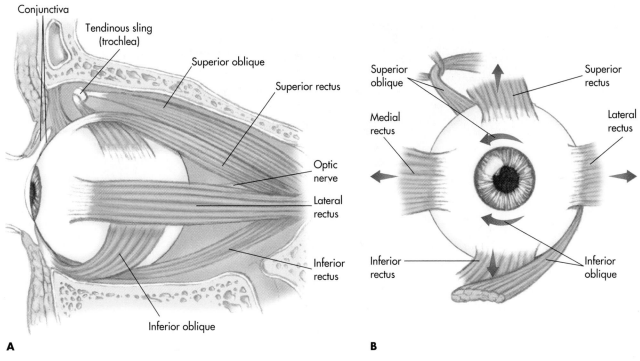

▶ **FIGURE 16–1**  Eye muscles. (A) lateral view, left eye and (B) anterior view, left eye.

see upper left and upper right, lower left and lower right. See Figure 16–1 ▲. The eye muscles also help maintain the shape of the eyeball.

## Eyelids

Each eye has a pair of **eyelids** that are continuous with the skin, cover the eyeball, and protect it from intense light, foreign particles, and impact. Through their blinking motion, eyelids keep the eyeball's surface lubricated and free from dust and debris. Known as the *superior* and *inferior palpebrae*, those movable *curtains* join to form a **canthus** or angle at either corner of the eye. The slit between the eyelids is called the **palpebral fissure** through which light reaches the inner eye.

The edges of the eyelids contain eyelashes that help protect the eyeball by preventing foreign particles, such as insects, from coming into contact with the eyeball. Along the inner margin of the thin skin of the lid, *meibomian glands* secrete sebum, an oily substance that helps keep the eyelids from sticking together. These glands are embedded in the tarsal plate of each eyelid and are called *tarsal glands* and *palpebral glands*.

## Conjunctiva

Lining the underside of each eyelid and reflected onto the anterior portion of the eyeball is a mucous membrane known as the **conjunctiva.** This membrane acts as a protective covering for the exposed surface of the eyeball.

## Lacrimal Apparatus

Included in the **lacrimal apparatus** are those structures that produce, store, and remove the tears that cleanse and lubricate the eye. These structures are the lacrimal gland, located in the outer corner of each eyelid, lacrimal canaliculi (ducts), the lacrimal sac, and the nasolacrimal duct, which empties into the nasal cavity (see Figure 16–2 ▶).

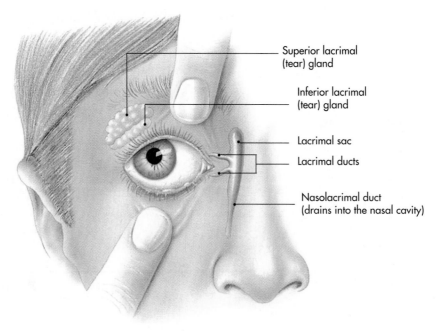

Superior lacrimal (tear) gland

Inferior lacrimal (tear) gland

Lacrimal sac

Lacrimal ducts

Nasolacrimal duct (drains into the nasal cavity)

▶ **FIGURE 16–2** Lacrimal glands and lacrimal canaliculi (ducts).

### Lacrimal Gland

Located above the outer corner of the eye, the **lacrimal gland** secretes tears through approximately 12 ducts onto the surface of the conjunctiva of the upper lid. This fluid washes across the anterior surface of the eye and is collected by the *lacrimal canaliculi* (ducts).

### Lacrimal Canaliculi

The **lacrimal canaliculi** are the two ducts at the inner corner of the eye that collect tears and drain into the lacrimal sac.

### Lacrimal Sac

The enlargement of the upper portion of the lacrimal duct is known as the **lacrimal sac.** Tears secreted by the lacrimal glands are pulled into this sac and subsequently forced into the nasolacrimal duct by the blinking action of the eyelids. The sac is dilated and pulls in fluid as the muscles associated with blinking close the lids. The sac constricts, forcing the fluid down the nasolacrimal duct as the lids are opened.

### Nasolacrimal Duct

The passageway draining lacrimal fluid into the nose is known as the **nasolacrimal duct.** The lacrimal sac is the enlarged upper portion of this duct.

## INTERNAL STRUCTURES OF THE EYE

The eyeball, its various structures, and the nerve fibers connecting it to the brain make up the internal eye (see Figure 16–3 ▶).

### Eyeball

The **eyeball** is the organ of vision. It is globe shaped and divided into two cavities. The space in front of the lens, called the **ocular cavity,** is further divided by the iris into

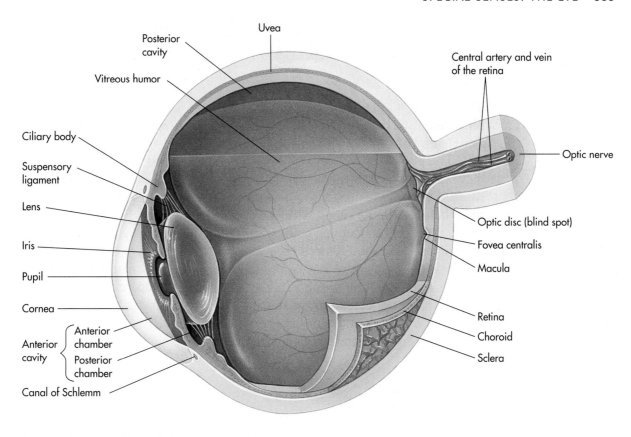

▶ FIGURE 16–3   Internal structure of the eye.

anterior and posterior chambers. The anterior chamber is filled with a watery fluid known as the aqueous humor. Behind the lens is a much larger cavity filled with a jelly-like material, the vitreous humor, which maintains the eyeball's spherical shape. The three layers forming the outer, middle, and inner surfaces of the eyeball as well as the lens and its functions are discussed here.

### Outer Layer

The eyeball's outer layer is composed of the sclera or white of the eye and the cornea or anterior transparent portion of the eye's fibrous outer surface. The curved surface of the cornea is important because it bends light rays and helps to focus them on the surface of the retina.

### Middle Layer

Known as the uvea, the middle layer of the eyeball, lying just below the sclera, consists of the iris, the ciliary body, and the choroid.

Iris.   The iris is a colored membrane attached to the ciliary body and suspended between the lens and the cornea in the aqueous humor. It has a circular opening in its center—the pupil—and two muscles that contract or dilate to regulate the amount of light admitted by the pupil.

Ciliary Body.   The ciliary body is a thickened portion of the vascular membrane to which the iris is attached. Smooth muscle forming a part of the ciliary body governs the convexity of the lens. The ciliary body secretes nutrient fluids (the *aqueous humor*) that nourish the cornea, the lens, and the surrounding tissues.

Choroid.    The **choroid** is a pigmented vascular membrane that prevents internal reflection of light.

### Inner Layer

The innermost layer of the eye, or **retina,** is richly supplied with blood vessels and contains photoreceptive cells that translate light waves focused on its surface into nerve impulses. See Figure 16–4 ▼.

The photosensitive cells of the retina are the **rods** and **cones.** Rods are sensitive to dim light and used for night vision. Cones are sensitive to bright light and color vision. Most of the approximately 6 million cone cells are grouped into a small area called the **macula lutea.** In the center of the macula lutea is a small depression, the **fovea centralis,** which is the central focusing point within the eye; it contains only cone cells. The eye contains approximately 120 million rods that are sensitive to dim light. They contain **rhodopsin,** a pigment necessary for night vision. The point at which nerve fibers from the retina converge to form the optic nerve is known as the **optic disk.** At the optic disk, fibers of the optic nerve extend to the thalamus and on to the visual cortical areas of the brain. The absence of rods and cones in the area of the optic disk creates a *blind spot* on the surface of the retina, located about 3 millimeters to the nasal side of the macula. It is the only part of the retina that is insensitive to light.

### Lens

A colorless crystalline body biconvex in shape and enclosed in a transparent capsule, the **lens** is suspended by ligaments just behind the iris. Contraction and relaxation of the ciliary muscle control the tension of the suspensory ligaments to change the shape of the lens. The function of the lens is to sharpen the focus of light on the retina. This process, called **accommodation** (ACC), is reflexive in nature and combines changes in the size of the pupil, the curvature of the lens, and the convergence of the optic axes to keep the image in the same place on both retinae. Accommodation occurs for both near and distant vision.

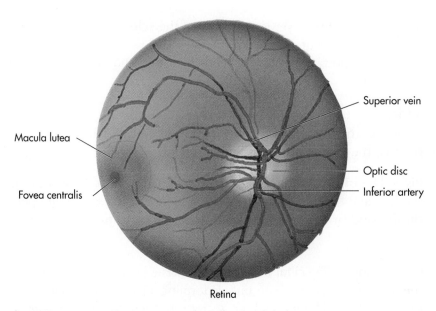

Macula lutea

Fovea centralis

Superior vein

Optic disc

Inferior artery

Retina

▶ FIGURE 16–4    Retina as seen through an ophthalmoscope.

# HOW SIGHT OCCURS

When a person views external objects, the light rays strike the eye and then pass through the cornea, pupil, aqueous humor, lens, and vitreous humor. They then reach the retina and stimulate the rods and cones. An upside-down image is relayed along nerve impulses to the optic nerve. The images are transferred to the brain, which turns the images into a right-side-up image. This image is the one that the person sees. See Figures 16–5 ▼ and 16–6 ▼.

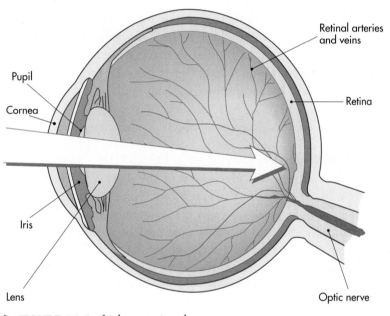

▶ **FIGURE 16–5**   Light entering the eye.

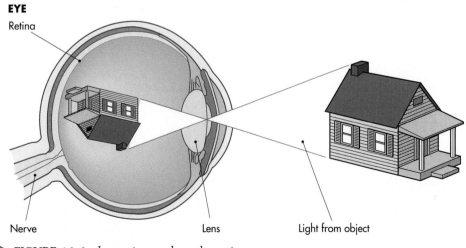

▶ **FIGURE 16–6**   Image inverted on the retina.

# LIFE SPAN CONSIDERATIONS

## ■ THE CHILD

The eyes begin to develop as an outgrowth of the forebrain in the 4-week-old embryo. At 24 weeks, the eyes are structurally complete. At 28 weeks, eyebrows and eyelashes are present, and the eyelids open. The newborn can see, and **visual acuity** is estimated to be around 20/400. Most newborns appear to have crossed eyes because their eye muscles are not fully developed. At first, the eyes appear to be blue or gray. Permanent coloring becomes fixed between 6 and 12 months of age. Tears do not appear until approximately 1 to 3 months because the lacrimal gland ducts are immature. Depth perception begins to develop around 9 months of age.

Every minute that an infant is awake, he or she is taking in the sights, sounds, smells, and feel of the surrounding world. For the 1- to 3-month-old, the human face is a favorite sight. By the second month, the baby's eye coordination has improved enough to follow something moving from one side of his or her face to the other. By the end of 3 months, brightly colored wall hangings or toys are favored.

Visual acuity improves with age and by the age of 2 or 3 years, it is around 20/30 or 20/20. Children are farsighted until about 5 years of age.

## ■ THE OLDER ADULT

Sensory decline alters one's perception of the world. Smells become more difficult to distinguish and detect. Eyes can need corrective lenses to adjust for decreasing ability to focus. As the ciliary muscles weaken, pupil size is decreased, reducing light to the retina. The lens becomes stiff, thicker, and more opaque and begins to yellow. These changes make the older adult sensitive to glare, and the ability to focus is impaired; therefore, **presbyopia,** or farsightedness, is common in the older adult. Night vision is impaired, and driving at night often becomes very difficult. The lens eventually can become opaque as **cataracts** develop. Vascular degeneration can affect the **retina,** which contains nerve cells for receiving images, and this condition causes permanent visual loss.

The leading cause of new cases of blindness in the older adult is age-related **macular degeneration,** a disease that affects the macula, the part of the eye that is responsible for sharp central vision. For the first time, researchers have linked gene defects to macular degeneration. The discovery could lead to the ability to identify people at high risk for the disorder and perhaps ways to treat or prevent vision loss.

# BUILDING YOUR MEDICAL VOCABULARY

This section provides the foundation for learning medical terminology. Review the following alphabetized word list. Note how common prefixes and suffixes are repeatedly applied to word roots and combining forms to create different meanings.

| | |
|---|---|
| P | Prefix |
| R | Root |
| CF | Combining form |
| S | Suffix |

| | |
|---|---|
| Pink words | Terms not built from word parts. |
| * | Indicates words covered in the Pathology Spotlights section. |
| (CD-ROM) | Check the CD-ROM for more information. |

| MEDICAL WORD | WORD PARTS (WHEN APPLICABLE) | | | DEFINITION |
|---|---|---|---|---|
| | **Part** | **Type** | **Meaning** | |
| **accommodation (Acc)** (ă-kŏm″ ō-dā′ shn) | | | | Process by which the eyes make adjustments to see objects at various distances |
| **amblyopia** (ăm″ blĭ-ō′ pĭ-ă) | ambly -opia | R S | dull vision | Dullness of vision; reduced or dimness of vision; also called *lazy eye* |
| **anisocoria** (ăn-ī″ sō-kŏ′ rĭă) | anis/o cor -ia | CF R S | unequal pupil condition | Condition in which the pupils are unequal |
| **aphakia** (ă-fā′ kĭ-ă) | a- phak -ia | P R S | lack of, without lentil, lens condition | Condition in which the crystalline lens is absent |
| **astigmatism** (ă-stĭg′ mă-tĭzm) | a- stigmat -ism | P R S | lack of, without point condition | Defect in the refractive powers of the eye in which a ray of light is not focused on the retina but is spread over an area. It is due to a misshapen curvature of the cornea and lens. |
| **bifocal** (bī-fō′ kăl) | bi- foc -al | P R S | two focus pertaining to | Pertaining to having two foci, as in bifocal glasses |
| **blepharitis** (blĕf″ ăr-ī′ tĭs) | blephar -itis | R S | eyelid inflammation | Inflammation of the hair follicles and glands along the edges of the eyelids |
| **blepharoptosis** (blĕf″ ă-rō-tō′ sĭs) | blephar/o -ptosis | CF S | eyelid prolapse, drooping | Drooping of the upper eyelid(s) |
| **cataract** (kăt″ ə răkt′) (CD-ROM) | | | | Opacity of the crystalline lens or its capsule; most often occurs in adults past middle age. See Figure 16–7 ▶. * See Pathology Spotlight: Cataract on page 549. |
| **chalazion** (kă-lā′ zĭ-ŏn) | | | | Small, hard, painless cyst of a sebaceous gland of the eyelids |
| **choroiditis** (kō″ royd-ī′ tĭs) | choroid -itis | R S | choroid inflammation | Inflammation of the vascular coat of the eye |

| MEDICAL WORD | WORD PARTS (WHEN APPLICABLE) | | | DEFINITION |
|---|---|---|---|---|
| | **Part** | **Type** | **Meaning** | |
| **conjunctivitis** (kŏn-junk″ tĭ-vi tĭs) | conjunctiv -itis | R S | to join together, conjunctiva inflammation | Inflammation of the conjunctiva caused by allergy, trauma, chemical injury, bacterial, viral, or rickettsial infection. The type called *pinkeye* is infectious and contagious. ✱ See Pathology Spotlight: Conjunctivitis on page 549. |
| **corneal** (kŏr′ nē-ăl) | corne -al | R S | cornea pertaining to | Pertaining to the cornea |
| **corneal transplant** (kŏr′ nē-ăl trăns′ plănt) | | | | Surgical process of transferring the cornea from a donor to a patient |
| **cryosurgery** (krī″ ō-sur′ jur-ē) | cry/o surgery | CF | cold surgery | Type of surgery that uses extreme cold to destroy tissue or to produce well-demarcated areas of cell injury; can be used in the removal of cataracts and in the repair of retinal detachment |
| **cycloplegia** (sī″ klō-plē′ jĭ-ă) | cycl/o -plegia | CF S | ciliary body stroke, paralysis | Paralysis of the ciliary muscle |
| **dacryoma** (dăk″ rī-ō′ mă) | dacry -oma | R S | tear, lacrimal duct, tear duct tumor | Tumorlike swelling caused by obstruction of the tear duct(s) |
| **diplopia** (dĭp-lō′ pĭ-ă) | dipl/o -opia | CF S | double sight, vision | Double vision. Note that the suffix begins with a vowel, so the "o" on the combining form dipl/o is dropped. |
| **electroretinogram** (ē-lĕk″ trō-rĕt′ ĭ-nō-grăm) | electr/o retin/o -gram | CF CF S | electricity retina mark, record | Record of the electrical response of the retina to light stimulation |
| **emmetropia (EM)** (ĕm″ ĕ-trō′ pĭ-ă) | em- metr -opia | P R S | in measure sight, vision | Normal or perfect vision. See Figure 16–8 ▶. |
| **entropion** (ĕn-trō-pē-ŏn) | en- trop -ion | P R S | in turn process | Turning inward of the margin of the lower eyelid |
| **enucleation** (ē-nū″ klē-ā′ shŭn) | enucleat -ion | R S | to remove the kernel of process | Process of removing an entire part or mass without rupture, as the eyeball from its orbit |

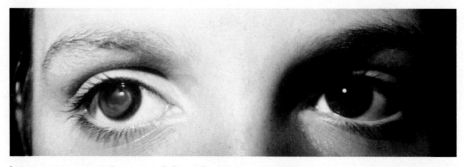

▶ FIGURE 16–7  Cataract of the right eye.

| MEDICAL WORD | WORD PARTS (WHEN APPLICABLE) | | | DEFINITION |
|---|---|---|---|---|
| | Part | Type | Meaning | |
| **esotropia (ST)**<br>(ĕs″ ō-trō′ pĭ-ă) | eso-<br>trop<br>-ia | P<br>R<br>S | inward<br>turn<br>condition | Condition in which the eye or eyes turn inward; *crossed eyes* |
| **exotropia (XT)**<br>(ĕks″ ō-trō′ pē-ă) | ex (o)-<br>trop<br>-ia | P<br>R<br>S | out<br>turn<br>condition | Turning outward of one or both eyes |
| **glaucoma**<br>(glaw-kō′ mă) | | | | Disease characterized by increased intraocular pressure, which results in atrophy of the optic nerve and blindness.<br>✷ See Pathology Spotlight: Glaucoma on page 551. |

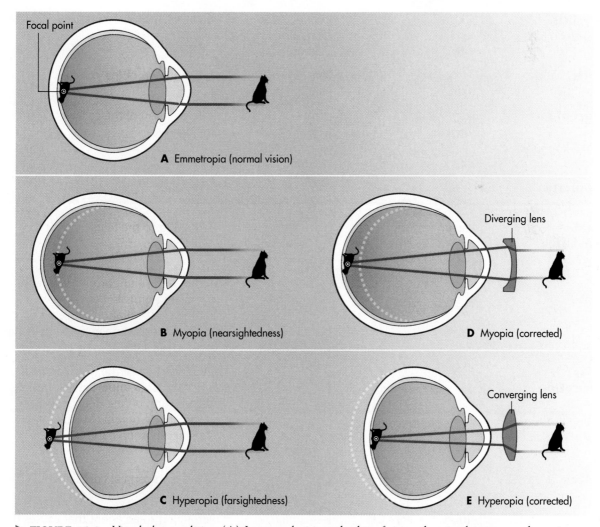

▶ **FIGURE 16–8**  Visual abnormalities. (A) In normal vision, the lens focuses the visual image on the retina. Common problems with the accommodation mechanism involve (B) myopia, the inability to lengthen the focal distance enough to focus the image of a distant object on the retina and (C) hyperopia, the inability to shorten the focal distance adequately for nearby objects. These conditions can be corrected by placing appropriately shaped lenses in front of the eyes. (D) Diverging lens is used to correct myopia and (E) converging lens is used to correct hyperopia.

| MEDICAL WORD | WORD PARTS (WHEN APPLICABLE) | | | DEFINITION |
|---|---|---|---|---|
| | Part | Type | Meaning | |
| **gonioscope**<br>(gō′ nĭ-ō-skōp) | goni/o<br>-scope | CF<br>S | angle<br>instrument for examining | Instrument used to examine the angle of the anterior chamber of the eye |
| **hemianopia**<br>(hĕm″ ē-ă-nŏ′ pē-ă) | hemi-<br>an-<br>-opia | P<br>P<br>S | half<br>lack of<br>sight, vision | Inability (blindness) to see half the field of vision |
| **hyperopia (HT)**<br>(hī″ pĕr-ō′ pĭ-ă) | hyper-<br>-opia | P<br>S | beyond<br>sight, vision | Vision defect in which parallel rays come to a focus beyond the retina; *farsightedness*. See Figure 16–8. |
| **intraocular**<br>(ĭn″ trăh-ŏk′ ū-lăr) | intra-<br>ocul<br>-ar | P<br>R<br>S | within<br>eye<br>pertaining to | Pertaining to within the eye |
| **iridectomy**<br>(ĭr″ ĭ-dĕk′ tō-mē) | irid<br>-ectomy | R<br>S | iris<br>surgical excision | Surgical excision of a portion of the iris |
| **iridocyclitis**<br>(ĭr″ ĭd-ō-sī-klī′ tĭs) | irid/o<br>cycl<br>-itis | CF<br>R<br>S | iris<br>ciliary body<br>inflammation | Inflammation of the iris and ciliary body |
| **keratitis**<br>(kĕr″ ă-tī′ tĭs) | kerat<br>-itis | R<br>S | cornea<br>inflammation | Inflammation of the cornea |
| **keratoconjunctivitis**<br>(kĕr″ ă-tō-kŏn-jŭnk″ tĭ-vī′ tĭs) | kerat/o<br>conjunctiv<br><br>-itis | CF<br>R<br><br>S | cornea<br>to join together, conjunctiva<br>inflammation | Inflammation of the cornea and the conjunctiva |
| **keratoplasty**<br>(kĕr′ ă-tō-plăs″ tē) | kerat/o<br>-plasty | CF<br>S | cornea<br>surgical repair | Surgical repair of the cornea |
| **lacrimal**<br>(lăk′ rĭm-ăl) | lacrim<br><br>-al | R<br><br>S | tear, lacrimal duct, tear duct<br>pertaining to | Pertaining to the tears |
| **laser**<br>(lā′ zĕr) | | | | Acronym for **l**ight **a**mplification by **s**timulated **e**mission of **r**adiation. ✳ See Pathology Spotlight: Glaucoma on page 551 for information about various types of laser eye surgery. |
| **macular degeneration**<br>(măk′ ū-lăr dē′ gēn-ĕr″ă-shŭn) | | | | Degeneration of the macular area of the retina, an area important in the visualization of fine details. ✳ See Pathology Spotlight: Macular Degeneration on page 552. |
| **microlens**<br>(mī′ krō-lĕns) | | | | Small, thin corneal contact lens |
| **miotic**<br>(mī-ŏt′ ĭk) | mi/o<br>-tic | CF<br>S | less, small<br>pertaining to | Pertaining to an agent that causes the pupil to contract |
| **mydriatic**<br>(mĭd″ rĭ-ăt′ ĭk) | mydriat<br>-ic | R<br>S | dilation, widen<br>pertaining to | Pertaining to an agent that causes the pupil to dilate |

| MEDICAL WORD | WORD PARTS (WHEN APPLICABLE) | | | DEFINITION |
|---|---|---|---|---|
| | Part | Type | Meaning | |
| **myopia (MY)**<br>(mī-ŏ′ pǐ-ă) | my<br>-opia | R<br>S | to shut<br>sight, vision | Vision defect in which parallel rays come to a focus in front of the retina; *nearsightedness*. See Figure 16–8. |
| **nyctalopia**<br>(nǐk″ tă-lō′ pǐ-ă) | nyctal<br>-opia | R<br>S | night<br>sight, vision | Condition in which the individual has difficulty seeing at night; *night blindness* |
| **nystagmus**<br>(nǐs-tăg′ mŭs) | | | | Involuntary, constant, rhythmic movement of the eyeball |
| **ocular**<br>(ŏk′ ū-lar) | ocul<br>-ar | R<br>S | eye<br>pertaining to | Pertaining to the eye |
| **ocular fundus**<br>(ŏk′ ū-lar fŭn-dŭs) | | | | Posterior inner part of the eye as seen with an ophthalmoscope |
| **ophthalmologist**<br>(ŏf″ thăl-mŏl′ ō-jǐst) | ophthalm/o<br>log<br>-ist | CF<br>R<br>S | eye<br>study of<br>one who specializes | Physician who specializes in the study of the eye |
| **ophthalmology**<br>(ŏf″ thăl-mŏl′ ō-jē) | ophthalm/o<br>-logy | CF<br>S | eye<br>study of | Study of the eye |
| **ophthalmoscope**<br>(ŏf″ thăl′ mō-skōp) | ophthalm/o<br>-scope | CF<br>S | eye<br>instrument for examining | Instrument used to examine the interior of the eye. See Figure 16–9 ▼. |
| **optic**<br>(op′ tǐk) | opt<br>-ic | R<br>S | eye<br>pertaining to | Pertaining to the eye |

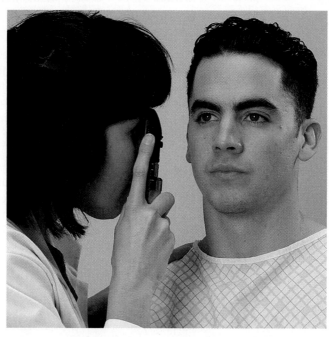

▶ FIGURE 16–9   Use of an ophthalmoscope to examine the interior of the eye.

| MEDICAL WORD | WORD PARTS (WHEN APPLICABLE) | | | DEFINITION |
|---|---|---|---|---|
| | Part | Type | Meaning | |
| **optician**<br>(ŏp-tĭsh′ ăn) | | | | One who specializes in making optical products and accessories. This person is not a physician. |
| **optometrist**<br>(ŏp-tŏm′ ĕ-trĭst) | opt/o<br>metr<br>-ist | CF<br>R<br>S | eye<br>measure<br>one who specializes | One who specializes in examining the eyes for refractive errors and providing appropriate corrective lenses. This person is not a physician but is trained and licensed as a doctor of optometry (OD). |
| **optomyometer**<br>(ŏp″ tō-mī-ŏm′ ĕt-ĕr) | opt/o<br>my/o<br>-meter | CF<br>CF<br>S | eye<br>muscle<br>instrument to measure | Instrument used to measure the strength of the muscles of the eye |
| **orthoptics**<br>(or-thŏp′ tĭks) | orth<br>opt<br>-ic (s) | R<br>R<br>S | straight<br>eye<br>pertaining to | Study and treatment of defective binocular vision resulting from defects in ocular musculature; also a technique of eye exercises for correcting defective binocular vision |
| **phacoemul-sification**<br>(făk″ ō-ē′ mŭl′ sĭ-fĭ-kā″ shŭn) | phac/o<br>emulsificat<br>-ion | CF<br>R<br>S | lens<br>disintegrate<br>process | Process of using ultrasound to disintegrate a cataract by inserting a needle through a small incision and aspirating the disintegrated cataract |
| **phacolysis**<br>(făk-ŏl″ ĭ-sĭs) | phac/o<br>-lysis | CF<br>S | lens<br>destruction, to separate | Surgical destruction and removal of the crystalline lens in the treatment of cataract |
| **phacosclerosis**<br>(făk″ ō-sklĕr-ō′ sĭs) | phac/o<br>scler<br>-osis | CF<br>R<br>S | lens<br>hardening<br>condition (usually abnormal) | Condition of hardening of the crystalline lens |
| **photocoagulation**<br>(fō″ tō-kō-ăg″ ū-lā′ shŭn) | phot/o<br>coagulat<br>-ion | CF<br>R<br>S | light<br>to clot<br>process | Process of altering proteins in tissue by the use of light energy such as the laser beam; used to treat retinal detachment, retinal bleeding, intraocular tumors, and/or macular degeneration (wet) |
| **photophobia**<br>(fō″ tō-fō′ bĭ-ă) | phot/o<br>-phobia | CF<br>S | light<br>fear | Unusual intolerance of light |
| **presbyopia**<br>(prĕz″ bĭ-ō′ pĭ-ă) | presby<br>-opia | R<br>S | old<br>sight, vision | Vision defect in which parallel rays come to a focus beyond the retina; occurs normally with aging; *farsightedness* |
| **pupillary**<br>(pū′ pĭ-lĕr-ē) | pupill<br>-ary | R<br>S | pupil<br>pertaining to | Pertaining to the pupil |
| **radial keratotomy**<br>(rā′ dē-ăl kĕr-ă′ tŏt′ ō-mē) | rad/i<br><br>-al<br>kerat/o<br>-tomy | CF<br><br>S<br>CF<br>S | radiating out from a center<br>pertaining to<br>cornea<br>incision | Surgical procedure that can be performed to correct nearsightedness *(myopia)*. Delicate spokelike incisions are made in the cornea to flatten it, thereby shortening the eyeball so that light reaches the retina. Vision is not improved for all patients, and complications could lead to blindness. |

| MEDICAL WORD | WORD PARTS (WHEN APPLICABLE) | | | DEFINITION |
|---|---|---|---|---|
| | Part | Type | Meaning | |
| **retinal detachment**<br>(rĕt′ ĭ-năl dē-tăch′mĕnt) | | | | Separation of the retina from the choroid layer of the eye that can be caused by trauma or can occur spontaneously. See Figure 16–10 ▼. |
| **retinitis**<br>(rĕt″ ĭ-nī′ tĭs) | retin<br>-itis | R<br>S | retina<br>inflammation | Inflammation of the retina |
| **retinitis pigmentosa**<br>(rĕt″ ĭ-nī′ tĭs pĭg″ mĕnt′ ŏsă) | | | | Chronic progressive disease marked by bilateral primary degeneration of the retina beginning in childhood and leading to blindness by middle age. Night blindness and a reduced field of vision are early clinical signs of this disease. |
| **retinoblastoma**<br>(rĕt″ ĭ-nō-blăs-tō′ mă) | retin/o<br>-blast<br>-oma | CF<br>S<br>S | retina<br>germ cell<br>tumor | Malignant tumor arising from the germ cell of the retina |
| **retinopathy**<br>(rĕt″ ĭn-ŏp′ ă-thē) | retin/o<br>-pathy | CF<br>S | retina<br>disease | Any disease of the retina. In the United States, *diabetic retinopathy* is the leading cause of new blindness in people age 20 to 74. See Figure 16–11 ▼. |
| **retrolental fibroplasia (RLF)**<br>(rĕt″ rō-lĕn-tăl fĭ-brō-plā-sē-ă) | retro-<br>lent<br>-al<br>fibr/o<br>-plasia | P<br>R<br>S<br>CF<br>S | behind<br>lens<br>pertaining to<br>fiber<br>formation | Disease of the retinal vessels present in premature infants; can be caused by excessive use of oxygen in the incubator; can cause retinal detachment and blindness |
| **scleritis**<br>(sklē-rī′ tĭs) | scler<br>-itis | R<br>S | sclera<br>inflammation | Inflammation of the sclera |

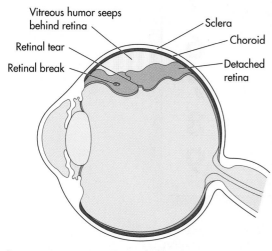

Vitreous humor seeps behind retina
Retinal tear
Retinal break
Sclera
Choroid
Detached retina

▶ FIGURE 16–10  Retinal detachment.

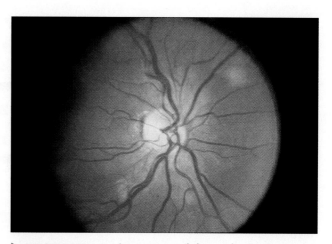

▶ FIGURE 16–11  Appearance of the ocular fundus in diabetic retinopathy. (Courtesy of the National Eye Institute, National Institutes of Health)

| MEDICAL WORD | WORD PARTS (WHEN APPLICABLE) | | | DEFINITION |
|---|---|---|---|---|
| | Part | Type | Meaning | |
| **Snellen chart** (sněl' ěn chart) | | | | Chart for testing visual acuity. It is printed with lines of black letters that are graduated in size from smallest, on the bottom to largest on the top. See Figure 16–12 ▼. |
| **strabismus** (stră-bĭz' mŭs) | strabism -us | R S | a squinting structure | Disorder of the eye in which the optic axes cannot be directed to the same object; also called a *squint* |
| **sty(e)** (stī) | | | | Inflammation of one or more of the sebaceous glands of the eyelid; also called a *hordeolum* |
| **tonography** (tō-nŏg' ră-fē) | ton/o -graphy | CF S | tone recording | Recording of intraocular pressure used in detecting glaucoma |

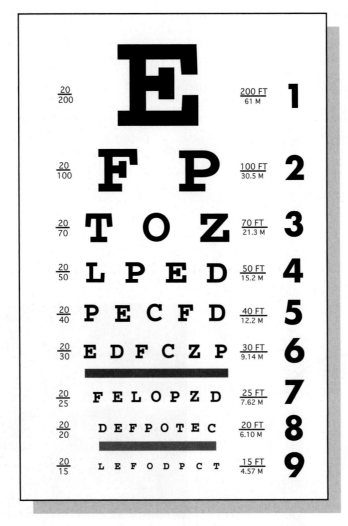

▶ FIGURE 16–12  Snellen eye chart. Individuals with normal vision can read line 8 of a full-sized chart at 20 feet (6.10 m).

| MEDICAL WORD | WORD PARTS (WHEN APPLICABLE) | | | DEFINITION |
|---|---|---|---|---|
| | **Part** | **Type** | **Meaning** | |
| **tonometer**<br>(tŏn-ŏm′ ĕ-tĕr) | ton/o<br>-meter | CF<br>S | tone<br>instrument to<br>measure | Instrument used to measure intraocular pressure. See Figure 16–13 ▼. |
| **trichiasis**<br>(trĭk-ī′ ăs-ĭs) | trich<br>-iasis | R<br>S | hair<br>condition | Condition of ingrowing eyelashes that rub against the cornea, causing a constant irritation to the eyeball |
| **trifocal**<br>(trĭ-fō′ căl) | tri-<br>foc<br>-al | P<br>R<br>S | three<br>focus<br>pertaining to | Pertaining to having three foci |
| **uveal**<br>(ū′ vē-ăl) | uve<br>-al | R<br>S | uvea<br>pertaining to | Pertaining to the second or vascular coat of the eye |
| **uveitis**<br>(ū-vē-ī′ tĭs) | uve<br>-itis | R<br>S | uvea<br>inflammation | Inflammation of the uvea (consists of the iris, ciliary body, and choroid, and forms the pigmented layer) |
| **xenophthalmia**<br>(zĕn″ ŏf-thăl′ mē-ă) | xen<br>ophthalm<br>-ia | R<br>R<br>S | foreign material<br>eye<br>condition | Inflamed eye condition caused by foreign material |
| **xerophthalmia**<br>(zē-rŏf-thăl′ mē-ă) | xer<br>ophthalm<br>-ia | R<br>R<br>S | dry<br>eye<br>condition | Eye condition in which the conjunctiva is dry |

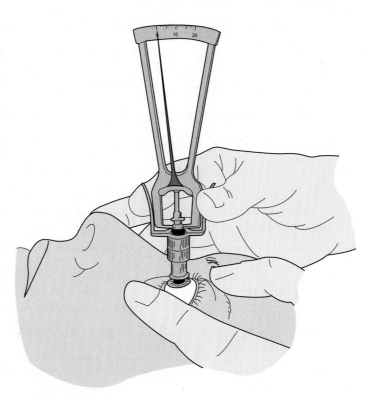

▶ **FIGURE 16–13**   Schiötz tonometer for measuring intraocular pressure.

# DRUG HIGHLIGHTS

| | |
|---|---|
| **Drugs used to treat glaucoma** | Either increase the outflow of aqueous humor, decrease its production, or produce both of these actions. |
| Prostaglandin analogues | Work by increasing the drainage of intraocular fluid, thereby decreasing intraocular pressure. |
| | *Examples: Travatan (travoprost ophthalmic solution 0.004%), Lumigan (bimatoprost ophthalmic solution 0.03%), and Xalatan (latanoprost)* |
| Adrenergic drugs | Increase drainage of intraocular fluid. |
| | *Examples: Epifin sterile ophthalmic solution and Propine ophthalmic solution, USP, 0.1% (epinephrine), and Dipivefin ophthalmic solution USP, 0.1%* |
| Alpha antagonist | Works both to decrease production of fluid and increase drainage. |
| | *Example: Alphagan (brimonide tartrate ophthalmic solution 0.2%)* |
| Beta blockers | Decrease production of intraocular fluid. |
| | *Examples: Akbeta (levobunolol HCl ophthalmic solution, USP), Carteleolo HCl (carteolo HCl ophthalmic solution), Timolol Maleate, Betoptic S (betaxolol HCl 0.25%), Betaxon (levobetaxolo ophthalmic suspension 0.5%), Betagan Liquifilm Sterile Ophthalmic Solution (levobunolol), OptiPranolol (metipranolol), Timoptic-XE (timolol maleate ophthalmic gel forming solution), Betimol (timolol hemihydrate), and Ocupress (carteolol HCl)* |
| Carbonic anhydrase inhibitors | Decrease production of intraocular fluid. |
| | *Examples: Azopt (brinzolamide ophthalmic suspension 1%), Diamox Sequels Sustained Release Capsules (acetazolomide), Trusopt (dorzolamide), and Neptazane (methazolamide)* |
| Cholinergic (miotic) | Increases drainage of intraocular fluid. |
| | *Examples: Ocusert Pilo-20 and Pilo-40 Ocular Therapeutic Systems (pilocarpine), and Pilocarpine HCl Ophthalmic Solution* |
| Cholinesterase | Increases drainage of intraocular fluid. |
| | *Example: Phospholine Iodide (echothiophate)* |
| Combination of beta blocker and carbonic anhydrase inhibitor | Decreases production of intraocular fluid. |
| | *Example: Cosopt (dorzolomide HCl timolol maleate ophthalmic solution)* |
| **Mydriatics** | Agents used to dilate the pupil (mydriasis) can be anticholinergics or sympathomimetics. |
| Anticholinergics | Dilate the pupil and interfere with the ability of the eye to focus properly (cycloplegia). They are used primarily as an aid in refraction, during internal examination of the eye, in intraocular surgery, and in the treatment of anterior uveitis and secondary glaucomas. |
| | *Examples: Atropisol (atropine sulfate), Hyoscine (scopolamine HBr), Mydriacyl (tropicamide)* |
| Sympathomimetics | Produce mydriasis without cycloplegia. Pupil dilation is obtained as the drug causes contraction of the dilator muscle of the iris. They also affect intraocular pressure by decreasing production of aqueous humor while increasing its outflow from the eye. |
| | *Examples: Propine (dipivefrin HCl), Naphcon (naphazoline HCl), Glaucon (epinephrine HCl), and neosynephrine (phenylephrine HCl)* |
| **Antibiotics** | Used to treat infectious diseases. Those used for the eye can be in the form of an ointment, cream, or solution. |
| | *Examples: Aureomycin Ophthalmic (chlortetracycline HCl) ointment 1%, erythromycin, bacitracin, tetracycline HCl, chloramphenicol, and polymyxin B sulfate* |

| | |
|---|---|
| Antifungal agent | *Natacyn (natamycin)* is used to treat fungal infections of the eye, such as blepharitis, conjunctivitis, and keratitis. |
| Antiviral agents | *Stoxil and Herplex (idoxuridine)* are potent antiviral agents used to treat keratitis caused by the herpes simplex virus. *Vira-A (vidarabine) and Viroptic (trifluridine)* are also used to treat viral infections of the eye and are effective in the treatment of herpes simplex infections. |

# DIAGNOSTIC AND LAB TESTS

| TEST | DESCRIPTION |
|---|---|
| **Color vision tests** | Use of polychromatic (multicolored) charts or an *anomaloscope* (a device for detecting color blindness) to assess an individual's ability to recognize differences in color. See Figure 16–14 ▼. |
| **Exophthalmometry** (ĕk″ sŏf-thăl-mŏm′ ĕ-tre) | Process of measuring the forward protrusion of the eye via an exophthalmometer; used to evaluate an increase or decrease in *exophthalmos* (abnormal protrusion of the eyeball). |
| **Gonioscopy** (gō″ nē-ŏs′ kō-pē) | Examination of the anterior chamber of the eye via a gonioscope; used for determining ocular motility and rotation. |
| **Keratometry** (kĕr″ ă-tŏm′ ĕ-trē) | Process of measuring the cornea via a keratometer. |
| **Ocular ultrasonography** (ŏk′ ū lăr ŭl-tră-sŏn-ŏg ră-fē) | Use of high-frequency sound waves (via a small probe placed on the eye) to measure for intraocular lenses (IOL) and to detect orbital and periorbital lesions; also used to measure the length of the eye and the curvature of the cornea in preparation for surgery. |
| **Ophthalmoscopy** (ŏf-thăl-mŏs′ kō-pē) | Examination of the interior of the eyes via an ophthalmoscope; used to identify changes in the blood vessels in the eye and to diagnose systemic diseases. |

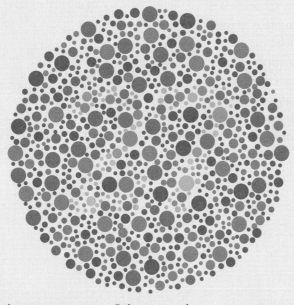

▶ **FIGURE 16–14**   Color vision chart.

| TEST | DESCRIPTION |
|------|-------------|
| **Tonometry** (tŏn-ŏm′ ĕ-trē) | Measurement of the intraocular pressure (IOP) of the eye via a tonometer; used to screen for and detect glaucoma. See Figure 16–13. |
| **Visual acuity (VA)** (vĭzh′ ū-ăl ă-kū′ ĭ-tē) | Acuteness or sharpness of vision. A Snellen eye chart can be used to test it; the patient reads letters of various sizes from a distance of 20 feet. Normal vision is 20/20. See Figure 16–15 ▼. |

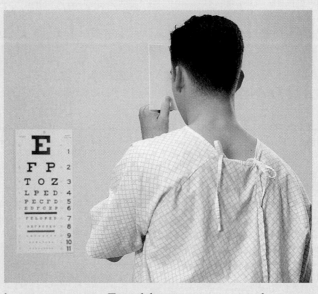

▶ **FIGURE 16–15** Test of distance vision using the Snellen eye chart.

# ABBREVIATIONS

| ABBREVIATION | MEANING | ABBREVIATION | MEANING |
|:------------:|---------|:------------:|---------|
| Acc | accommodation | RLF | retrolental fibroplasia |
| ALT | argon laser trabeculoplasty | RPE | retinal pigment epithelium |
| EM | emmetropia | SLT | selective laser trabeculoplasty |
| HT | hyperopia | ST | esotropia |
| IOL | intraocular lens | STDs | sexually transmitted diseases |
| IOP | intraocular pressure | VA | visual acuity |
| LPI | laser peripheral iridotomy | VF | visual field |
| MY | myopia | XT | exotropia |

# PATHOLOGY SPOTLIGHTS

## ✳ Cataract

A **cataract** is a clouding of the eye's lens. In its early stages, a cataract could cause no problems. The cloudiness can affect only a small part of the lens. However, over time, the cataract can grow and cloud more of the lens, making it more difficult to see. Because less light reaches the retina, the patient's vision can become dull and blurry. A cataract will not spread from one eye to the other, although many people develop cataracts in both eyes.

Following are the different types of cataracts:

- **Age-related cataract.** Most cataracts are related to aging. More than half of all Americans age 65 and older have a cataract.
- **Congenital cataract.** Some babies are born with cataracts or develop them in childhood, often in both eyes. These cataracts do not necessarily affect vision, but if they do, they can need to be removed.
- **Secondary cataract.** Cataracts are more likely to develop in people who have certain other health problems, such as diabetes. Also, cataracts are sometimes linked to steroid use.
- **Traumatic cataract.** Cataracts can develop soon after an eye injury or years later.

Although researchers are learning more about cataracts, no one knows for sure what causes them. Scientists think there could be several causes, including smoking, diabetes, and excessive exposure to sunlight.

The most common symptoms of a cataract follow:

- Cloudy or blurry vision.
- Problems with light, including headlights that seem too bright at night; glare from lamps or very bright sunlight; and seeing a halo around lights.
- Colors that seem faded.
- Poor night vision.
- Double or multiple vision.
- Frequent need for changes in eyeglass or contact lens prescription.

With an early cataract, vision can improve by using different eyeglasses, magnifying lenses, or stronger lighting. If these measures do not help, surgery is the only effective treatment. The most common surgery to remove a cataract is **phacoemulsification.**

Cataract removal is one of the most common operations performed in the United States today. It is also one of the safest and most effective. In about 90% of cases, people who have cataract surgery have better vision afterward. See Figure 16–16 ▶.

## ✳ Conjunctivitis

**Conjunctivitis,** often called *pinkeye,* is an inflammation of the conjunctiva, the tissue that lines the inside of the eyelid and helps keep the eyelid and eyeball moist. It is one of the most common and treatable eye infections in children and adults.

Conjunctivitis can be caused by a virus, bacteria, irritating substances (shampoos, dirt, smoke, and, especially, pool chlorine), allergens (substances that cause allergies), or sexually transmitted diseases (STDs). Types of pinkeye caused by bacteria, viruses, and STDs can spread easily from person to person but are not a serious health risk if diagnosed promptly.

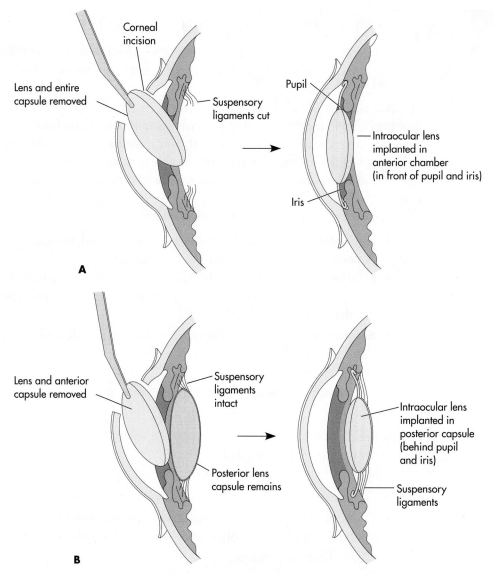

Corneal
incision

Lens and entire
capsule removed

Suspensory
ligaments cut

Pupil

Intraocular lens
implanted in
anterior chamber
(in front of pupil and iris)

Iris

**A**

Lens and anterior
capsule removed

Suspensory
ligaments
intact

Posterior lens
capsule remains

Intraocular lens
implanted in
posterior capsule
(behind pupil
and iris)

Suspensory
ligaments

**B**

▶ **FIGURE 16–16** Cataract removal with intraocular lens implant. (A) Intracapsular cataract extraction with removal of the entire lens and capsule. The intraocular lens is implanted in the eye's anterior chamber. (B) Extracapsular cataract extraction with removal of the lens and anterior capsule, leaving the posterior capsule intact. The intraocular lens is implanted within posterior capsule.

Following are the symptoms of conjunctivitis:

- Redness in the white of the eye or inner eyelid.
- Increased amount of tears.
- Thick yellow discharge that crusts over the eyelashes, especially after sleep (with conjunctivitis caused by bacteria).
- Other discharge (green or white) from the eyes.
- Itchy eyes (especially with conjunctivitis caused by allergies).
- Burning eyes (especially with conjunctivitis caused by chemicals and irritants).
- Blurred vision.
- Increased sensitivity to light.

An ophthalmologist or family physician diagnoses conjunctivitis by conducting an eye exam and perhaps taking a sample of fluid from the eyelid using a cotton swab. Bacteria or viruses that could have caused conjunctivitis, including STDs, can then be seen through a microscope.

Treatment is based on the cause. For example, antibiotic eye drops or ointments are used for conjunctivitis caused by a bacterial infection. If topical antibiotics do not solve the problem, oral antibiotics are used. Eye drops containing antihistamines, nonsteroidal anti-inflammatory agents, or corticosteroids are used if allergies are the cause. If foreign matter has caused the inflammation, it is removed.

## ⋆ Glaucoma

**Glaucoma** is a group of eye diseases characterized by *increased intraocular pressure* (IOP). See Figure 16–13 on page 545. The three major categories of glaucoma are closed-angle (acute), open-angle (chronic), and congenital glaucoma. See Figure 16–17 ▼. Glaucoma occurs when the aqueous humor is blocked and drains too slowly from the anterior chamber. This causes a buildup of intraocular pressure that is too high for the proper functioning of the optic nerve. When glaucoma is diagnosed early and managed properly, blindness can be prevented.

Glaucoma affects people of all ages and all races with an increased predisposition in those of African ancestry. Most patients have no symptoms from glaucoma; therefore, it is important to know the factors that predispose someone to glaucoma:

- Age of 60 years or more.
- African ancestry.
- Family member with glaucoma or diabetes.
- Previous eye injury.
- Use of steroid medication.
- Myopia.
- Thyroid disease.
- Diabetes.
- Hypertension.

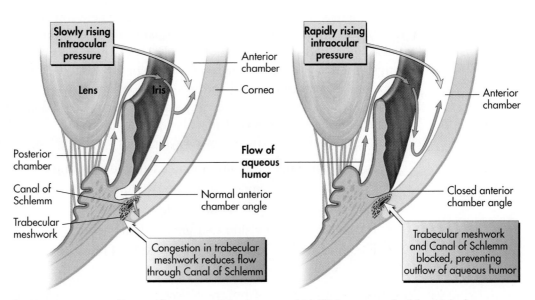

▶ **FIGURE 16–17**   Forms of primary adult glaucoma: (A) With open-angle (chronic) glaucoma, the anterior chamber angle remains open, but drainage of aqueous humor through the canal of Schlemm is impaired. (B) With closed-angle (acute) glaucoma, the angle of the iris and anterior chamber narrows, obstructing the outflow of aqueous humor.

Laser surgery can be used to treat glaucoma, including the following types:

1. Laser peripheral iridotomy (LPI) by which a small hole is made in the iris to allow it to fall back from the fluid channel and help the fluid drain.

2. Argon laser trabeculoplasty (ALT) by which a laser beam opens the fluid channels of the eye, helping the drainage system to work better.

3. Selective laser trabeculoplasty (SLT), a type of laser surgery that uses a combination of frequencies allowing the laser to work at very low levels. It treats specific cells selectively and leaves untreated portions of the trabecular meshwork (the meshlike drainage canals surrounding the iris) intact.

4. When medication and/or laser surgery does not lower the intraocular pressure of the eye, the doctor could recommend a procedure called *filtering microsurgery*. This procedure makes a tiny drainage hole in the sclera (*sclerostomy*). The new drainage hole allows fluid to flow out of the eye and thereby helps lower eye pressure. This prevents or reduces damage to the optic nerve.

 ## ✱ Macular Degeneration

**Macular degeneration** is an incurable eye disease that affects more than 10 million Americans. It is the leading cause of blindness for those ages 55 and older. Macular degeneration is caused by the deterioration of the central portion of the retina, the inside back layer of the eye that records the images a person sees and sends them via the optic nerve from the eye to the brain. The retina's central portion, known as *the macula*, is responsible for focusing central vision in the eye, and it controls the ability to read, drive a car, recognize faces or colors, and see objects in fine detail.

The two basic types of macular degeneration are dry and wet. Approximately 85% to 90% of the cases of macular degeneration are the dry (atrophic) type. In the dry type of macular degeneration, the deterioration of the retina is associated with the formation of small yellow deposits, known as *drusen*, under the macula. This phenomenon leads to a thinning and drying out of the macula. The amount of central vision loss is directly related to the location and amount of retinal thinning caused by the drusen. There is no known treatment or cure for the dry type of macular degeneration.

Approximately 10% of the cases of macular degeneration are the wet (exudative) type. In this type of macular degeneration, abnormal blood vessels (known as *subretinal neovascularization*) grow under the retina and macula. These new blood vessels can then bleed and leak fluid, thereby causing the macula to bulge or lift up, thus distorting or destroying central vision. This can cause rapid and severe vision loss. If vision is to be saved, immediate laser surgery should be done in the early stages of wet macular degeneration.

The signs and symptoms of macular degeneration vary depending on the type. Dry macular degeneration has the following symptoms:

- Increasingly bright illumination needed when reading or doing close work.
- Printed words that appear increasingly blurry.
- Colors that seem washed out and dull.
- Haziness of overall vision that gradually increases.
- Profound drop in central vision caused by a blind spot in the center of the visual field (VF).

With wet macular degeneration, the following symptoms can appear rapidly:

- Visual distortions, such as straight lines appearing wavy or crooked.
- Decreased central vision.
- Central blurry spot.

**Stargardt's disease,** also known as *juvenile macular degeneration*, is an inherited disease that affects 1 in 10,000 people. It usually manifests itself between the ages of 7 and 12. Scientists' current theory is that Stargardt's disease causes the eye's central vision to deteriorate because the rod cells just outside the macula erode, which eventually harms the retinal pigment epithelium (RPE). As the RPE fails, the disease can spread to the macula's cone cells, causing macular degeneration's characteristic loss of central vision. Vision loss is usually slow until the 20/40 level and then rapidly progresses to the 20/200 level. Unfortunately, in some cases, vision can degenerate to 10/200 in a period of months. Peripheral vision generally remains.

Presently there is no cure for Stargardt's disease, nor has any treatment been proven to improve visual loss or to retard the progression of the disease.

# ✓ PATHOLOGY CHECKPOINT

*Following is a concise list of the pathology-related terms that you have seen in the chapter. Review this checklist to make sure that you are familiar with the meaning of each term before moving to the next section.*

## Conditions and Symptoms

- ❏ amblyopia
- ❏ anisocoria
- ❏ aphakia
- ❏ astigmatism
- ❏ blepharitis
- ❏ blepharoptosis
- ❏ cataract
- ❏ chalazion
- ❏ choroiditis
- ❏ conjunctivitis
- ❏ cycloplegia
- ❏ dacryoma
- ❏ diplopia
- ❏ entropion
- ❏ esotropia
- ❏ exotropia
- ❏ glaucoma
- ❏ hemianopia
- ❏ hyperopia
- ❏ iridocyclitis
- ❏ keratitis
- ❏ keratoconjunctivitis
- ❏ macular degeneration

- ❏ myopia
- ❏ nyctalopia
- ❏ nystagmus
- ❏ phacosclerosis
- ❏ photophobia
- ❏ presbyopia
- ❏ retinal detachment
- ❏ retinitis
- ❏ retinitis pigmentosa
- ❏ retinoblastoma
- ❏ retinopathy
- ❏ retrolental fibroplasia
- ❏ scleritis
- ❏ Stargardt's disease
- ❏ strabismus
- ❏ sty(e)
- ❏ trichiasis
- ❏ uveitis
- ❏ xenophthalmia
- ❏ xerophthalmia

## Diagnosis and Treatment

- ❏ bifocal
- ❏ corneal transplant

- ❏ cryosurgery
- ❏ electroretinogram
- ❏ enucleation
- ❏ gonioscope
- ❏ iridectomy
- ❏ keratoplasty
- ❏ laser
- ❏ microlens
- ❏ miotic
- ❏ mydriatic
- ❏ ophthalmoscope
- ❏ optomyometer
- ❏ orthoptics
- ❏ phacoemulsification
- ❏ phacolysis
- ❏ photocoagulation
- ❏ radial keratotomy
- ❏ Snellen chart
- ❏ tonography
- ❏ tonometer
- ❏ trifocal

# STUDY AND REVIEW

*Write your answers to the following questions. Do not refer to the text.*

1. The external structures of the eye are the _____, _____,

    _____, _____, and the _____ _____.

2. The orbit is lined with _____ _____, which cushions the eye-ball.

3. The optic foramen is an opening for the _____ _____ and

    _____ _____.

4. State the functions of the muscles of the eye.

    a. _____

    b. _____

5. Each eye has a pair of eyelids that function to protect the eyeball from

    _____ _____, _____ _____, and

    _____.

6. Describe the conjunctiva and state its function. _____

    _____

7. Define *lacrimal apparatus*. _____

    _____

8. The internal structures of the eye are the _____, _____, and
    the _____ _____.

9. The eyeball is the organ of _____.

10. The point at which nerve fibers from the retina converge to form the optic nerve
    is known as the _____ _____.

11. Define *accommodation*. _____

    _____

12. Match the following terms and definitions by placing the correct letter on the line provided.

_____ 1. aqueous humor

_____ 2. vitreous humor

_____ 3. iris

_____ 4. sclera

_____ 5. uvea

_____ 6. pupil

_____ 7. retina

_____ 8. rods and cones

_____ 9. lens

_____ 10. cornea

a. White of the eye
b. Colored membrane attached to the ciliary body
c. Watery fluid
d. Opening in the center of the iris
e. Jelly-like material
f. Middle layer of the eyeball
g. Anterior transparent portion of the eyeball
h. Innermost layer of the eyeball
i. Photoreceptive cells
j. Colorless crystalline body

## Word Parts

1. In the spaces provided, write the definitions for the following prefixes, roots, combining forms, and suffixes. Do not refer to the listings of medical words. Leave blank those words you cannot define.

2. After completing as many as you can, refer to the medical word listings to check your work. For each word missed or left blank, write the word and its definition several times on the margins of these pages or on a separate sheet of paper.

3. To maximize the learning process, it is to your advantage to do the following exercises as directed. To refer to the word-building section before completing these exercises invalidates the learning process.

## PREFIXES

*Give the definitions of the following prefixes.*

1. a- _____

2. bi- _____

3. en- _____

4. em- _____

5. eso- _____

6. hyper- _____

7. intra- _____

8. tri- _____

9. ex(o)- _____

10. hemi- _____

11. an- _____

12. retro- _____

## ROOTS AND COMBINING FORMS

*Give the definitions of the following roots and combining forms.*

1. ambly _____

2. conjunctiv _____

3. anis/o _____

4. blephar _____

5. blephar/o _____

6. choroid _____

7. cry/o _____

8. cor _____

9. corne _____

10. cycl _____

11. cycl/o _____

12. enucleat _____

13. dacry _____

14. mi/o _____

15. electr/o _____

16. foc _____

17. goni/o _____

18. irid _____

19. irid/o _____

20. kerat _____

21. kerat/o _____

22. lacrim _____

23. log _____

24. metr _____

25. my _____

26. my/o _____

27. nyctal _____

28. ocul _____

29. ophthalm _____

30. ophthalm/o _____

31. opt _____

32. opt/o _____

33. phac/o _____

34. phak _____

35. phot/o _____

36. presby _____

37. pupill _____

38. retin _____

39. retin/o _____

40. scler _____

41. stigmat _____

42. ton/o _____

43. trop _____

44. uve _____

45. xen _____

46. xer _____

47. mydriat _____

48. orth _____

49. emulsificat _____

50. coagulat _____

51. rad/i _____

52. lent _____

53. fibr/o _____

54. strabism _____

55. trich _____

## SUFFIXES

*Give the definitions of the following suffixes.*

1. -al _____

2. -ar _____

3. -ary _____

4. -blast _____

5. -iasis _____

6. -ectomy _____

7. -gram _____

8. -graphy _____

9. -ia _____

10. -ic _____

11. -ion _____

12. -ism _____

13. -ist _____

14. -itis _____

15. -logy _____

16. -lysis _____

17. -plasia _____

18. -meter _____

19. -oma _____

20. -opia _____

21. -osis _____

22. -pathy _____

23. -phobia _____

24. -plasty _____

25. -plegia _____

26. -ptosis _____

27. -scope _____

28. -tic _____

29. -tomy _____

30. -us _____

## Identifying Medical Terms

*In the spaces provided, write the medical terms for the following meanings.*

1. _____ Dullness of vision

2. _____ Pertaining to having two foci

3. _____ Drooping of the upper eyelid

4. _____ Pertaining to the cornea

5. _____ Tumorlike swelling caused by obstruction of the tear duct

6. _____ Double vision

7. _____ Normal or perfect vision

8. _____ Pertaining to within the eye

9. _____ Inflammation of the cornea

10. _____ Surgical repair of the cornea

11. _____ Pertaining to tears

12. _____ Pertaining to the eye

13. _____ Unusual intolerance of light

## Spelling

*In the spaces provided, write the correct spelling of these misspelled words.*

1. atigmatism _____

2. cyloplegia _____

3. irdectomy _____

4. opthalmologist _____

5. pacosclerosis _____

6. pupilary _____

7. retinblastoma _____

8. sleritis _____

9. tonmeter _____

10. ueal _____

## Matching

*Select the appropriate lettered meaning for each of the following words.*

_____ 1. anomaloscope

_____ 2. entropion

_____ 3. cataract

_____ 4. hemianopia

_____ 5. phacoemulsification

_____ 6. photocoagulation

_____ 7. radial keratotomy

_____ 8. retrolental fibroplasia

_____ 9. strabismus

_____ 10. sty(e)

a. Squint

b. Disease of the retinal vessels present in premature infants

c. Process of using ultrasound to disintegrate a cataract

d. Use of a laser to treat retinal detachment and/or retinal bleeding

e. Device used to detect color blindness

f. Turning inward of the margin of the lower eyelid

g. Surgical procedure performed to correct myopia

h. Inability to see half of the field of vision

i. *Hordeolum*

j. Opacity of the crystalline lens or its capsule

k. Disease characterized by increased intraocular pressure

## Abbreviations

*Place the correct word, phrase, or abbreviation in the space provided.*

1. accommodation _____

2. EM _____

3. HT _____

4. intraocular lens _____

5. esotropia _____

6. MY _____

7. VA _____

8. IOP _____

9. visual field _____

10. XT _____

## Diagnostic and Laboratory Tests

*Select the best answer to each multiple choice question. Circle the letter of your choice.*

1. Process of measuring the forward protrusion of the eye.
   a. gonioscopy
   b. keratometry
   c. exophthalmometry
   d. tonometry

2. Process of measuring the cornea.
   a. gonioscopy
   b. keratometry
   c. exophthalmometry
   d. tonometry

3. Used to identify changes in the blood vessels in the eye and to diagnose systemic diseases.
   a. exophthalmometry
   b. gonioscopy
   c. ophthalmoscopy
   d. tonometry

4. Process of measuring the intraocular pressure of the eye.
   a. exophthalmometry
   b. gonioscopy
   c. ophthalmoscopy
   d. tonometry

5. Process used to measure the acuteness or sharpness of vision.
   a. color vision tests
   b. ultrasonography
   c. tonometry
   d. visual acuity

# PRACTICAL APPLICATION

## S O A P : Chart Note Analysis

*This exercise will make you aware of information, abbreviations, and medical terminology typically found in the chart of a patient who saw his primary care physician and was referred to an ophthalmologist.*

### Abbreviations Key

| | | | |
|---|---|---|---|
| **BP** | blood pressure | **P** | pulse |
| **c/o** | complains of | **PERRLA** | pupils equal, round, react to light and accommodation |
| **CTA** | clear to auscultation | | |
| **DOB** | date of birth | **phaco** | phacoemulsification |
| **EOM** | extra ocular movement | **R** | respiration |
| **F** | Fahrenheit | **SOAP** | subjective, objective, assessment, plan |
| **HEENT** | head, eyes, ears, nose, throat | | |
| **Ht** | height | **T** | temperature |
| **IOL** | intraocular lens | **TM** | tympanic membrane |
| **lb** | pound | **Wt** | weight |
| **NKDA** | no known drug allergies | **y/o** | year(s) old |

*Read the following chart note and then answer the questions that follow.*

**PATIENT:** Black, Edward E.                                                                                                   **DATE:** 7/29/07
**DOB:** 6/26/40     **AGE:** 67     **SEX:** Male
**INSURANCE:** 21st Century Health Co.

> **Vital Signs:**
> T: 98.6 F
> P: 82
> R: 20
> BP: 128/82
> Ht: 5' 11"
> Wt: 189 lb

**Allergies:** NKDA

**Chief Complaint:** Trouble driving at night, photophobia, blurred vision, feels like there is a film over his eyes, sees halos around lights.

**S** | **Subjective:** 67 y/o white male presents with "trouble driving at night." States "bright lights hurt my eyes." He c/o blurred vision while watching television and feels his glasses are dirty. Also, he feels there is a "film" over his eyes and occasionally he has seen halos around lights. He reports that, previously, he was told by his ophthalmologist that he was developing cataracts and that when the condition began to interfere with his lifestyle, he would be a candidate for surgery. He has come in today to discuss his overall health with Doctor Noble and get his recommendation about cataract surgery.

**O** | **Objective:**
**General Appearance:** Well groomed, pleasant and friendly. No obvious distress.
**HEENT:** Head: Normocephalic. Eyes: Snellen chart exam: left eye 20/50; right eye 20/70. Pupils round and equal in size. Brows and lashes present and normal bilaterally. Conjunctiva transparent and light pink in

**O** | color. Sclera appears opaque white. Gray coloration of the lens noted. Ears: TM pearly gray with landmarks intact. Nose: No discharge. Mucosa pink, no swelling. Throat: Mucosa pink, no lesions or exudate. Uvula rises midline on phonation. Gag reflex present.

**Heart:** Regular rate and rhythm, no murmurs, gallops, or rubs.

**Lungs:** CTA

**Skin:** Warm and dry. Turgor good.

**A** | **Assessment:** Cataracts.

**P** | **Plan:**
1. Ask Mr. Black to contact his ophthalmologist for further evaluation and then to notify this office of his plans.
2. To assist Mr. Black in deciding about surgery, explain the two types of cataract surgery: phacoemulsification (phaco) and extracapsular.
3. Teach the patient that, for a few days after surgery, he will be wearing an eye patch, using eye drops as prescribed by the ophthalmologist, and should not lift any heavy objects, run, jog, or ride a horse. He should also avoid sleeping on the operative side, rubbing his eyes, squeezing the eyelids shut, straining during a bowel movement, getting soap in his eyes, or engaging in sexual intercourse.

**FYI:** Phacoemulsification is a process in which a small incision is made on the side of the cornea. The doctor then inserts into the eye a tiny probe, which emits ultrasound waves that soften and break up the lens so that it can be removed by suction.

In extracapsular surgery, the doctor makes a longer incision on the side of the cornea and removes the cloudy core of the lens in one piece. The rest of the lens is removed by suction.

After the natural lens has been removed, it often is replaced by an artificial lens, an intraocular lens (IOL), which is a clear, plastic lens that requires no care and becomes a permanent part of the eye. Light is focused clearly by the IOL onto the retina, improving vision.

## Chart Note Questions
*Place the correct answer in the space provided.*

1. Mr. Black presented with complaints of trouble driving at night, photophobia, _____

   _____, film over his eyes, and seeing halos around lights.

2. Referral to a/an _____ was recommended.

3. Phacoemulsification uses _____ waves that soften and break up the lens so that it can be removed by suction.

4. The vision in Mr. Black's right eye is recorded as _____.

5. The abbreviation PERRLA means _____.

6. The conjunctiva was _____ and light pink in color.

7. The color of the lens noted in the objective analysis was _____.

8. The medical term for an unusual intolerance of light is called _____.

9. If surgical intervention is decided, the patient must understand that he should avoid

   _____ on the operative side.

10. An _____ is a clear, plastic lens that requires no care and becomes a permanent part of the eye.

# MULTIMEDIA PREVIEW

*Additional interactive resources and activities for this chapter can be found on the Companion Website. For videos, audio glossary, and review, access the accompanying CD-ROM in this book.*

## CD-ROM HIGHLIGHTS

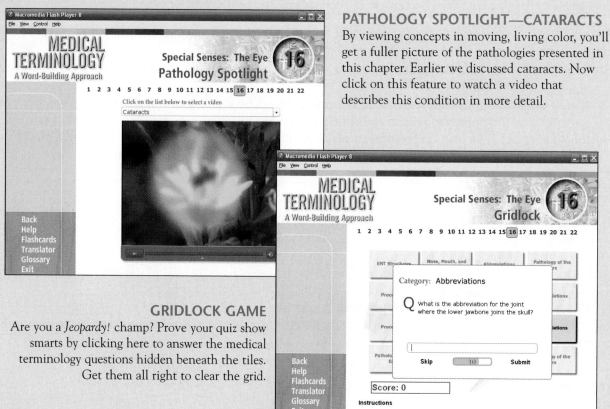

### PATHOLOGY SPOTLIGHT—CATARACTS

By viewing concepts in moving, living color, you'll get a fuller picture of the pathologies presented in this chapter. Earlier we discussed cataracts. Now click on this feature to watch a video that describes this condition in more detail.

### GRIDLOCK GAME

Are you a *Jeopardy!* champ? Prove your quiz show smarts by clicking here to answer the medical terminology questions hidden beneath the tiles. Get them all right to clear the grid.

## WEBSITE HIGHLIGHTS www.prenhall.com/rice

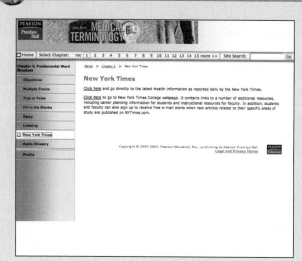

### MEDICINE IN THE NEWS

Click here and take advantage of the free-access on-line study guide that accompanies your textbook. You'll be able to stay current with a link to medical news articles updated daily by *The New York Times*. By clicking on this URL you'll also access a variety of quizzes with instant feedback, links to download mp3 audio reviews, and an audio glossary.

# Female Reproductive System

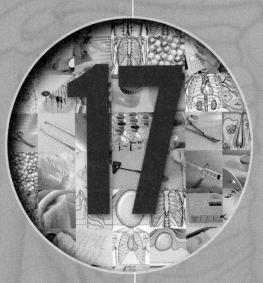

**17**

## ■ OBJECTIVES

*On completion of this chapter, you will be able to:*

- Describe the uterus and state its functions.
- Describe the fallopian tubes and state their functions.
- Describe the ovaries and state their functions.
- Describe the vagina and state its functions.
- Describe the breast.
- Describe the menstrual cycle.
- Analyze, build, spell, and pronounce medical words.
- Comprehend the drugs highlighted in this chapter.
- Describe diagnostic and laboratory tests related to the female reproductive system.
- Identify and define selected abbreviations.
- Describe each of the conditions presented in the Pathology Spotlights.
- Review the Pathology Checkpoint.
- Complete the Study and Review section and the Chart Note Analysis.

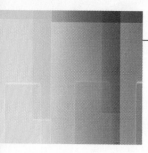

# Anatomy and Physiology Overview

The female reproductive system consists of a left and a right ovary, which are the female's primary sex organs, and the following accessory sex organs: two fallopian tubes, the uterus, the vagina, the vulva, and two breasts. See Figure 17–1 ▶. The vital function of the female reproductive system is to perpetuate the species through sexual or germ cell reproduction.

## Female Reproductive System

| Organ/Structure | Primary Functions |
| --- | --- |
| Uterus | Organ of the cyclic discharge of menses, provides place for the nourishment and development of the fetus; contracts during labor to help expel the fetus |
| Fallopian tubes | Serve as ducts for the conveyance of the ovum from the ovary to the uterus and for the conveyance of spermatozoa from the uterus toward the ovary |
| Ovaries | Produce ova and hormones |
| Vagina | Female organ of copulation (sexual intercourse), serves as a passageway for the discharge of menstruation and passageway for the birth of the fetus |
| Vulva | External female genitalia |
| *Mons pubis* | Provides pad of fatty tissue |
| *Labia majora* | Provides two folds of adipose tissue |
| *Labia minora* | Lying within the labia majora, encloses the vestibule |
| *Vestibule* | Serves as the entrance to the urethra, the vagina, and two excretory ducts of Bartholin's glands |
| *Clitoris* | Erectile tissue that is homologous to the penis of the male; produces pleasurable sensations during the sexual act |
| Breasts | Following childbirth, mammary glands produce milk |

# UTERUS

The **uterus** is a muscular, hollow, pear-shaped organ that is about 8 centimeters (cm) long, 5 cm wide, and 2.5 cm thick. The normal position of the uterus, known as **anteflexion,** is with the cervix pointing toward the lower end of the sacrum and the fundus toward the suprapubic region. See Figure 17–2 ▶. An average uterus weighs between 30 to 40 grams (g), which is 1 to 1.4 ounces (oz).

The uterus can be divided into two anatomical regions: the body and the cervix. The *uterine body* or *corpus* is the larger (upper) portion. The *fundus* is the rounded portion of the uterine body above the openings of the fallopian tubes. The body ends at a constricted central area known as the *isthmus.* The cervix is the lowermost cylindrical portion of the uterus that extends from the isthmus to the vagina.

The uterus is suspended in the anterior part of the pelvic cavity, halfway between the sacrum and the symphysis pubis, above the bladder, and in front of the rectum. A number of ligaments support the uterus and hold it in position: two broad ligaments, two round ligaments, two uterosacral ligaments, and the ligaments that are attached to the bladder. See Figure 17–3 ▶.

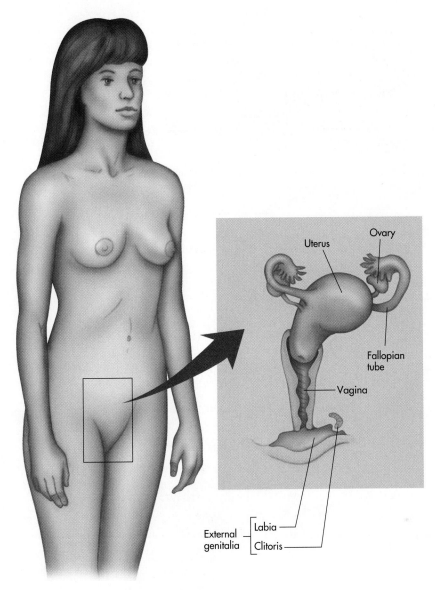

▶ **FIGURE 17–1** Female reproductive system.

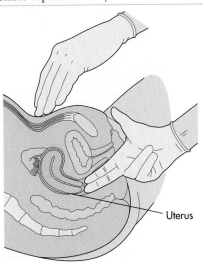

Anteflexion

▶ **FIGURE 17–2** Normal position of the uterus, called *anteflexion*.

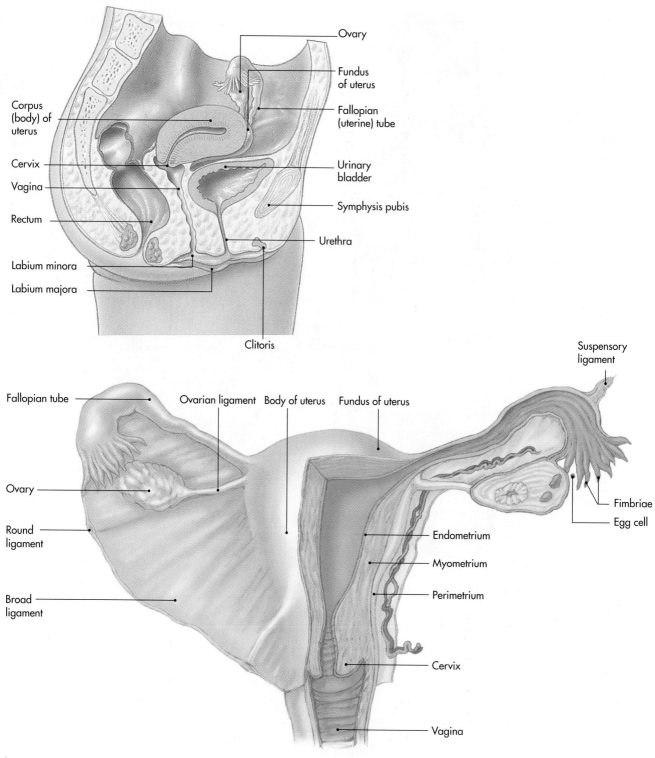

► **FIGURE 17–3** Female organs of reproduction and associated structures.

## Uterine Wall

The wall of the uterus consists of three layers: the **perimetrium** or outer layer, the **myometrium** or muscular middle layer, and the **endometrium,** which is the mucous membrane lining the inner surface of the uterus. See Figure 17–3. The endometrium is composed of columnar epithelium and connective tissue and is supplied with blood by both straight and spiral arteries. It undergoes marked changes in response to hormonal stimulation during the menstrual cycle.

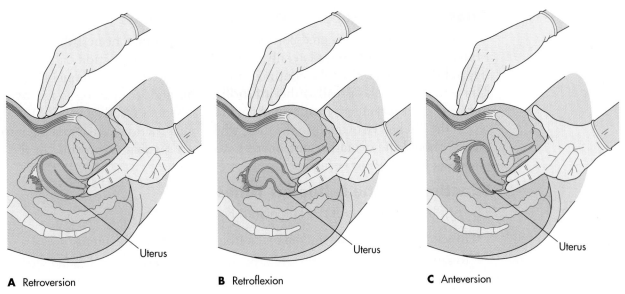

**A** Retroversion  **B** Retroflexion  **C** Anteversion

▶ **FIGURE 17-4** Displacement of the uterus within the uterine cavity. (A) Retroversion is a backward tilting. (B) Retroflexion is a backward bending. (C) Anteversion is a forward titling.

## Functions of the Uterus

Three primary functions are associated with the uterus:

• The organ of uterine cyclic changes that occur in the structure of the endometrium sheds the lining of the uterus every 21 to 40 days accompanied by bleeding (except during pregnancy and menopause).

• Provides a place for the protection and nourishment of the fetus during pregnancy.

• Contracts rhythmically and powerfully during labor to expel the fetus from the uterus.

## Abnormal Positions of the Uterus

The uterus can become malpositioned because of weakness of any of its supporting ligaments. Trauma, disease processes of the uterus, or multiple pregnancies can contribute to the weakening of the supporting ligaments. The following terms describe some of the abnormal positions (see Figure 17-4 ▲) of the uterus:

**Retroversion.** Turned backward with the cervix pointing forward toward the symphysis pubis.

**Retroflexion.** Bent backward at an angle with the cervix usually unchanged from its normal position.

**Anteversion.** Fundus turned forward toward the pubis with the cervix tilted up toward the sacrum.

## FALLOPIAN TUBES

Also called the **uterine tubes** or **oviducts,** the **fallopian tubes** extend laterally from either side of the uterus and end near each ovary. An average, normal fallopian tube is about 11.5 cm long and 6 mm wide. Its wall is composed of three layers: the **serosa** or outermost layer, composed of connective tissue; the **muscular layer,** containing inner circular and outer longitudinal layers of smooth muscle; and the **mucosa** or inner layer, consisting of simple columnar epithelium.

## Anatomical Features of the Fallopian Tubes

The **isthmus** is the constricted portion of the fallopian tube nearest the uterus. From the isthmus, the tube continues laterally and widens to form a section called the **ampulla.** Beyond the ampulla, the tube continues to expand and ends as a funnel-shaped opening. This end of the tube is called the **infundibulum,** and its opening is the **ostium.** Surrounding each ostium are **fimbriae** or *fingerlike structures* (see Figure 17–3) that work to propel the discharged ovum into the tube, where ciliary action aids in moving it toward the uterus. Should the ovum become impregnated by a spermatozoon while in the tube, the process of **fertilization** occurs.

## Functions of the Fallopian Tubes

The two basic functions of the fallopian tubes are as follows:

- To serve as ducts to convey the ovum from the ovary to the uterus.
- To serve as ducts to convey spermatozoa from the uterus toward each ovary.

# OVARIES

Located on either side of the uterus, the **ovaries** are almond-shaped organs attached to the uterus by the ovarian ligament. They lie close to the fimbriae of the fallopian tubes. The anterior border of each ovary is connected to the posterior layer of the broad ligament by the **mesovarium** (portion of the peritoneal fold). Each ovary is attached to the side of the pelvis by the **suspensory ligaments.** An average, normal ovary is about 4 cm long, 2 cm wide, and 1.5 cm thick. See Figure 17–5 ▼.

## Microscopic Anatomy

Each ovary consists of two distinct areas: the **cortex** or outer layer and the **medulla** or inner portion. The cortex contains small secretory sacs or follicles in three stages of development. These stages are known as **primary, growing,** and **graafian** or mature stage. The

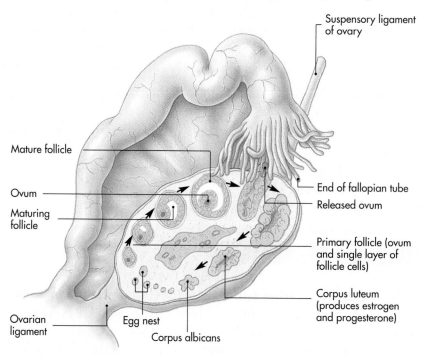

▶ FIGURE 17–5   Ovary.

ovarian medulla contains connective tissue, nerves, blood and lymphatic vessels, and some smooth muscle tissue in the region of the hilus.

### Function of the Ovaries

The anterior lobe of the pituitary gland, which produces the *gonadotropic hormones* FSH and LH, primarily control the functional activity of the ovaries. These abbreviations are for *follicle-stimulating hormone*, which is instrumental in the development of the ovarian follicles, and *luteinizing hormone*, which stimulates the development of the **corpus luteum,** a small yellow mass of cells that develops within a ruptured ovarian follicle.

Two functions have been identified for the ovary: the production of ova, female reproductive cells, and the production of hormones.

### Production of Ova

Each month a *graafian follicle* ruptures on the ovarian cortex, and an **ovum** (singular of ova) discharges into the pelvic cavity, where it enters the fallopian tube. This process is known as **ovulation.** In an average, normal woman more than 400 ova may be produced during her reproductive years (see Figure 17–5).

### Production of Hormones

The ovary is also an endocrine gland, producing **estrogen,** the female sex hormone secreted by the follicles, and **progesterone,** a steroid hormone secreted by the corpus luteum that is important in the maintenance of pregnancy. These hormones are essential in promoting growth and development and maintaining the female secondary sex organs and characteristics. These hormones also prepare the uterus for pregnancy, promote development of the mammary glands, and play a vital role in a woman's emotional well-being and sexual drive.

## VAGINA

The **vagina** is a musculomembranous tube extending from the vestibule to the uterus (see Figure 17–3). It is 10 to 15 cm in length and situated between the bladder and the rectum. It is lined by mucous membrane made up of *squamous epithelium.* A fold of mucous membrane, the **hymen,** partially covers the external opening of the vagina.

### Functions of the Vagina

The vagina has three basic functions:

- Receives the seminal fluid from the male penis; it is the female organ of copulation.
- Serves as a passageway for the discharge of menstruation.
- Serves as a passageway for the birth of the fetus.

## VULVA

The **vulva** consists of the following five organs that comprise the external female genitalia (see Figure 17–6 ▶):

**Mons pubis.** A pad of fatty tissue of triangular shape and, after puberty, covered with pubic hair. It may be referred to as the *mons veneris* or *mound of Venus* and is the rounded area over the symphysis pubis.

**Labia majora.** The two folds of adipose tissue, which are large liplike structures, lying on either side of the vaginal opening.

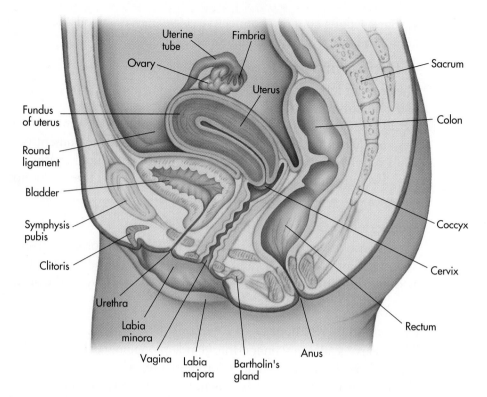

▶ **FIGURE 17–6** Sagittal section of the female pelvis showing organs of the reproductive system.

**Labia minora.** Two thin folds of skin that lie within the labia majora and enclose the vestibule.

**Vestibule.** The cleft between the labia minora. It is approximately 4 to 5 cm long and 2 cm wide. Four major structures open into it: the urethra, the vagina, and two excretory ducts of the Bartholin glands.

**Clitoris.** A small organ consisting of sensitive erectile tissue that is homologous to the penis of the male. It is located between the anterior labial commissure and partially hidden by the anterior portion of the labia minora.

The **perineum** is the region bounded by the inferior edges of the pelvis. In the female, it is located between the vulva and the anus. It is a muscular sheet that forms the pelvic floor and during childbirth it can be torn and cause injury to the anal sphincter. To avoid such an injury, an *episiotomy*, a surgical procedure to prevent tearing of the perineum and facilitate delivery of the infant, is usually performed. See Chapter 18 for more information on episiotomy.

## BREASTS

The **breasts** or mammary glands are compound alveolar structures consisting of 15 to 20 glandular tissue lobes separated by septa of connective tissue. Most women have two breasts that lie anterior to the pectoral muscles and curve outward from the lateral margins of the sternum to the anterior border of the axilla. The size of the breast can greatly vary according to age, heredity, and adipose (fatty) tissue present. The **areola** is the dark, pigmented

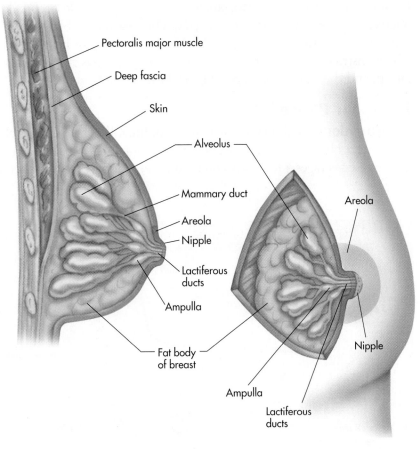

▶ FIGURE 17–7   Breast.

area found in the skin over each breast, and the *nipple* is the elevated area in the center of the areola. During pregnancy, the areola changes from its pinkish color to a dark brown or reddish color. The areola is supplied with a row of small sebaceous glands that secrete an oily substance to keep it resilient. The *lactiferous glands* consist of 20 to 24 glands in the areola of the nipple and, during lactation, secrete and convey milk to a suckling infant. See Figure 17–7 ▲. The hormone **prolactin,** which is produced by the anterior lobe of the pituitary, stimulates the mammary glands to produce milk after childbirth. Other hormones playing a role in milk production are insulin and glucocorticoids. **Colostrum,** a thin yellowish secretion, is the *first milk* and contains mainly serum and white blood cells. Suckling stimulates the production of **oxytocin** by the posterior lobe of the pituitary gland. It acts on the mammary glands to stimulate the release of milk and stimulates the uterus to contract during parturition.

# MENSTRUAL CYCLE

The menstrual cycle is a periodic recurrent series of changes occurring in the uterus, ovaries, vagina, and breasts. It is regulated by the complex interaction of hormones: luteinizing hormone (LH) and follicle-stimulating hormone (FSH), which are produced by the pituitary gland, and the female sex hormones estrogen and progesterone, which are produced by the ovaries. The onset of the **menstrual cycle,** *menarche,* occurs at the age of

**puberty** and ceases at **menopause.** The menstrual cycle occurs during a woman's reproductive years, except during pregnancy. The first day of bleeding is counted as the beginning of each menstrual cycle (day 1). The cycle ends just before the next menstrual period. The menstrual cycle occurs every 21 to 40 days and has three phases: follicular phase, ovulation, and the luteal phase. See Figure 17–8 ▼.

## Follicular Phase

**Menstruation,** which marks the first day of the follicular phase, is characterized by the discharge of a bloody fluid from the uterus accompanied by a shedding of the endometrium. This phase averages 4 to 5 days and is considered to be the first to the fifth days of the cycle.

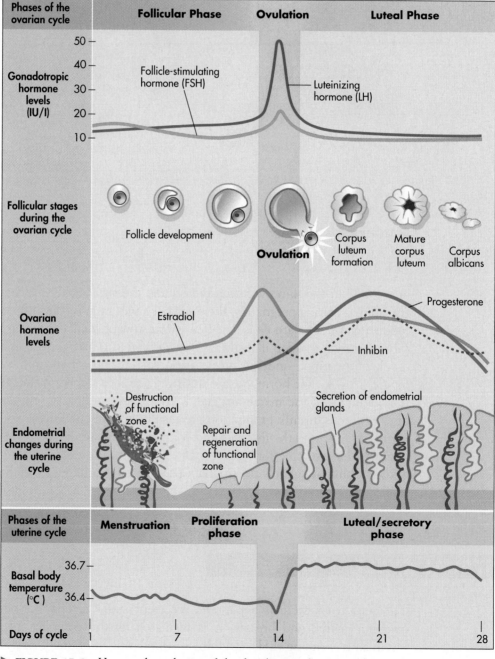

▶ **FIGURE 17–8**  Hormonal regulation of the female reproductive cycle.

## Ovulatory Phase

The **ovulatory phase** is characterized by the stimulation of estrogen, the thickening and vascularization of the endometrium, along with the maturing of the ovarian follicle. This phase begins about the fifth day and ends at the time of rupture of the graafian follicle (release of the egg), usually 36 hours after the surge in luteinizing hormone begins. About 12 to 24 hours after the egg is released, this surge can be detected by measuring the luteinizing hormone level in the urine. The egg can be fertilized at this time for about 12 hours. The ovulatory phase occurs about 14 days before the onset of menstruation.

## Luteal or Secretory Phase

The **luteal phase** follows ovulation. It last about 14 days, unless fertilization occurs, and ends just before a menstrual period. During this phase, the corpus luteum in the ovary is developing and secreting progesterone. The progesterone level is highest during this phase as the estrogen level decreases. The function of the corupus luteum is to prepare the uterus in case fertilization occurs. The progesterone produced causes the endometrium to thicken, filling with fluids and nutrients in preparation for a potential fetus. Progesterone causes the mucus in the cervix to thicken, making the entry of sperm or bacteria into the uterus less likely. It also causes the body temperature to increase slightly during the luteal phase and remain elevated until a menstrual period begins. This increase in temperature can be used to estimate whether ovulation has occurred. In the second part of the luteal phase, the estrogen level increases, also stimulating the endometrium to thicken. In response to the increase in estrogen and progesterone levels, the breasts may swell and become tender. If the egg is not fertilized, the corpus luteum degenerates after 14 days, and a new menstrual cycle begins.

## Premenstrual or Ischemic Time Period

During the **premenstrual** time period, the coiled uterine arteries become constricted, the endometrium becomes anemic and begins to shrink, and the corpus luteum decreases in functional activity. This time period lasts about 2 days and ends with the occurrence of menstruation. See Premenstrual Syndrome (PMS) in Pathology Spotlights on page 585 for information about a common condition that occurs during this time period.

# LIFE SPAN CONSIDERATIONS

### ■ THE CHILD

The sex of a child is determined at the time of **fertilization.** When a spermatozoon carrying the X sex chromosome fertilizes the X-bearing ovum, the result is a female child (X + X = female). When the X-bearing ovum is fertilized by the Y-bearing spermatozoon, a male child is produced (X + Y = male). Sex differentiation occurs early in the embryo. At 16 weeks, the external **genitals** of the fetus are recognizably male or female. This difference can be seen during ultrasonography. See Figure 17–9 ▶.

The genitals of the newborn are not fully developed at birth. They may be slightly swollen, and in the female infant, blood-tinged mucus may be discharged from the vagina. This is due to hormones transmitted from the mother to the infant. The labia minora may protrude beyond the labia majora.

The sex organs do not mature until the onset of **puberty.** At puberty, the female experiences breast development, vaginal secretions, and menarche. A study published

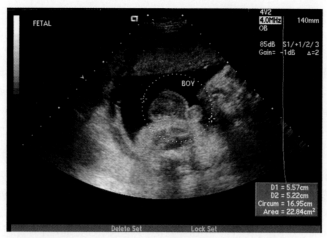

▶ **FIGURE 17–9**  Ultrasonogram showing a male fetus. (Courtesy of Nancy West)

several years ago in the *Journal of Pediatrics* revealed that many girls begin to develop sexually by age 8. This study involved 17,000 American girls ages 3 to 12, who were seen in 65 pediatric practices nationwide. At age 8, 48.3% of African American girls and 14.7% of Caucasian girls had begun developing breasts, pubic hair, or both. Among African American girls, menstruation began on average at 12.16 years; among Caucasian girls, the average was 12.88 years. The study raised questions about whether environmental estrogens—chemicals that mimic the female hormone estrogen—are bringing on puberty at an earlier age. The study also suggested that sex education should begin sooner than it often does.

### ■ THE OLDER ADULT

At about 50 years of age, men and women begin experiencing bodily changes that are directly related to **hormonal** production. In women, the ovaries cease to produce estrogen and progesterone. With decreased production of the female hormones, estrogen and progesterone, women enter the phase of life known as **menopause.** Natural menopause occurs in 25% of women by age 47, in 50% by age 50, 75% by age 52, and in 95% by age 55.

The symptoms of menopause vary from being hardly noticeable to being severe. Symptoms can include irregular periods, hot flashes, vaginal dryness, insomnia, joint pain, headache, emotional instability, irritability, and depression. Breast tissue can lose its firmness, and pubic and axillary hair becomes sparse. Without estrogen, the uterus becomes smaller, the vagina shortens, and vaginal tissues become drier. There can be loss of bone mass leading to **osteoporosis.**

# BUILDING YOUR MEDICAL VOCABULARY

This section provides the foundation for learning medical terminology. Review the following alphabetized word list. Note how common prefixes and suffixes are repeatedly applied to word roots and combining forms to create different meanings.

| | |
|---|---|
| P | Prefix |
| R | Root |
| CF | Combining form |
| S | Suffix |

| | |
|---|---|
| Pink words | Terms not built from word parts. |
| * | Indicates words covered in the Pathology Spotlights section. |
|  | Check the CD-ROM for more information. |

| MEDICAL WORD | WORD PARTS (WHEN APPLICABLE) | | | DEFINITION |
|---|---|---|---|---|
| | **Part** | **Type** | **Meaning** | |
| **adnexa**<br>(ăd-něk′să) | | | | Accessory parts of a structure. *Adnexa uteri* refers to the ovaries and fallopian tubes. |
| **amenorrhea**<br>(ă-měn″ō-rē′ a) | a-<br>men/o<br><br>-rrhea | P<br>CF<br><br>S | lack of<br>month, menses,<br>menstruation<br>flow | Lack of the monthly flow (menses or menstruation) |
| **bartholinitis**<br>(bar″ tō-lĭn-ī′ tĭs) | bartholin<br>-itis | R<br>S | Bartholin's glands<br>inflammation | Inflammation of Bartholin's glands. To check for swelling, redness, or tenderness, the Bartholin's gland is palpated at the posterior labia majora. See Figure 17–10 ▶. |
| **biotics**<br>(bī-ōt′ ĭks) | bi/o<br>-tic (s) | CF<br>S | life<br>pertaining to | Science of living organisms and the sum of knowledge regarding the life process |
| **cervicitis**<br>(sěr-vĭ-sī′ tĭs) | cervic<br>-itis | R<br>S | cervix<br>inflammation | Inflammation of the uterine cervix |
| **colposcope**<br>(kŏl′ pō-skōp) | colp/o<br>-scope | CF<br>S | vagina<br>instrument for examining | Instrument used to examine the vagina and cervix by means of a magnifying lens |
| **contraception**<br>(kŏn″ tră-sěp′ shŭn) | contra-<br>cept<br>-ion | P<br>R<br>S | against<br>receive<br>process | Process of preventing conception |
| **culdocentesis**<br>(kŭl″ dō-sěn-tē′ sĭs) | culd/o<br>-centesis | CF<br>S | cul-de-sac<br>surgical puncture | Surgical puncture of the cul-de-sac for removal of fluid |
| **cystocele**<br>(sĭs′ tō-sēl) | cyst/o<br>-cele | CF<br>S | bladder<br>hernia | Hernia of the bladder that protrudes into the vagina |
| **dysmenorrhea**<br>(dĭs″ měn-ō-rē′ ă) | dys-<br>men/o<br><br>-rrhea | P<br>CF<br><br>S | difficult, painful<br>month, menses,<br>menstruation<br>flow | Difficult or painful monthly flow (menses or menstruation) |

| MEDICAL WORD | WORD PARTS (WHEN APPLICABLE) | | | DEFINITION |
|---|---|---|---|---|
| | **Part** | **Type** | **Meaning** | |
| **dyspareunia**<br>(dĭs′ pă-rū′ nĭ-ă) | dys-<br>pareun<br><br>-ia | P<br>R<br><br>S | difficult, painful<br>lying beside,<br>sexual intercourse<br>condition | Difficult or painful sexual intercourse (copulation) |
| **endometriosis**<br>(ĕn″ dō-mē″ trĭ-ō′ sĭs) | endo-<br>metr/i<br>-osis | P<br>CF<br>S | within<br>uterus<br>condition (usually abnormal) | Condition in which endometrial tissue occurs in various sites in the abdominal or pelvic cavity. See Figure 17–11 ▼.<br>✳ See Pathology Spotlight: Endometriosis on page 583. |
| **fibroma**<br>(fī-brō′ mă) | fibr<br>-oma | R<br>S | fibrous tissue<br>tumor | Fibrous tissue tumor; also called *fibroid tumor,* most common benign tumor found in women. See *uterine fibroid.* |
| **genetics**<br>(jĕn-ĕt′ ĭks) | genet<br><br>-ic (s) | R<br><br>S | formation,<br>produce<br>pertaining to | Science of biology that studies the phenomenon of heredity and the laws governing it |
| **genitalia**<br>(jĕn-ĭ-tăl′ ĭ-ă) | genital<br>-ia | R<br>S | belonging to birth<br>condition | Male or female reproductive organs. See Figure 17–12 ▶. |
| **gynecologist**<br>(gī″ nĕ-kŏl′ ō-jĭst) | gynec/o<br>log<br>-ist | CF<br>R<br>S | female<br>study of<br>one who specializes | Physician who specializes in the study of the female, especially the diseases of the female reproductive organs and the breasts |
| **gynecology (GYN)**<br>(gī″ nĕ-kŏl′ ō-jē) | gynec/o<br>-logy | CF<br>S | female<br>study of | Study of the female, especially the diseases of the female reproductive organs and the breasts |

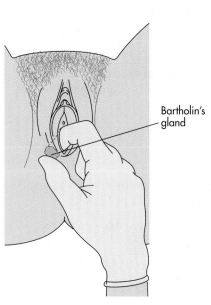

▶ **FIGURE 17–10** Palpating Bartholin's glands.

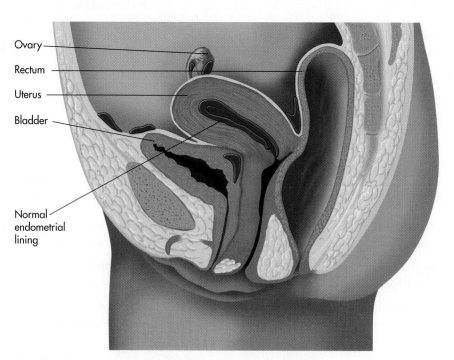

▶ **FIGURE 17–11** Locations of endometriosis outside the uterus are shown in red.

| MEDICAL WORD | WORD PARTS (WHEN APPLICABLE) | | | DEFINITION |
|---|---|---|---|---|
| | Part | Type | Meaning | |
| **hymenectomy**<br>(hī" mĕn-ĕk' tō-mē) | hymen<br>-ectomy | R<br>S | hymen<br>surgical excision | Surgical excision of the membranous fold of tissue (the hymen) that partially or completely covers the vaginal opening |
| **hysterectomy**<br>(hĭs" tĕr-ĕk' tō-mē) | hyster<br>-ectomy | R<br>S | womb, uterus<br>surgical excision | Surgical excision of the uterus.<br>✱ See Pathology Spotlight: Hysterectomy on page 583. |
| **hysteroscope**<br>(hĭs' tĕr-ō-skōp) | hyster/o<br>-scope | CF<br>S | womb, uterus<br>instrument for examining | Instrument used in the biopsy of uterine tissue before 12 weeks of gestation. This tissue is then analyzed for chromosome arrangement, DNA sequence, and genetic defects. |
| **hysterotomy**<br>(hĭs" tĕr-ŏt' ō-mē) | hyster/o<br>-tomy | CF<br>S | womb, uterus<br>incision | Incision into the uterus; also called a *cesarean section* |
| **intrauterine**<br>(ĭn' tră-ū' tĕr-ĭn) | intra-<br>uter<br>-ine | P<br>R<br>S | within<br>uterus<br>pertaining to | Pertaining to within the uterus |
| **laser ablation**<br>(lā' zĕr ăb-lā' shŭn) | | | | Procedure that uses a laser to destroy the uterine lining. A biopsy is performed before the procedure to make sure no cancer is present. This procedure can be used for disabling menstrual bleeding. *It causes sterility.* |
| **laser laparoscopy**<br>(lā' zĕr lăp-ăr-ŏs' kō-pē) | | | | Procedure that uses a long, telescopelike instrument equipped with a laser, lights, and a tiny video camera. It can be used to explore the abdominal area and to treat ectopic pregnancy. |

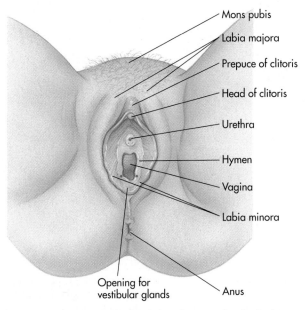

▶ FIGURE 17–12  External female genitalia (vulva).

| MEDICAL WORD | WORD PARTS (WHEN APPLICABLE) | | | DEFINITION |
|---|---|---|---|---|
| | Part | Type | Meaning | |
| **laser lumpectomy** (lā-zĕr lŭm-pĕk′ tō-mē) | | | | Use of a contact Yag laser to remove a tumor from the breast. It appears to cause less pain for the patient and decreases time in the hospital. |
| **lumpectomy** (lŭm-pĕk′ tō-mē) | lump -ectomy | R S | lump surgical excision | Surgical removal of a tumor from the breast. This procedure removes only the tumor, no other tissue or lymph nodes; usually not considered for large tumors, although the latest strategy involves shrinking large tumors with chemotherapy so that they become small enough to be removed by this method. See Figure 17–13 ▼. |
| **mammoplasty** (măm′ ō-plăs″ tē) | mamm/o -plasty | CF S | breast surgical repair | Surgical repair of the breast |
| **mastectomy** (măs-tĕk′ tō-mē) | mast -ectomy | R S | breast surgical excision | Surgical excision of the breast. See Figure 17–14 ▼. |
| **menarche** (mĕn-ar′ kē) | men -arche | R S | month, menses, menstruation beginning | Beginning of the monthly flow (menses, menstruation) |
| **menopause** (mĕn′ ō-pawz) | men/o pause | CF R | month, menses, menstruation cessation | Cessation of the monthly flow; also called *climacteric* |
| **menorrhagia** (mĕn″ ō-rā′ jĭ-ă) | men/o -rrhagia | CF S | month, menses, menstruation to burst forth | Excessive uterine bleeding at the time of a menstrual period, either in number of days or amount of blood or both. Causes include uterine fibroid tumors and pelvic inflammatory disease; also may be caused by an endocrine imbalance. |

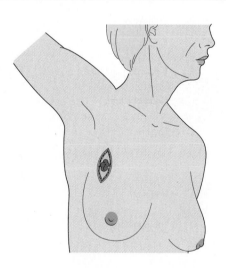

Lumpectomy

▶ **FIGURE 17–13**   A lumpectomy removes only the tumor and a small margin of surrounding tissue.

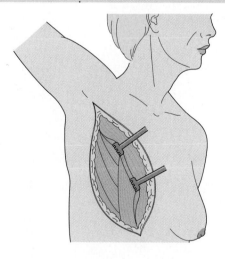

Modified radical mastectomy

▶ **FIGURE 17–14**   A modified radical mastectomy removes all breast tissue and the underarm lymph nodes but leaves the underlying muscles.

| MEDICAL WORD | WORD PARTS (WHEN APPLICABLE) | | | DEFINITION |
|---|---|---|---|---|
| | Part | Type | Meaning | |
| **menorrhea**<br>(mĕn″ ō-rē′ ă) | men/o<br><br>-rrhea | CF<br><br>S | month, menses,<br>menstruation<br>flow | Normal monthly flow (menses,<br>menstruation) |
| **mittelschmerz**<br>(mĭt′ ĕl-shmārts) | | | | Abdominal pain midway between the<br>menstrual periods, which occurs at the<br>time of ovulation and at the site of<br>ovulation |
| **myometritis**<br>(mī″ ō-mē-trī′ tĭs) | my/o<br>metr<br>-itis | CF<br>R<br>S | muscle<br>womb, uterus<br>inflammation | Inflammation of the muscular wall of the<br>uterus |
| **oligomenorrhea**<br>(ŏl″ ī-gō-mĕn″ ō-rē′ ă) | oligo-<br>men/o<br><br>-rrhea | P<br>CF<br><br>S | scanty<br>month, menses,<br>menstruation<br>flow | Scanty monthly flow (menses,<br>menstruation) |
| **oogenesis**<br>(ō″ ō-jĕn′ ĕ-sĭs) | o/o<br>-genesis | CF<br>S | ovum, egg<br>formation,<br>produce | Formation of the ovum |
| **oophorectomy**<br>(ō″ ŏf-ō-rĕk′ tō-mē) | oophor<br>-ectomy | R<br>S | ovary<br>surgical excision | Surgical excision of an ovary |
| **ovulation**<br>(ŏv″ ū-lā′ shŭn) | ovulat<br>-ion | R<br>S | little egg<br>process | Process in which an ovum is discharged<br>from the cortex of the ovary; periodic<br>ripening and rupture of a mature<br>graafian follicle and the discharge of an<br>ovum from the cortex of the ovary.<br>Occurs approximately 14 days before the<br>onset of the next menstrual period. See<br>Figure 17–15 ▼. |
| **pelvic inflammatory<br>disease (PID)**<br>(pĕl′ vĭk ĭn-flăm′ ă-tŏr′ ē<br>dĭ-zēz) | | | | Infection of the upper genital area; can<br>affect the uterus, ovaries, and fallopian<br>tubes. ✱ See Pathology Spotlight: Pelvic<br>Inflammatory Disease on page 584. |
| **perimenopause**<br>(pĕr-ĭ-mĕn′ ō-pawz) | peri-<br>men/o<br><br>pause | P<br>CF<br><br>R | around<br>month, menses,<br>menstruation<br>cessation | Period of gradual changes that lead into<br>menopause affecting a woman's<br>hormones, body, and feelings. It can be a<br>stop-start process that can take months<br>or years. Hormone levels fluctuate,<br>thereby causing changes in the<br>menstrual cycle, which becomes<br>irregular. |

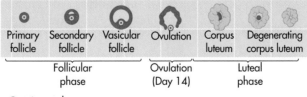

Ovarian cycle

▶ **FIGURE 17–15**  Changes in the ovarian follicles during
the 28-day ovarian cycle.

| MEDICAL WORD | WORD PARTS (WHEN APPLICABLE) | | | DEFINITION |
|---|---|---|---|---|
| | **Part** | **Type** | **Meaning** | |
| **postcoital**<br>(pōst-kō' ĭt-ăl) | post-<br>coit<br>-al | P<br>R<br>S | after<br>a coming together<br>pertaining to | Pertaining to after sexual intercourse |
| **premenstrual syndrome (PMS)**<br>(prē-měn-stroo-ăl sĭn-drŏm) | | | | Condition that affects certain women and can cause distressful symptoms such as constipation, diarrhea, nausea, appetite cravings, headache, backache, muscular aches, edema, insomnia, clumsiness, irritability, indecisiveness, mental confusion, and depression. ✳ See Pathology Spotlight: Premenstrual Syndrome on page 585. |
| **rectovaginal**<br>(rěk" tō-văj' ĭ-năl) | rect/o<br>vagin<br>-al | CF<br>R<br>S | rectum<br>vagina<br>pertaining to | Pertaining to the rectum and vagina |
| **retroversion**<br>(rět" rō-vur' shŭn) | retro-<br>vers<br>-ion | P<br>R<br>S | backward<br>turning<br>process | Process of being turned backward, such as the displacement of the uterus with the cervix pointed forward. See Figure 17–4 on page 567. |
| **salpingectomy**<br>(săl" pĭn-jěk' tō-mē) | salping<br>-ectomy | R<br>S | fallopian tube<br>surgical excision | Surgical excision of a fallopian tube |
| **salpingitis**<br>(săl" pĭn-jī' tĭs) | salping<br>-itis | R<br>S | fallopian tube<br>inflammation | Inflammation of a fallopian tube |
| **salpingo-oophorectomy**<br>(săl' pĭng" gō-ō" ŏf-ō-rēk' tō-mē) | salping/o<br>oophor<br>-ectomy | CF<br>R<br>S | fallopian tube<br>ovary<br>surgical excision | Surgical excision of an ovary and a fallopian tube |
| **toxic shock syndrome (TSS)**<br>(tŏk' sĭk shŏk sĭn' drōm) | | | | Poisonous *Staphylococcus aureus* infection that can strike young, menstruating women |
| **uterine fibroid**<br>(ū' těr-ĭn fī-broyd) | uter<br>-ine<br>fibr<br>-oid | R<br>S<br>R<br>S | uterus<br>pertaining to<br>fiber<br>resemble | Benign fibrous tumor of the uterus made up of muscle cells and other tissues that grow within the wall of the uterus; also called *uterine leiomyoma*. ✳ See Pathology Spotlight: Uterine Fibroids on page 586 and Figure 17–18. |
| **vaginitis**<br>(văj" ĭn-ī' tĭs) | vagin<br>-itis | R<br>S | vagina<br>inflammation | Inflammation of the vagina |
| **venereal**<br>(vē-nē' rē-ăl) | venere<br>-al | R<br>S | sexual intercourse<br>pertaining to | Pertaining to or resulting from sexual intercourse |

# DRUG HIGHLIGHTS

**Female hormones**

Estrogens

Used for a variety of conditions including amenorrhea, dysfunctional uterine bleeding (DUB), and hirsutism as well as in palliative therapy for breast cancer in women and prostatic cancer in men. They are also used as hormone replacement therapy (HRT) in the treatment of uncomfortable symptoms that are related to menopause.

*Examples: Premarin (conjugated estrogens, USP), DES (diethylstilbestrol), Estrace (estradiol), Estraderm (estradiol) transdermal system, Ogen (estropipate), and Menest (esterified estrogens)*

Progestogens/progestins

Synthetic progesterones used to prevent uterine bleeding; combined with estrogen for treatment of amenorrhea. They may be used in cases of infertility and threatened or habitual miscarriage. Progesterone is responsible for changes in the uterine endometrium during the second half of the menstrual cycle, development of maternal placenta after implantation, and development of mammary glands.

*Examples: Provera (medroxyprogesterone acetate), Norlutin and Norlutate (norethindrone acetate), Ovrette (norgestrel), and Prometrium (natural progesterone)*

**Contraceptives**

Birth control pills (BCP)

Oral contraceptives (OC) containing mixtures of estrogen and progestin in various levels of strength that are nearly 100% effective when used as directed. The estrogen in the pill inhibits ovulation, and the progestin inhibits pituitary secretion of luteinizing hormone (LH), causes changes in the cervical mucus that renders it unfavorable to penetration by sperm, and alters the nature of the endometrium.

*Examples: Ortho-Novum 10/11, Triphasil, Micronor, Brevicon, Demulen, Lo/Ovral, Ovrette, Nelova 10/11, Alesse, and Nor-QD*

Birth control patch

*Ortho Evra* is the first transdermal birth control patch that continuously delivers two synthetic hormones, progestin (norelgestromin) and estrogen (ethinyl estradiol). The patch impedes pregnancy by preventing the ovaries from releasing eggs (ovulation) and thickening the cervical mucus. The patch is applied directly to the skin (buttocks, abdomen, upper torso, or upper outer arm) and has an effectiveness rate of 95%.

Injectable

*Depo-Provera* is an injectable contraceptive that is given four times a year. It contains medroxyprogesterone acetate, a synthetic drug that is similar to progesterone. Depo-Provera prevents pregnancy by stopping the ovaries from releasing eggs (ovulation) and thickens the cervical mucus. When used correctly, it can prevent pregnancy over 99% of the time.

Intrauterine device (IUD)

Small device that is placed within the uterus to prevent pregnancy. It is usually made of soft, flexible, ultralight plastic and is 99.2% to 99.9% effective as birth control. Two types are available: ParaGard and Mirena. ParaGard uses copper around the plastic. Anyone allergic to copper should not use it. Mirena releases small amounts of a synthetic progesterone over time and can be left in place for up to 5 years. IUDs do not protect against sexually transmitted diseases (STDs) or the human immunodeficiency virus (HIV). See Figure 17–16 ▼.

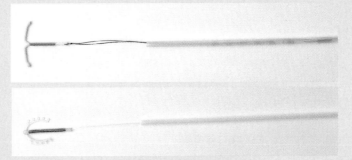

▶ **FIGURE 17–16**   Examples of intrauterine devices (IUDs).

# DIAGNOSTIC AND LAB TESTS

| TEST | DESCRIPTION |
| --- | --- |
| Breast examination | Visual inspection and manual examination of the breast for changes in contour, symmetry, dimpling of skin, retraction of the nipple(s), and the presence of lumps. |
| Colposcopy (kŏl-pŏs′ kō-pē) | Visual examination of the vagina and cervix via a colposcope. Abnormal results can indicate cervical or vaginal erosion, tumors, and dysplasia. |
| Culdoscopy (kŭl-dŏs′ kō-pē) | Direct visual examination of the viscera of the female pelvis through a culdoscope. The instrument is introduced into the pelvic cavity through the posterior vaginal fornix. Can be used in suspected ectopic pregnancy and unexplained pelvic pain and to check for pelvic masses. |
| Estrogen (es′ trō-jĕns) | Urine or blood serum test to determine the level of estrone, estradiol, and estriol. |
| Hysterosalpingography (HSG) (hĭs″ tĕr-ō-săl″ pĭn-gŏg′ ră-fē) | X-ray of the uterus and fallopian tubes after the injection of a radiopaque substance. Size and structure of the uterus and fallopian tubes can be evaluated. Uterine tumors, fibroids, tubal pregnancy, and tubal occlusion can be observed. Also used for treatment of an occluded fallopian tube. |
| Laparoscopy (lăp-ăr-ŏs′ kō-pē) | Visual examination of the abdominal cavity. A flexible, lighted instrument (laparoscope) is inserted through a periumbilical incision to examine the ovaries and fallopian tubes. |
| Mammography (măm-ŏg′ ră-fē) | Process of obtaining images of the breast by use of x-rays to locate breast tumors before they grow to 1 cm. It is the most effective means of detecting early breast cancers. |
| Papanicolaou (Pap smear) (păp′ ăh-nĭk″ ō-lă′ oo) | Screening technique to aid in the detection of cervical/uterine cancer and cancer precursors. It is not a diagnostic procedure. Both false-positive and false-negative results have been experienced with Pap smears. Any lesion should be biopsied unless not indicated clinically. The Pap smear should not be used as a sole means to diagnose or exclude malignant and premalignant lesions. It is a screening procedure only.<br><br>Pap smear results are generally reported as within normal limits (WNL), abnormal squamous cells of undetermined significance (Ascus), mild dysplasia (CIN [cervical intraepithelial neoplasia] I), moderate dysplasia (CIN II), and severe dysplasia and/or carcinoma in-situ (CIN III). |
| Pregnanediol (prĕg″ nān-dī-ŏl) | Urine test to determine menstrual disorders or possible abortion. |
| Wet mat or wet-prep | Examination of vaginal discharge for the presence of bacteria and yeast. Vaginal smear placed on a microscopic slide, wet with normal saline, and then viewed under a microscope by the physician. |

# ABBREVIATIONS

| ABBREVIATION | MEANING | ABBREVIATION | MEANING |
| --- | --- | --- | --- |
| AH | abdominal hysterectomy | HSG | hysterosalpingography |
| Ascus | atypical squamous cells of undetermined significance | IUD | intrauterine device |
| | | HIV | human immunodeficiency virus |
| BCP | birth control pill | LH | luteinizing hormone |
| CIN | cervical intraepithelial neoplasia | OC | oral contraceptive |
| cm | centimeter | OTC | over-the-counter |
| D&C | dilation and curettage | PID | pelvic inflammatory disease |
| DES | diethylstilbestrol | PMS | premenstrual syndrome |
| DUB | dysfunctional uterine bleeding | STDs | sexually transmitted diseases |
| HRT | hormone replacement therapy | TSS | toxic shock syndrome |

# PATHOLOGY SPOTLIGHTS

## ✳ Endometriosis

The *endometrium* is the tissue that lines the inside of the uterus. **Endometriosis** is a condition in which endometrial tissue occurs in various sites in the abdominal or pelvic cavity. This tissue responds to cyclic hormonal signals. Because it is outside the uterus and cannot be cast off each month, the tissue causes bleeding, with the formation of scars and adhesions. This is generally what causes daily or monthly cyclic pain.

Symptoms of endometriosis include hematuria (blood in the urine), dysuria (difficulty in urinating), **dyspareunia** (painful intercourse), **menorrhagia** (excessive menstrual bleeding), irregular or more frequent periods, nausea and vomiting, pain with bowel movements, and spotty bleeding just before the onset of the period. The most common symptom of endometriosis is **dysmenorrhea** or increasingly painful periods. The woman can experience a steady dull or severe pain in the lower abdomen, vagina, and/or back. This pain can begin 5 to 7 days before a period. After **menopause,** the symptoms subside as the abnormal tissue shrinks.

The cause of endometriosis is unknown. Diagnosis of endometriosis begins with a complete medical history and physical exam, including a pelvic exam. A **laparoscopy** can be performed to confirm the diagnosis.

Early diagnosis and treatment can limit cell growth and help prevent adhesions while pregnancy, oral contraceptives, and other hormones seem to delay the onset of endometriosis. Treatment with medications include analgesic therapy for the relief of the discomfort of the disease. This therapy is usually indicated for women with mild to moderate premenstrual pain and no pelvic examination abnormalities. Surgery is usually reserved for women with severe endometriosis.

## ✳ Hysterectomy

A **hysterectomy** is a surgical procedure to remove a woman's uterus. When the entire uterus, including the cervix, fallopian tubes, and ovaries are removed, it is referred to as a *panhysterosalpingo-oophorectomy*. If a woman has not yet reached menopause, a hysterectomy stops menstruation (monthly periods), as well as ending her ability to become pregnant.

There are several types of hysterectomy:

- A *complete* or *total hysterectomy* removes the cervix as well as the uterus. This is the most common type of hysterectomy.
- A *partial* or *subtotal hysterectomy* (also called a *supracervical hysterectomy*) removes the upper part of the uterus and leaves the cervix in place.
- A *radical hysterectomy* removes the uterus, the cervix, the upper part of the vagina, and supporting tissues. This is done in some cases of cancer.

Often one or both ovaries and fallopian tubes are removed at the same time a hysterectomy is done. When both ovaries and both tubes are removed, it is called a *bilateral salpingo-oophorectomy*. This procedure causes *surgical menopause* in women who are premenopausal.

Hysterectomies are done through a cut in the abdomen (abdominal hysterectomy [AH]) or the vagina (vaginal hysterectomy). Sometimes a laparoscope is used to view inside the abdomen. The type of surgery that is done depends on the reason for the surgery. Abdominal hysterectomies are more common than vaginal hysterectomies and usually require a longer recovery time. Hysterectomies are most often performed because of uterine fibroids and endometriosis. A type of surgery to remove only the fibroids without removing the uterus is called a *myomectomy*.

Endometrial cancer, uterine sarcoma, cervical cancer, and cancer of the ovaries or fallopian tubes often require hysterectomy, but cancers affecting the pelvic organs account for only about 10% of all hysterectomies. Depending on the type and extent of the cancer, other kinds of treatment such as radiation and hormonal therapy can be used as well.

Other reasons for hysterectomies include chronic pelvic pain, heavy bleeding during or between periods, and chronic pelvic inflammatory disease.

## ★ Pelvic Inflammatory Disease

The most common and serious complication of sexually transmitted diseases (STDs) among women is **pelvic inflammatory disease** (PID). This condition is an infection of the upper genital area and occurs when disease-causing organisms migrate upward from the vagina and cervix into the upper genital area. PID can affect the uterus, ovaries, and fallopian tubes. If untreated, this disease can cause scarring, which can lead to infertility, tubal pregnancy, chronic pelvic pain, and other serious consequences. Infertility occurs in approximately 20% of women who have had PID.

Each year in the United States, more than 1 million women experience an episode of acute PID, with the rate of infection highest among teenagers. More than 100,000 women become infertile each year as a result of this condition, and a large proportion of the 70,000 **ectopic** pregnancies (occurring elsewhere than in the uterus) occurring every year are due to the consequences of PID.

Many different organisms can cause PID, but most cases are associated with gonorrhea and genital chlamydial infections, two very common STDs. Scientists have found that bacteria normally present in small numbers in the vagina and cervix also can play a role.

The major symptoms of PID are lower abdominal pain and abnormal vaginal discharge. Other symptoms such as fever, painful intercourse, and irregular menstrual bleeding can occur. Particularly when caused by chlamydial infection, PID can produce only minor symptoms or no symptoms at all, even though it can seriously damage the reproductive organs.

To distinguish between PID and other serious problems that mimic PID, tests such as a sonogram, endometrial biopsy, or laparoscopy are ordered. The treatment consists of two antibiotics that are effective against a wide range of infectious agents. The antibiotics must be taken as ordered to acquire an effective cure.

About one-fourth of women with suspected PID must be hospitalized. The physician can recommend this if the patient is severely ill; if she cannot take oral medication and needs intravenous antibiotics; if she is pregnant; if she is an adolescent; if the diagnosis is uncertain and includes an abdominal emergency such as appendicitis; or if she is infected with HIV.

## ✱ Premenstrual Syndrome

**Premenstrual syndrome** (PMS) is a condition that affects certain women and cause distressful symptoms such as constipation, diarrhea, nausea, anorexia, appetite cravings, headache, backache, muscular aches, edema, insomnia, clumsiness, malaise, irritability, indecisiveness, mental confusion, and depression. These symptoms may begin 2 weeks before the onset of menstruation. Although the exact cause of this syndrome has not been determined, it could be due to the amount of prostaglandin produced, a deficient or excessive amount of estrogen or progesterone, or an interrelationship between these factors. The multisystem effects of premenstrual syndrome are presented in Figure 17–17 ▼.

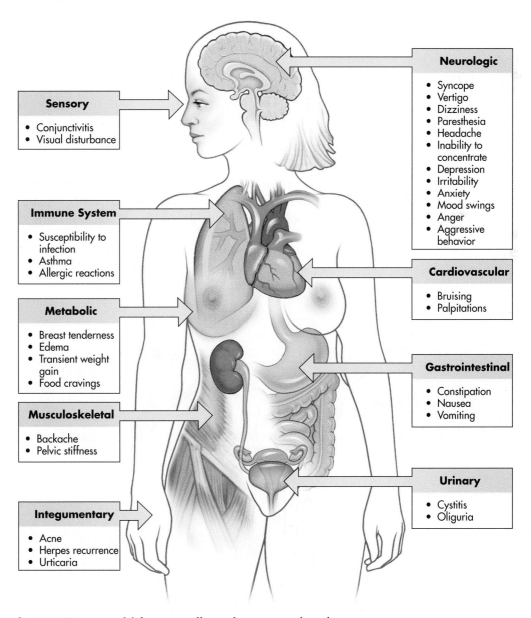

▶ **FIGURE 17–17**   Multisystem effects of premenstrual syndrome.

## ✴ Uterine Fibroids

**Uterine fibroids** are benign tumors or growths made up of muscle cells and other tissues that grow within the wall of the uterus. Fibroids can grow as a single growth or in clusters (groups). Their size can vary from small such as an apple seed (or less than one inch or 2½ cm) to even larger than a grapefruit (or eight inches or 20 cm across or more). The cause of fibroids is not known.

Uterine fibroids are the most common benign tumors in women of childbearing age. Fibroids are classified into three groups based on where they grow, such as just underneath the lining of the uterus, between the muscles of the uterus, or on the outside of the uterus. Most fibroids grow within the wall of the uterus, some grow on stalks (called *peduncles*) that grow out from the surface of the uterus or into the cavity of the uterus. See Figure 17–18 ▼.

Most fibroids do not cause any symptoms, but some women with fibroids experience the following:

- Heavy bleeding or painful periods.
- Bleeding between periods.
- Feeling of fullness in the pelvic area (lower abdomen).
- Frequent urination.
- Pain during sex.
- Lower back pain.
- Reproductive problems, such as infertility, or early onset of labor during pregnancy.

Treatment for women with fibroids who have mild symptoms may only involve pain medication. Over-the-counter (OTC) anti-inflammatory drugs (such as Advil or Motrin) or other medications (Tylenol) can be used for mild pain. Other drugs used to treat fibroids, called *gonadotropin releasing hormone agonists (GnRHa)*, can decrease the fibroid size. Sometimes they are used before surgery to shrink the fibroids, making them easier to remove.

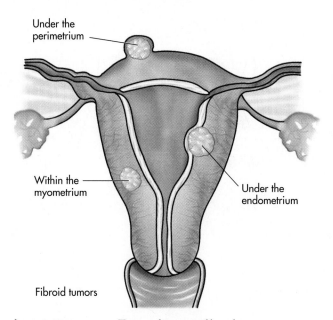

Under the perimetrium

Within the myometrium

Under the endometrium

Fibroid tumors

▶ **FIGURE 17–18**   Types of uterine fibroid tumors.

These drugs offer only temporary relief from the symptoms of fibroids; once the drug therapy is discontinued, the fibroids often grow back.

Following are the types of surgery used to treat fibroids:

- *Dilation and curettage* (D&C) is a procedure that involves enlarging the cervix (dilation) and then scraping (curettage) out portions of the lining of the uterus. It is considered to be minor surgery performed in a hospital, ambulatory surgery center, or clinic. When used for fibroids or polyps, D&C can stop bleeding for a while, usually 2 to 6 months. It is mainly performed to take tissue samples or remove tissue following an incomplete miscarriage.

- *Myomectomy* is a surgery to remove fibroids without taking out the healthy tissue of the uterus. A surgeon can perform this procedure in many ways. It can be major surgery (with an abdominal incision) or minor surgery. The type, size, and location of the fibroids determine what type of procedure is done.

- *Hysterectomy* is a surgery to remove the uterus and is the only sure way to cure uterine fibroids. This surgery is used when a woman's fibroids are large or if she has heavy bleeding and is either near or past menopause and/or does not want to become pregnant in the future.

# ✔ PATHOLOGY CHECKPOINT

*Following is a concise list of the pathology-related terms that you have seen in the chapter. Review this checklist to make sure that you are familiar with the meaning of each term before moving to the next section.*

## Conditions and Symptoms

- ❏ amenorrhea
- ❏ bartholinitis
- ❏ cervicitis
- ❏ cystocele
- ❏ dysmenorrhea
- ❏ dyspareunia
- ❏ endometriosis
- ❏ fibroma
- ❏ menorrhagia
- ❏ menorrhea
- ❏ mittelschmerz
- ❏ myometritis
- ❏ oligomenorrhea

- ❏ pelvic inflammatory disease
- ❏ premenstrual syndrome
- ❏ retroversion
- ❏ salpingitis
- ❏ toxic shock syndrome
- ❏ uterine fibroid
- ❏ vaginitis
- ❏ venereal disease

## Diagnosis and Treatment

- ❏ colposcope
- ❏ culdocentesis
- ❏ genetics
- ❏ hymenectomy

- ❏ hysterectomy
- ❏ hysteroscope
- ❏ hysterotomy
- ❏ laser ablation
- ❏ laser laparoscopy
- ❏ laser lumpectomy
- ❏ lumpectomy
- ❏ mammoplasty
- ❏ mastectomy
- ❏ oophorectomy
- ❏ salpingectomy
- ❏ salpingo-oophorectomy

# STUDY AND REVIEW

## Anatomy and Physiology

*Write your answers to the following questions. Do not refer to the text.*

1. List the primary and accessory sex organs of the female reproductive system.

   a. _____     b. _____

   c. _____     d. _____

   e. _____     f. _____

2. State the vital function of the female reproductive system. _____

   _____

3. The normal position of the uterus is known as _____

4. Define *fundus.* _____

   _____

5. Name the ligaments that support the uterus and hold it in position.

   a. _____     b. _____

   c. _____     d. _____

6. Name the three layers of the uterine wall.

   a. _____     b. _____

   c. _____

7. State the three primary functions associated with the uterus.

   a. _____

   b. _____

   c. _____

8. Define the following terms:

   a. *Retroflexion* _____

   _____

   b. *Anteversion* _____

   _____

   c. *Retroversion* _____

   _____

9. The fallopian tubes are also called the _____ _____ or

   _____.

10. Name the three layers of the fallopian tubes.

    a. _____     b. _____

    c. _____

11. Define *fimbriae*. _____

    _____

12. Should the ovum become impregnated by a spermatozoon while in the fallopian

    tube, the process of _____ occurs.

13. State two functions of the fallopian tubes.

    a. _____     b. _____

14. Describe the ovaries. _____

    _____

15. Name the three stages of an ovarian follicle.

    a. _____     b. _____

    c. _____

16. The functional activity of the ovary is controlled by the _____.

17. State the two functions of the ovary.

    a. _____     b. _____

18. The vagina is a _____ tube extending from the _____ to the
    uterus.

19. State the three functions of the vagina.

    a. _____     b. _____

    c. _____

20. Name the organs that comprise the external female genitalia.

    a. _____     b. _____

    c. _____     d. _____

    e. _____

21. The breasts or _____ _____ are compound alveolar
    structures.

22. The _____ is the dark pigmented area found in the skin over each

    breast, and the _____ is the elevated area in its center.

23. Name the three hormones that play a role in milk production.

    a. _____        b. _____

    c. _____

24. Define *colostrum*. _____

_____

25. Name the three phases of the menstrual cycle.

    a. _____        b. _____

    c. _____

26. Define *premenstrual syndrome*. _____

_____

_____

## Word Parts

1. In the spaces provided, write the definitions of these prefixes, roots, combining forms, and suffixes. Do not refer to the listings of medical words. Leave blank those words you cannot define.

2. After completing as many as you can, refer to the medical word listings to check your work. For each word missed or left blank, write the word and its definition several times on the margins of these pages or on a separate sheet of paper.

3. To maximize the learning process, it is to your advantage to do the following exercises as directed. To refer to the word-building section before completing these exercises invalidates the learning process.

## PREFIXES

*Give the definitions of the following prefixes.*

1. a- _____    2. contra- _____

3. dys- _____    4. endo- _____

5. intra- _____    6. oligo- _____

7. peri- _____    8. post- _____

9. retro- _____

## ROOTS AND COMBINING FORMS

*Give the definition of the following roots and combining forms:*

1. bartholin _____
2. cept _____
3. cervic _____
4. coit _____
5. colp/o _____
6. culd/o _____
7. cyst/o _____
8. fibr _____
9. genital _____
10. gynec/o _____
11. bi/o _____
12. hymen _____
13. hyster _____
14. hyster/o _____
15. log _____
16. mamm/o _____
17. mast _____
18. men _____
19. men/o _____
20. metr _____
21. metr/i _____
22. my/o _____
23. o/o _____
24. oophor _____
25. ovulat _____
26. par _____
27. pause _____
28. rect/o _____
29. salping _____
30. salping/o _____
31. genet _____
32. uter _____
33. vagin _____
34. venere _____
35. vers _____
36. lump _____
37. pareun _____

## SUFFIXES

*Give the definitions of the following suffixes.*

1. -al _____
2. -arche _____
3. -cele _____
4. -centesis _____
5. -ectomy _____
6. -genesis _____
7. -ia _____
8. -ine _____
9. -ion _____
10. -ist _____
11. -itis _____
12. -oma _____
13. -osis _____
14. -plasty _____
15. -rrhagia _____
16. -rrhea _____
17. -scope _____
18. -ic _____
19. -oid _____
20. -tic(s) _____

## Identifying Medical Terms

*In the spaces provided, write the medical terms for the following meanings.*

1. _____ Inflammation of the uterine cervix

2. _____ Difficult or painful monthly flow

3. _____ Fibrous tissue tumor

4. _____ Study of the female

5. _____ Surgical excision of the hymen

6. _____ Surgical repair of the breast

7. _____ Normal monthly flow

8. _____ Formation of the ovum

9. _____ Difficult or painful sexual intercourse

10. _____ Male or female reproductive organs

## Spelling

*In the spaces provided, write the correct spelling of these misspelled words.*

1. bartolinitis _____

2. hystrotomy _____

3. menorhagia _____

4. oophritis _____

5. salpinitis _____

6. vajinitis _____

7. veneral _____

8. menache _____

9. oligomenorhea _____

10. postcotal _____

## Matching

*Select the appropriate lettered meaning for each of the following words.*

_____ 1. laser ablation

_____ 2. lumpectomy

_____ 3. menarche

_____ 4. mittelschmerz

_____ 5. ovulation

_____ 6. gynecologist

_____ 7. contraception

_____ 8. perimenopause

_____ 9. hysterotomy

_____ 10. rectovaginal

a. Beginning of the monthly flow (menses, menstruation)
b. Surgical removal of a tumor from the breast
c. Abdominal pain that occurs midway between the menstrual periods at ovulation
d. Process in which an ovum is discharged from the cortex of the ovary
e. Procedure that uses a laser to destroy the uterine lining
f. Pertaining to the rectum and vagina
g. Period of gradual changes that lead into menopause
h. Physician who specializes in the study of the female
i. Also called cesarean section
j. Process of preventing conception
k. Lack of the monthly flow (menses, menstruation)

## Abbreviations

*Place the correct word, phrase, or abbreviation in the space provided.*

1. AH _____

2. DES _____

3. birth control pill _____

4. intrauterine device _____

5. pelvic inflammatory disease _____

6. cervical intraepithelial neoplasia _____

7. DUB _____

8. PMS _____

9. dilation and curettage _____

10. toxic shock syndrome _____

## Diagnostic and Laboratory Tests

*Select the best answer to each multiple choice question. Circle the letter of your choice.*

1. X-ray of the uterus and fallopian tubes after the injection of a radiopaque substance.
   a. hysterosalpingography
   b. laparoscopy
   c. culdoscopy
   d. mammography

2. Used to examine the ovaries and fallopian tubes.
   a. colposcopy
   b. culdoscopy
   c. laparoscopy
   d. mammography

3. Process of obtaining pictures of the breast by use of x-rays.
   a. colposcopy
   b. culdoscopy
   c. laparoscopy
   d. mammography

4. Screening technique to aid in the detection of cervical/uterine cancer and cancer precursors.
   a. colposcopy
   b. Papanicolaou (Pap smear)
   c. estrogens
   d. mammography

5. Urine test that determines menstrual disorders or possible abortion.
   a. wet mat or wet-prep
   b. culdoscopy
   c. Pap smear
   d. pregnanediol

# PRACTICAL APPLICATION

## S O A P : Chart Note Analysis

*This exercise will make you aware of information, abbreviations, and medical terminology typically found in a gynecology patient's chart note.*

### Abbreviations Key

| | | | |
|---|---|---|---|
| ABD | abdomen | mg | milligram |
| ASAP | as soon as possible | MS | musculoskeletal |
| BP | blood pressure | NSSC | normal size, shape, and |
| CBC | complete blood count | | consistency |
| CTA | clear to auscultation | P | pulse |
| DOB | date of birth | Pap | Papanicolaou (smear) |
| F | Fahrenheit | R | respiration |
| FROM | full range of motion | R/O | rule out |
| FSH | follicle stimulating hormone | SOAP | subjective, objective, assessment, |
| GYN | gynecology | | plan |
| Ht | height | T | temperature |
| JVD | jugular vein distention | TSH | thyroid stimulating hormone |
| lb | pound | WNL | within normal limits |
| LMP | last menstrual period | Wt | weight |
| mcg | microgram | y/o | year(s) old |

*Read the following chart note and then answer the questions that follow.*

**PATIENT:** Smith, Ann M.                                                    **DATE:** 2/21/07
**DOB:** 01/24/1955      **AGE:** 52      **SEX:** Female
**INSURANCE:** Best Care Insurance

   **Vital Signs:**
      **T:** 98.8 F
      **P:** 70
      **R:** 16
      **BP:** 120/78
      **Ht:** 5′ 3″
      **Wt:** 135 lb

**Allergies:** Penicillin

**Chief Complaint:** Patient presents with irregular menses, hot flashes, insomnia, dyspareunia and moodiness

**S** **Subjective:** 52 y/o white female presents with complaints of irregular periods, hot flashes, and trouble sleeping. She states, "Sex with my husband has become uncomfortable and I am very moody. I am really having trouble with hot flashes. I wake up in the middle of the night soaked—especially my hair and neck." When asked about her children, she indicates that she has two children, one daughter who is an English teacher and one son who is a pharmacist. She also states that she has never had an abortion. Her LMP was 11/21/06.

**O**   Objective:

**General Appearance:** Attractive, well-groomed, and pleasant. Noted a slight nervousness and concern during initial interview.

**Neck:** No bruits or JVD, full range of motion, no pain, trachea midline

**Lungs:** CTA

**Heart:** Normal rate and rhythm

**ABD:** Bowel sounds all 4 quadrants, soft, no masses or tenderness

**MS:** FROM, joints and muscles symmetric, no swelling, masses, or deformity. Normal spinal curvature

**Skin:** Warm to touch, dry, and smooth. Skin tone good, no lesions

**Rectal exam:** No fissures, hemorrhoids, or skin lesions in perianal area. Sphincter tone good, no prolapse. No masses or tenderness.

**GYN:**

> Breasts: Symmetrical, no palpable masses or tenderness, no dimpling or skin changes
> External genitalia: No lesions or inflammation, normal hair distribution with thinning
> Cervix: Pink, smooth, no cervical motion tenderness
> Adnexa uteri: Nontender, no masses
> Uterus: NSSC, noted retroversion position, firm, slightly enlarged, with possible uterine fibroid tumor
> Pregnancies: Gravida 2 Para 2 Abortions 0

**A**   **Assessment:** Perimenopause

**P**   **Plan:** Patient elected the nonprescription treatment for 6 months. To be reevaluated August 2007.

1. Schedule mammogram ASAP. If WNL, then annually.
2. Review results of Pap smear with maturation index. If WNL, follow up with annual Pap.
3. Advised to use over-the-counter water-soluble vaginal lubricant for intercourse and moisturizer for vaginal dryness.
4. Advised to go to the laboratory for CBC, cholesterol, triglycerides, and glucose. Check TSH, FSH, and estradiol levels to R/O thyroid disorder and obtain hormone baseline levels.
5. Recommended she take a multivitamin and mineral complex that contains 400 mcg of folic acid. Also, take 1500 mg of calcium with Vitamin D daily and an antioxidant.
6. Schedule a pelvic ultrasound to R/O uterine fibroid tumor, ASAP.
7. Recommend a bone density study before reevaluation in August.

**Nonprescription Regimen**

- ***Exercise.*** Aerobic, weight-bearing, and/or stretching exercises at least 30 minutes to an hour, 4 to 5 times a week.
- ***Diet.*** High in fruits and vegetables and low in saturated fat. To include 4 to 6 servings of soy products, foods such as soybeans, tofu, soymilk, and roasted soy nuts daily. Reduce intake of caffeine, alcohol, hot beverages, and spicy foods.

**FYI:** Soy contains phytoestrogens that are similar to estrogen and isoflavones. Blueberries and cherries also contain bioflavonoids that are a source of phytoestrogens. Flaxseeds and flaxseed oil are lignans—also phytoestrogens—and can help relieve hot flashes and vaginal dryness. These lignans also can have a stabilizing effect on hormone-related mood swings.

**Note:** *Phyto* is the combining form for plant. The phytoestrogens, isoflavones, and lignans are important secondary nutrients contained in soybeans and linseed. Isoflavones are a type of phytoestrogen, compounds that have weak estrogenic activity. Isoflavones are found in chickpeas and legumes. The legume soy has the most concentrated amount. Lignans are often considered a type of fiber but are more appropriately considered as a type of phytoestrogen or a plant compound with estrogenlike activity. Bioflavonoids refers to a class of water-soluble plant pigments believed to have favorable medicinal qualities.

## Chart Note Questions
*Place the correct answer in the space provided.*

1.  What is the abbreviation for gynecology? _____

2.  What does the statement, "I wake up in the middle of the night soaked—especially my hair and neck," indicate? _____

3.  Lignans and phytoestrogens can help relieve _____ and vaginal dryness.

4.  Are the patient's vital signs WNL? _____

5.  What does the abbreviation R/O stand for? _____

6.  What is the medical word for difficult or painful sexual intercourse? _____

7.  Phytoestrogens, isoflavones, and lignans are important secondary nutrients contained in _____ and linseed.

8.  What is the abbreviation for jugular vein distention? _____

9.  Is the cervix described as normal or abnormal? _____

10. Why is a pelvic ultrasound recommended? _____

# MULTIMEDIA PREVIEW

*Additional interactive resources and activities for this chapter can be found on the Companion Website. For videos, audio glossary, and review, access the accompanying CD-ROM in this book.*

## CD-ROM HIGHLIGHTS

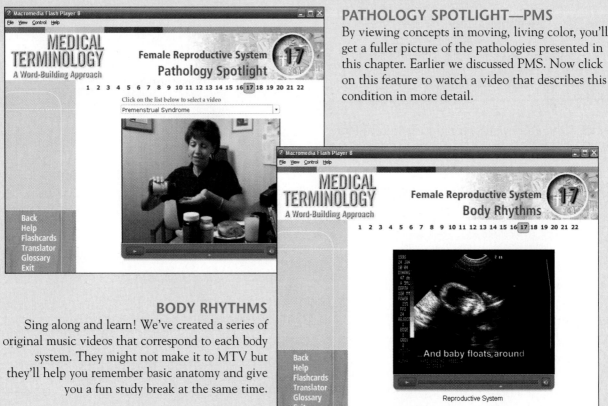

## PATHOLOGY SPOTLIGHT—PMS

By viewing concepts in moving, living color, you'll get a fuller picture of the pathologies presented in this chapter. Earlier we discussed PMS. Now click on this feature to watch a video that describes this condition in more detail.

## BODY RHYTHMS

Sing along and learn! We've created a series of original music videos that correspond to each body system. They might not make it to MTV but they'll help you remember basic anatomy and give you a fun study break at the same time.

## WEBSITE HIGHLIGHTS—www.prenhall.com/rice

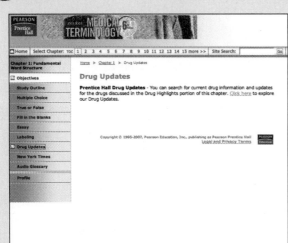

## DRUG UPDATES

Click here and take advantage of the free-access on-line study guide that accompanies your textbook. You'll find a feature that allows you to search for current information on the drugs discussed in this chapter. By clicking on this URL you'll also access links to download mp3 audio reviews, current news articles, review questions, and an audio glossary.

# Obstetrics

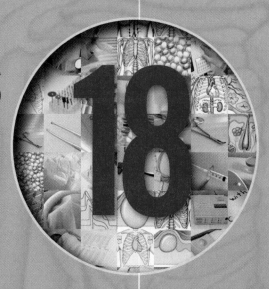

## ■ OUTLINE

## ■ OBJECTIVES

*On completion of this chapter, you will be able to:*

- Define obstetrics.
- Define pregnancy and describe its four stages.
- Describe prenatal care.
- Describe the three stages of labor.
- Analyze, build, spell, and pronounce medical words.
- Provide the description of diagnostic and laboratory tests related to pregnancy.
- Identify and define selected abbreviations.
- Describe each of the conditions presented in the Pathology Spotlights.
- Review the Pathology Checkpoint.
- Complete the Study and Review section and the Chart Note Analysis.

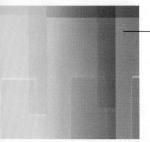

# Overview of Obstetrics

**Obstetrics** (OB) is the branch of medicine that pertains to the care of women during pregnancy, childbirth, and the postpartum period, which is also called the **puerperium.** A physician specializing in this medical field is known as an **obstetrician.**

## FERTILIZATION

**Fertilization** is the process in which a sperm penetrates an ovum and unites with it. See Figure 18–1 ▼. At this time, the 23 chromosomes from the male combine with the 23 chromosomes from the female to make a new life. Fertilization generally occurs within 24 hours following ovulation and usually takes place in the fallopian tube. A single sperm penetrates the ovum, and the resulting cell is called a **zygote.** See Figure 18–2 ▶.

By this event, called **conception,** the gender and other biologic traits of the new individual are determined. The fertilized ovum or zygote is genetically complete and immediately begins to divide, forming a solid mass of cells called a **morula.** The cells of the morula continue to divide, and by the time the developing **embryo** (the term for the stage of development between weeks 2 and 8) reaches the uterus, it is a hollow ball of cells known as a **blastocyst,** which consists of an outer layer of cells and an inner cell mass. As the blastocyst develops, it forms a structure with two cavities, the **yolk sac** and **amniotic cavity.** In humans, the yolk sac is the site of formation of the first red blood cells and the cells that will become ovum and sperm.

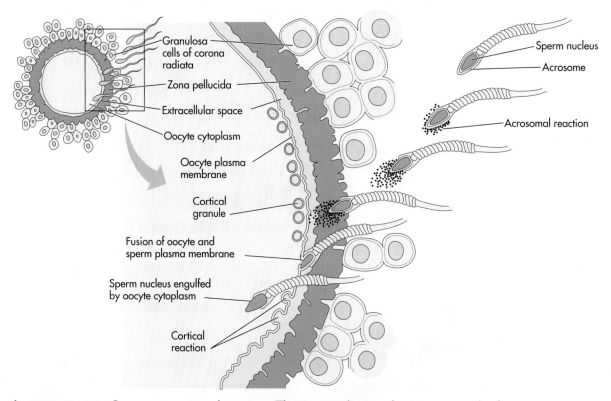

Granulosa cells of corona radiata

Zona pellucida

Extracellular space

Oocyte cytoplasm

Oocyte plasma membrane

Cortical granule

Fusion of oocyte and sperm plasma membrane

Sperm nucleus engulfed by oocyte cytoplasm

Cortical reaction

Sperm nucleus

Acrosome

Acrosomal reaction

▶ **FIGURE 18–1**　Sperm penetration of an ovum. The sequential steps of oocyte penetration by a sperm are depicted moving from top to bottom.

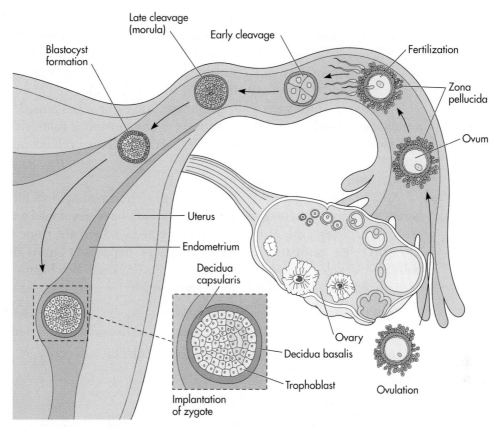

▶ **FIGURE 18–2** During ovulation, the ovum leaves the ovary and enters the fallopian tube. Subsequent changes in the fertilized ovum from conception to implantation are depicted.

The amniotic cavity is the fluid-filled cavity of the **amnion,** the inner transparent sac that holds the fetus suspended in the **amniotic fluid.** This liquid protects the **fetus** (the term for the stage of development from the third month until birth) from injury. It also helps maintain an even temperature, prevents formation of adhesions between the amnion and the skin of the fetus, and prevents conformity of the sac to the fetus. The amniotic fluid is constantly being absorbed and renewed at a rapid rate. About one-third of the water in the amniotic fluid is replaced each hour.

The **placenta** is composed of tissues from the mother and the child. It anchors the developing fetus to the uterus and provides the means by which the fetus receives its nourishment and oxygen. It also functions as an excretory, respiratory, and endocrine organ, which produces human chorionic gonadotropin (hCG). The placenta consists of a fetal portion and a maternal portion. The fetal portion has a shiny, slightly grayish appearance and is formed by a coming together of chorionic villi in which the umbilical vein and arteries intertwine to form the **umbilical cord.** The maternal portion develops from the decidual basalis of the uterus. It has a red, beefy-looking appearance. The mature placenta is 15 to 18 centimeters (cm) (6 to 7 inches) in diameter and weighs approximately 450 grams (about 1 pound). When expelled following **parturition** (the act of giving birth), it is known as the **afterbirth.**

## PREGNANCY

**Pregnancy** may be defined as a temporary condition that occurs within a woman's body from the time of conception through the embryonic and fetal periods to birth. The normal term of pregnancy is approximately 40 weeks (280 days); this equals 10 lunar months or

9⅓ calendar months. The length of pregnancy is called the **gestation period** and is divided into three segments of three months each called **trimesters.**

Human development follows three stages: the *preembryonic stage* is the first 14 days of development after the ovum is fertilized; the *embryonic stage* begins in the third week after fertilization; and the *fetal stage* begins in the ninth week. See Figure 18–3 ▼.

During the fifth week of development, the embryo has a marked C-shaped body and a rudimentary tail. At 7 weeks, the head of the embryo is rounded and nearly erect. The eyes have shifted forward and are closer together and the eyelids begin to form. At 9 weeks, every organ system and external structure are present, and the developing embryo is now called a *fetus*. See Figure 18–4 ▶.

At 14 weeks, the skin of the fetus is so transparent that blood vessels are visible beneath it. More muscle tissue and body skeleton have developed and holds the fetus more erect. At 20 weeks, the fetus weighs approximately 435 to 465 g and measures about 19 cm. The skin is less transparent due to subcutaneous deposits of brown fat. Fingernails and toenails have developed and "woolly" hair covers the head. See Figure 18–5 ▶.

Pregnancy is divided into four stages:

- **Prenatal stage,** the time period between conception and onset of labor, refers to both the care of the woman during pregnancy and the growth and development of the fetus.

- **Labor,** the last phase of pregnancy to the time of delivery.

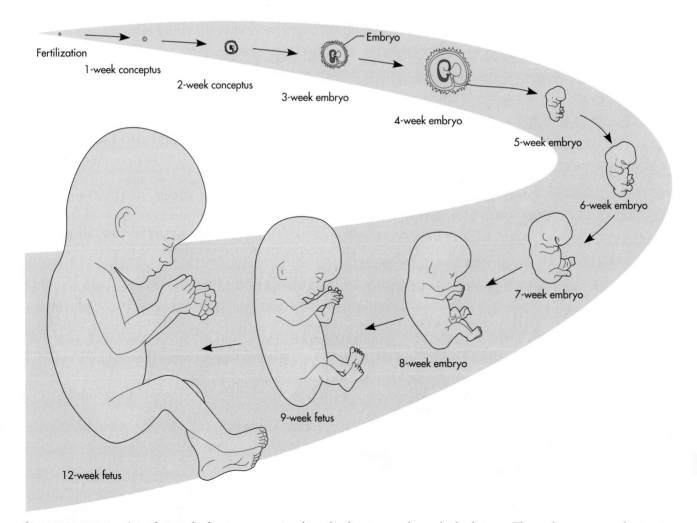

▶ **FIGURE 18–3**   Actual size of a human conceptus from fertilization to the early fetal stage. The embryonic stage begins in the 3rd week after fertilization; the fetal stage begins in the 9th week.

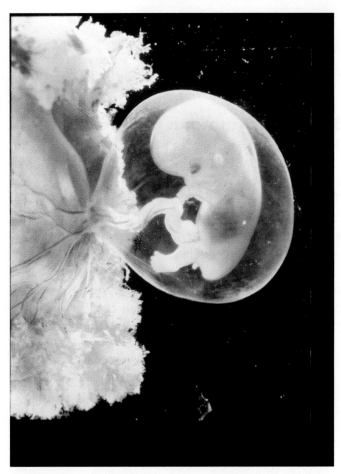

▶ **FIGURE 18–4**   Fetus at 9 weeks. Every organ system and external structure is present. (Source: Lennart Nilsson and Albert Bonniers Förlag AB, *A Child Is Born*, New York: Dell Publishing)

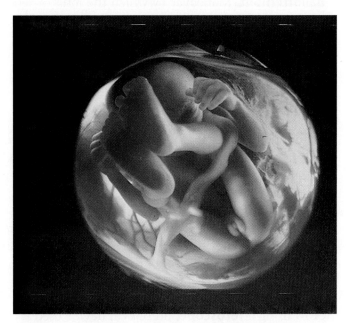

▶ **FIGURE 18–5**   Fetus at 20 weeks. The fetus weighs approximately 435 to 465 g and measures about 19 cm. Subcutaneous deposits of brown fat make the skin less transparent. "Woolly" hair covers the head, and nails have developed on the fingers and toes. (Source: Lennart Nilsson/Albert Bonniers Förlag AB, *A Child Is Born*, New York: Dell Publishing)

- **Parturition,** the act of giving birth, also known as **childbirth** or **delivery.**
- **Postpartum period** or **puerperium,** the 6 weeks following childbirth and expulsion of the placenta. The female reproductive organs usually return to an essentially prepregnant condition in which *involution of the uterus* (return of the uterus to normal size after childbirth) occurs.

## Signs and Symptoms of Pregnancy

The signs and symptoms of pregnancy are divided into three general groups: subjective (presumptive), objective (probable), and diagnostic (positive). **Subjective signs** are those experienced by the expectant mother, that suggest pregnancy but are not positive signs. These early signs include amenorrhea, nausea and sometimes vomiting, breast changes, pigmentation changes, frequency and urgency of urination, fatigue and drowsiness, and quickening. **Quickening** is the movement of the fetus felt in the uterus, generally beginning in weeks 16 to 20 of pregnancy.

**Objective signs** of pregnancy are those that are observable by the examiner. Even though the following signs are stronger indicators of pregnancy, they can be caused by other *conditions** and are not considered to be positive signs of pregnancy.

- **Goodell's sign.** Softening of the cervix and vagina caused by increased vascular congestion. **Can also be caused by hormonal imbalance or infection.*
- **Chadwick's sign.** Purplish or bluish discoloration of the cervix, vagina, and vulva caused by increased vascular congestion. **Can also be caused by hormonal imbalance or infection.*
- **Hegar's sign.** Softening of the lower uterine segment.
- **Abdominal and uterine enlargement.**
- **Braxton Hicks contractions.** Irregular, painless uterine contractions (UC) that begin in the second trimester and can occur throughout the pregnancy. **Can also be caused by uterine fibroids.*
- **Ballottement.** Maneuver by which the fetus or fetal part rebounds when displaced by a light tap of the examining finger on the cervix. **Can also be caused by uterine or cervical polyps.*
- **Fetal outline.** Identified by palpation after week 24. **Could also be a tumor of the uterus.*
- **Abdominal striae.** Commonly known as *stretch marks,* the fine, pinkish-white or purplish-gray lines that some women develop when the elastic tissue of the skin has been stretched to its capacity.
- **Pregnancy tests.** Tests using maternal blood or urine to determine the presence of hCG (human chorionic gonadotropin) hormone produced by the chorionic villi of the placenta that is secreted during pregnancy and detectable in the urine about 10 days after conception.

The **diagnostic** or **positive signs** of pregnancy are the only absolute indicators of a developing fetus. They include the presence of fetal heart activity, fetal movements felt by an examiner, and visualization of the fetus with ultrasound.

- **Fetal heartbeat.** Can be detected by ultrasound at approximately 10 weeks gestation, or by using a **fetoscope,** an optical device used for direct visualization of the fetus in the uterus, at approximately 18 to 20 weeks of pregnancy.
- **Fetal movements.** Can be felt by the examiner in the second trimester and can be observed by using **ultrasonography,** high-frequency sound waves that visualize a

structure or produce a record of ultrasonic echoes as they strike tissues of different densities.

- **Visualization of the fetus.** Using ultrasound, this is possible as early as 4 to 5 weeks of gestation with 100% reliability, providing the earliest positive confirmation of pregnancy.

# PRENATAL CARE

**Prenatal care** (sometimes called *antepartal care*) is the care of the woman during the period of gestation. It should begin as soon as a woman suspects that she is pregnant. The care of the mother during her entire pregnancy is essential to her well-being and that of her fetus. It consists of periodic examinations to determine blood pressure, weight, changes in the size of the uterus, and the condition of the fetus. Also included are laboratory tests such as urinalysis and blood analysis; instruction in nutritional requirements and care of the newborn; and suggestions and support to deal with the discomforts of pregnancy.

On the first prenatal visit, a medical history is taken, and a complete physical examination is performed. For an uncomplicated pregnancy, the recommended schedule for prenatal visits is:

- Conception to 28 weeks: every 4 weeks.
- 29 to 36 weeks: every 2 to 3 weeks.
- 37 weeks to birth: weekly.

## Determination of the Estimated Date of Delivery

The average duration of a term pregnancy is 40 weeks (280 days) after the last normal menstrual period (LMP). The date of delivery can be determined in several ways. Näegele's rule, a gestational wheel, or other means may be used to determine the estimated date of delivery.

### Näegele's Rule to Determine the Estimated Date of Delivery (EDD)
- Determine the first day of the last normal menstrual period.
- Count backward 3 months.
- Add 7 days.

  Consider the following example.

  First day of the LMP: June 25
  Count backward 3 months: March 25
  Add 7 days: April 1 is the EDD

*Note:* The following abbreviations are also used to describe the estimated date of delivery: EDC (estimated date of confinement) and EDB (estimated date of birth).

## Prenatal Tests

Certain diagnostic and laboratory tests are done on the first or second prenatal visit; other tests can be performed at specific times during pregnancy. Several tests are commonly done for all pregnant women; others are based on the presence of specific risk factors or complications of pregnancy. See Diagnostic and Laboratory Tests for more information on the tests that may be used during pregnancy.

## LABOR AND DELIVERY

**Parturition** is the act of giving birth. It is also known as **childbirth** or **delivery. Labor** is the process by which forceful contractions move the fetus down the birth canal and expel it from the uterus. The signs and symptoms that labor is about to start can occur from hours to weeks before the actual onset of labor. Signs of impending labor include Braxton Hicks contractions, increased vaginal discharge, lightening, bloody show, rupture of the membranes, energy spurt, and weight loss.

- **Braxton Hicks contractions.** Irregular contractions that begin in the second trimester and intensify as full term approaches.

- **Increased vaginal discharge.** Normally clear and nonirritating discharge caused by fetal pressure.

- **Lightening.** The descent of the baby into the pelvis. The expectant mother will notice that she can breathe easier and often states, "The baby has dropped." This may occur 2 to 3 weeks before the first stage of labor begins.

- **Bloody show.** Thick mucus mixed with pink or dark-brown blood. As the cervix softens, effaces, and dilates, the mucous plug that has sealed the uterus during pregnancy is dislodged from the cervix and small capillaries are torn, producing the bloody show.

- **Rupture of the membranes.** Occurs when the amniotic sac (bag of waters) ruptures.
    *Note: When the membranes do not rupture on their own, they will be ruptured by the attending physician or midwife. This is known as* **AROM:** *artificial rupture of membranes.*

- **Energy spurt or nesting.** Occurs in many women shortly before the onset of labor. They may suddenly have the energy to clean their houses and do things that they have not had the energy to do previously.

- **Weight loss.** Loss of 1 to 3 pounds shortly before labor can occur as hormone changes cause excretion of extra body water.

### Stages and Phases of Labor

True labor is characterized by rhythmic contractions that develop a regular pattern and are more frequent, more intense, and last longer. A general feeling of discomfort is felt in the lower back and lower abdomen. A bloody show is often present, and progressive effacement and dilation of the cervix occur. Labor is divided into three stages (See Figure 18–6 ▶):

- **First stage.** Begins with the onset of true labor and lasts until the cervix is fully dilated to 10 cm. This is the stage of dilation.

- **Second stage.** Continues after the cervix is dilated to 10 cm until the delivery of the baby. This is the stage of expulsion.

- **Third stage.** Delivery of the placenta.

### First Stage

The first stage of labor describes the time from the onset of labor until full dilation of the cervix. It is generally the longest phase for both **nulliparas,** women who have borne no offspring, and **multiparas,** women who have borne more than one child. It is broken down into three phases:

Early Labor or Latent Phase.   This phase starts with the onset of labor and lasts until the cervix is dilated to 3 cm. Duration is about 8 to 12 hours; contractions last about 30 to 45 seconds, with about 5 to 30 minutes of rest between contractions. Contractions are typically mild, somewhat irregular, but progressively become stronger and closer together. The *bag of waters* can break any time during the first phase.

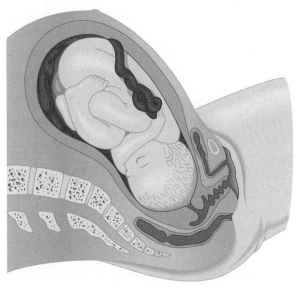

DILATION STAGE:
First uterine contraction to dilation of cervix

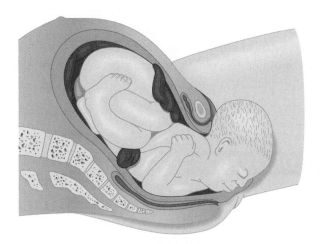

EXPULSION STAGE:
Birth of baby or expulsion

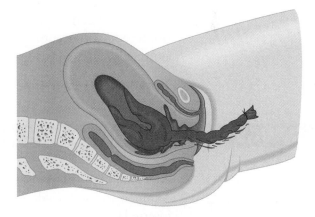

PLACENTAL STAGE:
Delivery of placenta

▶ **FIGURE 18–6** Three stages of labor and delivery.

**Active Labor Phase.**   This phase continues until the cervix is dilated to 7 cm. Duration is about 3 to 5 hours. Contractions during this phase last about 45 to 60 seconds with 3 to 5 minutes rest between contractions. *Effacement,* the shortening of the vaginal portion of the cervix and thinning of its walls as it is stretched and dilated by the fetus during labor, is completed.

**Transition Phase.**   This phase continues until the cervix is fully dilated to 10 cm. Duration is about 30 minutes to 2 hours. Contractions during this phase last about 60 to 90 seconds with rest periods of 30 seconds to 2 minutes. Contractions are long, strong, intense, and may overlap.

### Second Stage
The second stage of labor is from the time of full cervical dilation (10 cm) until the birth of the baby. The entire process lasts anywhere from 20 minutes to 2 hours or longer. Contractions last about 45 to 90 seconds with a 3- to 5-minute rest between contractions. There is a strong natural urge to push with a feeling of pressure on the rectum. The second stage ends with the arrival of the baby. Generally, the head of the baby appears first; this is known as **crowning.**

The newborn baby usually has a cone-shaped or molded head due to its journey down the birth canal. It is covered with **vernix caseosa,** a protective cheesy substance that covers the fetus during intrauterine life. The baby will present with **lanugo,** fine downy hair that covers the body, especially the shoulders, back, forehead, and temple. The external **genitalia,** the male or female reproductive organs, are usually enlarged.

The first assessment of the newborn involves using the Apgar score. It is performed immediately following the birth of the baby. This method was developed by Virginia Apgar (U.S. anesthesiologist, 1909–1974) as the first objective evaluation of newborns in 1952 and since then, the Apgar score has become the standard tool for assessing newborn babies. The five assessments of the Apgar score are a mnemonic based upon Virginia's last name. Ratings are based on **A**ppearance (color), **P**ulse (heartbeat), **G**rimace (reflex), **A**ctivity (muscle tone), and **R**espiration (breathing). The score is taken at 1 and 5 minutes after birth, the high score being 10 and the low score being one. See Table 18–1.

### Third Stage

The third and shortest stage is the delivery of the placenta. The time it takes to deliver the placenta is anywhere from 5 to 30 minutes. The placenta is expelled in one or two ways: the **Schultze mechanism,** with the fetal surface presenting, or the **Duncan mechanism** presenting the maternal surface. The placenta is examined to be certain that all of it has been expelled. Any small portion of the placenta that remains in the uterus could interfere with uterine contractions after the birth of the baby and contribute to infection. To control bleeding from the vessels that supplied the placenta during pregnancy, the uterus must contract and remain contracted after placental expulsion.

## DRUGS USED DURING LABOR AND DELIVERY

An epidural block can be used to reduce the discomfort and pain of contractions. This is a common method of administering anesthesia during labor. A small amount of anesthesia is inserted through a narrow catheter that is threaded through a needle inserted into the dura space near the spinal cord. Local anesthetics or a pudendal block (a procedure that provides regional pain relief in the perineum area during birth) can be used to numb the vaginal area in preparation for an **episiotomy.**

Drugs that selectively stimulate contraction of the myometrium, the muscular middle layer of the uterus, are known as oxytocic agents or uterine stimulants. These agents act to increase the strength and frequency of contractions. They can be used in obstetrics to induce labor at term and to control postpartum hemorrhage. An example is *Pitocin* (*oxytocin*).

TABLE 18–1  **The Apgar Score**

| Sign | 0 | 1 | 2 |
|------|---|---|---|
| Heart rate | Absent | Less than 100/min | More than 100/min |
| Respiratory effort | Absent | Slow, irregular | Regular or crying |
| Reflex irritability | No response | Grimace, frown | Cry, cough |
| Muscle tone | Limp | Some motion, some flexion of extremities, some resistance to extension of extremities | Active, spontaneous flexion, good tone |
| Color | Cyanotic or pale | Body pink, extremities cyanotic | Completely pink |

# BREASTFEEDING

Breastfeeding is the act of providing milk to a baby from the mother's breasts. Mature mother's milk and its precursor, colostrum (the *first milk*), are considered to be the most balanced foods available for normal infants. Breast milk is sterile, easily digested, nonallergenic, and transmits maternal antibodies that protect against various infections and illnesses. In addition, the baby's suckling causes the release of oxytocin in the mother, which stimulates uterine contractions and promotes the return of the uterus to a normal nonpregnant size and state.

The American Academy of Pediatrics currently recommends the following:

*Pediatricians and parents should be aware that exclusive breastfeeding is sufficient to support optimal growth and development for approximately the first 6 months of life and provides continuing protection against diarrhea and respiratory tract infection. Breastfeeding should be continued for at least the first year of life and beyond for as long as mutually desired by mother and child.*

Some of the noted advantages of breastfeeding and breast milk are:

- Provides an ideal food for most newborn babies.
- Provides essential nutrients for growth and development.
- Is virtually free from harmful bacteria.
- Does not need to be prepared.
- Costs nothing to make and is in ready supply.
- Is good for the environment because there are no bottles, cans, and boxes to put in the garbage.
- Can help prevent dehydration. Continued breastfeeding during an infant's diarrhea may reduce the severity, duration, and negative nutritional consequences of diarrhea.
- Can help pregnancy spacing because exclusive breastfeeding can reduce potential fertility.
- Helps to bond mother and child.

After the first 2 weeks, the nursing mother may produce 1 or more pints of milk per day. Milk production can be affected by emotions, food, fluid intake, physical health, and medications. Breastfeeding can burn 500 calories a day in the nursing mother.

# LIFE SPAN CONSIDERATIONS

## ■ THE CHILD

Worldwide there are more than 15 million births to females under the age of 20. Potential risk factors for becoming pregnant at an early age include early dating, smoking, alcohol and substance abuse, low academic interest, single-parent families, and poverty. Those who seek early prenatal care are at no greater risk during pregnancy than women over 20 years of age. However, many adolescents do not seek early prenatal care, placing themselves and their unborn children at risk. As a result, adolescent pregnancy is associated with adverse maternal and fetal effects.

Maternal complications due to adolescent pregnancy include iron deficiency anemia, preeclampsia, eclampsia, sexually transmitted diseases (STDs), premature labor and delivery, and cephalopelvic disproportion (CPD), in which the size of the maternal pelvis and of the presenting fetal head differs. If the maternal pelvis diameters are less than average, or if the fetus is very large or is in a malpresentation or malpositon, CPD is said to be present, and vaginal birth is not possible.

The most common complications concerning the infant of an adolescent are related to preterm births, low birth weight (LBW), infection, chemical dependence (due to maternal substance abuse), and sudden infant death syndrome (SIDS).

## ■ THE OLDER ADULT

According to the National Center for Health Statistics, between 1978 and 2000, the birth rates for women age 35 to 39 and 40 to 44 more than doubled. Women in their late 30s and 40s are likely to have healthy babies, but they often face particular risks.

Besides the increased risk of diabetes and high blood pressure, women over 35 have an increased risk of placental problems. The most common placental difficulty is placenta previa, in which the placenta covers part or all of the opening of the cervix. See Figures 18–13 on page 618 and 18–16 on page 635. A 2002 Canadian study found that women over age 35 were 20% to 40% more likely than younger women to have a low birth weight baby (less than 5½ pounds), and 20% more likely to have a premature delivery (born at less than 37 full weeks of pregnancy). These risks appear to rise modestly but progressively with a woman's age, even if she does not have age-related chronic health problems such as diabetes and high blood pressure.

A Danish study found that women over age 35 had an increased risk of ectopic pregnancy (in which the fertilized egg implants outside of the uterus, usually in the fallopian tube). See Figure 18–10 on page 614. The Danish and Canadian studies also found a slightly increased risk of stillbirth, though other studies did not.

The newborns of mothers in their 40s can suffer more complications (such as asphyxia and brain bleeds) than those of younger mothers, according to a University of California at Davis study. However, in spite of the increased risk of complications, there were no more deaths among babies of older mothers than of younger ones, and the vast majority of babies recovered from early difficulties and progressed normally.

Pregnant women who are 35 or older face some special risks, but many of them can be managed effectively with good prenatal care.

# BUILDING YOUR MEDICAL VOCABULARY

This section provides the foundation for learning medical terminology. Review the following alphabetized word list. Note how common prefixes and suffixes are repeatedly applied to word roots and combining forms to create different meanings.

| | | | |
|---|---|---|---|
| **P** | Prefix | | |
| **R** | Root | | |
| **CF** | Combining form | | |
| **S** | Suffix | | |

| | |
|---|---|
| Pink words | Terms not built from word parts. |
| * | Indicates words covered in the Pathology Spotlights section. |
| (CD-ROM) | Check the CD-ROM for more information. |

| MEDICAL WORD | WORD PARTS (WHEN APPLICABLE) | | | DEFINITION |
|---|---|---|---|---|
| | **Part** | **Type** | **Meaning** | |
| **abortion (AB)**<br>(a-bōr'shŭn) | abort<br>-ion | R<br>S | to miscarry<br>process | Process of miscarrying; termination of the pregnancy before the fetus is viable.<br>*See Pathology Spotlight: Spontaneous Abortion on page 625. |
| **abruptio placentae**<br>(ă-brŭp'shē-ō plă-sĕn'tă) | | | | Premature separation of a normally situated placenta after the 20th week of gestation |
| **amniocentesis**<br>(ăm"nĭ-ō-sĕn-tĕ'sĭs) | amni/o<br>-centesis | CF<br>S | amniotic fluid<br>surgical puncture | Surgical puncture of the amniotic sac to obtain a sample of amniotic fluid from which it can be determined whether the fetus has Down syndrome, neural tube defects, Tay-Sachs disease, or other genetic defects. See Figure 18–7 ▶. |
| **antepartum**<br>(ăn'tē pär'tŭm) | ante-<br>partum | P<br>R | before<br>labor | Time between conception and before the onset of labor; used to describe the period during which a woman is pregnant; also referred to as *prenatal period* |
| **breech presentation** | | | | Presentation during birth of the buttocks or with one or both feet first. See Figure 18–8 ▶. |
| **cerclage**<br>(sār-klŏzh') | | | | Suturing an incompetent cervix to keep it from dilating prematurely during pregnancy. The sutures are removed near the end of the pregnancy. An incompetent cervix is a painless dilatation of the cervix without contractions due to a functional or structural defect. |
| **cesarean section (CS, C-section)**<br>(sē-sār'ē-ăn sĕk shŭn) | | | | Delivery of the fetus by means of an incision through the abdominal cavity and then into the uterus. Elective C-section is indicated for known cephalopelvic (head to pelvis) disproportion, malpresentations, and active herpes infection. Fetal distress is the most common cause for an emergency C-section. |

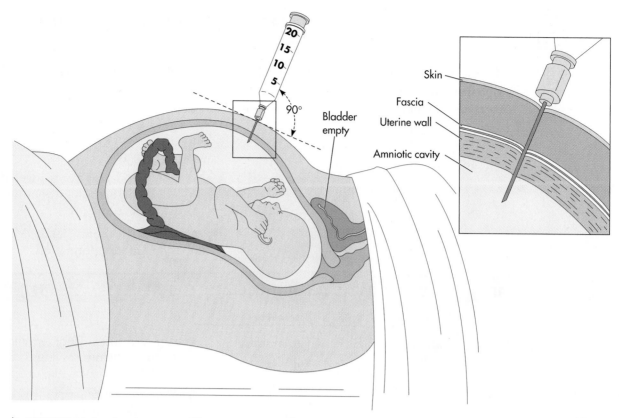

▶ **FIGURE 18–7**  Amniocentesis. The woman is usually scanned by ultrasound to determine the placental site and to locate a pocket of fluid. As the needle is inserted, three levels of resistance are felt when the needle penetrates the skin, fascia, and uterine wall. When the needle is placed within the amniotic cavity, amniotic fluid is withdrawn.

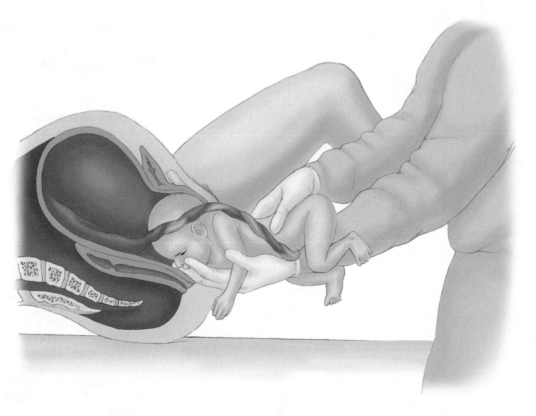

▶ **FIGURE 18–8**  Breech presentation.

| MEDICAL WORD | WORD PARTS (WHEN APPLICABLE) | | | DEFINITION |
|---|---|---|---|---|
| | **Part** | **Type** | **Meaning** | |
| **chloasma** (klō-ăz′mă) | | | | Brownish pigmentation of the face, often occurring in pregnancy; usually disappears after delivery; also called the *mask of pregnancy* |
| **cleavage** (klē′věj) | | | | Division of a fertilized egg into many smaller cells |
| **cord blood** | | | | Blood rich in stem cells present in the umbilical cord at the time of birth |
| **cordocentesis** (kor-dō-sēn-tē′sĭs) | cord/o -centesis | CF S | cord surgical puncture | Process of obtaining a sample of blood from the umbilical cord while the fetus is in utero |
| **decidua** (dē-sĭd′ū-ă) | | | | Name applied to the endometrium (lining) of the uterus after implantation of the fertilized ovum |
| **diagnostic ultrasound** (di″ ăg-nŏs′ tĭk ŭl′trăh-sŏund) | dia- gnost -ic ultra- -sound | P R S P S | through knowledge pertaining to beyond sound | Use of extremely high-frequency sound waves for diagnosing genetic defects and hydrocephalic conditions in the unborn fetus |
| **Doppler ultrasound** (däp′lər ŭl′trăh-sŏund) | | | | Procedure using an audio transformation of high-frequency sounds to monitor the fetal heartbeat. See Figure 18–9 ▼. |
| **dystocia** (dĭs-tŏ′sĭ-ă) | dys- toc -ia | P R S | difficult, painful birth condition | Condition of a difficult and painful childbirth |
| **eclampsia** (ě-klămp′sē-ă) | ec- lamp (s) -ia | P R S | out to shine condition | Complication of severe preeclampsia that involves seizures; also known as *toxemia* or *pregnancy-induced hypertension* (PIH). ✱ See Pathology Spotlight: Preeclampsia and Eclampsia on page 623. |

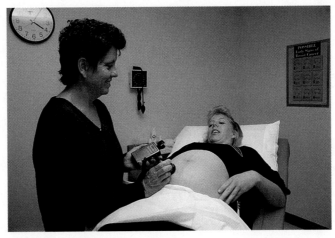

▶ **FIGURE 18–9** Listening to the fetal heartbeat with a Doppler device.

| MEDICAL WORD | WORD PARTS (WHEN APPLICABLE) | | | DEFINITION |
|---|---|---|---|---|
| | Part | Type | Meaning | |
| **ectopic pregnancy** (ĕk-tŏp′ĭk prĕg′năn-sē) | ectop -ic | R S | displaced pertaining to | Pregnancy that occurs when the fertilized egg is implanted in one of various sites, most commonly a fallopian tube; also referred to as a *tubal pregnancy*. See Figure 18–10 ▼. This type of pregnancy is life threatening to the mother and almost always fatal to the fetus. It is the leading cause of pregnancy-related death in African American women. |
| **electronic fetal monitor (EFM)** | | | | Electronic instrument used to record fetal heartbeat and contractions of the mother's uterus during labor |
| **embryo** (ĕm′brē-ō) | | | | Stage of development between the 2nd and 8th week |
| **episiotomy** (ĕ-pĭs″ē-ŏt′-mē) | episi/o -tomy | CF S | vulva, pundenda incision | Surgical procedure performed during labor to prevent tearing of the perineum and to facilitate delivery of the fetus. See Figure 18–11 ▶. |
| **false labor** | | | | Condition in which the expectant mother experiences regular, painful contractions that do not dilate or thin the cervix; often difficult to differentiate from *true labor* |
| **fetal distress** | | | | Evidence that the fetus is in jeopardy, such as not getting adequate oxygen; can be noted by changes in fetal heart rate (FHR) or fetal activity/movement |

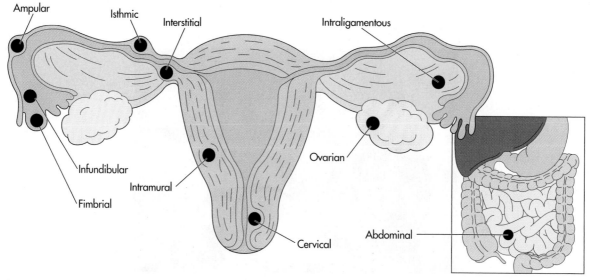

▶ **FIGURE 18–10**  Various implantation sites in ectopic pregnancy. The most common site is within the fallopian tube, hence the name *tubal pregnancy*.

| MEDICAL WORD | WORD PARTS (WHEN APPLICABLE) | | | DEFINITION |
|---|---|---|---|---|
| | Part | Type | Meaning | |
| **fetal scalp electrode** (fē′ tăl skălp ē-lĕk′trōd) | | | | Instrument used to monitor the fetus's heartbeat while it is still in the uterus. The device is placed just under the skin of the fetus's scalp. |
| **gestational diabetes** (jĕs-tā′shŭn-ăl dī″ă-bē′tēz) | | | | Form of diabetes that appears during pregnancy (gestation); condition may or may not remain after the birth |
| **gravida** (grăv′ĭ-dă) | | | | Refers to any pregnancy, regardless of duration, including the present one; when used in the recording of an obstetrical history, indicates the number of pregnancies |
| **group B streptococcus (GBS)** (strĕp″tō-kŏk′ŭs) | | | | Type of bacterium commonly found in the vagina and intestinal tract; found in 10% to 25% of all pregnant women; it can cause life-threatening infections in the newborn |

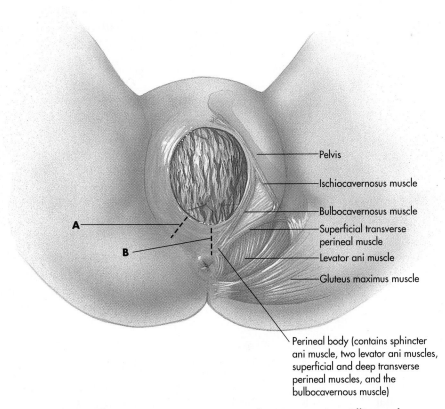

▶ **FIGURE 18–11** The two most common types of episiotomy are midline and mediolateral. (A) Right mediolateral. (B) Midline.

| MEDICAL WORD | WORD PARTS (WHEN APPLICABLE) | | | DEFINITION |
|---|---|---|---|---|
| | **Part** | **Type** | **Meaning** | |
| **hydatidiform mole** (hī" dă-tĭd'ĭ-form mōl) | | | | Intrauterine condition with multiple cysts of grapelike, enlarged chorionic villi that occurs in 1 in 1500 pregnancies in the United States; also called *hydatid mole* or spelled *hydatiform*. Signs include a fundal height higher than gestational age, absence of fetal heart sounds, dark brown or bright red vaginal discharge or bleeding, expulsion of cystic vesicles, edema, and hypertension. |
| **hyperemesis gravidarum** (hī-per-em'ĕ-sis grav-i-dā'rŭm) | hyper- | P | excessive | Excessive nausea and vomiting in pregnancy; can cause severe dehydration in the mother and fetus |
| | -emesis | S | vomiting | |
| | gravidar | R | pregnancy | |
| | -um | S | tissue | |
| **induced labor** | | | | Labor begun by intervention, such as artificial rupture of the membranes (AROM) or using an IV drip of oxytocin (Pitocin) |
| **Kegel exercises** (Ke'gul) | | | | Exercises that can be done during pregnancy to help strengthen the pelvic floor before delivery; consist of contracting and holding the muscles used to stop the flow of urine |
| **Lamaze method** (Lah-māz') | | | | Childbirth preparation method in which the expectant mother is instructed in breathing techniques that help her to facilitate delivery by relaxing at the proper time |
| **linea nigra** (lĭn'ē-ă nĭ'gră) | | | | Dark line on the abdomen that runs from above the umbilicus to the pubis during pregnancy. See Figure 18–12 ▶. |
| **lochia** (lō'kē-ă) | | | | Vaginal discharge occurring after childbirth. At first it is blood-tinged (*rubra*); then, after 3 or 4 days, it becomes pink and brown-tinged (*serosa*); after that, it becomes yellow and then turns to white (*alba*). Lochia typically last 2 to 4 weeks. |
| **meconium** (mĕ-kō'nē-ŭm) | | | | First stool of the newborn infant. A mixture of amniotic fluid and secretions of the intestinal glands that is thick and sticky, and dark green in color. Usually passed 8 to 24 hours following birth. |
| **multipara** (mŭl-tĭp'ă-ră) | multi- | P | many | Woman who has given birth to two or more children |
| | para | R | to bear | |
| **neonatal** (nē"ō-nā'tăl) | neo- | P | new | Pertaining to the first 4 weeks of an infant's life |
| | nat | R | birth | |
| | -al | S | pertaining to | |

| MEDICAL WORD | WORD PARTS (WHEN APPLICABLE) | | | DEFINITION |
|---|---|---|---|---|
| | Part | Type | Meaning | |
| **nulligravida**<br>(nŭl-ĭ′ grăv′ĭ-dă) | nulli-<br>gravida | P<br>R | none<br>pregnancy | Woman who has never been pregnant; *Gravida 0* |
| **nullipara**<br>(nŭl-ĭ′ p′ă-ră) | nulli-<br>para | P<br>R | none<br>to bear | Woman who has not given birth after more than 20 weeks of gestation; *Para 0* |
| **ovum transfer**<br>(ō′vum trăns′fer) | | | | Method of fertilization for women who cannot conceive a child. A donor ovum is impregnated within the donor's body by artificial insemination and later transferred to the recipient female. |
| **para**<br>(p′ă-ră) | | | | Means to bear or bring forth; refers to a woman who has given birth after 20 weeks gestation, regardless of whether the infant is born alive or dead. When used in the recording of an obstetrical history, *para* or *Para* is used to indicate the number of births. |
| **pelvimetry**<br>(pĕl-vĭm′ĕt-rē) | pelv/i<br>-metry | CF<br>S | pelvis<br>measurement | Measurement of the expectant mother's pelvic dimensions to determine whether it will be possible to deliver a fetus through the normal vaginal route |
| **perinatology**<br>(pĕr″ĭ-nă-tŏl′ō-jē) | peri-<br>nat/o<br>-logy | P<br>CF<br>S | around<br>birth<br>study of | Study of the fetus and infant from 20 to 29 weeks of gestation to 1 to 4 weeks after birth |
| **placenta**<br>(plă-sen′tă) | | | | Highly vascular organ that anchors the developing fetus to the uterus and provides the means by which the fetus receives its nourishment and oxygen |

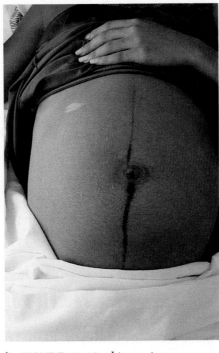

▶ **FIGURE 18–12** Linea nigra.

| MEDICAL WORD | WORD PARTS (WHEN APPLICABLE) | | | DEFINITION |
|---|---|---|---|---|
| | **Part** | **Type** | **Meaning** | |
| **placenta previa**<br>(plă-sen'tă prē'vē-ă) | | | | In this condition, the placenta is improperly implanted in the lower uterine segment. The fetus receives less oxygen and the expectant mother has an increased risk of hemorrhage and infection. See Figure 18–13 ▼. ✻ See Pathology Spotlight: Placenta Previa on page 623. |
| **polyhydramnios**<br>(pŏl"ē-hī-drăm'nē-ŏs) | poly-<br>hydr<br>amni/o (s) | P<br>R<br>CF | excessive<br>water<br>amniotic fluid | Excessive amniotic fluid in the bag of waters during pregnancy |
| **postpartum**<br>(pōst păr'tŭm) | | | | After childbirth |
| **postterm labor**<br>(pōst "tĕrm) | | | | Labor that occurs after 42 weeks of gestation |
| **preeclampsia**<br>(prē"ē-klămp'sē-ă) | pre-<br>ec-<br>lamp (s)<br>-ia | P<br>P<br>R<br>S | before<br>out<br>to shine<br>condition | Complication of pregnancy characterized by increasing hypertension, proteinuria (abnormal concentrations of urinary protein), and edema, also known as *toxemia* or *pregnancy-induced hypertension* (PIH) ✻ See Pathology Spotlight: Preeclampsia and Eclampsia on page 623. |
| **prenatal**<br>(prē-nā'tl) | pre-<br>nat<br>-al | P<br>R<br>S | before<br>birth<br>pertaining to | Pertaining to the fetus/infant before birth |
| **preterm labor** | | | | Premature labor that occurs after 20 weeks but before the completion of 37 weeks of gestation |

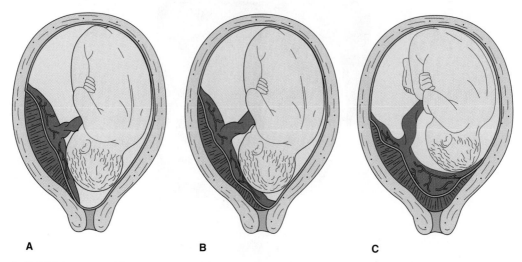

A              B              C

▶ **FIGURE 18–13**   Placenta previa. (A) Low placental implantation. (B) Partial placenta previa. (C) Total placenta previa.

| MEDICAL WORD | WORD PARTS (WHEN APPLICABLE) | | | DEFINITION |
|---|---|---|---|---|
| | Part | Type | Meaning | |
| **primigravida** (prī-mĭ-grăv'vĭ-dă) | primi- gravida | P R | first pregnancy | Refers to a woman who is pregnant for the first time; first pregnancy—*Gravida 1* |
| **primipara** (prī-mĭp'ă-ră) | primi- para | P R | first to bear | Refers to a woman who has had one birth at more than 20 weeks gestation, regardless of whether the infant is born alive or dead—*Para 1* |
| **pseudocyesis** (sū"dō-sī-ē'sĭs) | pseudo- -cyesis | P S | false pregnancy | False pregnancy |
| **pudendal** (pū-dĕn'dăl) | pudend -al | R S | external genitals pertaining to | Pertaining to the external female genitalia |
| **puerperium** (pū"ĕr-pē'rĭ-ŭm) | | | | Time period of six weeks following childbirth and expulsion of the placenta, when the female reproductive organs usually return to an essentially prepregnant condition |
| **secundines** (sĕk'ŭn-dīnz) | second -ine (s) | R S | second pertaining to | Afterbirth consisting of the placenta, umbilical cord, and the fetal membranes |
| **stillbirth** | | | | Fetus born dead after 20 weeks of gestation |
| **surrogate mother** | surrog -ate | R S | substitute use | Female who contracts to bear a child for another. Pregnancy may occur as a result of artificial insemination. |
| **term** | | | | Normal duration of pregnancy, which is 40 weeks (280 days) |
| **toxoplasmosis** (tŏks-ō-plăs-mō'sĭs) | | | | Condition caused by a protozoan, *Toxoplasma gondii,* which is found in many mammals (such as cats) and birds. Transplacental transmission can occur during an acute infection of the mother and is very serious in the fetus. The congenital form is characterized by destructive lesions of the central nervous system, jaundice, anemia, and generalized lymphadenopathy. |
| **trimester** | tri- mester | P R | three month | Period of 3 months |
| **umbilical cord blood retrieval** (ūm-bĭl'ĭ-kăl) | | | | Process of collecting the blood from a baby's umbilical cord at birth. It may be donated to a cord blood bank or, if properly frozen, be available for a bone marrow transplant should it be needed by the baby or a family member. |

# DIAGNOSTIC AND LAB TESTS

| TEST | DESCRIPTION |
| --- | --- |
| **Amniocentesis** (ăm″nĭ-ō-sĕn-tĕ′sĭs) | Determines chromosomal abnormalities and biochemical disorders. |
| **Blood groupings (A, B, AB, and O)** | Determines blood type. |
| **Chorionic villus sampling (CVS)** (kō″rē-ŏn-ĭk vĭl′ŭs sām′plĭng) | Determines chromosomal abnormalities and biochemical disorders (Down syndrome, Tay-Sachs disease, and cystic fibrosis). |
| **Complete blood count** | Test for anemia, infection, or cell abnormalities. |
| **Cordocentesis** (kor-dō-sĕn-tē′sĭs) (also known as fetal blood sampling, percutaneous umbilical blood sampling (PUBS), and umbilical vein sampling) | Examination of the blood from the fetus to detect fetal abnormalities (Down syndrome and fetal blood disorders). |
| **Group B streptococcus (GBS) screening** (grüp B strĕp″tō-kŏk′ŭs skrēn′ĭng) | Test for vaginal strep B infection performed between the 35th and 37th week of pregnancy. Any time other than this will not be significant to show whether the expectant mother is carrying GBS during her time of delivery. *Note: When the expectant mother tests positive, intravenous antibiotics are recommended during delivery to reduce the chance of the baby becoming infected with GBS.* |
| **Hematocrit** (hē-măt′ ō-krĭt) | Test for anemia during pregnancy. |
| **Hemoglobin** (hē″ mō-glō′ bĭn) | Test for anemia during pregnancy. |
| **Hepatitis B screen** (hĕp″ă-tī′tĭs B skrēn ) | Test to identify carriers of hepatitis. |
| **Human chorionic gonadotropin (hCG)** (hyü-mən kō″rē-ŏn-ĭk gŏn″ă-dō-trō′ĭn) | Test to determine the presence of hCG, which is secreted by the placenta. A positive result usually indicates pregnancy. |
| **Human immuno-deficiency virus (HIV) screen** (hyü-mən ĭm″ū-nō-dĕ-fĭsh′ĕn-sē vī′rŭs skrēn) | Test to identify HIV infection. |
| **Maternal blood glucose** | Test to screen for gestational diabetes. If the level of glucose is moderately elevated, a more conclusive glucose tolerance test (GTT) can be ordered. |

| TEST | DESCRIPTION |
|------|-------------|
| **Nonstress test (NST)** | Test to identify fetal compromise in conditions with poor placenta function, such as hypertension, diabetes mellitus, or postterm gestation (pregnancy lasts beyond 42 weeks). |
| **Papanicolaou (PAP) smear** (păp′ ăh-nĭk″ ō-lă′ oo smīr) | Test to screen for cervical cancer. |
| **Rh factor (positive or negative)** | Test to determine risk for maternal-fetal blood incompatibility. |
| **Rubella (German measles) titer** (roo-bĕl′lă tĭ′tēr) | Test to determine immunity to rubella. |
| **TORCH panel** (tōrch) | Test to screen for toxoplasmosis, rubella, cytomegalovirus (CMV), and herpes simplex virus (HSV). |
| **Toxoplasmosis screen** (tŏks-ō-plăs-mō′sĭs) | Test to determine toxoplasmosis infection. |
| **Quad marker screen (AFP, hCG, UE, and inhibin-A)** (kwod) | Test to assess probabilities of potential genetic disorders by measuring high and low levels of alpha-fetoprotein (AFP), a protein produced by the baby's liver, and abnormal levels of human chorionic gonadotropin (hCG), a hormone produced by the placenta; unconjugated estriol (UE), a hormone produced in the placenta and in the baby's liver; and inhibin-A, a hormone produced by the placenta. |
| **Ultrasound** (ŭl′tră-sŏund) | Test to confirm viable pregnancy, fetal heartbeat (FHB), ectopic pregnancy, molar pregnancy (hydatidiform mole or hydatid mole), multiple pregnancies, and intrauterine death; to measure the crown-rump length or gestational age; to assess abnormal gestation; to diagnose fetal malformation and structural abnormalities; to determine gender of the baby; to identify placenta location and uterine and pelvic abnormalities of the mother during pregnancy; and to observe fetal presentation and movements |
| **Urinalysis** (ū′ rĭ-năl′ i-sĭs) | Test that checks for infection, renal disease, or diabetes. |
| **Venereal Disease Research Laboratory (VDRL)** (vē-nē′ rē-ăl) | Test to screen for syphilis. Another blood test that is used to screen for syphilis is the RPR (rapid plasma reagin). |

# ABBREVIATIONS

| ABBREVIATION | MEANING | ABBREVIATION | MEANING |
|---|---|---|---|
| ACOG | American College of Obstetrics and Gynecology | HDN | hemolytic disease of the newborn |
| AFP | alpha-fetoprotein | HIV | human immunodeficiency virus |
| AROM | artificial rupture of membranes | HSV | herpes simplex virus |
| cm | centimeter | LBW | low birth weight |
| CMV | cytomegalovirus | LMP | last menstrual period |
| CPD | cephalopelvic disproporiton | NST | nonstress test |
| | | OB | obstetrics |
| CS | cesarean section | Pap | Papanicolaou (smear) |
| CVS | chorionic villus sampling | PIH | pregnancy-induced hypertension |
| D&C | dilation (dilatation) and curettage | PUBS | percutaneous umbilical blood sampling |
| EFM | electronic fetal monitor | RPR | rapid plasma reagin |
| EDB | estimated date of birth | SAB | spontaneous abortion |
| EDC | estimated date of confinement (delivery) | SIDS | sudden infant death syndrome |
| EDD | estimated date of delivery | STDs | sexually transmitted diseases |
| FHB | fetal heartbeat | UC | uterine contractions |
| GBS | group B streptococcus | UE | unconjugated estriol |
| GTT | glucose tolerance test | VDRL | venereal disease research laboratory |
| hCG | human chorionic gonadotropin | | |

# PATHOLOGY SPOTLIGHTS

## ✶ Mastitis

**Mastitis** is an inflammation of the breast, a condition that occurs most commonly in women who are breastfeeding. It is caused by bacteria that enter through a crack or abrasion of the nipple. Infection begins in one lobule but can extend to other areas of the breast.

The signs and symptoms of mastitis can include both general symptoms of infection and localized symptoms involving the breast. Generalized symptoms include fever, chills, and headache. Localized symptoms include breast pain, redness, tenderness, and swelling. Usually there is difficulty in getting the milk to flow and pain in the nipple. If the breastfeeding mother has any of the mentioned symptoms, she should contact her physician promptly.

Treatment includes application of local heat to the affected area and appropriate antibiotics (usually for a 10-day period) and anti-inflammatory drugs to reduce inflammation and relieve pain. The patient is advised to rest as much as possible, to drink plenty of fluids, and to breastfeed more often, especially from the breast that is infected. Breastfeeding will help keep the breast emptied and relieve the fullness. If breastfeeding is too painful or it does not relieve the fullness, a breast pump may be used. The use of an electric breast pump can generally empty the breast.

If symptoms are not better within 48 hours after starting antibiotics or a tender breast lump develops that is not relieved by nursing, the patient should contact her physician. Also, the pediatrician should be contacted if the baby develops a yeast infection that can occur due to antibiotics taken by the mother. Antibiotics can change the normal body flora, thereby making the suckling baby more susceptible to *Candida albicans*. The most common type of yeast infection seen in a child is thrush, which is characterized by fever, creamy, white, curdlike patches of exudate on an inflamed tongue or buccal mucosa.

## ✷ Placenta Previa

**Placenta previa** is a displaced attachment of the placenta over the cervical os (opening of the cervix). In this condition, the fetus receives less oxygen, and the expectant mother has an increased risk of hemorrhage and infection. Placenta previa is classified as one of four degrees:

1. **Total placenta previa.** The placenta completely covers the internal os.
2. **Partial placenta previa.** The placenta partially covers the internal os.
3. **Marginal placenta previa.** The edge of the placenta is at the margin of the internal os.
4. **Low-lying placenta.** The placenta is implanted in the lower segment but does not reach the internal os, although it is in close proximity to it.

The most common symptom of placenta previa is painless uterine bleeding during the second half of pregnancy. Bleeding can be scanty or profuse (hemorrhage). When this occurs, the expectant mother is advised to go to the hospital.

To determine a diagnosis, a transabdominal ultrasound examination is performed to pinpoint the placenta's location. See Figure 18–16 on page 635. A vaginal examination usually is avoided because it could trigger heavy bleeding. A woman who has been diagnosed with placenta previa may need to stay in the hospital until delivery. If the bleeding stops, as it often does, her physician continues to monitor the expectant mother and her baby.

Treatment involves delaying birth, if possible, until 37 weeks of gestation to allow the fetus to mature. During hospitalization, recommendations include bed rest; no vaginal examinations; monitoring blood loss, pain, and uterine contractility; evaluation of fetal heart rate (FHR) with external monitor; monitoring maternal vital signs (V/S), intake, and output (I&O); assessing blood tests (hemoglobin and hematocrit) for anemia; and administration of IV fluids (Ringer's solution). Also, two units of cross-matched blood should be made available for possible transfusion. Emotional support for the patient and her family are very important. *Note: A cesarean section (C-section, CS) is indicated if severe and life-threatening hemorrhage occurs or fetal distress is apparent.*

## ✷ Preeclampsia and Eclampsia

**Preeclampsia** is a complication of pregnancy characterized by increasing hypertension, proteinuria, and edema. It is also known as **toxemia** or **pregnancy-induced hypertension** (PIH). Preeclampsia develops in approximately 5% of pregnant women and usually occurs after the 20th week of pregnancy. The condition can be mild or severe.

Some experts believe that a problem with the placenta causes preeclampsia. The mother has spasms of the blood vessels, which increase her blood pressure, impairing the blood flow to the placenta. The high blood pressure can also affect the woman's brain, kidneys, liver, and lungs.

The symptoms of preeclampsia include agitation and confusion, changes in mental status, decreased urine output, headaches, nausea and vomiting, pain in the right upper part of the abdomen, shortness of breath, sudden weight gain over 1 to 2 days and weight gain of more than 2 pounds per week, swelling of the face or hands, and visual impairment.

Factors that increase a woman's risk of preeclampsia are: African American ethnicity, age younger than 20 or older than 35, first pregnancy, low socioeconomic status, and multiple gestation such as twins or triplets. Additional factors that increase the risk of preeclampsia include preeclampsia or eclampsia in previous pregnancies, diabetes, high blood pressure before pregnancy, underlying kidney disease, and if the baby's mother or father was born of a pregnancy in which the expectant mother developed preeclampsia or eclampsia.

There are no known ways to prevent preeclampsia. All pregnant women should have early prenatal care, and blood pressure changes should be watched closely.

**Eclampsia** is a complication of severe preeclampsia that involves seizures and possibly coma. One in 200 pregnant women who have preeclampsia develop eclampsia. Usually the seizures of eclampsia start before the baby is born. However, about 20% to 25% of the time, seizures begin within the first 24 hours after the baby is born, and in a few cases, continue up to 3 weeks. There usually are no clues or warning signs before a seizure, which can cause muscle spasms, loss of consciousness, and short-term memory problems. During or after a seizure, a woman could bite her tongue, break bones, breathe fluids into her lungs, develop fluid and swelling in her lungs that make it difficult to breathe, experience a detached retina in the eye, or harm her head. Afterward, the woman can breathe very rapidly to make up for the lack of oxygen during the seizure itself. A fever at this point is a sign of serious trouble.

It is not known why some women with preeclampsia develop the seizures associated with eclampsia. Theories about the cause of seizures during pregnancy involve small clots that block blood vessels in the brain and restrict oxygen, narrowing of tiny arteries in the brain, areas of bleeding in the brain, high blood pressure, dietary risks, genetic risks, and a problem with the brain or nervous system.

## ✱ Rh Incompatibility

The presence of a substance called an *agglutinogen* (a gluing or clumping together) in the red blood cells is responsible for what is known as the *Rh factor*. About 85% of the population have the Rh factor and are called *Rh-positive* (+). The other 15% lack the Rh factor and are designated *Rh-negative* (⁻).

A pregnant woman who is Rh-negative can become sensitized by blood of an Rh-positive fetus. Sensitization can also occur if an Rh-negative woman has had a previous miscarriage, induced abortion, or ectopic pregnancy. There is also a slight chance that a woman could develop antibodies after having amniocentesis done later in pregnancy. These are all cases in which fetal blood (that might be Rh-positive) could mix with maternal blood, resulting in the production of antibodies that could complicate a subsequent pregnancy. In subsequent pregnancies, if the fetus is Rh-positive, Rh antibodies produced in maternal blood may cross the placenta and destroy fetal cells, producing hemolytic disease of the newborn (HDN). See Figure 18–14 ▶. Today, hemolytic disease can, for the most part, be prevented if the Rh-negative woman has not already made antibodies against the Rh factor from an earlier pregnancy or blood transfusion.

RhoGAM (Rh₀ (D) immunoglobulin) is an injectable blood product that can safely prevent sensitization of an Rh-negative mother by suppressing her ability to respond to Rh-positive red cells and protect an Rh-positive fetus from antibodies by its Rh-negative mother. With its use, sensitization can be prevented almost always, although RhoGAM is not helpful if the mother has already been sensitized. The idea underlying RhoGAM is that if anti-Rh antibody is given soon after delivery, it will block the sensitization of the mother

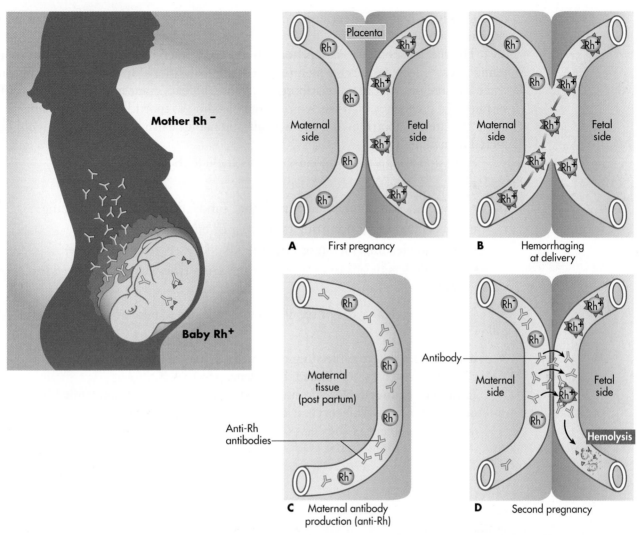

▶ **FIGURE 18–14** Rh factors and pregnancy: When an Rh-negative woman has her first Rh-positive child, fetal and maternal blood mix at delivery when the placenta breaks down. The appearance of Rh-positive blood cells in the maternal bloodstream sensitizes the mother, stimulating the production of anti-Rh antibodies. If another pregnancy occurs with an Rh-positive fetus, maternal anti-Rh antibodies can cross the placenta and attack fetal blood cells, producing hemolytic disease of the newborn (HDN).

and prevent Rh disease from occurring in the woman's next Rh-positive child. RhoGAM is now given routinely to an Rh-negative woman after a pregnancy in which she carried an Rh-positive fetus. This will prevent the mother's immune system from reacting to the Rh-positive blood of any subsequent fetuses.

## ✳ Spontaneous Abortion

A **spontaneous abortion** (SAB), commonly called a *miscarriage,* is the loss of a fetus as the result of natural causes occurring during the first 20 weeks of gestation. Pregnancy losses after the 20th week of gestation are categorized as *preterm deliveries.* Miscarriage is the most common type of pregnancy loss, according to the American College of Obstetrics and Gynecology (ACOG). It is estimated that up to 50% of all fertilized eggs die and are aborted spontaneously, usually before the woman knows that she is pregnant. Studies reveal that anywhere from 10% to 25% of all clinically recognized pregnancies will end in miscarriage. Most miscarriages occur during the first 13 weeks of pregnancy. Among the most common causes are chromosomal abnormalities of the embryo, abnormalities of the placenta, endocrine disturbances, acute infectious diseases, severe trauma, and shock. Other causes include lifestyle situations such as the use of certain drugs, alcohol, or excessive caffeine.

The risk for spontaneous abortion is higher in women over age 35, in women with systemic diseases such as diabetes mellitus or thyroid conditions, and women with a history of three or more prior spontaneous abortions. When an expectant mother is having difficulty sustaining a pregnancy, signs such as vaginal bleeding or spotting may occur. This is generally a threatened abortion, and the woman's prenatal health care provider should be contacted immediately.

Signs and symptoms of miscarriage may include these:

- Nausea.
- Low back pain or abdominal pain that can be dull, sharp, or cramping.
- True contractions occurring every 5 to 20 minutes.
- Vaginal bleeding: brown or bright red blood or spotting with or without cramps.
- Passing clots or bits of tissue from the vagina (these should be saved for laboratory analysis).

There are several types of spontaneous abortions or miscarriages. These include the following.

**Threatened.** Uterine bleeding or spotting is accompanied by cramping or low-back pain. The cervix is not dilated. See Figure 18–15A ▼.

**Imminent or inevitable.** Uterine bleeding or spotting is accompanied by cramping or low back pain. The cervix is dilated. Miscarriage is inevitable when there is dilation or effacement of the cervix or rupture of the membranes. See Figure 18–15B.

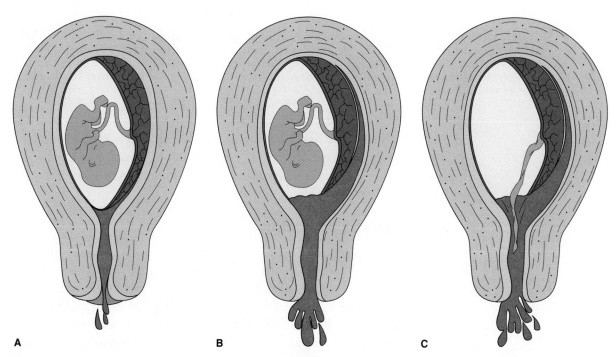

A                    B                    C

▶ **FIGURE 18–15**    Types of spontaneous abortion. (A) Threatened: The cervix is not dilated, and the placenta is still attached to the uterine wall, but some bleeding occurs. (B) Imminent: The placenta has separated from the uterine wall, the cervix has dilated, and the amount of bleeding has increased. (C) Incomplete: The embryo/fetus has passed out of the uterus; however, the placenta remains.

**Incomplete.**  Some products of conception have been expelled, but some remain in the uterus. Bleeding and cramps may persist when the miscarriage is not complete. See Figure 18–15C.

**Complete.**  All of the products of conception are expelled. A completed miscarriage can be confirmed by an ultrasound.

**Missed.**  This is a pregnancy demise in which nothing is expelled. It is not known why this occurs. Signs of this would be a loss of pregnancy symptoms and the absence of fetal heart tones.

**Recurrent miscarriage (RM).**  This is defined as 3 or more consecutive first trimester miscarriages. Also referred to as habitual abortion.

Treatment during or after a miscarriage includes measures to prevent hemorrhage and infection. With any type of miscarriage, the patient should see her health care provider as soon as possible. If the abortion is incomplete and not all tissue has been expelled, a dilation and curettage (D&C), which is an expansion of the cervical canal and scraping of the uterine wall, is usually performed.

# ✔ PATHOLOGY CHECKPOINT

*Following is a concise list of the pathology-related terms that you have seen in the chapter. Review this checklist to make sure that you are familiar with the meaning of each term before moving to the next section.*

## Conditions and Symptoms

- ❏ abortion
- ❏ abruptio placentae
- ❏ dystocia
- ❏ eclampsia
- ❏ ectopic pregnancy
- ❏ fetal distress
- ❏ gestational diabetes
- ❏ hydatidiform mole
- ❏ hyperemesis gravidarum
- ❏ incompetent cervix
- ❏ mastitis
- ❏ miscarriage
- ❏ placenta previa
- ❏ polyhydramnios
- ❏ preeclampsia
- ❏ pregnancy-induced hypertension
- ❏ preterm labor
- ❏ pseudocyesis

- ❏ Rh incompatibility
- ❏ spontaneous abortion
- ❏ stillbirth
- ❏ toxemia
- ❏ toxoplasmosis

## Diagnosis and Treatment

- ❏ amniocentesis
- ❏ blood groupings (A, B, AB, and O)
- ❏ cerclage
- ❏ cesarean section (C-section)
- ❏ chorionic villus sampling
- ❏ complete blood count
- ❏ cordocentesis
- ❏ diagnostic ultrasound
- ❏ Doppler ultrasound
- ❏ electronic fetal monitor
- ❏ episiotomy

- ❏ group B streptococcus screening
- ❏ hematocrit
- ❏ hemoglobin
- ❏ hepatitis B screen
- ❏ human immunodeficiency virus screen
- ❏ maternal blood glucose
- ❏ nonstress test
- ❏ pelvimetry
- ❏ Rh factor
- ❏ RhoGAM
- ❏ rubella titer
- ❏ TORCH panel
- ❏ toxoplasmosis screen
- ❏ Quad marker screen
- ❏ urinalysis
- ❏ venereal disease research laboratory

# STUDY AND REVIEW

## Overview of Obstetrics

*Write your answers to the following questions. Do not refer to the text.*

1. _____ is the branch of medicine that pertains to the care of women during pregnancy, childbirth, and the postpartum period.

2. _____ is the process in which a sperm penetrates an ovum.

3. The fertilized ovum is also known as a _____

4. As the blastocyst develops, it forms a structure with two cavities, the

   _____ and _____

5. The _____ is composed of tissues from the mother and the child.

6. Pregnancy is divided into four stages. Describe each of these stages.

   a. Prenatal stage _____

   b. Labor _____

   c. Parturition _____

   d. Postpartum period _____

7. The signs and symptoms of pregnancy are divided into three general groups. Define each of the following:

   a. Subjective or presumptive signs _____

   b. Objective or probable signs _____

   c. Diagnostic or positive signs _____

8. Certain diagnostic and laboratory tests are performed during pregnancy. Give the purpose of the following test.

   a. Blood groupings _____

   b. Rh factor _____

   c. Urinalysis _____

   d. Maternal blood glucose _____

   e. Cordocentesis _____

   f. Chorionic villus sampling _____

   g. Amniocentesis _____

   h. Group B streptococcus screening _____

9. Labor is divided into three stages. Describe each of these stages.

    a. First stage _____

       _____

    b. Second stage _____

       _____

    c. Third stage _____

10. A(n) _____ can be used to reduce the discomfort and pain of contractions during labor.

## Word Parts

1. In the spaces provided, write the definitions of these prefixes, roots, combining forms, and suffixes. Do not refer to the listings of medical words. Leave blank those words you cannot define.

2. After completing as many as you can, refer to the medical word listings to check your work. For each word missed or left blank, write the word and its definition several times on the margins of these pages or on a separate sheet of paper.

3. To maximize the learning process, it is to your advantage to do the following exercises as directed. To refer to the word-building section before completing these exercises invalidates the learning process.

## PREFIXES

*Give the definitions of the following prefixes.*

1. ante- _____

2. dia- _____

3. dys- _____

4. ec- _____

5. hyper- _____

6. neo- _____

7. peri- _____

8. poly- _____

9. pre- _____

10. primi- _____

11. pseudo- _____

12. tri- _____

13. ultra- _____

## ROOTS AND COMBINING FORMS

*Give the definitions of the following roots and combining forms.*

1. abort _____

2. amni/o _____

3. cord/o _____

4. ectop _____

5. gnost _____

6. gravida _____

7. gravidar _____

8. hydr _____

9. lamp(s) _____

10. mester _____

11. nat _____

12. nat/o _____

13. para _____

14. pelv/i _____

15. pudend _____

16. second _____

17. surrog _____

18. toc _____

## SUFFIXES

*Give the definitions of the following suffixes.*

1. -al _____

2. -ate _____

3. -centesis _____

4. -cyesis _____

5. -emesis _____

6. -ia _____

7. -ic _____

8. -ine(s) _____

9. -ion _____

10. -logy _____

11. -metry _____

12. -sound _____

13. -um _____

## Identifying Medical Terms

*In the spaces provided, write the medical terms for the following meanings.*

1. _____ Process of miscarrying

2. _____ Time before the onset of labor

3. _____ Called the *mask of pregnancy*

4. _____ Obtaining a sample of fetal umbilical cord blood

5. _____ Difficult and painful childbirth

6. _____ Discoloration of the abdomen seen in pregnancy

7. _____ Pertaining to the first 4 weeks after birth

8. _____ Displaced attachment of the placenta

9. _____ Pertaining to before birth

10. _____ Refers to a woman during her first pregnancy

11. _____ Woman who is bearing her first child

12. _____ False pregnancy

13. _____ Pertaining to the external female genitalia

14. _____ Afterbirth

15. _____ Period of 3 months

## Spelling

*In the spaces provided, write the correct spelling of these misspelled words.*

1. amiocentesis _____

2. ceclage _____

3. cloasma _____

4. dytocia _____

5. eclampia _____

6. locia _____

7. polyhydranios _____

8. primigavida _____

9. pudedal _____

10. secudines _____

## Matching

*Select the appropriate lettered meaning for each of the following words.*

_____ 1. lightening

_____ 2. amniotic sac

_____ 3. nullipara

_____ 4. multipara

_____ 5. effacement

_____ 6. transition phase

_____ 7. crowning

_____ 8. lanugo

_____ 9. quickening

_____ 10. puerperium

a. Fine, downy hair

b. Continues until the cervix is fully dilated to 10 cm

c. Movement of the fetus felt in the uterus

d. Descent of baby into the pelvis

e. 6 weeks following childbirth and expulsion of the placenta

f. Woman who has borne no offspring

g. Shortening and thinning of the cervix and its walls

h. Woman who has borne more than one child

i. Head of the baby appears first

j. Bag of waters

## Abbreviations

*Place the correct word, phrase, or abbreviation in the space provided.*

1. AFP _____

2. AROM _____

3. C-section _____

4. chorionic villus sampling _____

5. EFM _____

6. EDD _____

7. group B streptococcus _____

8. OB _____

9. SAB _____

10. uterine contractions _____

## Diagnostic and Laboratory Tests

*Select the best answer to each multiple choice question. Circle the letter of your choice.*

1. Test performed to screen for gestational diabetes.
   a. TORCH panel
   b. Quad marker
   c. maternal blood glucose
   d. cordocentesis

2. Blood test to check for anemia during pregnancy.
   a. hemoglobin
   b. cordocentesis
   c. blood groupings
   d. Quad marker

3. Test performed to identify fetal compromise in conditions with poor placenta function.
   a. Rh factor
   b. rubella titer
   c. toxoplasmosis screen
   d. nonstress test

4. Positive result of this test usually indicates pregnancy.
   a. chorionic villus sampling
   b. human chorionic gonadotropin
   c. amniocentesis
   d. cordocentesis

5. Test used to check for anemia, infection, or cell abnormalities.
   a. hematocrit
   b. hemoglobin
   c. complete blood count
   d. hepatitis B screen

# PRACTICAL APPLICATION

## S O A P : Chart Note Analysis

*This exercise will make you aware of information, abbreviations, and medical terminology typically found in an obstetric patient's chart note.*

### Abbreviations Key

| | | | |
|---|---|---|---|
| AB | abortion | I & O | intake & output |
| Abd | abdomen | IV | intravenous |
| BP | blood pressure | lb | pound |
| CBC | complete blood count | NKDA | no known drug allergies |
| C-section | cesarean section | P | pulse |
| CTA | clear to auscultation | SOAP | subjective, objective, assessment, plan |
| DOB | date of birth | | |
| F | Fahrenheit | T | temperature |
| FHR | fetal heart rate | V/S | vital signs |
| Hct | hematocrit | WNL | within normal limits |
| Hgb | hemoglobin | Wt | weight |
| Ht | height | y/o | year(s) old |

*Read the following chart note and then answer the questions that follow.*

**PATIENT:** Brown, Susie A.      **DATE:** 07/16/2007

**DOB:** 02/12/1972     **AGE:** 35     **SEX:** Female

**INSURANCE:** Best Care Insurance

**Vital Signs:**
- T: 98.9 F
- P: 88
- R: 16
- BP: 140/90
- Ht: 5' 6"
- Wt: 175 lb

**Allergies:** NKDA

**Chief Complaint:** Profuse amount of painless vaginal bleeding (hemorrhage); apprehensive and anxious

**S**   **Subjective:** 35 y/o white female, 34 weeks gestation, presents with passing a large amount of "bright red blood" when she went to the bathroom early this morning. She became very apprehensive and contacted her physician who instructed her to go to Mercy Hospital. Patient denies pain or history of previous bleeding with this pregnancy.

**O**   **Objective:**

**General Appearance:** The patient appears to have been crying. Expression of sadness apparent. Voiced concern about the welfare of her baby. Anxious about the outcome of this pregnancy. Her overall state of health appeared to be WNL.

**Lungs:** CTA

**Heart:** Slightly elevated rate with normal rhythm

**Abd:** Reddish, wavy, depressed streaks (striae) present over the abdomen. Fundal height slightly higher than 34 weeks of gestation.

**Skin:** Cool, moist, and smooth to touch. Irregular pigmentation of checks, forehead, and nose. Striae over abdomen and breasts bilaterally.

**GYN:** Vaginal exam deferred due to possible hemorrhage. Multiparity: Gravida 3 Para 2 AB 0

**A**  **Assessment:** Placenta previa as indicated by transabdominal ultrasound

**P**  **Plan:**

1. Delay birth if possible, until 37 weeks of gestation to allow the fetus to mature.
2. Provide education and emotional support for the patient and her family.
3. Have two units of cross-matched blood available for possible transfusion if hemorrhage persists or becomes more severe, and results of blood test indicate the need for a transfusion.
4. Bed rest with bathroom privileges only.
5. No vaginal examinations, no sexual intercourse, and no douching due to potential for hemorrhage. Monitor blood loss, pain, and uterine contractility. Evaluate FHR with external monitor; monitor maternal V/S every 15 minutes until bleeding subsides then every 30 minutes until stable. Monitor I&O. Assess blood tests results of CBC along with Hgb and Hct, for anemia. Administration of IV fluids (Ringer's Lactate solution) until assessment is completed and determination is made on status of patient and fetus.
6. A C-section will be performed if severe and life-threatening hemorrhage occurs or fetal distress is apparent.

**FYI:** The cause of placenta previa can be unknown in a patient, although factors associated are multiparity (multiple births), increasing age (35 y/o and older), defective development of blood vessels in the decidua, prior cesarean birth, smoking, a recent spontaneous or induced abortion, and a large placenta. See Figure 18–16 ▶ for an ultrasound showing placenta previa.

**Note:** V/S may be WNL as a pregnant woman may lose up to 40% of blood volume before showing signs of shock. When used in the recording of a medical history, Para is used to indicate the number of births, and Gravida is used to indicate the number of pregnancies.

## Chart Note Questions
*Place the correct answer in the space provided.*

1. What is the medical term for a profuse amount of vaginal bleeding? _____

2. The diagnosis of placenta previa was determined by a _____

3. Why is it important to try to delay birth until 37 weeks of gestation? _____

4. Which blood tests are used to assess the patient for anemia? _____ and _____

5. When would a C-section be indicated for this patient? _____

6. What is the medical term for having borne more than one child? _____

7. A(n) _____ monitor is used to monitor FHR when the patient is diagnosed with placenta previa.

8. Why are vaginal exams avoided with placenta previa?

_____

9. What is the rationale for having two units of cross-matched blood available?

_____

10. Name five of the seven factors associated with placenta previa.

_____    _____    _____

_____    _____

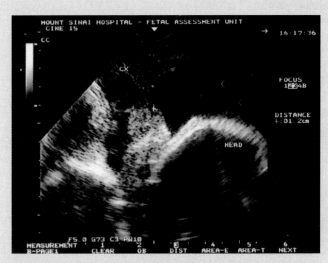

**FIGURE 18–16**   Ultrasound of placenta previa.

# MULTIMEDIA PREVIEW

*Additional interactive resources and activities for this chapter can be found on the Companion Website. For videos, audio glossary, and review, access the accompanying CD-ROM in this book.*

 **CD-ROM HIGHLIGHTS**

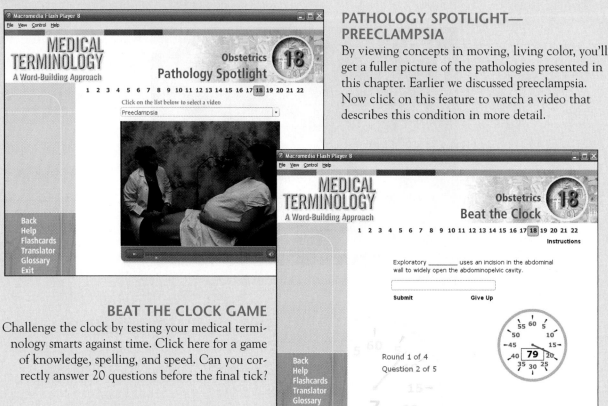

## PATHOLOGY SPOTLIGHT— PREECLAMPSIA

By viewing concepts in moving, living color, you'll get a fuller picture of the pathologies presented in this chapter. Earlier we discussed preeclampsia. Now click on this feature to watch a video that describes this condition in more detail.

## BEAT THE CLOCK GAME

Challenge the clock by testing your medical terminology smarts against time. Click here for a game of knowledge, spelling, and speed. Can you correctly answer 20 questions before the final tick?

 **WEBSITE HIGHLIGHTS—www.prenhall.com/rice**

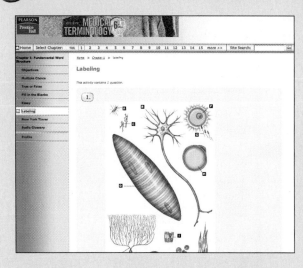

## LABELING EXERCISE

Click here and take advantage of the free-access online study guide that accompanies your textbook. You'll find an image labeling question that corresponds to the concepts in this chapter. By clicking on this URL you'll also access links to download mp3 audio reviews, current news articles, and an audio glossary.

# Male Reproductive System

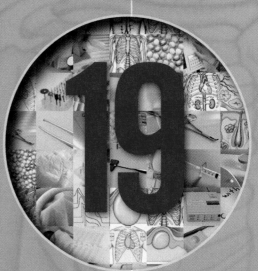

**19**

## ■ OUTLINE

## ■ OBJECTIVES

*On completion of this chapter, you will be able to:*

- Describe and state the functions of the male's external organs of reproduction.
- Describe and state the functions of the male's internal organs of reproduction.
- Analyze, build, spell, and pronounce medical words.
- Comprehend the drugs highlighted in this chapter.
- Provide the description of diagnostic and laboratory tests related to the male reproductive system.
- Identify and define selected abbreviations.
- Describe each of the conditions presented in the Pathology Spotlights.
- Review the Pathology Checkpoint.
- Complete the Study and Review section and the Chart Note Analysis.

# Anatomy and Physiology Overview

The male reproductive system consists of the testes, various ducts, the urethra, and the following accessory glands: bulbourethral, prostate, and the seminal vesicles. The supporting structures and accessory sex organs are the scrotum and the penis (see Figure 19–1 ▼). The vital function of the male reproductive system is to provide the sperm cells necessary to fertilize the ovum, thereby perpetuating the species. The following is a general overview of the organs and functions of this system.

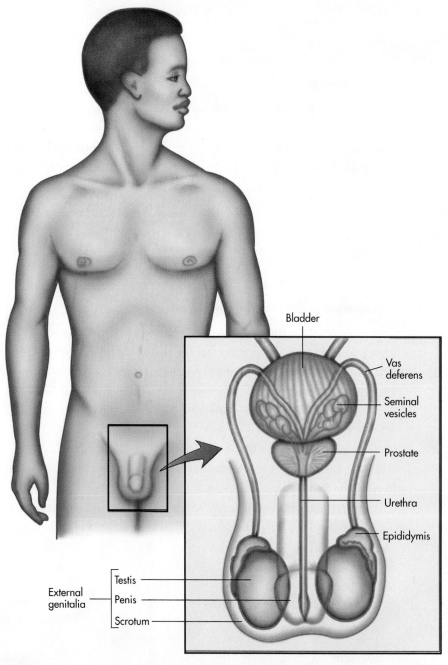

▶ **FIGURE 19–1**   Male reproductive system: seminal vesicles, prostate, urethra, vas deferens, epididymis, and external genitalia.

## Male Reproductive System

| Organ/Structure | Primary Functions |
| --- | --- |
| Scrotum | Houses testes and connecting tubes; brings the testes closer to the perineum through contractile action to absorb sufficient body heat to maintain the viability of the spermatozoa |
| Penis | Acts as male organ of copulation; site of the orifice for the elimination of urine and semen from the body |
| Testes | Provide the male sex hormone, testosterone, provided by cells within them; contain seminiferous tubules that are the site of the development of spermatozoa; |
| Epididymis | Acts as storage site for the maturation of sperm |
| Vas Deferens | Acts as excretory duct of the testis |
| Seminal Vesicles | Produce a slightly alkaline fluid that becomes a part of the seminal fluid or semen |
| Prostate Gland | Secretes an alkaline fluid that aids in maintaining the viability of spermatozoa |
| Bulbourethral or Cowper's Glands | Produce a mucous secretion before ejaculation, which becomes a part of the semen |
| Urethra | Transmits urine and semen out of the body |

# EXTERNAL ORGANS

In the male, the scrotum and the penis are the external organs of reproduction.

## Scrotum

The **scrotum** is a pouchlike structure located behind the penis. It is suspended from the perineal region and is divided by a septum into two sacs, each containing one of the testes along with its connecting tube called the **epididymis.** Within the tissues of the scrotum are fibers of smooth muscle that contract in the absence of sufficient heat, giving the scrotum a wrinkled appearance. This contractile action brings the testes closer to the perineum where they can absorb sufficient body heat to maintain the viability of the **spermatozoa.** Under normal conditions, the walls of the scrotum are generally free of wrinkles, and it hangs loosely between the thighs (see Figure 19–1).

## Penis

The **penis** is the external male sex organ and is composed of erectile tissue covered with skin. The size and shape of the penis varies, with an average erect penis being 15 to 20 cm in length. The penis has three longitudinal columns of erectile tissue that are capable of significant enlargement when engorged with blood, as is the case during sexual stimulation. Two of these columns, located side by side, form the greater part of the penis. These columns are known as the *corpora cavernosa penis.* The third longitudinal column, the *corpus spongiosum,* has the same function as the first two columns but is transversed by the penile portion of the urethra and tends to be more elastic when in an erectile state. The *corpus spongiosum,* at its distal end, expands to form the *glans penis,* the cone-shaped head of the penis, and is the site of the urethral orifice. It is covered with loose skin folds called the **foreskin** or prepuce. See Figure 19–2 ▶. The foreskin contains glands that secrete a lubricating fluid called *smegma.* The foreskin can be removed by a surgical procedure known as **circumcision.** See Figure 19–5 on page 644.

The erectile state in the penis results when sexual stimulation causes large quantities of blood from dilated arteries supplying the penis to fill the cavernous spaces in the erectile tissue. When the arteries constrict, the pressure on the veins in the area is reduced, thus allowing more blood to leave the penis than enters, and the penis returns to its normal state. The functions of the penis are to serve as the male organ of **copulation** (sexual intercourse) and as the site of the orifice for the elimination of urine and semen from the body.

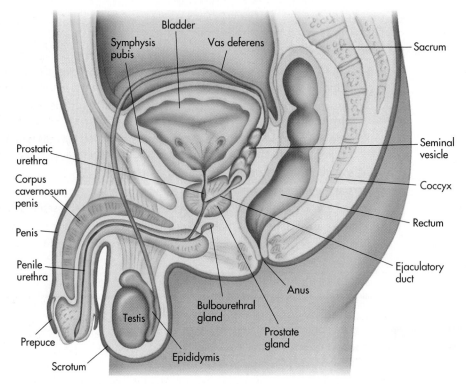

► **FIGURE 19–2**   Sagittal section of the male pelvis, showing the organs of the reproductive system.

## INTERNAL ORGANS

In the male, the testes, the epididymis, the vas deferens, the seminal vesicles, the prostate gland, the bulbourethral glands, and the urethra are the internal organs of reproduction.

### Testes

The male has two ovoid-shaped organs, the **testes,** located in the scrotum. See Figure 19–3 ►. Each testis is about 4 cm long and 2.5 cm wide. The interior of each testis is divided into about 250 wedge-shaped lobes by fibrous tissues. Coiled within each lobe are one to three small tubes called the **seminiferous tubules,** which are the site of the development of male reproductive cells, the **spermatozoa.** Cells within the testes also produce the male sex hormone, **testosterone,** which is responsible for the development of secondary male characteristics during puberty. Testosterone is essential for normal growth and development of the male accessory sex organs. It plays a vital role in the erection process of the penis and thus is necessary for the reproductive act, copulation. Additionally, it affects the growth of hair on the face, muscular development, and vocal timbre. The *seminiferous tubules* form a plexus or network called the rete testis from which 15 to 20 small ducts, the efferent ductules, leave the testis and open into the epididymis (see Figures 19–1 and 19–2).

### Epididymis

Each testis is connected by efferent ductules to an **epididymis,** which is a coiled tube laying on the posterior aspect of the testis. The epididymis is between 13 and 20 feet in length but is coiled into a space less than 2 inches (5 cm) long and ends in the ductus deferens. Each epididymis functions as a storage site for the maturation of **sperm** (see Figure

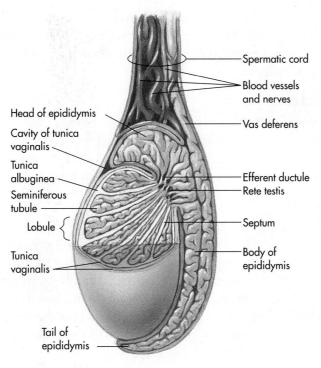

Spermatic cord

Blood vessels and nerves

Head of epididymis

Cavity of tunica vaginalis

Vas deferens

Tunica albuginea

Seminiferous tubule

Efferent ductule

Rete testis

Lobule {

Septum

Tunica vaginalis

Body of epididymis

Tail of epididymis

▶ **FIGURE 19–3** Sagittal view of the testes showing interior anatomy.

19–4 ▼) and as the first part of the duct system through which sperm pass on their journey to the urethra (see Figures 19–1 and 19–2).

## Vas Deferens

The **vas deferens,** also called the **ductus deferens,** is a slim muscular tube, about 45 cm in length, and is a continuation of the epididymis. It has been described as the *excretory duct* of the testis and extends from a point adjacent to the testis to enter the abdomen through

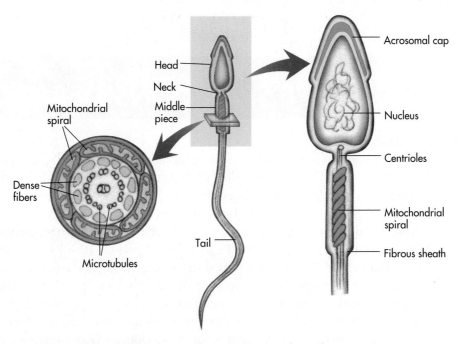

Mitochondrial spiral

Head

Neck

Middle piece

Dense fibers

Microtubules

Tail

Acrosomal cap

Nucleus

Centrioles

Mitochondrial spiral

Fibrous sheath

▶ **FIGURE 19–4** Basic structure of a spermatozoon (sperm).

the inguinal canal. It is later joined by the duct from the seminal vesicle. Between the testis and the part of the abdomen known as the *internal inguinal ring*, the vas deferens is contained within a structure known as the **spermatic cord** that also contains arteries, veins, lymphatic vessels, and nerves.

## Seminal Vesicles

There are two **seminal vesicles,** each connected by a narrow duct to a vas deferens, which then forms a short tube, the **ejaculatory duct,** which penetrates the base of the prostate gland and opens into the prostatic portion of the urethra. The seminal vesicles produce a slightly alkaline fluid that becomes a part of the seminal fluid or semen.

## Prostate Gland

The **prostate gland** is about 4 cm wide and weighs about 20 g. It is composed of glandular, connective, and muscular tissue and lies behind the urinary bladder. It surrounds the first 2.5 cm of the urethra and secretes an alkaline fluid that aids in maintaining the viability of spermatozoa. Enlargement of the prostate, called **benign prostatic hyperplasia** (BPH), is a condition that sometimes occurs in older men. In this condition, the prostate obstructs the urethra and interferes with the normal passage of urine. When this occurs, a **prostatectomy** can be performed to remove a part of the gland. The prostate gland can also be a site for cancer in older men.

## Bulbourethral Glands

The **bulbourethral glands,** or Cowper's glands, are two small pea-sized glands located below the prostate and on either side of the urethra. A duct about 2.5 cm long connects them with the wall of the urethra. The bulbourethral glands produce a mucous secretion before ejaculation, which becomes a part of the semen.

## Urethra

The male **urethra** is approximately 20 cm long and is divided into three sections: prostatic, membranous, and penile. It extends from the urinary bladder to the external urethral orifice at the head of the penis. It serves the function of transmitting urine and semen out of the body.

# LIFE SPAN CONSIDERATIONS

## ■ THE CHILD

In the newborn, the **testicles** can appear large at birth. They can fail to descend into the scrotum, causing a condition called **cryptorchidism.** The foreskin of the penis can be tight at birth, causing **phimosis,** a condition of narrowing of the opening of the prepuce wherein the foreskin cannot be drawn back over the glans penis. Congenital defects such as **epispadias** (urethra opens on the dorsum of the penis) and **hypospadias** (urethra opens on the underside of the penis) can be present. See Figure 19–7 on page 645.

**Puberty** is defined as a period of rapid change in the lives of boys and girls during which time the reproductive systems mature and become functionally capable of reproduction. In the male, puberty begins around 12 years of age when the genitals start to increase in size and the shoulders broaden and become muscular. As testosterone is released, secondary sexual characteristics develop, such as pubic and axillary hair, increase in size of the penis and testes, voice changes, facial hair, erections, and nocturnal emissions.

### ■ THE OLDER ADULT

With aging, the prostate gland enlarges and its glandular secretions decrease, the testes become smaller and firmer, the production of testosterone gradually decreases, and pubic hair becomes sparser and stiffer. This period of change in the male has been referred to as the *male climacteric* and can be associated with symptoms such as hot flashes, feelings of suffocation, insomnia, irritability, and emotional instability. Testosterone replacement therapy may be recommended for those experiencing the male climacteric.

In a healthy, normal male, **spermatogenesis** and the ability to have erections last a lifetime. However, sexual arousal can be slowed with a longer refractory period between erections. In men, a *refractory period* is the time span after one orgasm during which they are not physically able to have another one. See Pathology Spotlight: Erectile Dysfunction on page 652 for more information.

# BUILDING YOUR MEDICAL VOCABULARY

This section provides the foundation for learning medical terminology. Review the following alphabetized word. Note how common prefixes and suffixes are repeatedly applied to word roots and combining forms to create different meanings.

| P | Prefix |
|---|---|
| R | Root |
| CF | Combining form |
| S | Suffix |

| Pink words | Terms not built from word parts. |
|---|---|
| * | Indicates words covered in the Pathology Spotlights section. |
| 💿 | Check the CD-ROM for more information. |

| MEDICAL WORD | WORD PARTS (WHEN APPLICABLE) | | | DEFINITION |
|---|---|---|---|---|
| | **Part** | **Type** | **Meaning** | |
| **anorchism**<br>(ăn-ōr′ kĭzm) | an-<br>orch<br>-ism | P<br>R<br>S | lack of<br>testicle<br>condition | Condition in which there is a lack of one or both testes |
| **artificial insemination**<br>(ăr″ tĭ-fĭsh′ ăl ĭn-sĕm″ ĭn-ā′ shŭn) | artific/i<br>-al<br>in-<br>seminat<br>-ion | CF<br>S<br>P<br>R<br>S | not natural<br>pertaining to<br>into<br>semen, seed<br>process | Process of artificially placing semen into the vagina so that conception can take place. *Artificial insemination homologous (AIH)* means using the husband's semen and *artificial insemination heterologous* refers to using sperm from a donor other than the husband. |
| **aspermia**<br>(ă-spĕr′ mē-ă) | a-<br>sperm<br>-ia | P<br>R<br>S | lack of<br>seed<br>condition of | Condition of lack of sperm or failure to ejaculate sperm |
| **azoospermia**<br>(ă-zō″ ō-spĕr′ mē-ă) | a-<br>zo/o<br>sperm<br>-ia | P<br>CF<br>R<br>S | lack of<br>animal<br>seed<br>condition | Condition in which the semen lacks spermatozoa |

| MEDICAL WORD | WORD PARTS (WHEN APPLICABLE) | | | DEFINITION |
|---|---|---|---|---|
| | Part | Type | Meaning | |
| **balanitis** (băl″ ă-nī′ tĭs) | balan -itis | R S | glans inflammation | Inflammation of the glans penis |
| **benign prostatic hyperplasia (BPH)** (bē-nīn′ prŏs-tăt′-ĭk hī″ pĕr-plā′zē-a) | | | | Enlargement of the prostate gland. ✳ See Pathology Spotlight: Benign Prostatic Hyperplasia on page 651 and Figure 19–11. |
| **castrate** (kăs′ trāt) | castr -ate | R S | to prune use | To remove the testicles in a man or ovaries in a woman; *to geld; to spay* |
| **circumcision** (sĕr″ kŭm-sĭ′ shŭn) | circum- cis -ion | P R S | around to cut process | Surgical process of removing the foreskin of the penis. See Figure 19–5 ▼. |
| **cloning** (klōn′ ing) | | | | Process of creating a genetic duplicate of an individual organism through asexual reproduction |
| **coitus** (kō′ ĭ-tŭs) | | | | Sexual intercourse between a man and a woman; *copulation* |
| **condom** (kŏn′ dŭm) | | | | Thin, flexible protective sheath, usually rubber, worn over the penis during copulation to help prevent impregnation or venereal disease (VD) |
| **condyloma** (kŏn″ dĭ-lō′ mă) | | | | Wartlike growth on the skin, most often seen on the external genitalia; either viral or syphilitic in origin. See Figure 19–6 ▼. |

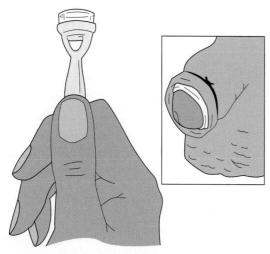

▶ **FIGURE 19–5** Circumcision using the Plastibell. The bell is fitted over the glans. A suture is tied around the bell's rim, and then the excess prepuce is cut away. The plastic rim remains in place for 3 to 4 days until healing occurs. The bell may be allowed to fall off; it is removed if still in place after 8 days.

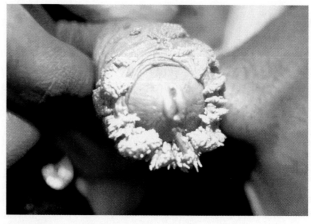

▶ **FIGURE 19–6** Genital warts. (Courtesy of the Centers for Disease Control and Prevention)

| MEDICAL WORD | WORD PARTS (WHEN APPLICABLE) | | | DEFINITION |
|---|---|---|---|---|
| | Part | Type | Meaning | |
| **cryptorchidism** (krĭpt-ōr′ kĭzm) | crypt orchid -ism | R R S | hidden testicle condition | Condition in which the testes fail to descend into the scrotum |
| **ejaculation** (ē-jăk″ ū-lā′ shŭn) | ejaculat -ion | R S | to throw out process | Process of expulsion of seminal fluid from the male urethra |
| **epididymitis** (ĕp″ ĭ-dĭd″ ĭ-mī′ tĭs) | epi- didym -itis | P R S | upon testis inflammation | Inflammation of the epididymis |
| **epispadias** (ĕp″ ĭ-spā′ dĭ-ăs) | epi- spadias | P R | upon a rent, an opening | Congenital defect in which the urethra opens on the dorsum of the penis. See Figure 19–7A ▼. |
| **erectile dysfunction (ED)** (ĕ-rĕk′ tĭl dĭs-fŭnk′ shŭn) | | | | Inability to achieve and maintain penile erection sufficient to complete satisfactory intercourse. ⚹ See Pathology Spotlight: Erectile Dysfunction on page 652. |
| **Ericsson sperm separation method** (er′ ik-son sperm sĕp″ ă-rā′ shŭn mĕth od) | | | | Process of separating the Y-chromosome sperm from the X-chromosome sperm. A sperm sample is taken and placed in a tube of albumin. Those that survive are Y-chromosome sperm, which make male babies. Women inseminated with these sperm have a 75% to 80% chance of producing a male child. |
| **eugenics** (ū-jĕn′ ĭks) | eu- -genic(s) | P S | good formation, produce | Study and control of the bringing forth of offspring as a means of improving genetic characteristics of future generations |
| **gamete** (găm′ ēt) | | | | Mature reproductive cell of the male or female; *a spermatozoon* or *ovum* |

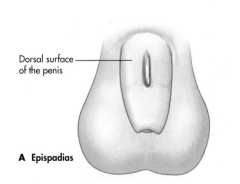
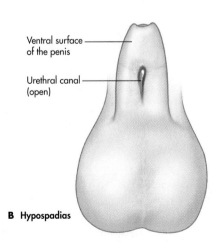

▶ **FIGURE 19–7** Hypospadias and epispadias. (A) In epispadias the canal is open on the dorsal surface. (B) In hypospadias the urethral canal is open on the ventral surface of the penis.

| MEDICAL WORD | WORD PARTS (WHEN APPLICABLE) | | | DEFINITION |
|---|---|---|---|---|
| | Part | Type | Meaning | |
| **gonorrhea (GC)** (gŏn″ ŏ-rē′ ă) | gon/o -rrhea | CF S | genitals flow | Highly contagious venereal disease of the genital mucous membrane of either sex, the infection is transmitted by the gonococcus *Neisseria gonorrhoeae*. ✱ See Pathology Spotlight: Sexually Transmitted Diseases on page 654. |
| **gynecomastia** (ji″ nĕ-kō-măs′ tĭ-ă) | gynec/o mast -ia | CF R S | female breast condition | Condition of excessive development of the mammary glands in the male |
| **herpes genitalis** (hĕr′ pēz jĕn-ĭ-tăl′ ĭs) | | | | Highly contagious venereal disease of the genitalia of either sex; caused by herpes simplex virus-2 (HSV-2). ✱ See Pathology Spotlight: Sexually Transmitted Diseases on page 654. |
| **heterosexual** (hĕt″ ĕr-ō-sĕk′ shū-ăl) | hetero- sexu -al | P R S | different sex pertaining to | Pertaining to the opposite sex; refers to an individual who has a sexual preference for the opposite sex |
| **homosexual** (hō″ mō-sĕks′ ū-ăl) | homo- sexu -al | P R S | similar, same sex pertaining to | Pertaining to the same sex; refers to an individual who has a sexual preference for the same sex |
| **hydrocele** (hī′ drō-sēl) | hydro- -cele | P S | water hernia, swelling, tumor | Accumulation of fluid in a saclike cavity. One that occurs during prenatal development is caused by a failure of the closure of the canal between the peritoneal cavity and the scrotum. See Figure 19–8 ▼. |
| **hypospadias** (hī″ pō-spă′ dĭ-ăs) | hypo- spadias | P R | under a rent, an opening | Congenital defect in which the urethra opens on the underside of the penis. See Figure 19–7B ◄. |
| **infertility** (ĭn″ fĕr-tĭl′ ĭ-tē) | | | | Inability to produce a viable offspring |

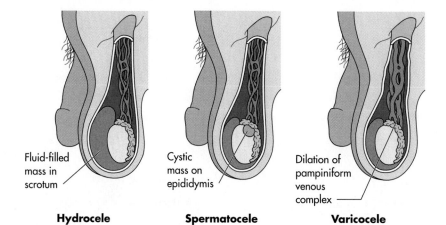

Fluid-filled mass in scrotum

Cystic mass on epididymis

Dilation of pampiniform venous complex

**Hydrocele**      **Spermatocele**      **Varicocele**

▶ FIGURE 19–8   Common disorders of the scrotum. Hydroceles and spermatoceles do not usually require treatment unless they become large and cause pain. Varicoceles are usually treated to prevent infertility.

| MEDICAL WORD | WORD PARTS (WHEN APPLICABLE) | | | DEFINITION |
|---|---|---|---|---|
| | **Part** | **Type** | **Meaning** | |
| **mitosis**<br>(mī-tō′ sĭs) | mit<br>-osis | R<br>S | thread<br>condition (usually abnormal) | Ordinary condition of cell division |
| **oligospermia**<br>(ŏl″ ĭ-gō-spĕr′ -mĭ-ă) | oligo-<br>sperm<br>-ia | P<br>R<br>S | scanty<br>Seed<br>condition | Condition in which there is a scanty amount of spermatozoa in the semen |
| **orchidectomy**<br>(or″ kĭ-dĕk′ tō-mē) | orchid<br>-ectomy | R<br>S | testicle<br>surgical excision | Surgical excision of a testicle |
| **orchidotomy**<br>(or″ kĭd-ŏt′ ō-mē) | orchid/o<br>-tomy | CF<br>S | testicle<br>incision | Incision into a testicle |
| **orchiditis**<br>(or-kī′ tĭs) | orchid<br>-itis | R<br>S | testicle<br>inflammation | Inflammation of a testicle |
| **parenchyma**<br>(păr-ĕn′ kĭ-mă) | par-<br>enchyma | P<br>R | beside<br>to pour | Essential cells of a gland or organ that are concerned with its function |
| **phimosis**<br>(fĭ-mō′ sĭs) | phim<br>-osis | R<br>S | a muzzle<br>condition (usually abnormal) | Narrowing of the opening of the prepuce wherein the foreskin cannot be drawn back over the glans penis |
| **prepuce**<br>(prē′ pūs) | | | | Foreskin over the glans penis in the male |
| **prostate cancer**<br>(prŏs′ tāt kăn′ sĕr) | | | | Malignant tumor of the prostate gland. ✱ See Pathology Spotlight: Prostate Cancer on page 653. |
| **prostatectomy**<br>(prŏs″ tă-tĕk′ tō-mē) | prostat<br>-ectomy | R<br>S | prostate<br>surgical excision | Surgical excision of the prostate |
| **prostatitis**<br>(prŏs″ tă-tī′ tĭs) | prostat<br>-itis | R<br>S | prostate<br>inflammation | Inflammation of the prostate |
| **puberty**<br>(pū′ ber-tē) | | | | Stage of development in the male and female when secondary sex characteristics begin to develop and become functionally capable of reproduction |
| **semen**<br>(sē′ mĕn) | | | | Fluid-transporting medium for spermatozoa discharged during ejaculation |
| **spermatoblast**<br>(spĕr-măt′ ō-blăst) | spermat/o<br>-blast | CF<br>S | seed, sperm<br>immature cell, germ cell | Sperm germ cell |
| **spermatocele**<br>(spĕr-măt′ ō-sēl) | spermat/o<br>-cele | CF<br>S | seed, sperm<br>hernia, swelling, tumor | Cystic swelling of the epididymis that contains spermatozoa; is mobile, usually painless, and requires no treatment. See Figure 19–8. |
| **spermatogenesis**<br>(spĕr″ măt-ō-jĕn′ ĕ-sĭs) | spermat/o<br>-genesis | CF<br>S | seed, sperm<br>formation, produce | Formation of spermatozoa |
| **spermatozoon**<br>(spĕr″ măt-ō-zō′ ŏn) | spermat/o<br>zoon | CF<br>R | seed, sperm<br>life | Male sex cell; plural form is *spermatozoa* |

| MEDICAL WORD | WORD PARTS (WHEN APPLICABLE) | | | DEFINITION |
|---|---|---|---|---|
| | **Part** | **Type** | **Meaning** | |
| **spermicide** (spĕr′ mĭ-sīd) | sperm/i -cide | CF S | seed, sperm to kill | Agent that kills sperm |
| **syphilis** (sĭf′ ĭ-lĭs) | | | | Chronic infectious venereal disease caused by *Treponema pallidum,* which is transmitted sexually. ✳ See Pathology Spotlight: Sexually Transmitted Diseases on page 654. |
| **testicular** (tĕs-tĭk′ ū-lar) | testicul -ar | R S | testicle pertaining to | Pertaining to a testicle |
| **trisomy** (trī′ sōm-ē) | tri- som -y | P R S | three body pertaining to | Genetic condition of having three chromosomes instead of two that causes various birth defects, such as Down syndrome. See Figure 19–9 ▼. |
| **varicocele** (văr′ ĭ-kō-sēl) | varic/o -cele | CF S | twisted vein hernia, swelling, tumor | Enlargement and twisting of the veins of the spermatic cord. See Figure 19–8. |
| **vasectomy** (văs-ĕk′ tō-mē) | vas -ectomy | R S | vessel surgical excision | Surgical procedure in which the vas deferens are tied off and cut apart, providing permanent sterility by preventing transport of sperm out of the testes. See Figure 19–10 ▼. ✳ See Pathology Spotlight: Vasectomy on page 656. |
| **vesiculitis** (vĕ-sĭk″ ū-lī′ tĭs) | vesicul -itis | R S | seminal vesicle inflammation | Inflammation of a seminal vesicle |

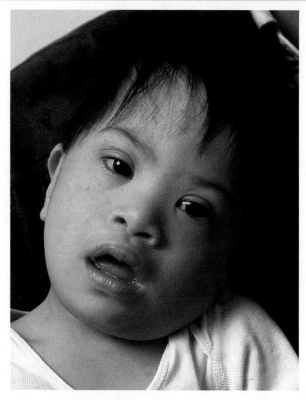

▶ **FIGURE 19–9** Child with Down syndrome, a birth defect caused by trisomy.

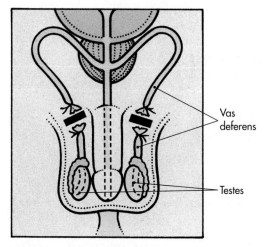

▶ **FIGURE 19–10** Vasectomy.

Vas deferens

Testes

# DRUG HIGHLIGHTS

| | |
|---|---|
| **Testosterone** | Responsible for growth, development, and maintenance of the male reproductive system and secondary sex characteristics. |
| Therapeutic use | As replacement therapy in primary hypogonadism and to stimulate puberty in carefully selected males. It can be used to relieve symptoms of the male climacteric due to androgen deficiency and to help stimulate sperm production in oligospermia and impotence due to androgen deficiency. It can also be used with advanced inoperable metastatic breast cancer in women who are 1 to 5 years postmenopausal.<br><br>*Examples: Andro 100 and AndroGel (testosterone), DepoTestosterone (testosterone cypionate in oil), Delatestryl (testosterone enanthate in oil), Testex (testosterone propionate in oil), and Testoderm and Androderm (testosterone transdermal systems).* |
| Patient teaching | Educate the patient to be aware of possible adverse reactions and report any of the following to the physician. *All patients:* nausea, vomiting, jaundice, edema. *Males:* frequent or persistent erection of the penis. *Females:* hoarseness, acne, changes in menstrual periods, growth of hair on face and/or body. |
| Special considerations | Testosterone can decrease blood glucose and insulin requirements in diabetic patients.<br><br>Testosterone can decrease the anticoagulant requirements of patients receiving oral anticoagulants. These patients require close monitoring when testosterone therapy is begun and then when it is stopped. Individuals who seek to increase muscle mass, strength, and overall athletic ability can abuse anabolic steroids (testosterone). This form is illegal; signs of abuse include flulike symptoms; headaches; muscle aches; dizziness; bruises; needle marks; increased bleeding (nosebleeds, petechiae, gums, conjunctiva); enlarged spleen, liver, and/or prostate; edema; and in the female increased facial hair, menstrual irregularities, and enlarged clitoris. |

# DIAGNOSTIC AND LAB TESTS

| TEST | DESCRIPTION |
|---|---|
| **Fluorescent treponemal antibody absorption (FTA-ABS)** (floo-ō-rĕs′ ĕnt trĕp″ ō-nē măl ăn′ tĭ-bŏd″ ē ab-sorp′ shŭn) | Test performed on blood serum to determine the presence of *Treponema pallidum* to detect syphilis. |
| **Paternity** (pă-tĕr′ nĭ-tē) | Test to determine whether a certain man is the father of a specific child. The most common and accurate test used is the DNA test, which compares a child's DNA pattern with that of the alleged father to check for evidence of inheritance. Result is either an exclusion (not the father) or inclusion (is the father). The mother's participation helps exclude half of the child's DNA, leaving the other half for comparison with the alleged father's DNA. A buccal (cheek) sample is taken from each participating person. Most states have laws that require an unmarried couple to fill out an Acknowledgement of Paternity (AOP) form to legally establish the identity of the father of a child. |

| TEST | DESCRIPTION |
|------|-------------|
| Prostate-specific antigen (PSA) immunoassay (prŏs′ tāt-spĕ-sĭf′ ĭk ăn′ tĭ-jĕn ĭm″ ū-nō-ăs′ sā) | Blood test that measures concentrations of a special type of protein known as *prostate-specific antigen*. An increased level indicates prostate disease or possibly prostate cancer. |
| Semen (sē′ mĕn) | Test performed on semen that looks at the volume, pH, sperm count, sperm motility, and morphology to evaluate infertility in men. |
| Testosterone toxicology (tĕs-tŏs′ tĕr-ōn tŏks″ ĭ-kŏl′ ō-jē) | Test performed on blood serum to identify the level of testosterone; increased level can indicate benign prostatic hyperplasia; decreased level can indicate hypogonadism, testicular hypofunction, hypopituitarism, and/or orchidectomy. |
| Venereal disease research laboratory (VDRL) (vē-nē′ rē-ăl) | Test performed on blood serum to determine the presence of *Treponema pallidum* to detect syphilis. |

# ABBREVIATIONS

| ABBREVIATION | MEANING | ABBREVIATION | MEANING |
|--------------|---------|--------------|---------|
| AIH | artificial insemination homologous | PID | pelvic inflammatory disease |
| AOP | Acknowledgement of Paternity | PSA | prostate-specific antigen |
| BPH | benign prostatic hyperplasia (also denotes benign prostatic hypertrophy) | STDs | sexually transmitted diseases |
| | | TUIP | transurethral incision of the prostate |
| CAM | complementary and alternative medicines | TUMT | transurethral microwave thermotherapy |
| DHT | dihydrotestosterone | TUNA | transurethral needle ablation |
| ED | erectile dysfunction | TUR | transurethral resection |
| FDA | Food and Drug Administration | TURP | transurethral resection of the prostate |
| FTA-ABS | fluorescent treponemal antibody absorption | VCD | vacuum constriction device |
| GC | gonorrhea | VD | venereal disease |
| HPV | human papillomavirus | VDRL | venereal disease research laboratory |
| HSV-2 | herpes simplex virus-2 | | |
| NGU | nongonococcal urethritis | | |

# PATHOLOGY SPOTLIGHTS

## ✷ Benign Prostatic Hyperplasia

**Benign prostatic hyperplasia** (BPH), also called *benign prostatic hypertrophy,* is an enlargement of the prostate gland that can occur in men who are 50 years of age and older. A microscopic exam of the prostate tissue reveals whether the prostate is enlarged due to the enlargement of individual cells (hypertrophy) or to the presence of more cells. By age 60, four of five men have an enlarged prostate.

As the prostate enlarges, it compresses the urethra, thereby restricting the normal flow of urine. See Figure 19–11 ▼. This restriction generally causes a number of symptoms and can be referred to as prostatism.

**Prostatism** is any condition of the prostate gland that interferes with the flow of urine from the bladder. Symptoms usually include these:

- Weak or difficult-to-start urine stream.
- Feeling that the bladder is not empty.
- Need to urinate often, especially at night.
- Feeling of urgency (a sudden need to urinate).
- Abdominal straining; decrease in size and force of the urinary stream.
- Interruption of the stream.
- Acute urinary retention.
- Recurrent urinary infections.

Treatment for benign prostatic hyperplasia includes drug therapy, nonsurgical procedures, and/or surgery.

- **Drug therapy.** Proscar (finasteride) is an oral medication prescribed to help relieve the symptoms of BPH. It lowers the levels of dihydrotestosterone (DHT), which is a major factor in enlargement of the prostate. Other medications used in the treatment of BPH include terazosin (Hytrin), doxazosin (Cardura), and tamsulosin (Flomax). All three drugs act by relaxing the smooth muscle of the prostate and bladder neck to improve urine flow and to reduce bladder outlet obstruction.

- **Nonsurgical treatment.** Because drug therapy is not effective in all cases, researchers in recent years have developed a number of procedures that relieve the symptoms of BPH and are less invasive than surgery. Two of these procedures follow:

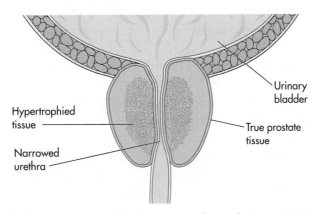

▶ FIGURE 19–11   Benign prostatic hyperplasia.

1. **Transurethral microwave.** This procedure uses a device, Prostatron, that employs microwaves to heat and destroy excess prostate tissue. In the procedure, called *transurethral microwave thermotherapy (TUMT)*, the Prostatron sends computer-regulated microwaves through a catheter to heat-selected portions of the prostate to at least 111 degrees Fahrenheit. A cooling system protects the urinary tract during the procedure. The procedure takes about 1 hour and can be performed on an outpatient basis without general anesthesia. It has been reported that this procedure does not lead to impotence or incontinence.

2. **Transurethral needle ablation.** The transurethral needle ablation (TUNA) system is a minimally invasive treatment for BPH. It delivers low-level radio-frequency energy through twin needles to burn away a well-defined region of the enlarged prostate. Shields protect the urethra from heat damage. The TUNA system improves urine flow and relieves symptoms with fewer side effects when compared with transurethral resection of the prostate (TURP). No incontinence or impotence has been observed.

- **Surgery**

   1. **Transurethral resection of the prostate (TURP or TUR).** This is the most common form of surgery used for benign prostatic hyperplasia. During this procedure, an endoscopic instrument that has ocular and surgical capabilities is introduced directly through the urethra to the prostate and small pieces of the prostate gland are removed by using an electrical cutting loop.

   2. **Transurethral incision of the prostate (TUIP).** Used to widen the urethra by making a few small cuts in the bladder neck where the urethra joins the bladder and in the prostate gland itself.

   3. **Open surgery.** This surgery is used when a transurethral procedure cannot be done. It is often done when the gland is greatly enlarged, when there are complicating factors, or when the bladder has been damaged and needs to be repaired.

   4. **Laser surgery.** This surgery employs side-firing laser fibers and ND: YAG (Neodimium Doped Yttrium Aluminum Garnet) lasers to vaporize obstructing prostate tissue.

 ## ✱ Erectile Dysfunction

**Erectile dysfunction** (ED) is the inability to achieve or maintain an erection sufficient for sexual intercourse. It occurs when not enough blood is supplied to the penis, when the smooth muscle in the penis fails to relax, or when the penis does not retain the blood that flows into it. According to studies by the National Institutes of Health, 5% of men have some degree of erectile dysfunction at age 40 and approximately 15% to 25% at age 65 or older. Although the likelihood of erectile dysfunction increases with age, it is not an inevitable part of aging. About 80% of erectile dysfunction has a physical cause. See Table 19–1 for physical causes of erectile dysfunction.

Risk factors for ED include hypertension, hyperlipidemia, endocrine disorders, low testosterone (such as patients receiving hormonal therapy for prostate cancer or patients with hypogonadotropic hypogonadism), thyroid disease, diabetes, coronary artery disease, peripheral vascular disease, anemia, medications, smoking, alcohol abuse, surgical procedures, vascular surgeries, radical prostatectomy, neurological conditions, psychiatric illness, anxiety disorder, depression, obsessive-compulsive disorder, and injury.

Treatment includes counseling or sex therapy for men whose erectile dysfunction stems from emotional problems. Treatments for physical causes are based on the cause. For

## TABLE 19–1  Some Physical Causes of Erectile Dysfunction

| | |
|---|---|
| Vascular diseases | Arteriosclerosis, hypertension, high cholesterol, and other conditions that can cause obstruction of blood flow to the penis |
| Diabetes | Can alter nerve function and blood flow to the penis |
| Prescription drugs | Certain antihypertensive and cardiac medications, antihistamines, psychiatric medications, and other prescription drugs |
| Substance abuse | Excessive smoking, alcohol, and illegal drugs that constrict blood vessels |
| Neurologic diseases | Multiple sclerosis, Parkinson's disease, and other diseases that interrupt nerve impulses to the penis |
| Surgery | Prostate, colon, bladder, and other types of pelvic surgery that damage nerves and blood vessels |
| Spinal Injury | Interruptions of nerve impulses from the spinal cord to the penis |
| Other | Hormonal imbalance, kidney failure, dialysis, and reduced testosterone levels |

example, if ED is caused by a medication, the man should consult with his physician about changing medications. Mixing medications and/or not following instructions are common causes of ED.

Many treatment options for ED are available today. These include the vacuum constriction device (VCD); oral medications such as Viagra (sildenafil), Levitra (vardenafil), and Cialis (tadalafil); medication patches and gels; urethral and penile injection therapies; and surgical therapies including penile prostheses (implants).

## ✴ Prostate Cancer

**Prostate cancer** is a malignant tumor that grows in the prostate gland. It is the most common type of cancer found in American men. By age 50, up to one in four men have some cancerous cells in the prostate gland. By age 80, the ratio increases to one in two. In the United States, the average age at diagnosis is 70. Diagnosis of prostate cancer can be confirmed with a medical history, physical examination, including a rectal exam, and results of a PSA blood test. The physician performs a digital rectal exam to assess the size and condition (firm, soft, hard) of the prostate gland.

Prostate cancer is the second leading cause of cancer death in men, exceeded only by lung cancer. While 1 man in 6 will have prostate cancer during his lifetime, only 1 man in 32 will die of this disease. A man is more likely to die *with* prostate cancer than to die *from* prostate cancer.

Some men with prostate cancer have no symptoms. Others notice symptoms such as dull pain in the lower pelvic area; general pain in the lower back, hips, or upper thighs; blood in the urine or semen; dribbling when urinating; erectile dysfunction; frequent urination, especially at night; painful urination and/or ejaculation; a smaller stream of urine and/or an urgent need to urinate; and loss of appetite and weight. If the cancer has spread to other parts of the body, such as the bones, the man could have persistent bone pain, occasional nerve paralysis, or loss of bladder function.

Prostate cancer is graded and staged for aggressiveness based on how far it has spread throughout the body. CT scans and bone scans help in staging, but sometimes it becomes clear only at the time of surgery. Following are the stages of prostate cancer:

- Stages A and B are confined to the prostate gland.
- Stage C has spread to other tissues near the prostate gland.
- Stage D has spread to lymph nodes or sites in the body a distance away from the prostate.

The proper management of the many stages of prostate cancer is controversial. Depending on the grade and stage of the cancer, some options are as follows:

- Chemotherapy.
- Cryosurgery to freeze cancer cells.
- External radiation to the prostate and pelvis.
- Hormone therapy.
- Radioactive implants put directly into the prostate, which slowly kill cancer cells.
- Surgery to remove part or all of the prostate and surrounding tissue.
- Surgical removal of the testicles to block testosterone production.
- Watchful waiting and monitoring only.

A significant number of prostate cancer patients use *complementary and alternative medicines* (CAM) as part of their treatment according to a new study, but many of those men do not tell their doctors about these therapies, which could have a negative effect on their care.

 ✴ **Sexually Transmitted Diseases**

**Sexually transmitted diseases** (STDs) can occur in men, women, and children. They are passed from person to person through sexual contact or from mother to child. The following is a summary of the most common sexually transmitted diseases:

| Disease | Cause | Symptoms | Treatment |
|---------|-------|----------|-----------|
| Chlamydia (klă-mĭd′ ē-ă) | *Chlamydia trachomatis* (bacterium) | Can be asymptomatic or exhibit the following: **MALE:** Mucopurulent discharge from penis, burning, itching in genital area, dysuria, swollen testes; can cause nongonococcal urethritis (NGU) and sterility **FEMALE:** Mucopurulent discharge from vagina, cystitis, pelvic pain, cervicitis; can lead to pelvic inflammatory disease (PID) and sterility **NEWBORN:** Eye infection, pneumonia; can cause death | Antibiotics—tetracycline or erythromycin |
| Genital warts (jĕn′ ĭ-tăl worts) | Human papillomavirus (HPV) | **MALE:** Cauliflowerlike growths on the penis and perianal area **FEMALE:** Cauliflowerlike growths around vagina and perianal area | Laser surgery, chemotherapy, cryosurgery, cauterization **Note:** Recently the first vaccine developed to prevent cervical cancer and other diseases in females caused by certain types of *genital human papillomavirus (HPV)* was licensed by the Food and Drug Administration (FDA) for use in girls/women, ages 9–26 years. The vaccine, Gardasil®, protects against four HPV types, which are responsible for 70% of cervical cancers and 90% of genital warts. |

| Disease | Cause | Symptoms | Treatment |
|---------|-------|----------|-----------|
| Gonorrhea (gŏn" ŏ-rē' ā) | *Neisseria gonorrhoeae* (bacterium) | **MALE:** Purulent urethral discharge, dysuria, urinary frequency<br>**FEMALE:** Purulent vaginal discharge, dysuria, urinary frequency, abnormal menstrual bleeding, abdominal tenderness; can lead to PID and sterility<br>**NEWBORN:** Gonorrheal ophthalmia neonatorum, purulent eye discharge; can cause blindness | Antibiotics—penicillin or tetracycline |
| Herpes genitalis (hĕr' pēz jĕn-ĭ-tāl' ĭs) | Herpes simplex virus-2 (HSV-2) | **ACTIVE PHASE**<br>**MALE:** Fluid-filled vesicles (blisters) on penis; caused by acute pain and itching<br>**FEMALE:** Blisters in and around vagina<br>**NEWBORN:** Can be infected during vaginal delivery; severe infection, physical and mental damage<br>**GENERALIZED:** Flulike symptoms, fever, headache, malaise, anorexia, muscle pain | No cure; antiviral drug acyclovir (Zovirax) can be used to relieve symptoms during acute phase |
| Syphilis (sĭf' ĭ-lĭs) | *Treponema pallidum* (bacterium) | **PRIMARY STAGE:** Chancre at point of infection; see Figure 19–12 ▼<br>**MALE:** penis, anus, rectum<br>**FEMALE:** vagina, cervix<br>**BOTH:** lips, tongue, fingers, nipples<br>**SECONDARY STAGE:** Flulike symptoms with a skin rash over moist, fatty areas of the body; see Figure 19–13 ▼ | Antibotics—penicillin, tetracycline, or erythromycin |

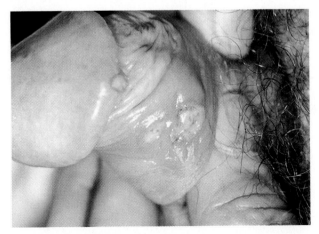

▶ **FIGURE 19–12** Chancre. (Courtesy of Jason L. Smith, MD)

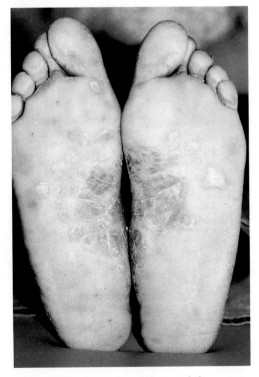

▶ **FIGURE 19–13** Secondary syphilis. (Courtesy of Jason L. Smith, MD)

| Disease | Cause | Symptoms | Treatment |
|---------|-------|----------|-----------|
| | | **LATE STAGE:** Difficulty coordinating muscle movements, paralysis, numbness, gradual blindness, and dementia; this damage can be serious enough to cause death | |
| | | **NEWBORN:** Congenital syphilis— heart defect, bone or other deformities | |
| Trichomoniasis (trĭk″ ō-mō-nī′ ă-sĭs) | *Trichomonas* (parasitic protozoa) | **MALE:** Usually asymptomatic; can lead to cystitis, urethritis, prostatitis, and nongonococcal urethritis (NGU) | Metronidazole (Flagyl) |
| | | **FEMALE:** White frothy vaginal discharge, burning and itching of vulva; can lead to cystitis, urethritis, vaginitis | |

 ✴ **Vasectomy**

A **vasectomy** is a surgery in which the vas deferens are tied off and cut apart. This causes permanent sterility by preventing transport of sperm out of the testes. See Figure 19–10 on page 648. A vasectomy is usually done in the surgeon's office while the patient is awake using local anesthesia. After the surgery, the patient is able to return home immediately and to work the next day (if the job is sedentary) and can resume strenuous physical activity in 3 to 7 days.

This surgery does not affect a man's ability to achieve orgasm, ejaculate, or achieve erections. There is still a fluid ejaculate, but no sperm is in this fluid, so the man cannot impregnate his partner.

Vasectomy provides permanent sterilization. It is not recommended as a temporary or reversible procedure. After vasectomy, the sperm count gradually decreases. After 4 to 6 weeks, sperm are no longer present in the semen. A semen specimen must be examined and found to be totally free of sperm a month or more after vasectomy before the patient can rely on the vasectomy for birth control. Continued use of contraception is recommended until 2 to 3 sperm count tests are negative, indicating that the patient is sterile.

# ✓PATHOLOGY CHECKPOINT

*Following is a concise list of the pathology-related terms that you have seen in the chapter. Review this checklist to make sure that you are familiar with the meaning of each term before moving to the next section.*

## Conditions and Symptoms

- ❏ anorchism
- ❏ aspermatism
- ❏ azoospermia
- ❏ balanitis
- ❏ benign prostatic hyperplasia
- ❏ condyloma
- ❏ cryptorchidism
- ❏ epididymitis
- ❏ epispadias
- ❏ erectile dysfunction
- ❏ gonorrhea
- ❏ gynecomastia
- ❏ herpes genitalis
- ❏ hydrocele
- ❏ hypospadias
- ❏ infertility
- ❏ oligospermia
- ❏ orchiditis
- ❏ phimosis
- ❏ prostate cancer
- ❏ prostatitis
- ❏ spermatocele
- ❏ syphilis
- ❏ trisomy
- ❏ varicocele
- ❏ vesiculitis

## Diagnosis and Treatment

- ❏ artificial insemination
- ❏ castrate
- ❏ circumcision
- ❏ Ericsson sperm separation method
- ❏ orchidectomy
- ❏ orchidotomy
- ❏ prostatectomy
- ❏ spermicide
- ❏ vasectomy

# STUDY AND REVIEW

## Anatomy and Physiology

*Write your answers to the following questions. Do not refer to the text.*

1. List the primary and accessory glands of the male reproductive system.

   a. _____   b. _____

   c. _____   d. _____

   e. _____   f. _____

2. Name the supporting structure and accessory sex organs of the male reproductive system.

   a. _____   b. _____

3. State the vital function of the male reproductive system.

   _____

4. Describe the scrotum.

   _____

5. The _____ _____ _____ and the _____

   _____ are names of the three longitudinal columns of erectile tissue in the penis.

6. The average erect penis measures _____ to _____ cm in length.

7. The _____ _____ is the cone-shaped head of the penis.

8. Define *prepuce*.

   _____

9. Define *smegma*.

   _____

10. State two functions of the penis.

    a. _____   b. _____

11. Describe the testes.

    _____

    _____

12. _____ _____ is the site of the development of spermatozoa.

13. List five effects of testosterone regarding male development.

    a. _____    b. _____

    c. _____    d. _____

    e. _____

14. Name the plexus that the seminiferous tubules form. _____

15. Describe the epididymis.

    _____

16. State two functions of the epididymis.

    a. _____    b. _____

17. The excretory duct of the testes is known by two names, _____

    _____ or _____ _____.

18. The spermatic cord contains five types of structures and connects the testes with organs in the abdomen. Name these five structures.

    a. _____    b. _____

    c. _____    d. _____

    e. _____

19. State the function of the seminal vesicles.

    _____

20. Describe the prostate gland.

    _____

21. Define the condition known as *benign prostatic hyperplasia.*

    _____

22. The two small pea-sized glands located below the prostate and on either side of

    the urethra are known as the _____ glands or as _____ glands.

23. Name the three sections of the male urethra.

    a. _____    b. _____

    c. _____

24. State a function of the male urethra. _____

25. The male urethra is approximately _____ cm long.

## Word Parts

1. In the spaces provided, write the definitions of these prefixes, roots, combining forms, and suffixes. Do not refer to the listings of medical words. Leave blank those words you cannot define.

2. After completing as many as you can, refer to the medical word listings to check your work. For each word missed or left blank, write the word and its definition several times on the margins of these pages or on a separate sheet of paper.

3. To maximize the learning process, it is to your advantage to do the following exercises as directed. To refer to the word-building section before completing these exercises invalidates the learning process.

## PREFIXES

*Give the definitions of the following prefixes.*

1. a- _____

2. an- _____

3. circum- _____

4. epi- _____

5. hydro- _____

6. hypo- _____

7. oligo- _____

8. par- _____

9. in- _____

10. eu- _____

11. heter- _____

12. homo- _____

13. tri- _____

## ROOTS AND COMBINING FORMS

*Give the definitions of the following roots and combining forms.*

1. balan _____

2. cis _____

3. crypt _____

4. artific/i _____

5. didym _____

6. enchyma _____

7. orch _____

8. orchid _____

9. orchid/o _____

10. phim _____

11. prostat _____

12. castr _____

13. spadias _____

14. sperm _____

15. seminat _____

16. spermat/o _____

17. sperm/i _____

18. testicul _____

19. varic/o _____

20. vas _____

21. vesicul _____

22. zo/o _____

23. zoon _____

24. ejaculat _____

25. gon/o _____

26. gynec/o _____

27. mast _____

28. sexu _____

29. mit _____

30. som _____

## SUFFIXES

*Give the definitions of the following suffixes.*

1. -al _____

2. -ar _____

3. -blast _____

4. -cele _____

5. -cide _____

6. -ectomy _____

7. -genesis _____

8. -ia _____

9. -ion _____

10. -ism _____

11. -itis _____

12. -ate _____

13. -osis _____

14. -genic(s) _____

15. -rrhea _____

16. -tomy _____

17. -y _____

## Identifying Medical Terms

*In the spaces provided, write the medical terms for the following meanings.*

1. _____  Inflammation of the glans penis

2. _____  Surgical excision of the epididymis

3. _____  Surgical excision of a testicle

4. _____  Foreskin over the glans penis

5. _____  Accumulation of fluid in a saclike cavity

6. _____  Wartlike growth on the skin

7. _____  Sperm germ cell

8. _____  Male sex cell

9. _____  Agent that kills sperm

10. _____  Pertaining to a testicle

## Spelling

*In the spaces provided, write the correct spelling of these misspelled words.*

1. crptorchism _____

2. hyospadias _____

3. orchdotomy _____

4. ugenics _____

5. tisomy _____

## Matching

*Select the appropriate lettered meaning for each of the following words.*

_____ 1. circumcision

_____ 2. coitus

_____ 3. condom

_____ 4. gamete

_____ 5. genital warts

_____ 6. gonorrhea

_____ 7. infertility

_____ 8. prepuce

_____ 9. syphilis

_____ 10. trichomoniasis

a. Caused by the bacterium *Treponema pallidum*
b. Mature reproductive cell of the male or female
c. Sexual intercourse between a man and a woman
d. Caused by a parasitic protozoa
e. Surgical process of removing the foreskin of the penis
f. Thin, flexible protective sheath worn over the penis during copulation to help prevent impregnation or venereal disease
g. Disease caused by the human papillomavirus
h. Inability to produce a viable offspring
i. Causes purulent urethral discharge in the male and purulent vaginal discharge in the female
j. Caused by the bacterium *Chlamydia trachomatis*
k. The foreskin over the glans penis in the male

## Abbreviations

*Place the correct word, phrase, or abbreviation in the space provided.*

1. benign prostatic hyperplasia _____

2. GC _____

3. human papillomavirus _____

4. HSV-2 _____

5. STDs _____

6. erectile dysfunction _____

7. TURP _____

8. NGU _____

9. venereal disease _____

10. prostate-specific antigen _____

## Diagnostic and Laboratory Tests

*Select the best answer to each multiple choice question. Circle the letter of your choice.*

1. Test performed on blood serum to detect syphilis.
   a. paternity
   b. semen
   c. FTA-ABS
   d. HSV-2

2. Test to determine whether a certain man is the father of a specific child.
   a. paternity
   b. semen
   c. FTA-ABS
   d. HSV-2

3. Increased level indicates prostate disease or possibly prostate cancer.
   a. fluorescent treponemal antibody
   b. prostate-specific antigen
   c. semen
   d. testosterone toxicology

4. Used to determine infertility in men.
   a. paternity
   b. prostate-specific antigen
   c. semen
   d. testosterone toxicology

5. Increased level can indicate benign prostatic hyperplasia.
   a. fluorescent treponemal antibody
   b. prostate-specific antigen
   c. testosterone toxicology
   d. venereal disease research laboratory

# PRACTICAL APPLICATION

## S O A P : Chart Note Analysis

*This exercise will make you aware of information, abbreviations, and medical terminology typically found in a patient's chart at a family practice office.*

### Abbreviation Key

| | | | |
|---|---|---|---|
| α | alpha | lb | pound |
| Abd | abdomen | mg | milligram |
| BP | blood pressure | NKDA | no known drug allergies |
| BPH | benign prostatic hyperplasia (hypertrophy) | P | pulse |
| | | PM | evening |
| c/o | complains of | PO | orally, by mouth |
| cm | centimeter | PSA | prostate-specific antigen |
| CTA | clear to auscultation | R | respiration |
| DHT | dihydrotestosterone | SOAP | subjective, objective, assessment, plan |
| DOB | date of birth | T | temperature |
| DRE | digital rectal examination | Wt | weight |
| F | Fahrenheit | y/o | year(s) old |
| Ht | height | | |

*Read the following chart note and then answer the questions that follow.*

**PATIENT:** Rowe, Ralph A.                                                                 **DATE:** 01/30/2007

**DOB:** 01/01/47     **AGE:** 60     **SEX:** Male

**INSURANCE:** Excel Healthcare

**Vital Signs:**
T: 98.8 F
P: 82
R: 20
BP: 146/89
Ht: 5' 11''
Wt: 192 lb

**Allergies:** NKDA

**Chief Complaint:** Frequency, urgency, and decrease in amount and force of urinary stream

**S** | **Subjective:** 60 y/o male c/o difficulty with urination. "I am having to urinate more frequently, especially at night. I feel this urgency and then I have trouble starting my stream. I pee only a little."

**O** | **Objective:**

**General Appearance:** Appears uncomfortable. Hesitant in talking about symptoms.

**Heart:** Regular rate and rhythm. No murmurs, gallops, or rubs.

**Lungs:** CTA

**Abd:** Bowel sounds heard all 4 quadrants. No masses or tenderness noted. No distention of bladder or renal tenderness.

**Prostate:** DRE revealed enlarged prostate, approximately 5.5 cm, projecting 1.5 cm into the rectum. Smooth without normal central groove, no nodules or indurations, tender, firm to rubbery consistency.

**A**   **Assessment:** Benign prostatic hyperplasia (BPH)

**P**   **Plan:**

1. Advised to go to the laboratory for a complete urinalysis and a PSA test.
2. Prescribed Proscar (finasteride) 5 mg PO once a day for 6 months.
3. Instruct to limit fluid intake during the PM hours, especially alcohol and caffeine, to reduce the need for night-time urination.
4. Educate that side effects of Proscar can include impotence and decreased sexual desire.
5. Inform that Proscar can alter the PSA test that is used to screen for prostate cancer.
6. Educate that women who are pregnant or of child bearing age should not touch Proscar tablets, particularly crushed or broken tablets, because of possible adverse effects to unborn child or damage to ovaries if medicine is absorbed through their skin.
7. Schedule follow-up visit for 6 months.

**FYI:** Proscar (finasteride) is a 5α-reductase inhibitor that lowers the levels of DHT, the major factor in enlargement of the prostate. Shrinkage of the enlarged prostate usually occurs in 6 to 12 months with medication therapy. Note: Proscar (5 mg) is one brand of finasteride that is prescribed for BPH while Propecia (1 mg) is another brand of finasteride that is prescribed for male pattern baldness.

## Chart Note Questions

*Place the correct answer in the space provided.*

1. Signs and symptoms of BPH include increased frequency, _____, and decrease in size and force of urinary stream.

2. DRE is an abbreviation for _____ _____ _____

3. The medication of choice for an enlarged prostates is _____ a 5α-reductase inhibitor.

4. This medication can alter the _____ test that is used to screen for prostate cancer.

5. Side effects of Proscar can include _____ and decreased sexual desire.

6. Upon DRE, Mr. Rowe's enlarged prostate was approximately _____ cm.

7. The enlarged prostate projected _____ cm into the rectum.

8. What is considered as a major factor in the enlargement of the prostate? _____

9. Limiting PM fluids, especially alcohol and caffeine, should help _____ the need for night-time urination.

10. To evaluate the effectiveness of drug therapy, a follow-up is recommended in _____ months.

# MULTIMEDIA PREVIEW

*Additional interactive resources and activities for this chapter can be found on the Companion Website. For videos, audio glossary, and review, access the accompanying CD-ROM in this book.*

## CD-ROM HIGHLIGHTS

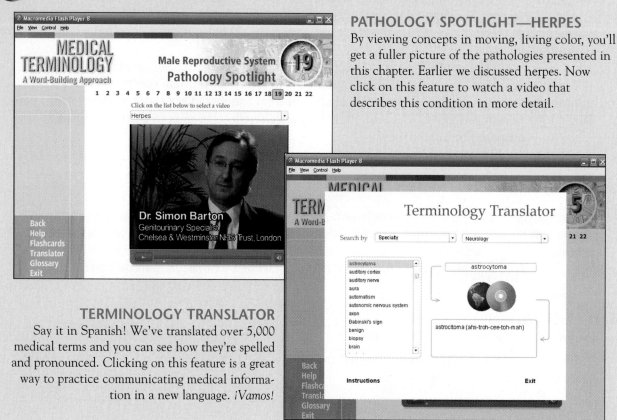

## PATHOLOGY SPOTLIGHT—HERPES

By viewing concepts in moving, living color, you'll get a fuller picture of the pathologies presented in this chapter. Earlier we discussed herpes. Now click on this feature to watch a video that describes this condition in more detail.

## TERMINOLOGY TRANSLATOR

Say it in Spanish! We've translated over 5,000 medical terms and you can see how they're spelled and pronounced. Clicking on this feature is a great way to practice communicating medical information in a new language. *¡Vamos!*

## WEBSITE HIGHLIGHTS—www.prenhall.com/rice

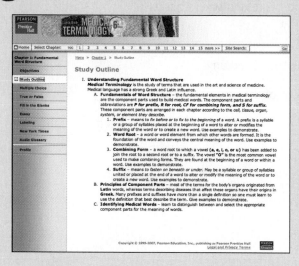

## STUDY OUTLINES

Click here and take advantage of the free-access on-line study guide that accompanies your textbook. You'll find outline summaries of each chapter to give you a snapshot of the important concepts. By clicking on this URL you'll also access a variety of quizzes with instant feedback, links to download mp3 audio reviews, news updates, and an audio glossary.

# Oncology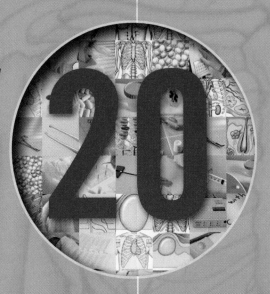

## ■ OBJECTIVES

*On completion of this chapter, you will be able to:*

- Describe cancer.
- Describe cell differentiation.
- Identify the staging system that evaluates the spread of a tumor.
- Describe methods that can be used in diagnosing cancer.
- List the various forms of treatment for cancer.
- Define *radiation therapy*.
- Describe important factors that must be considered when determining the use of radiotherapy for the cancer patient.
- Analyze, build, spell, and pronounce medical words.
- Identify and define selected abbreviations.
- Describe each of the conditions presented in the Pathology Spotlights.
- Review the Pathology Checkpoint.
- Complete the Study and Review section and the Chart Note Analysis.

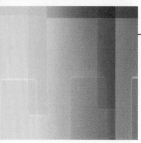

# Overview of Cancer

**Cancer** (CA), a Latin word meaning **crab,** was first identified around 400 BC during the time of Hippocrates. Early reports on cancer compared the disease to a crab because of its tendency to stretch out and spread like the crab's four pairs of legs. Today, cancer refers to any malignant tumor (neoplasm, oncoma). More than 200 different types of cancer have been identified.

The incidence of cancer is now five times higher than it was 100 years ago. Cancer will strike 1 of every 3 Americans, according to recent statistics from the American Cancer Society (ACS). However, there is hope for those afflicted. Cancer has become one of the most curable of the major diseases in the United States, and those tumors that cannot be cured can be controlled through treatment, thereby giving the patient an extended life span. With early detection followed by immediate treatment, the cure rate for cancer is now 1 in every 2. Highly advanced **surgical techniques** are being used to remove cancerous tissue, and it is usually possible to excise all the cancer cells when the malignancy is discovered in its earliest stages (St). **Chemotherapy** (chemo) and **radiation therapy** are the other two principal means of treatment for patients with cancer. These treatments employ agents to kill cancerous cells that remain after surgery or in malignancies deemed inoperable. **Immunotherapy** and **photodynamic therapy** are two newer methods employed in the treatment of cancer.

Although the exact cause or causes remain unknown, research has shown that some cancers can be prevented, especially those associated with environmental factors. Oncologists searching for the causes of cancer have identified numerous factors that play a role in the development of cancer. See Figure 20–1 ▼. These factors are generally grouped under three main classifications: environmental, hereditary, and biological.

The American Cancer Society recommends various safeguards against cancer, which encourages individuals to take specific steps to safeguard their health and aid in the early

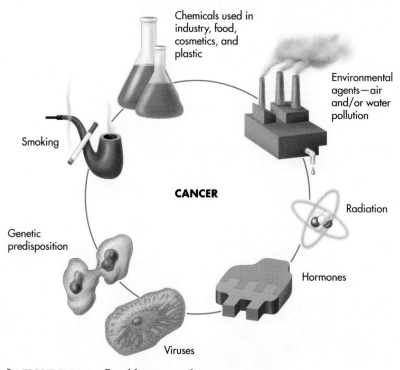

▶ **FIGURE 20–1**  Possible causes of cancer.

detection of cancer (see the following table). Some of these recommendations, according to site and action, are listed here for you. For additional information, go to www.cancer.org.

| Site | Action |
|------|--------|
| Breast | Routine monthly breast self-examination; professional exam every 3 years from age 20 to 39 and yearly thereafter; screening mammography every year from age 40 |
| Uterus | Yearly pelvic exam and Pap smear test for sexually active females over 18; less often for women with three consecutive negative results |
| Lung | Regular chest x-ray for smokers |
| Skin | Regular skin check for those who are frequently exposed to the sun |
| Colon-rectum | Proctoscopy annually, especially after 40; colonoscopy after 50 |
| Mouth | Exams regularly |
| Whole body | Annual health checkup including chest x-ray and various laboratory tests |
| Prostate | Annual digital rectal exam; PSA test yearly beginning at age 50 (men at higher risk should begin at 40) |
| Testicles | Monthly testicular self-examination |

# CLASSIFICATION OF CANCER

Classification of cancer helps determine appropriate treatment and prognosis. Tumors are classified according to their anatomic site of origin, grading, and staging.

## Anatomic Site

The anatomic site indicates where the cancer originated in the body. **Carcinomas** make up the great majority of all cancers and are malignant tumors of epithelial tissues. Epithelial tissue lines body surfaces including those of glands and organs; therefore, carcinomas make up the majority of the glandular cancers and are generally found in the breast, stomach, uterus, tongue, and skin. They are named according to the type of epithelial cell in which the malignancy occurs or the primary site of the tumor. For instance, a cancer of squamous epithelium is called a **squamous carcinoma** (see Figure 20–2 ▼ and Figure 5–32 in Chapter 5 on page 88), and a type of skin cancer is called a **basal cell carcinoma** (see Figure 20–4 on page 682). Likewise a cancer originating in the bronchus of the respiratory tract is a **bronchogenic carcinoma.**

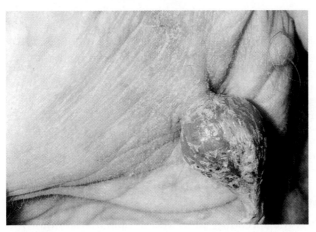

▶ **FIGURE 20–2** Squamous cell carcinoma. (Courtesy of Jason L. Smith, MD)

**Sarcomas** originate in connective or supportive tissues of the body such as the muscles, tendons, fat, joints, and bone. They are named by adding the suffix -oma (tumor) with the root sarc (flesh) to the word part that identifies the tissue of origin. A cancer of the bone, for examples, is an **osteosarcoma:** osteo (CF), bone; sarc (R), flesh; and -oma (S), tumor.

Cancers of lymphatic tissue, bone marrow, and blood cells are called **leukemias, lymphomas,** and **myelomas.** Leukemias are cancers of the blood-forming tissues. Lymphomas are cancers of lymphoid tissue, and myelomas are cancers of the bone marrow.

# CELL DIFFERENTIATION AND GRADING

Normal cells reproduce themselves through **mitosis,** an orderly process that ensures growth, tissue repair, and cell reproduction. Normal cells have a distinct appearance and a specialized function. In normal cell development, immature cells undergo normal changes as they mature and assume their specialized functions. This process is called **differentiation.** Knowledge of cell differentiation allows a pathologist or histologist to identify the body area from which the tissue was removed by looking at a sample of tissue through a microscope. In cancer, an abnormal process in which a cell or group of cells undergoes changes and no longer carries on normal cell functions occurs. This failure of immature cells to develop specialized functions is called **dedifferentiation.** It is believed that this process involves a disturbance in the DNA of the affected cells. **Malignant cells** usually multiply rapidly, forming a mass of abnormal cells that enlarges, ulcerates, and sheds malignant cells that invade surrounding tissues. This process destroys the normal cells, and malignant cells take their places. Microscopic analysis of a malignant cell reveals a loss of differentiation, anaplasia, nuclei of various sizes that are hyperchromatic, and cells in the process of rapid and disorderly division.

Based on microscopic analysis, malignant tumors are further classified as grades I, II, III, or IV. The following describes each of the four grades of tumors in this system:

**Grade I.** The most differentiated and the least malignant tumors. Only a few cells are undergoing mitosis; however, some abnormality does exist.

**Grade II.** Moderately undifferentiated. More cells are undergoing mitosis, and the pattern is fairly irregular.

**Grade III.** Many undifferentiated cells. Tissue origin can be difficult to recognize. Many cells are undergoing mitosis.

**Grade IV.** The least differentiated and high degree of malignancy.

This system of grading tumors is used to report the prognosis of the disease and to determine whether the tumor is likely to respond to radiation therapy.

# INVASIVE PROCESS

Two ways in which malignant cells spread to body parts are by invasive growth and metastasis.

## Invasive Growth

**Invasive growth** is the spreading process of a malignant tumor into adjacent normal tissue (see Figure 20–8 on page 687). Young malignant cells divide at the periphery of the tumor and spread by active migration or direct extension. In **active migration,** the malignant cells break away from the neoplasm (new growth), invade surrounding tissue, divide, form secondary neoplasms, and then reunite with the primary tumor as growth continues. In **direct extension,** multiplication of malignant cells is rapid, and subsequently spread into surrounding tissues via the interstitial spaces accompanied by engulfment and destruction of normal cells. As a tumor's mass enlarges, its weight is supported by connective fibers that attach to surrounding structures. These fibers invade adjacent veins and lymph vessel and become pathways for the spread of malignant cells.

### Metastasis

**Metastasis** is the process whereby cancer cells are spread from a primary site to distant secondary sites elsewhere in the body. This process usually occurs when malignant cells invade the bloodstream or lymph system and are transported to a secondary site where they become lodged and form a neoplasm. Malignant cells carried in the bloodstream can lodge in highly vascular organs such as the lungs or liver, and the development of a secondary neoplasm depends on the viability and the receptivity of the organ.

## STAGING

Further reporting of the development and spread of cancer cells may be made through the use of a system that evaluates the spread of the tumor. The staging system uses the letters **T** (tumor), **N** (node), and **M** (metastasis) to indicate spread and uses numerical subscripts to indicate degree of tumor involvement. For example, $T_2N_1M_0$ indicates a primary tumor at stage II, abnormality of regional lymph nodes at stage I, and no evidence of distant metastasis.

A numerical system is also used to classify the staging of cancer. This system describes the various stages according to the extent of the spreading process.

| | |
|---|---|
| **Stage 0** | Cancer in situ (limited to inner lining surface of the organ and not invading the organ) |
| **Stage I** | Cancer limited to the tissue of origin and has not spread past the tissue or organ where it started |
| **Stage II** | Limited local spread of cancerous cells, sometimes to lymph nodes |
| **Stage III** | Extensive local and regional spread of cancer, usually to draining lymph nodes |
| **Stage IV** | Distant metastasis, has spread beyond the regional lymph nodes to distant parts of the body |

## CHARACTERISTICS OF NEOPLASMS

**Neoplasms** or *tumors,* as they are commonly called, may be **benign** or **malignant.** See page 672 for characteristics that distinguish the differences between benign and malignant neoplasms.

As malignant cells proliferate and begin the invasive process, the patient is unaware of the development of the cancer. In its early stages, cancer is said to be silent; however, cytologic changes are occurring that could be detected if a tissue sample were taken and analyzed by a pathologist. With the proliferation of malignant cells and the continuation of the invasive process, tissues, organs, and surrounding structures become compressed, and ischemia can occur, causing necrosis, inflammation, ulceration, and bleeding. This bleeding is usually **occult** (*hidden*). The enlarging tumor eventually causes sufficient pressure on

| Benign Tumors | Malignant Tumors |
|---|---|
| Grow slowly | Grow rapidly |
| Are encapsulated | Are not encapsulated |
| Have cells that resemble the normal cells from which they arose | Have cells that undergo permanent change, abnormal rapid proliferation |
| Grow by expansion and cause pressure on surrounding tissue | Have invasive growth and metastasis |
| Remain localized | Spread via the bloodstream |
| Do not recur when surgically removed | Can recur when surgically removed if invasive growth has occurred |
| Have minimal tissue destruction | Have extensive tissue destruction if invasive growth has occurred |
| Have no cachexia | Have cachexia (extreme weakness, fatigue, wasting, and malnutrition) |
| Are usually not a threat to life | Are threats to life unless detected early and properly treated |

surrounding tissues and organs to create a feeling of numbness, tingling, and pain. Because the tumor itself does not have nerve endings, pain is not an early symptom of its development. Because of the silent development of cancer, the patient does not usually become aware of its symptoms until its systemic effects are evident. These systemic effects depend on the site and type of cancer but usually result in an imbalance in the patient's physiology, leading to subtle but noticeable changes that can warn of the disease.

The American Cancer Society lists seven warning signals of cancer. The first letters of each warning signal combine to spell the word CAUTION, and persons who develop any of the following symptoms should bring it to the attention of a physician immediately:

- **C**hange in bowel or bladder habits.
- **A** sore that does not heal.
- **U**nusual bleeding or discharge.
- **T**hickening or lump in breast or elsewhere.
- **I**ndigestion or difficulty in swallowing.
- **O**bvious change in a wart or mole.
- **N**agging cough or hoarseness.

# DIAGNOSIS

A variety of *diagnostic tools* and *procedures* is used to detect the possible presence of cancer. Principal among these are examination, visualization by endoscopy, laboratory analysis, biopsy (Bx), and diagnostic radiology.

## Examination

An *annual physical examination* could be the best means to protect a person's state of health. The American Cancer Society publishes a cancer detection examination that recommends certain tests be included in an annual physical examination in addition to the medical history and usual tests. For more specific information visit the American Cancer Society's Web site at www.cancer.org.

## Visualization by Endoscopy

**Endoscopy** provides the physician a direct view of certain portions of the body. The following is a list of endoscopic procedures used to assess specific locations within the body:

**Sigmoidoscopy.** Use of a sigmoidoscope to examine the lower 10 inches of the large intestines

**Laryngoscopy.** Use of a laryngoscope to examine the interior of the larynx.

**Bronchoscopy.** Use of a bronchoscope to examine the bronchi

**Gastroscopy.** Use of a gastroscope to examine the interior of the stomach

**Cystoscopy.** Use of a cystoscope to examine the bladder

**Colposcopy.** Use of a colposcope to examine the cervix and vagina

**Proctoscopy.** Use of a proctoscope to examine the anus and rectum

**Colonoscopy.** Use of a colonoscope to examine the colon

**Laparoscopy.** Use of a laparoscope to examine the abdomen

## Laboratory Analysis

**Laboratory analysis** plays a key role in detecting specific types of cancer. The following are some of the laboratory tests that may be used to diagnose cancer:

**Pap smear/test.** Cytologic screening test developed by Dr. George Papanicolaou and used to detect the presence of abnormal or cancerous cells from the cervix and vagina.

**Fecal occult blood test.** Test to detect occult (hidden) blood; can be used to check for cancer of the colon.

**Sputum cytology test.** Microscopic examination of sputum to detect abnormal or cancerous cells of the bronchi and lungs.

**Blood serum test.** Analysis of blood serum to obtain useful information about certain proteins synthesized by cancer; two such tests are the AFP and HCG.

**Alpha-fetoprotein (AFP) test.** Test to diagnose or monitor fetal distress or fetal abnormalities, diagnose some liver disorders, and screen for and monitor some cancers; higher than normal levels can indicate cancer in testes, ovaries, biliary tract, stomach, or pancreas.

**Human chorionic gonadotropin (HCG) test.** Test in which abnormal results can indicate ectopic pregnancy, miscarriage, testicular cancer, or trophoblastic tumor. It is used to monitor treatment in certain patients with cancer. During therapy, a falling HCG level indicates that the cancer is responding to treatment; rising levels can indicate that the cancer is not responding to therapy. Increased levels after treatment can indicate a recurrence of disease.

**Bone marrow study.** A test to detect abnormal bone marrow cells, which can indicate leukemia.

**Urine assay test.** Test providing useful information about catecholamines, which can indicate pheochromocytoma of the adrenal medulla.

**Cancer antigen 125 (CA-125).** Test that measures the amount of this protein in the blood. CA-125 is found on the surface of many ovarian cancer cells. It also can be found in other cancers and in small amounts in normal tissue.

**Carcinoembryonic antigen (CEA).** Test that measures the amount of a protein that can appear in the blood of some people who have certain kinds of cancers, especially large intestine (colon and rectal) cancer; also can be present in people with cancer of the pancreas, breast, ovary, or lung.

**Human epidermal growth factor receptor-2 (HER-2/neu).** Tests can be performed on breast cancer cells to determine the presence of HER-2/neu protein, a genetic protein that is in part responsible for how certain cancer cells grow, divide, and repair themselves. This information is useful when making treatment decisions.

**Prostate-specific antigen (PSA).** Blood test that measures the amount of PSA, a substance produced by the prostate gland; should be offered every year to men 50 years of age or older. The American Cancer Society recommends that screening tests start at the age of 40 years for African American men or men with a family history of prostate cancer.

## Biopsy

The surgical removal of a small piece of tissue for microscopic examination is known as biopsy (Bx). It is the method of providing the proof of cancer in the diagnosis of the disease. The following different types of biopsy can be used for tissue removal:

**Excisional biopsy.** Surgical removal of a piece of tissue from the suspected body site.

**Incisional biopsy.** Surgical incision to remove a section or wedge of tissue from the suspected body site.

**Needle biopsy.** Puncture of a tumor for the removal of a core of tissue through the lumen of a needle.

**Fine needle aspiration (FNA).** Form of breast biopsy in which a small needle is used to withdraw a sample of cells from the breast lump. If the lump is a cyst, removal of the fluid will cause the cyst to collapse. If the lump is solid, cells can be smeared onto slides for examination.

**Stereotactic biopsy.** Alternative to traditional surgical biopsy; the procedure, which uses a mammogram-guided needle, is performed by a radiologist and assisted by mammography technologists. It is most helpful when mammography shows a mass, a cluster of microcalcifications (tiny calcium deposits that are closely grouped together), or an area of abnormal tissue change but no lump can be felt on careful breast examination.

**Core biopsy.** Large-bore needle removal of a generous sample of breast tissue and a vacuum-assisted needle biopsy device (VAD), which uses vacuum suction to obtain a tissue sample.

**Cone biopsy.** Removal of a cone of tissue from the uterine cervix.

**Sternal biopsy.** Removal of a piece of bone marrow from the sternum.

**Endoscopic biopsy.** Removal of a piece of tissue through an endoscope.

**Punch biopsy.** Removal of a plug of tissue (epidermis, dermis, and subcutaneous tissue) from the skin.

**Sentinel node biopsy.** Process by which a physician pinpoints the first lymph node into which a tumor drains (the sentinel node) and removes only the nodes most likely to contain cancer cells. To locate the sentinel node, the physician injects a radioactive tracer in the area around the tumor. The tracer travels the same path to the lymph nodes that cancer cells would take, making it possible for the surgeon to determine the one or two nodes most likely to test positive. The surgeon then removes the nodes most likely to be cancerous.

## Diagnostic Radiology

Encompassing a wide range of tests and procedures, **diagnostic radiology** can reveal tumors that were not detected by other diagnostic procedures (see Chapter 21, Radiology and Nuclear Medicine, on page 707).

## TREATMENT

The treatment of cancer can employ any one or a combination of the following methods: surgery, chemotherapy, radiation therapy, immunotherapy, or photodynamic therapy (PDT). The treatment of choice depends on the type of cancer, its location, its invasive process, and the patient's state of health. The ultimate goal of treatment is to kill every cancer cell. Therefore, the need to treat tumors at an early stage is critical. For example, a 1-cm breast tumor can contain 1 billion cancer cells before it is detected. A drug killing 99% of these cells would be considered an excellent drug, but 10 million cancer cells would still remain in the body. The relationship between cell kill and chemotherapy is shown in Figure 20–3 ▼.

## Surgery

**Surgery** can be the treatment of choice when the tumor is small and localized and the surrounding tissue is accessible for removal. The aim of surgery is to remove all cancerous tissue plus some of the surrounding normal tissue. Surgery is also used to alleviate some of the complications of cancer, such as the obstruction of an area caused by the enlargement of a tumor.

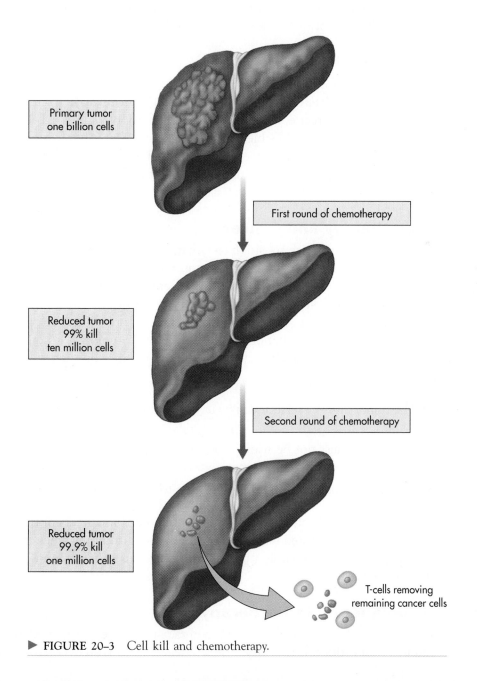

Primary tumor
one billion cells

First round of chemotherapy

Reduced tumor
99% kill
ten million cells

Second round of chemotherapy

Reduced tumor
99.9% kill
one million cells

T-cells removing
remaining cancer cells

▶ **FIGURE 20–3**   Cell kill and chemotherapy.

## Chemotherapy

**Chemotherapy** (chemo) can be the treatment of choice when the cancer is disseminated (wide spread) and cannot be surgically removed. It is also used when a tumor fails to respond to radiation therapy. Antineoplastic drugs injure individual cells, interfere with their vital functions, and kill or destroy malignant cells. In rendering cancerous cells harmless, certain normal cells could also be destroyed. The normal cells with the greatest sensitivity to destruction are the hematopoietic cells, epithelial cells, and the hair follicles. The plan of treatment for patients undergoing chemotherapy is individualized. The aim of chemotherapy is to put the patient in remission so that life can continue without **exacerbation** of symptoms.

Combination chemotherapy (the combination of certain antineoplastic agents) has proven to be effective in treating acute leukemia; Hodgkin's disease; non-Hodgkin's lymphoma; carcinoma of the breast, testis, and ovary; childhood neuroblastoma; Wilms' tumor; and osteogenic sarcoma. The physician who prescribes combination chemotherapy weighs the anticipated benefits against the possible additive toxic effects of the drugs. Examples include TPE—Taxol (paclitaxel), Platinol (cisplatin), and VePesid (etoposide).

## Radiation Therapy

The treatment of disease by the use of ionizing radiation is called **radiotherapy, x-ray therapy, cobalt treatment,** or simply **radiation therapy.** In all cases, this treatment seeks to deliver a precise, calculated dose of radiation to diseased tissue, such as a tumor, while causing the least possible damage to surrounding normal tissue. **Radiation** can be defined as the process whereby energy is beamed from its source through space and matter to a selected target area. See Figure 20–6 on page 685. Substances that emit radiation are said to be *radioactive*.

## Radiotherapy and Cancer

Malignant cells are more sensitive to radiation than are normal cells. They seem less able to repair themselves; therefore, radiation is frequently used treating patients with cancer as either a *curative* or a *palliative* mode of therapy. Certain types of cancer cells can be destroyed by radiation therapy, thus preventing the unrestrained growth of such tumors. In other cancers, radiation has only a palliative effect, preventing cell growth, reducing pain, pressure, and bleeding but not providing complete tumor destruction. Important factors that must be considered when determining the use of radiotherapy for the cancer patient include the following:

- The tumor must be surrounded by normal tissue that can tolerate the radiation and then repair itself.
- The tumor must not be widely spread. If the tumor has metastasized, radiation can be used as a palliative form of treatment.
- The tumor must be moderately sensitive to radiation (a radiosensitive tumor).

Radiotherapy is often the treatment of choice for cancers of the skin, uterus, cervix, or larynx or those located within the oral cavity. With other types of cancer, radiotherapy is frequently used in combination with other forms of treatment, including surgery and chemotherapy.

## Techniques of Radiotherapy

The two methods for the administration of radiation are **external radiation therapy** (ERT) and **internal radiation therapy** (IRT). The following is an overview of these two methods.

### External Radiation Therapy

With the **ERT** method, the patient receives calculated doses of radiation from a machine located at some distance from the site of the tumor. The patient is carefully prepared for treatment by a radiation therapist, sometimes assisted by the **dosimetrist** or a radiation physicist. The precise size and location of the tumor are determined, and the **port,** or point of entry for the radiation, is marked using a dye or tattoo. In formulating the treatment plan, a computer is used to calculate the radiation dosage needed to effect maximal destruction of malignant cells and minimal damage to surrounding normal tissue. Special lead blockers or shields can be constructed by a radiation physicist to protect surrounding normal tissue from the harmful effects of radiation.

### Internal Radiation Therapy

The **IRT** method of treatment can have two forms of administration known as **sealed** and **unsealed radiation therapy.** Sealed radiation therapy involves the implantation of sealed containers of radioactive material near the tumor site within the body. Unsealed radiation therapy involves the introduction of a liquid containing a radioactive substance into the patient through the mouth, via the bloodstream, or by instillation into a body cavity.

**Sealed Radiation Therapy.** Radioactive material such as *radium, cesium-137, cobalt-60,* and *iridium-192* is sealed in small gold containers called *seeds* or within molds, plaques, needles, or other devices designed to hold the radioactive substance near the malignancy. In some cases, the radiation source is implanted within the diseased tissue. In other cases, special devices or applicators have been designed to hold the implant in position for the desired period of treatment.

**Unsealed Radiation Therapy.** *Radioactive iodine-131, radioactive phosphorus-32,* and *radioactive gold-198* are some of the substances used in the unsealed form of internal radiation therapy. *Phosphorus-32* may be intravenously administered for use in the treatment of leukemia or lymphoma. *Gold-198* and/or *phosphorus-32* is placed in colloidal suspension and instilled in a body cavity for the palliative treatment of certain malignancies. *Iodine-131* can be orally administered, usually in conjunction with a thyroidectomy.

## Side Effects of Radiation

Because radiotherapy unavoidably affects normal tissue while destroying malignant cells, patients usually experience some unpleasant **side effects.** The degree of severity associated with the side effects depends on the individual, the cancer, its location, and the amount of radiation. The following are some side effects that can occur as a result of radiation therapy: anorexia, nausea, vomiting, diarrhea, malaise, mild erythema, edema, ulcers, alopecia, taste blindness, stomatitis, mucositis, and xerostomia.

## Immunotherapy

**Immunotherapy** is the treatment of disease by stimulation of the body's immune system. It may be used as an adjuvant to other types of treatment. There are three types of immunotherapy: **active specific** (the use of various agents to produce a specific host–immune response), **passive** (the use of serum or other products from an immunocompetent individual that are given to an immunodeficient individual to produce an immune response), and **adoptive** (the process of transferring a form of specific immune response from a donor to a recipient).

### Photodynamic Therapy

**Photodynamic therapy** (PDT), a type of laser therapy, involves the use of a special chemical that is injected into the bloodstream and absorbed by cells all over the body. The chemical rapidly leaves normal cells but remains in cancer cells for a longer time. A *laser* light aimed at the cancer activates the chemical, which then kills the cancer cells that have absorbed it. Photodynamic therapy can be used to reduce symptoms of lung cancer, for example, to control bleeding or to relieve breathing problems due to blocked airways when the cancer cannot be removed through surgery. Photodynamic therapy can also be used to treat very small tumors in patients for whom the usual treatments for lung cancer are not appropriate.

## PREVENTION OF CANCER

### Stop Smoking or Don't Start

**Smoking** is the most preventable cause of death in humans. In the United States, tobacco use is responsible for more than 1 in 6 deaths. Cigarette smoking is responsible for 90% of lung cancer among men and 79% among women. Smoking accounts for about 30% of all cancer deaths According to the World Health Organization (WHO), approximately 2.5 million people each year worldwide die as a result of smoking.

### Stop Using Smokeless Tobacco or Don't Start

There has been a resurgence in the use of all forms of smokeless tobacco. The greatest cause of concern centers on the increased use of *dipping snuff*. In this practice, tobacco that has been processed into a coarse, moist powder is placed between the cheek and gum, and nicotine, along with a number of carcinogens, is absorbed through the oral mucosa. Use of chewing tobacco or snuff increases the risk of cancer of the mouth, larynx, pharynx, and esophagus.

### Avoid Direct Sunlight and/or Use Protective Sunscreen

Epidemiologic evidence shows that sun exposure is a major factor in the development of melanoma and that incidence increases for those living near the equator. Almost all of the more than 700,000 cases of basal and squamous cell skin cancer diagnosed each year in the United States are sun related (ultraviolet radiation).

### Avoid Ionizing Radiation and/or Limit Exposure

Excessive exposure to ionizing radiation can increase cancer risk. Excessive radon exposure in homes, schools, and the workplace can increase the risk of lung cancer, especially in cigarette smokers.

#### Proper Nutrition and Diet

More and more evidence shows that **proper nutrition** and **diet** can help prevent disease. The risk of cancer can be reduced by the following:

- **Maintaining desirable weight.** Individuals 40% or more overweight increase their risk of colon, breast, prostate, gallbladder, ovary, and uterine cancer.
- **Eat a variety of vegetables and fruits each day.** The National Cancer Institute (NCI) suggests eating at least 5 servings of fruits and vegetables each day. Studies have shown

that daily consumption of vegetables and fruits can decrease the risk of lung, prostate, esophagus, colorectal, and stomach cancers.

- **Eat more foods that are high in fiber.** These include whole grains, breads, vegetables, and fruits. High-fiber diets may reduce the risk of colon cancer.
- **Cut down on total fat intake.** It is recommended that only 30% or less of a person's daily intake be from fat. A high-fat diet can contribute to breast, colon, and prostate cancer.
- **Limit the consumption of alcohol to a minimum.**
- **Limit the consumption of salt-cured, smoked, and nitrite-cured foods.** Areas of the world where salt-cured and smoked foods are eaten frequently have a higher incidence of cancer of the esophagus and stomach.

## Avoid Occupational Hazards

Exposure to several different **industrial agents** (nickel, chromate, asbestos, vinyl chloride, etc.) increases risk of various cancers. Risk of lung cancer from **asbestos** is greatly increased when combined with cigarette smoking.

# LIFE SPAN CONSIDERATIONS

### ■ THE CHILD

When a child is diagnosed with cancer, the issue of how much to tell the child about the cancer arises. The impact of a diagnosis of cancer can be very distressing, not only to the parents and other family members but also to the child. How much information and the best way to relate information on cancer depends on the child's age and level of understanding. Being gentle, open, and honest is best.

Children up to 2 years of age do not understand cancer, but they worry about being away from their parents. Children between 2 and 7 can link events to themselves and think that their cancers are caused by their misbehavior. Children 7 to 12 years of age are starting to understand links between things and events and are less likely to think that cancer is caused by anything they did. Children over 12 years old can often understand complicated relationships between events. The following are suggestions for talking to children about cancer or other serious illnesses.

- Communicate at the level of the child's understanding.
- Do not overload the child with too much information at one time.
- Tell the child about his or her disease soon after the diagnosis. The child usually knows that something is wrong and can imagine worse things than the truth.
- Encourage the child to ask questions, and answer the questions openly and honestly.
- Plan ahead how to answer questions about what the child can expect over the course of the illness, treatments, and outcome.
- As long as possible, keep the child involved in daily living and helping activities. These are good times to talk about the child's illness and to explain the treatment program. When the time is right, explain about hair loss, medicines, radiation therapy, and surgery.
- Give the child lots of love with hugs and kisses.

- Tape-record some favorite stories that can be played while the child is in the hospital for surgery or treatment. Have siblings participate in this project.

- Keep household routines as normal as possible; this provides stability to all family members.

## ■ THE OLDER ADULT

More than 60% of cancers in the United States occur in people over the age of 65. It is estimated that by the year 2050, 79 million people will be older than 65. Cancers of the skin, breast, bladder, colon, rectum, lung, pancreas, prostate, and stomach are the most common cancers in people over 65.

Older adults with cancer frequently have distinctive medical, emotional, physical, and financial issues. It is important for the older adult to be fully informed about his or her diagnosis, treatment regimen, and follow-up care. There may be financial limitations because older adults are more likely to have limited resources, which can cause them to refuse procedures or treatment due to cost. Other considerations for the older adult with cancer follow:

- Diagnosis and treatment can be more difficult because of multiple health conditions, such as heart disease, hypertension, arthritis, and diabetes.

- Anxiety and depression should be anticipated and treated.

- Modifications in lifestyle can be challenging to accomplish.

- Getting adequate nutrition can be difficult, especially for those living alone.

- Finding a responsible caregiver can be difficult and cause anxiety.

- Loss of personal independence can trigger depression or despair.

- Arranging transportation to appointments and treatments can be difficult.

Planning for additional needs after surgery, chemotherapy, and discharge from a hospital should include information on supportive services, such as home health aides, visiting nurses, physical therapy, social work, support groups, and community resource referrals.

# BUILDING YOUR MEDICAL VOCABULARY

This section provides the foundation for learning medical terminology. Review the following alphabetized word. Note how common prefixes and suffixes are repeatedly applied to word roots and combining forms to create different meanings.

| | |
|---|---|
| **P** | Prefix |
| **R** | Root |
| **CF** | Combining form |
| **S** | Suffix |

| | |
|---|---|
| Pink words | Terms not built from word parts. |
| ✳ | Indicates words covered in the Pathology Spotlights section. |
| 💿 | Check the CD-ROM for more information. |

| MEDICAL WORD | WORD PARTS (WHEN APPLICABLE) | | | DEFINITION |
|---|---|---|---|---|
| | **Part** | **Type** | **Meaning** | |
| **adenocarcinoma (Adeno-CA)** (ăd″ ĕ-nō-kăr″ sĭn-ō′ mă) | aden/o<br>carcin<br>-oma | CF<br>R<br>S | gland<br>cancer<br>tumor | Malignant tumor arising in a glandular organ |
| **adjuvant therapy** (ăd′ jū-vănt thĕr′ ă-pē) | | | | Treatment given following the primary treatment to enhance the effectiveness of the primary treatment. In breast cancer, adjuvant therapy includes chemotherapy, radiation therapy, or hormone therapy. |
| **anaplasia** (ăn″ ă-plā′ zĭ-ă) | ana-<br><br><br>-plasia | P<br><br><br>S | up, apart, backward<br><br>formation | Characteristic of most cancerous cells in which there is a loss of differentiation and an irreversible alteration in adult cells toward more embryonic cell types |
| **astrocytoma** (ăs″ trō-sī-tō′ mă) | astro-<br>cyt<br>-oma | P<br>R<br>S | star-shaped<br>cell<br>tumor | Tumor composed of star-shaped neuroglial cells |
| **betatron** (bā′ tă-trŏn) | | | | Megavoltage machine used in administering external radiation therapy |
| **brachytherapy** (brăk″ ĭ thĕr′ ă-pē) | brachy-<br>-therapy | P<br>S | short<br>treatment | Radiation therapy in which the radioactive substance is inserted into a body cavity or organ. The source of radiation is located a short distance from the body area being treated. |
| **Burkitt's lymphoma** (bŭrk′ ĭtz lĭm-fō′ mă) | | | | Malignant tumor, most commonly found in Africa, that affects children; the characteristic symptom is a massive, swollen jaw |
| **carcinogen** (kăr″ sĭn′ ō-jĕn) | carcin/o<br>-gen | CF<br>S | cancer<br>formation, produce | Agent or substance that incites or produces cancer |
| **carcinoid** (kăr′ sī-nōīd) | carcin<br>-oid | R<br>S | cancer<br>resemble | Tumor derived from the argentaffin cells in the intestinal tract, bile duct, pancreas, bronchus, or ovary |

| MEDICAL WORD | WORD PARTS (WHEN APPLICABLE) | | | DEFINITION |
|---|---|---|---|---|
| | Part | Type | Meaning | |
| **carcinoma** (kăr″ sĭ-nō′ mă) | carcin -oma | R S | cancer tumor | Malignant tumor arising in epithelial tissue. See Figure 20–4 ▼. |
| **chondrosarcoma** (kŏn″ drō-săr-kō′ mă) | chondr/o sarc -oma | CF R S | cartilage flesh tumor | Cancerous tumor derived from cartilage cells |
| **choriocarcinoma** (kō″ rĭ-ō-kăr″ sĭ-nō′ mă) | chori/o carcin -oma | CF R S | chorion cancer tumor | Cancerous tumor of the uterus or at the site of an ectopic pregnancy |
| **cyclotron** (sī′ klō-trŏn) | | | | Megavoltage machine used in administering external radiation therapy |
| **dedifferentiation** (dē-dĭf″ ĕr-ĕn′ shē-ā′ shŭn) | | | | Process by which normal cells lose their specialization (differentiation) and become malignant |
| **deoxyribonucleic acid (DNA)** (dē-ŏk″ sĭ-ri″ bō- nū-klē′ ĭk ăs′ ĭd) | | | | Complex protein of high molecular weight found in the nucleus of every cell; controls all of the cell's activities and the genetic material necessary for the organism's heredity |
| **differentiation** (dĭf″ ĕr-ĕn″ shē-ā″ shŭn) | | | | Process by which normal cells have a distinct appearance and specialized function |
| **ductal carcinoma in situ (DCIS)** (dŭk-tăl kăr′ sĭ-nō′ mă ĭn sī′ too) | duct -al carcin -oma in- situ | R S R S P R | to lead pertaining to cancer tumor in place | Abnormal cells that involve only the lining of a duct and have not spread outside the duct to other tissues in the breast; also called *intraductal carcinoma*. ⭐ See Pathology Spotlight: Breast Cancer on page 690. |
| **encapsulated** (ĕn-kăp″ sū-lā′ tĕd) | en- capsul -ate(d) | P R S | in a little box use, action | Enclosed within a site, sheath, or capsule |

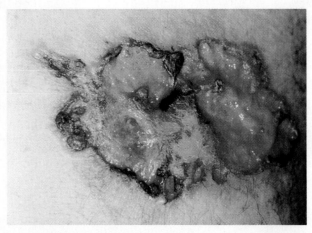

▶ **FIGURE 20–4**   Basal cell carcinoma. (Courtesy of Jason L. Smith, MD)

| MEDICAL WORD | WORD PARTS (WHEN APPLICABLE) | | | DEFINITION |
|---|---|---|---|---|
| | Part | Type | Meaning | |
| **Ewing's sarcoma**<br>(ū' ingz săr-kō' mă) | | | | Primary bone cancer occurring in the pelvic area or in one of the long bones; occurs mostly in children and adolescents |
| **exacerbation**<br>(ĕks-ăs" ĕr-bā' shŭn) | | | | Process of increasing the severity of symptoms; a time when the symptoms of a disease are most prevalent |
| **external radiation**<br>ĕk-stur' năl rā-dĭ-ā' shŭn) | | | | Process of administering radiation to the patient via a radiation machine located outside the body |
| **fibrosarcoma**<br>(fī" brō-săr-kō' mă) | fibr/o<br>sarc<br>-oma | CF<br>R<br>S | fiber<br>flesh<br>tumor | Cancerous tumor arising in collagen-producing fibroblasts |
| **fungating**<br>(fŭn' gāt-ĭng) | | | | Process of growing rapidly, like a fungus |
| **glioblastoma**<br>(glī' ō-blăs-tō' mă) | gli/o<br>-blast<br>-oma | CF<br>S<br>S | glue<br>immature cell<br>tumor | Cancerous tumor of the brain, usually of the cerebral hemispheres |
| **glioma**<br>(gli-ō' mă) | gli<br>-oma | R<br>S | glue<br>tumor | Cancerous tumor of the brain. |
| **hemangiosarcoma**<br>(hē-măn" jĭ-ō-săr-kō' mă) | hem<br>angi/o<br>sarc<br>-oma | R<br>CF<br>R<br>S | blood<br>vessel<br>flesh<br>tumor | Cancerous tumor originating in blood vessels |
| **Hodgkin's disease (HD)**<br>(hŏj' kĭns dĭ-zēz") | | | | Form of lymphoma that occurs in young adults. See Figure 20–5 ▶. ✳ See Pathology Spotlight: Hodgkin's Disease on page 692. |
| **human T-cell leukemia-lymphoma virus (HTLV)**<br>(hū' măn tē' sĕl lū-kē' mĭ-ă lĭm-fō' mă vī' rŭs) | | | | First virus known to cause cancer in humans |
| **hyperplasia**<br>(hī" pĕr-plā' zĭ-ă) | hyper-<br>-plasia | P<br>S | excessive<br>formation | Excessive formation and growth of normal cells |
| **immunosuppression**<br>(ĭm" ū-nō-sŭ-prĕsh' ŭn) | immun/o<br>suppress<br>-ion | CF<br>R<br>S | safe, immunity<br>suppress<br>process | Process of preventing formation of the immune response |
| **immunotherapy**<br>(ĭm" mū-nō-thĕr' ă pē) | immun/o<br>-therapy | CF<br>S | safe, immunity<br>treatment | Treatment of disease by active, passive, or adoptive immunity |
| **infiltrative**<br>(ĭn' fĭl-trā" tĭve) | in-<br>filtrat<br>-ive | P<br>R<br>S | into<br>to strain through<br>nature of | Pertaining to the process of extending or growing into normal tissue; invasive |

| MEDICAL WORD | WORD PARTS (WHEN APPLICABLE) | | | DEFINITION |
|---|---|---|---|---|
| | **Part** | **Type** | **Meaning** | |
| **in situ**<br>(ĭn sī′ too) | | | | Within a site; refers to tumor cells that remain at a site and have not invaded adjacent tissue |
| **interstitial**<br>(ĭn″ tĕr-stĭsh′ ăl) | | | | Pertaining to between spaces |
| **invasive** | | | | Pertaining to the spreading process of a malignant tumor into normal tissue |
| **Kaposi's sarcoma (KS)**<br>(kăp′ ō-sēz săr-kō′ mă) | | | | Malignant neoplasm that causes violaceous (purplish discoloration) vascular lesions and general lymphadenopathy; often seen in patients who have AIDS |
| **leiomyosarcoma**<br>(lī″ ō-mī″ ō-săr-kō′ mă) | lei/o<br>my/o<br>sarc<br>-oma | CF<br>CF<br>R<br>S | smooth<br>muscle<br>flesh<br>tumor | Cancerous tumor of smooth muscle tissue |
| **lesion**<br>(lē′ zhŭn) | | | | Wound; an injury, altered tissue, or a single infected patch of skin |
| **leukemia**<br>(lū-kē′ mĭ-ă) | leuk<br>-emia | R<br>S | white<br>blood condition | Disease of the blood characterized by overproduction of leukocytes; cancer of the blood-forming tissues. ✳ See Pathology Spotlight: Leukemia on page 693. |

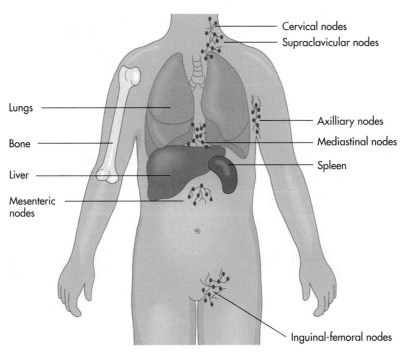

▶ **FIGURE 20–5**  Lymph nodes and organs affected in Hodgkin's disease in children.

| MEDICAL WORD | WORD PARTS (WHEN APPLICABLE) | | | DEFINITION |
|---|---|---|---|---|
| | **Part** | **Type** | **Meaning** | |
| **leukoplakia**<br>(lū" kō-plā' kĭ-ă) | leuk/o<br>-plakia | CF<br>S | white<br>plate | White, thickened patches formed on the mucous membranes of the cheeks, gums, or tongue that tend to become cancerous |
| **linear accelerator**<br>(lĭn' ē-ar ăk-sĕl' ĕr-ā" tŏr) | | | | Megavoltage machine used in administering external radiation therapy. See Figure 20–6 ▼. |
| **liposarcoma**<br>(lĭp" ō-săr-kō' mă) | lip/o<br>sarc<br>-oma | CF<br>R<br>S | fat<br>flesh<br>tumor | Cancerous tumor of fat cells |
| **lobular carcinoma in situ (LCIS)**<br>(lŏb' ū-lăr kăr' sĭ-nō' mă ĭn sī' too) | lobul<br>-ar<br>carcin<br>-oma<br>in-<br>situ | R<br>S<br>R<br>S<br>P<br>R | small lobe<br>pertaining to<br>cancer<br>tumor<br>in<br>place | Abnormal cells found in the lobules of the breast. This condition seldom becomes invasive cancer. However, having lobular carcinoma in situ increases the risk of developing cancer in either breast; also called *LCIS*. |
| **lymphangiosarcoma**<br>(lĭm-făn" jē-ō-săr-kō' mă) | lymph<br>angi/o<br>sarc<br>-oma | R<br>CF<br>R<br>S | lymph<br>vessel<br>flesh<br>tumor | Cancerous tumor of lymphatic vessels |
| **lymphoma**<br>(lĭm-fō' mă) | lymph<br>-oma | R<br>S | lymph<br>tumor | Cancerous tumor of the lymph nodes |
| **lymphosarcoma**<br>(lĭm" fō-săr-kō' mă) | lymph/o<br>sarc<br>-oma | CF<br>R<br>S | lymph<br>flesh<br>tumor | Cancerous disease of lymphatic tissue; also called *lymphoblastoma* |
| **malignant**<br>(mă-lĭg' nănt) | malign<br>-ant | R<br>S | bad kind<br>forming | Pertaining to a bad wandering; refers to the spreading process of cancer from one area of the body to another |

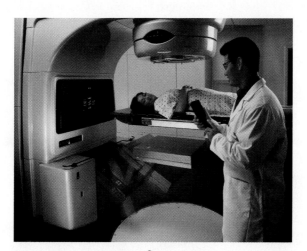

▶ **FIGURE 20–6**   Clinac® 23 EX linear accelerator. Used for the delivery of computer-driven intensity-modulated radiation therapy (IMRT), as well as conventional therapy in the treatment of cancer. (Courtesy of Varian Medical Systems of Palo Alto, CA. © 1999, Varian Medical Systems. All rights reserved.)

| MEDICAL WORD | WORD PARTS (WHEN APPLICABLE) | | | DEFINITION |
|---|---|---|---|---|
| | Part | Type | Meaning | |
| **medulloblastoma**<br>(mĕ-dŭl″ ō-blăs-tō′ mă) | medull/o<br>-blast<br>-oma | CF<br>S<br>S | marrow<br>immature cell<br>tumor | Cancerous tumor of the brain, the fourth ventricle, and the cerebellum |
| **melanoma**<br>(mĕl″ ă-nō′ mă) | melan<br>-oma | R<br>S | black<br>tumor | Cancerous black mole or tumor. See Figure 20–7 ▼. |
| **meningioma**<br>(mĕn-ĭn″ jĭ-ō′ mă) | mening/i<br><br>-oma | CF<br><br>S | meninges,<br>membrane<br>tumor | Cancerous tumor originating in the arachnoidal (meninges) membrane of the brain |
| **metastasis**<br>(mĕ-tăs′ tă-sis) | meta-<br>-stasis | P<br>S | beyond<br>control | Spreading process of cancer from a primary site to a secondary site See Figure 20–10 on page 691. Similarly, *invasive growth* is the spreading process of a malignant tumor into adjacent normal tissue. See Figure 20–8 ▶. |
| **mucositis**<br>(mū″ kō-sī′ tĭs) | mucos<br>-itis | R<br>S | mucus<br>inflammation | Inflammation of the oral mucosa caused by exposure to high-energy beams delivered by radiation therapy |
| **mutagen**<br>(mū′ tă-jĕn) | muta<br>-gen | R<br>S | to change<br>formation,<br>produce | Agent that causes a change in the genetic structure of an organism |
| **mutation**<br>(mū-tā′ shŭn) | mutat<br>-ion | R<br>S | to change<br>process | Process by which the genetic structure is changed |
| **mycotoxin**<br>(mī″ kō-tŏk′ sĭn) | myc/o<br>tox<br>-in | CF<br>R<br>S | fungus<br>poison<br>substance | Substance produced by fungus growing in food or animal feed that, if ingested, can cause cancer |
| **myeloma**<br>(mī″ ĕ-lō′ mă) | myel<br>-oma | R<br>S | bone marrow<br>tumor | Tumor arising in the hemopoietic portion of the bone marrow |
| **myosarcoma**<br>(mī″ ō-săr-kō′ mă) | my/o<br>sarc<br>-oma | CF<br>R<br>S | muscle<br>flesh<br>tumor | Cancerous tumor of muscle tissue |

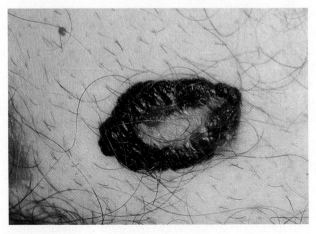

▶ **FIGURE 20–7** Melanoma. (Courtesy of Jason L. Smith, MD)

| MEDICAL WORD | WORD PARTS (WHEN APPLICABLE) | | | DEFINITION |
|---|---|---|---|---|
| | Part | Type | Meaning | |
| **neoplasm** (nē′ ō-plăzm) | neo- -plasm | P S | new a thing formed | New thing formed, such as an abnormal growth or tumor |
| **nephroblastoma** (něf″ rō-blăs-tō′ mă) | nephr/o -blast -oma | CF S S | kidney immature cell tumor | Cancerous tumor of the kidney; also called *Wilms' tumor;* most often found in children 2 to 3 years of age |
| **neuroblastoma** (nū″ rō-blăs-tō′ mă) | neur/o -blast -oma | CF S S | nerve immature cell tumor | Cancerous tumor composed chiefly of neuroblasts; can appear anywhere but usually in the abdomen as a swelling; most often diagnosed during the first year of life |
| **oligodendro-glioma** (ŏl″ ĭ-gō-děn″ drō-glī-ō′ mă) | oligo- dendr/o gli -oma | P CF R S | little tree glue tumor | Cancerous tumor composed chiefly of neuroglial cells and located in the cerebrum |
| **oncogenes** (ŏng″ kō-jēn z′) | onc/o -genes | CF S | tumor formation, produce | Cancer-causing genes; genes in a virus that can induce tumor formation |
| **oncogenic** (ŏng″ kō-jēn′ ĭk) | onc/o -genic | CF S | tumor formation, produce | Pertaining to the formation of tumors, especially cancerous ones |
| **osteogenic sarcoma** (ŏs″ tē-ō-jěn′ ĭk săr-kō′ mă) | oste/o -genic sarc -oma | CF S R S | bone formation, produce flesh tumor | Cancerous tumor composed of osseous tissue |

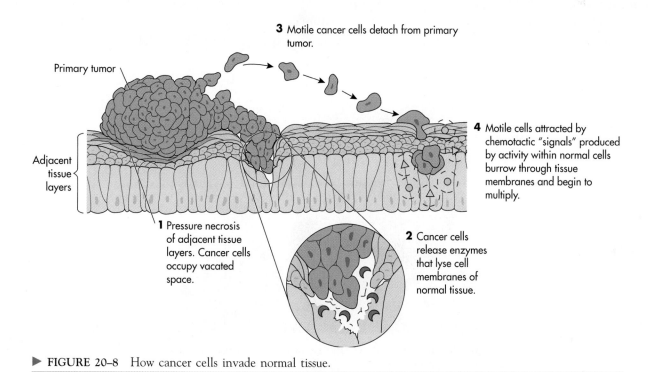

**3** Motile cancer cells detach from primary tumor.

Primary tumor

Adjacent tissue layers

**4** Motile cells attracted by chemotactic "signals" produced by activity within normal cells burrow through tissue membranes and begin to multiply.

**1** Pressure necrosis of adjacent tissue layers. Cancer cells occupy vacated space.

**2** Cancer cells release enzymes that lyse cell membranes of normal tissue.

▶ **FIGURE 20–8** How cancer cells invade normal tissue.

| MEDICAL WORD | WORD PARTS (WHEN APPLICABLE) | | | DEFINITION |
|---|---|---|---|---|
| | Part | Type | Meaning | |
| **Paget's disease** (păj′ ĕts dĭ-zēz′) | | | | Inflammatory bone disease that can precede the development of bone cancer; characteristics include softening and bowing of the long bones of the legs. Paget's disease of the nipple is also known as nipple cancer and is associated with carcinoma in deeper breast tissue. See Figure 20–9 ▼. |
| **palliative** (păl′ ĭ-ā-tĭv) | palliat -ive | R S | cloaked nature of | Pertaining to a form of treatment to relieve or alleviate symptoms without curing |
| **port** | | | | In radiation therapy, refers to the skin area of entry for the radiation |
| **precancerous** (prē-kăn′ sĕr-ŭs) | pre- cancer -ous | P R S | before crab, cancer pertaining to | Pertaining to the state of a growth or condition before the onset of cancer |
| **primary site** | | | | Original, initial, or principal site |
| **proliferation** (prō-lĭf″ ĕr-ā′ shŭn) | | | | Process of rapid production; growth by multiplying |
| **remission** (rē- mĭsh′ ŭn) | remiss -ion | R S | remit process | Process of lessening the severity of symptoms; time when symptoms of a disease are at rest |
| **reticulosarcoma** (rĕ-tĭk″ ū-lō-săr-kō′ mă) | reticul/o sarc -oma | CF R S | net flesh tumor | Cancerous tumor of the lymphatic system |
| **retinoblastoma** (rĕt″ ĭ-nō-blăs-tō′ mă) | retin/o -blast -oma | CF S S | retina immature cell tumor | Cancerous tumor of the retina. Although relatively rare, it accounts for 5% of childhood blindness. |

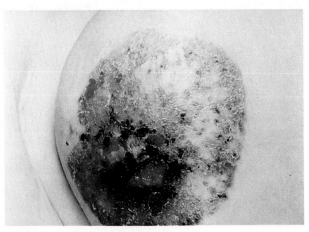

► **FIGURE 20–9**  Paget's disease of the breast. (Courtesy of Jason L. Smith, MD)

| MEDICAL WORD | WORD PARTS (WHEN APPLICABLE) | | | DEFINITION |
|---|---|---|---|---|
| | Part | Type | Meaning | |
| **rhabdomyo-sarcoma**<br>(răb″ dō-mī″ ō-săr-kō′ mă) | rhabd/o<br>my/o<br>sarc<br>-oma | CF<br>CF<br>R<br>S | rod<br>muscle<br>flesh<br>tumor | Cancerous tumor originating from the same embryonic cells that develop into striated muscles. It is the most common soft tissue sarcoma in children. |
| **ribonucleic acid (RNA)**<br>(rī″ bō-nū′ klē′ ĭk ăs′ ĭd) | | | | Nucleic acid found in all living cells; responsible for protein synthesis |
| **sarcoma**<br>(săr-kō′ mă) | sarc<br>-oma | R<br>S | flesh<br>tumor | Cancerous tumor arising in connective tissue |
| **secondary site**<br>(sĕk′ ăn-dĕr″ ē sīt) | | | | Second site usually derived from the primary site |
| **seminoma**<br>(sĕm″ ĭ-nō′ mă) | semin<br>-oma | R<br>S | seed<br>tumor | Cancerous tumor of the testis |
| **tamponade (cardiac)**<br>(tam′ pŏn-ād [kăr′ dē-ăk]) | | | | Pathologic condition of the heart in which there is accumulation of excess fluid in the pericardium; can be caused by advanced cancer of the lung or a tumor that has metastasized to the pericardium |
| **teletherapy**<br>(tĕl″ ĕ-thĕr′ ă-pē) | | | | Radiation therapy in which the radioactive substance is at a distance from the body area being treated |
| **teratoma**<br>(tĕr″ ă-tō′ mă) | terat<br>-oma | R<br>S | monster<br>tumor | Cancerous tumor of the ovary or testis; can contain embryonic tissues of hair, teeth, bone, or muscle |
| **thymoma**<br>(thī-mō′ mă) | thym<br>-oma | R<br>S | thymus<br>tumor | Tumor of the thymus gland |
| **trismus**<br>(trĭz′ mŭs) | trism<br>-us | R<br>S | grating<br>pertaining to | Pertaining to the inability to open the mouth fully; occurs in patients with oral cancer who undergo a combination of surgery and radiation therapy |
| **tumor**<br>(tū′ mor) | | | | Abnormal growth, swelling, or enlargement |
| **viral**<br>(vī′ răl) | vir<br>-al | R<br>S | virus (poison)<br>pertaining to | Pertaining to a virus, which means *poison* in Latin; minute organism that could be responsible for 50% of all diseases |
| **Wilms' tumor**<br>(vĭlmz tū′ mor) | | | | Cancerous tumor of the kidney occurring mainly in children |
| **xerostomia**<br>(zē″ rō-stō′ mē-ă) | xer/o<br>stom<br>-ia | CF<br>R<br>S | dry<br>mouth<br>condition | Condition of dryness of the mouth; oral change caused by radiation therapy or chemotherapy |

# ABBREVIATIONS

| ABBREVIATION | MEANING | ABBREVIATION | MEANING |
|---|---|---|---|
| ACS | American Cancer Society | HCC | hepatocellular carcinoma |
| Adeno-CA | adenocarcinoma | HD | Hodgkin's disease |
| AFP | alpha-fetoprotein | HER-2/neu | human epidermal growth factor receptor-2 |
| AIDS | acquired immunodeficiency syndrome | HTLV | human T-cell leukemia-lymphoma virus |
| ALL | acute lymphocytic leukemia | | |
| AML | acute myeloid leukemia | IRT | internal radiation therapy |
| BRCA | breast cancer gene | KS | Kaposi's sarcoma |
| BSE | breast self-examination | LCIS | lobular carcinoma in situ |
| Bx | biopsy | mL | milliliter |
| CA | cancer | NCI | National Cancer Institute |
| CA-125 | cancer antigen 125 | NHL | non-Hodgkin's lymphoma |
| CEA | carcinoembryonic antigen | PDT | photodynamic therapy |
| chemo | chemotherapy | PSA | prostate-specific antigen |
| CIS | carcinoma in situ | RNA | ribonucleic acid |
| CLL | chronic lymphocytic leukemia | St | stage (of disease) |
| CML | chronic myelocytic leukemia | TC | testicular cancer |
| CT | computed tomography | TNM | tumor, node, metastasis |
| DCIS | ductal carcinoma in situ | TSE | testicular self-examination |
| DNA | deoxyribonucleic acid | TPE | Taxol, Platinol, and VePesid |
| ERT | external radiation therapy | VAD | vacuum-assisted needle biopsy device |
| ETS | environmental tobacco smoke | | |
| FNA | fine needle aspiration | WHO | World Health Organization |

# PATHOLOGY SPOTLIGHTS

## ∗ Breast Cancer

In 2006, approximately 211,300 women and approximately 1,300 men were diagnosed with **breast cancer.** It kills about 39,800 women a year and is the leading cause of death in women between the ages of 32 and 52.

Early detection of breast cancer is extremely important. The 5-year survival rate for women with localized and properly treated breast cancer is 92%. If cancer is not detected and treated early, it will continue to grow, invade, and destroy adjacent tissue and spread into surrounding lymph nodes. See Figure 20–10 ▶. It can be carried by the lymph and/or blood to other areas of the body. Once this process, known as *metastasis*, has occurred, the cancer is usually advanced and/or disseminated and the 5-year survival rate is low.

Approximately 50% of malignant tumors of the breast appear in the upper, outer quadrant and extend into the armpit. Eighteen percent of breast cancers occur in the nipple area, 11% in the lower outer quadrant, and 6% in the inner quadrant.

Signs and symptoms of breast cancer are generally insidious and can include these:

- Unusual secretions from the nipple.
- Changes in the nipple's appearance.

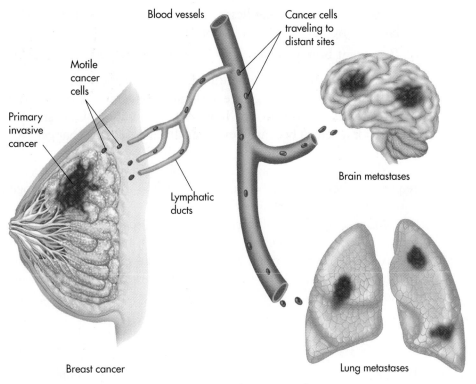

Blood vessels

Cancer cells traveling to distant sites

Motile cancer cells

Primary invasive cancer

Lymphatic ducts

Brain metastases

Breast cancer

Lung metastases

▶ **FIGURE 20–10**   Invasion and metastasis by cancer cells.

- Nontender, movable lump.
- Well-localized discomfort that may be described as burning, stinging, or aching sensation.
- Dimpling or *peau d'orange* (orange-peel appearance) may be present over the area of cancer of the breast.
- Asymmetry and an elevation of the affected breast.
- Nipple retraction.
- Pain in the later stages.

Stages of breast cancer, according to the American Cancer Society, indicate the size of a tumor and how far the cancer has spread within the breast, to nearby tissues, and to other organs. Specific treatment is most often determined by the following stages of the disease:

**Carcinoma in situ (CIS).**   Cancer is confined to the lobules (milk-producing glands) or ducts (passages connecting milk-producing glands to the nipple) and has not invaded nearby breast tissue; also referred to as *ductal carcinoma in situ (DCIS)*.

**Stage I.**   Tumor is smaller than or equal to 2 cm in diameter and axillary (underarm) lymph nodes test negative for cancer.

**Stage II.**   Tumor is between 2 and 5 cm in diameter with or without positive lymph nodes or is more than 5 cm without positive lymph nodes.

**Stage III.**   This stage is divided into substages known as IIIA and IIIB.

- **IIIA.**   Tumor is larger than 5 cm with positive movable lymph nodes or is any size with lymph nodes that adhere to one another or surrounding tissue.
- **IIIB.**   Tumor of any size has spread to the skin, chest wall, or internal mammary lymph nodes (located beneath the breast and inside the chest).

**Stage IV.** Tumor, regardless of size, has metastasized (spread) to distant sites such as bones, lungs, or lymph nodes not near the breast.

**Recurrent breast cancer.** The disease has returned despite initial treatment.

Two genes have been identified as breast cancer genes: BRCA-1 and BRCA-2 are genes that, when changed, place a woman at greater risk of developing breast cancer compared to women who do not have either mutation. One single genetic mishap is not enough for a cell to become cancerous. It takes several changes. Women who have inherited mutations within the BRCA-1 and BRCA-2 genes are at higher risk for breast cancer than those who do not have the mutations. However, for cancer to occur in these women requires further events. Internal factors, such as the hormone estrogen, and external factors can contribute to this chain of events.

More than 90% of all breast lumps are discovered by women themselves. The majority of these lumps are benign (noncancerous), but for those that are not, early detection and treatment are essential. A woman should examine her breasts every month (Breast Self-Examination [BSE]); see Figure 20–11 ▶). Check for appearance, size, shape, symmetry, tenderness, thickening, and texture changes. See Chapter 21, Chart Note Analysis, on page 735 for more information about breast cancer.

## ✱ Hodgkin's Disease

**Hodgkin's disease** (HD), sometimes called *Hodgkin's lymphoma*, is a cancer (lymphoma) that starts in lymphatic tissue. The two kinds of lymphoma are *Hodgkin's disease* (named after Dr. Thomas Hodgkin, who first recognized it in 1832) and *non-Hodgkin's lymphoma*.

Because lymphatic tissue is present in many parts of the body, Hodgkin's disease can start almost anywhere, but most often starts in lymph nodes in the upper part of the body. The most common sites are in the chest, neck, or under the arms. Hodgkin's disease enlarges the lymphatic tissue, which can then cause pressure on important structures. It can spread through the lymphatic vessels to other lymph nodes. Most Hodgkin's disease spreads to nearby lymph node sites in the body, not distant ones. It rarely gets into the blood vessels, but when it does, it can spread to almost any other site in the body, including the liver and lungs.

The cancer cells in Hodgkin's disease are called *Reed-Sternberg cells* after the two doctors who first described them in detail. Under a microscope, they look different from cells of non-Hodgkin's lymphomas and other cancers. Most scientists now believe that Reed-Sternberg cells are a type of malignant *B lymphocyte*. Normal B lymphocytes are the cells that make antibodies that help fight infections.

Before 1970, few people with diagnosed Hodgkin's disease recovered. Today, more than 80% of people who receive initial treatment experience a complete remission. Advances in diagnosis, staging, and treatment of Hodgkin's disease have helped to make this once uniformly fatal disease highly treatable with potential for full recovery.

**Non-Hodgkin's lymphoma** (NHL) is cancer that begins in the lymphatic system, usually in a B cell in a lymph node. The abnormal cell divides and makes copies of itself. The new cells divide again and again, making more and more abnormal (cancer) cells. The cancer cells can spread to nearly any other part of the body.

Symptoms of non-Hodgkin's lymphoma include swollen, painless lymph nodes in the neck, armpits, or groin; unexplained weight loss; fever; soaking night sweats; coughing, trouble breathing, or chest pain; weakness and tiredness that does not go away; and pain, swelling, or a feeling of fullness in the abdomen. Diagnosis is confirmed by either an *excisional biopsy* (entire lymph node is removed) or *incisional biopsy* (only part of a lymph node is removed). When lymphoma is found, the pathologist reports the type. The most common types are *diffuse large B-cell lymphoma* and *follicular lymphoma*. Lymphomas can also be grouped by how quickly they are likely to grow: indolent (low-grade) lymphomas grow

**WHY DO THE BREAST SELF-EXAM?**

There are many good reasons for doing a breast self-exam each month. One reason is that it is easy to do and the more you do it, the better you will get at it. When you get to know how your breasts normally feel, you will quickly be able to feel any change, and early detection is the key to successful treatment and cure.

REMEMBER: A breast self-exam could save your breast – and save your life. Most breast lumps are found by women themselves, but in fact, most lumps in the breast are not cancer. Be safe, be sure.

**WHEN TO DO BREAST SELF-EXAM**

The best time to do breast self-exam is right after your period, when breasts are not tender or swollen. If you do not have regular periods or sometimes skip a month, do it on the same day every month.

**NOW, HOW TO DO BREAST SELF-EXAM**

1. Lie down and put a pillow under your right shoulder. Place your right arm behind your head.

2. Use the finger pads of your three middle fingers on your left hand to feel for lumps or thickening. Your finger pads are the top third of each finger.

3. Press firmly enough to know how your breast feels. If you're not sure how hard to press, ask your health care provider. Or try to copy the way your health care provider uses the finger pads during a breast exam. Learn what your breast feels like most of the time. A firm ridge in the lower curve of each breast is normal.

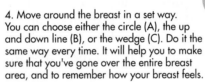

A    B    C

4. Move around the breast in a set way. You can choose either the circle (A), the up and down line (B), or the wedge (C). Do it the same way every time. It will help you to make sure that you've gone over the entire breast area, and to remember how your breast feels.

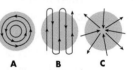

5. Now examine your left breast using your right hand finger pads.

6. If you find any changes, see your doctor right away.

**FOR ADDED SAFETY:**

You should also check your breasts while standing in front of a mirror right after you do your breast self-exam each month. See if there are any changes in the way your breasts look: dimpling of the skin, changes in the nipple, or redness or swelling.

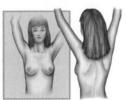

You might also want to do a breast self-exam while you're in the shower. Your soapy hands will glide over the wet skin, making it easy to check how your breasts feel.

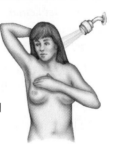

▶ FIGURE 20–11   Breast self-examination.

slowly; aggressive (intermediate-grade and high-grade) lymphomas grow and spread more quickly.

Non-Hodgkin's lymphoma is more common than Hodgkin's disease. Survival rates are good with early diagnosis.

## ∗ Leukemia

Leukemia is cancer that usually affects the white blood cells, which develop from stem cells in the bone marrow. Leukemia results when something goes wrong with the process of maturation from stem cell to white blood cell and a cancerous change occurs. The change often involves a rearrangement of pieces of chromosomes. Because the chromosomal rearrangements disturb the normal control of cell division, the affected cells multiply without restraint, becoming cancerous. They ultimately occupy the bone marrow, replacing the cells that produce normal blood cells. These leukemic (cancer) cells can also invade other organs, including the liver, spleen, lymph nodes, kidneys, and brain.

There are four major types of leukemia named for how quickly they progress and the type of white blood cell they affect. Acute leukemias progress rapidly; chronic leukemias progress slowly. Lymphocytic leukemias affect lymphocytes; myeloid (myelocytic) leukemias affect myelocytes.

**Acute lymphocytic leukemia** (ALL) is a life-threatening disease in which the cells that normally develop into lymphocytes become cancerous and rapidly replace normal cells in the bone marrow. About 3,970 new cases of ALL are diagnosed each year in the United States. It is the most common type of leukemia in children and young people under the age of 19. Children are most likely to develop the disease, but it can occur at any age. ALL has several names, including *acute lymphoid leukemia* and *acute lymphoblastic leukemia*.

**Acute myeloid leukemia** (AML) is a life-threatening disease in which myelocytes become cancerous and rapidly replace normal cells in the bone marrow. This type of leukemia affects people of all ages but mostly adults. Exposure to large doses of radiation and use of some cancer chemotherapy drugs increase the likelihood of developing AML, which also has several names, including *myelocytic, myelogenous, myeloblastic,* and *myelomonocytic leukemia*.

**Chronic lymphocytic leukemia** (CLL), also referred to as *chronic lymphoid leukemia,* strikes nearly 9,730 people in the United States yearly. CLL is characterized by a large number of cancerous mature lymphocytes (a type of white blood cell) and enlarged lymph nodes. More than three-fourths of the people who have this type of leukemia are over age 60; it affects men two to three times more often than women.

**Chronic myelocytic leukemia** (CML) is a disease in which a cell in the bone marrow becomes cancerous and produces a large number of abnormal granulocytes. This disease affects people of any age and of either sex but is uncommon in children under 10 years old. Chronic myelocytic leukemia is also referred to as *myeloid, myelogenous,* and *granulocytic leukemia*.

## ✳ Lung Cancer

Cancers that begin in the lungs are divided into two major types, **nonsmall cell lung cancer** and **small cell lung cancer**, depending on how the cells look under a microscope. Each type of lung cancer grows and spreads in different ways and is treated differently. There are three main types of nonsmall cell lung cancer. They are named for the type of cells in which the cancer develops: squamous cell carcinoma (also called *epidermoid carcinoma*), adenocarcinoma, and large cell carcinoma. Small cell lung cancer, sometimes called *oat cell cancer,* is less common than nonsmall cell lung cancer. This type of lung cancer grows more quickly and is more likely to spread to other organs in the body. See Figure 20–12 ▶ for the effects of lung cancer throughout the body.

Common signs and symptoms of lung cancer include the following:

- Cough that does not go away and gets worse over time.
- Constant chest pain.
- Coughing up blood.
- Shortness of breath, wheezing, or hoarseness.
- Repeated problems with pneumonia or bronchitis.
- Swelling of the neck and face.

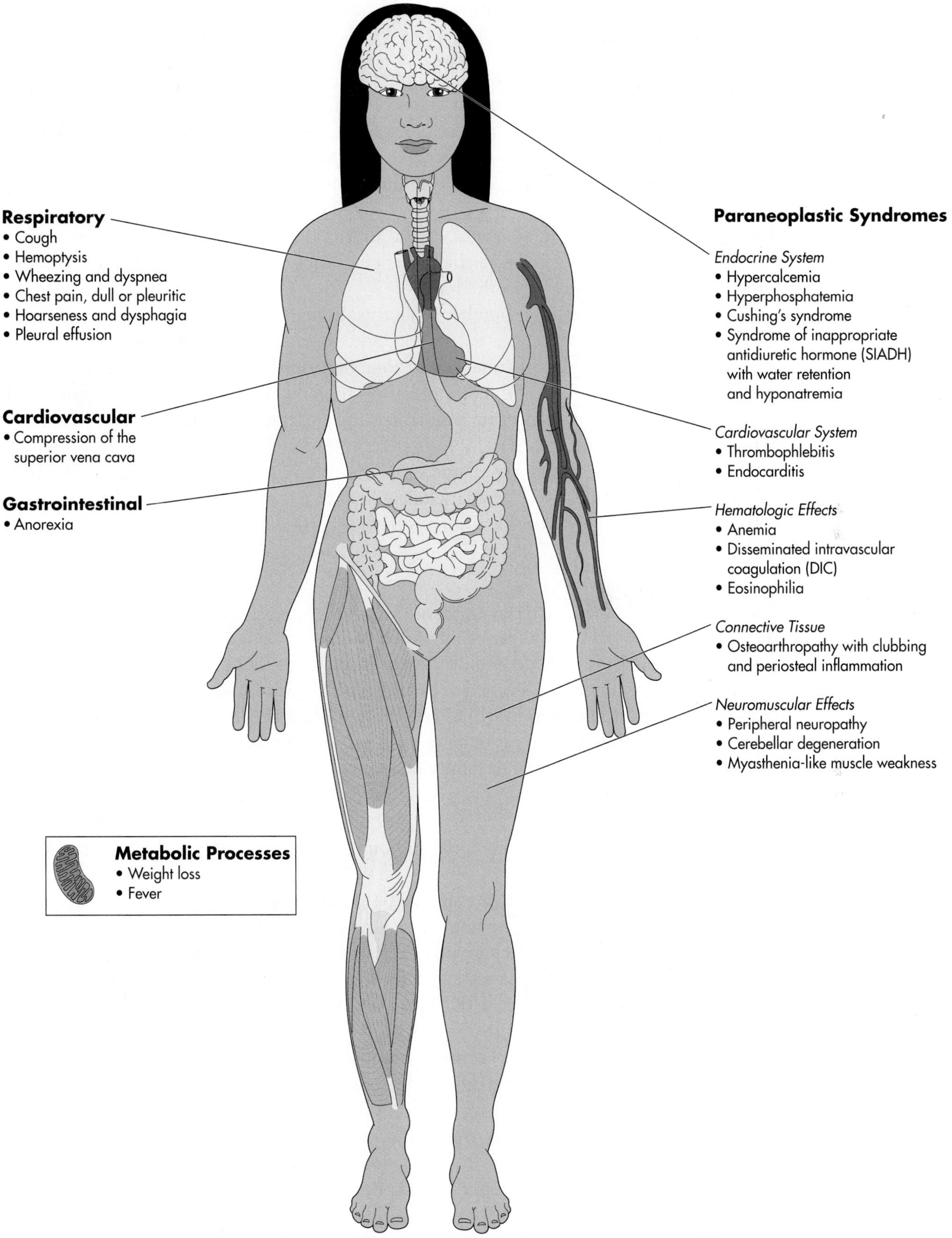

**Respiratory**
- Cough
- Hemoptysis
- Wheezing and dyspnea
- Chest pain, dull or pleuritic
- Hoarseness and dysphagia
- Pleural effusion

**Cardiovascular**
- Compression of the superior vena cava

**Gastrointestinal**
- Anorexia

**Metabolic Processes**
- Weight loss
- Fever

**Paraneoplastic Syndromes**

*Endocrine System*
- Hypercalcemia
- Hyperphosphatemia
- Cushing's syndrome
- Syndrome of inappropriate antidiuretic hormone (SIADH) with water retention and hyponatremia

*Cardiovascular System*
- Thrombophlebitis
- Endocarditis

*Hematologic Effects*
- Anemia
- Disseminated intravascular coagulation (DIC)
- Eosinophilia

*Connective Tissue*
- Osteoarthropathy with clubbing and periosteal inflammation

*Neuromuscular Effects*
- Peripheral neuropathy
- Cerebellar degeneration
- Myasthenia-like muscle weakness

▶ **FIGURE 20–12**   Multisystem effects of lung cancer.

- Loss of appetite or weight loss.
- Fatigue.

*Note:* These symptoms can be caused by lung cancer or by other conditions. It is important to see a physician if any of these symptoms persist.

To diagnose lung cancer, the doctor evaluates a person's medical history, smoking history, exposure to environmental and occupational substances, and family history of cancer. The doctor also performs a physical exam and can order a chest x-ray and other tests. If lung cancer is suspected, sputum cytology (the microscopic examination of cells obtained from a deep-cough sample of mucus in the lungs) is a simple test that can be useful in detecting lung cancer. To confirm the presence of lung cancer, the doctor must perform a biopsy and examine tissue from the lung.

Treatment depends on a number of factors, including the type of lung cancer (nonsmall or small cell lung cancer), size, location, and extent of the tumor and the patients general health. Many different treatments and combinations of treatments can be used for lung cancer, such as surgery, chemotherapy, radiation therapy, or photodynamic therapy (PDT).

The best way to prevent lung cancer is to quit (or never start) smoking. Researchers have discovered several causes of lung cancer; most are related to the use of tobacco, such as smoking cigarettes, cigars, pipes, and exposure to environmental tobacco smoke (ETS) or secondhand smoke. Other causes include exposure to radon, asbestos, and pollution. See Chapter 21, Life Span Considerations, on page 716 for more information about lung cancer.

## ✷ Testicular Cancer

**Testicular cancer** (TC) is a disease in which malignant cells form in the tissues of one or both testicles. It is the most common cancer in men age 20 to 35. In a given year, about 7,500 American men are diagnosed with this type of cancer. For unknown reasons, TC is about 4 times more common in white men than in black men. Some risk factors associated with TC include having had an undescended testicle, having had abnormal development of the testicles, and a personal or family history of testicular cancer.

Most testicular tumors are discovered by patients themselves, either by accident or while performing a testicular self-examination (TSE). See Figure 20–13 ▶. It is most important that TC be diagnosed early, so young men should be taught how to examine their testicles.

The most common presenting sign of testicular cancer is an enlarged, painless lump or swelling in either testicle. The lump typically is pea sized but sometimes it can be as big as a marble or even an egg. Occasionally there is pain. Besides lumps, if a man notices any other abnormality—an enlarged testicle, a feeling of heaviness or sudden collection of fluid in the scrotum, or a dull ache in the lower abdomen or groin—he should seek medical attention immediately. The origin and nature of scrotal masses must be determined as soon as possible because most testicular masses are malignant. Prognosis depends on the histology and extent of the tumor. With early detection, the survival rates for testicular cancer are approximately 95% at 5 years for seminomas and nonseminomas localized to the testis.

Nearly all testicular tumors stem from germ cells, the special sperm-forming cells within the testicles. These tumors fall into one of two types, seminomas or nonseminomas. Other forms of TC, such as sarcomas or lymphomas, are extremely rare.

Testicular cancer is diagnosed by a medical history and physical examination, ultrasound, serum tumor marker test, and a radical inguinal orchidectomy including a tissue biopsy. Imaging tests such as chest x-ray, computed tomography, magnetic resonance imaging, lymphangiogram, and positron emission tomography are often utilized to assess the spread of the disease and the staging of the cancer. Staging allows the doctor to plan the most appropriate treatment for each patient. Stages of TC are as follows:

**Stage I.** Cancer confined to the testicle.

**Stage II.** Disease spread to retroperitoneal lymph nodes, located in the rear of the body below the diaphragm.

**Stage III.** Cancer spread beyond the lymph nodes to remote sites in the body, such as the lungs and/or liver.

**Recurrent.** Recurrent disease means that the cancer has come back after it has been treated. It may come back in the same place or in another part of the body.

No one treatment works for all testicular cancers. Seminomas and nonseminomas differ in their tendency to spread, spread patterns, and response to radiation therapy. Thus, they often require different treatment strategies, which doctors choose based on the type of tumor and the stage of disease.

Because they are slow growing and tend to stay localized, seminomas generally are diagnosed in Stage I or II. Treatment could be a combination of testicle removal, radiation, or chemotherapy. Stage III seminomas are usually treated with a combination of chemotherapy drugs. Because certain treatments can cause infertility, the patient who wishes to have children should consider sperm banking before beginning treatment.

For more information on testicular cancer, visit the Lance Armstrong Foundation Web site at www.livestrong.org.

**Testicular Self-Examination**

- Examine testicles while taking a warm shower or bath, or just after if using a mirror to compare size.

- The scrotum, testicles, and hands should be soapy to allow easy manipulation of the tissue.

- Gently roll each testicle between the thumb and fingers of each hand. If one testicle is substantially larger than the other, or if any hard lumps are detected, consult a physician immediately.

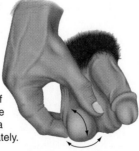

- Normal scrotal contents may be confusing. Just above and behind the testicle is the epididymis. It feels soft and tender overall, although parts of it may be rather firm. This is normal. The spermatic cord, a small, round, moveable tube, extends up from the epididymis. It feels firm and smooth. Of greatest concern is any hard lump felt directly on the testicle, even if it is painless.

- Choose a day out of each month on which to examine yourself. Most men choose an easy day to remember, such as the first or last day of the month.

**FIGURE 20–13**  Procedure for testicular self-examination.

# ✔ PATHOLOGY CHECKPOINT

*Following is a concise list of the pathology-related terms that you have seen in the chapter. Review this checklist to make sure that you are familiar with the meaning of each term before moving to the next section.*

## Conditions and Symptoms

- ❏ acute lymphocystic leukemia
- ❏ acute myeloid leukemia
- ❏ adenocarcinoma
- ❏ anaplasia
- ❏ astrocytoma
- ❏ basal cell carcinoma
- ❏ breast cancer
- ❏ bronchogenic carcinoma
- ❏ Burkitt's lymphoma
- ❏ carcinoma
- ❏ carcinoma in situ
- ❏ chondrosarcoma
- ❏ choriocarcinoma
- ❏ chronic lymphocytic leukemia
- ❏ chronic myelocytic leukemia
- ❏ ductal carcinoma in situ
- ❏ Ewing's sarcoma
- ❏ fibrosarcoma
- ❏ glioblastoma
- ❏ glioma
- ❏ hemangiosarcoma
- ❏ Hodgkin's disease
- ❏ hyperplasia
- ❏ Kaposi's sarcoma
- ❏ leiomyosarcoma
- ❏ leukemia
- ❏ leukoplakia
- ❏ liposarcoma
- ❏ lobular carcinoma in situ
- ❏ lung cancer
- ❏ lymphangiosarcoma
- ❏ lymphoma

- ❏ lymphosarcoma
- ❏ medulloblastoma
- ❏ melanoma
- ❏ meningioma
- ❏ mucositis
- ❏ myeloma
- ❏ myosarcoma
- ❏ neoplasm
- ❏ nephroblastoma
- ❏ neuroblastoma
- ❏ non-Hodgkin's lymphoma
- ❏ oligodendroglioma
- ❏ osteogenic sarcoma
- ❏ Paget's disease
- ❏ reticulosarcoma
- ❏ retinoblastoma
- ❏ rhabdomyosarcoma
- ❏ sarcoma
- ❏ seminoma
- ❏ squamous carcinoma
- ❏ tamponade (cardiac)
- ❏ teratoma
- ❏ testicular cancer
- ❏ thymoma
- ❏ trismus
- ❏ tumor
- ❏ Wilms' tumor
- ❏ xerostomia

## Diagnosis and Treatment

- ❏ adjuvant therapy
- ❏ blood serum test
- ❏ bone marrow study
- ❏ bronchoscopy

- ❏ cancer antigen 125
- ❏ carcinoembryonic antigen
- ❏ chemotherapy
- ❏ colonoscopy
- ❏ core biopsy
- ❏ cystoscopy
- ❏ diagnostic radiology
- ❏ endoscopic biopsy
- ❏ endoscopy
- ❏ excisional biopsy
- ❏ fecal occult blood test
- ❏ gastroscopy
- ❏ human chorionic gonadotropin
- ❏ human epidermal growth factor receptor–2
- ❏ immunotherapy
- ❏ incisional biopsy
- ❏ laparoscopy
- ❏ laryngoscopy
- ❏ needle biopsy
- ❏ Pap smear test
- ❏ photodynamic therapy
- ❏ proctoscopy
- ❏ prostate-specific antigen
- ❏ punch biopsy
- ❏ radiation therapy
- ❏ sentinel node biopsy
- ❏ sigmoidoscopy
- ❏ sputum cytology test
- ❏ stereotactic biopsy
- ❏ sternal biopsy
- ❏ surgery
- ❏ urine assay test

# STUDY AND REVIEW

## Overview of Oncology

*Write your answers to the following questions. Do not refer to the text.*

1. Name the three main classifications of cancer.

   a. _____   b. _____

   c. _____

2. Define *cell differentiation*. _____

   _____

3. Define *dedifferentiation*. _____

   _____

4. Name three ways that malignant cells spread to body parts.

   a. _____   b. _____

   c. _____

5. List the seven warning signals for cancer.

   a. _____   b. _____

   c. _____   d. _____

   e. _____   f. _____

   g. _____

6. Name four methods used in the treatment of cancer.

   a. _____   b. _____

   c. _____   d. _____

## Spelling

*In the spaces provided, write the correct spelling of these misspelled words.*

1. anplasia _____   2. fibrsarcoma _____

3. lymphsarcoma _____   4. myloma _____

5. oncgenic _____   6. semioma _____

## Word Parts

1. In the spaces provided, write the definitions of these prefixes, roots, combining forms, and suffixes. Do not refer to the listings of medical words. Leave blank those words you cannot define.

2. After completing as many as you can, refer to the medical word listings to check your work. For each word missed or left blank, write the word and its definition several times on the margins of these pages or on a separate sheet of paper.

3. To maximize the learning process, it is to your advantage to do the following exercises as directed. To refer to the word-building section before completing these exercises invalidates the learning process.

## PREFIXES

*Give the definitions of the following prefixes.*

1. ana- _____

2. astro- _____

3. hyper- _____

4. neo- _____

5. oligo- _____

6. pre- _____

7. en- _____

8. in- _____

9. meta- _____

10. brachy- _____

## ROOTS AND COMBINING FORMS

*Give the definitions of the following roots and combining forms.*

1. aden/o _____

2. angi/o _____

3. cancer _____

4. carcin _____

5. carcin/o _____

6. chondr/o _____

7. chori/o _____

8. cyt _____

9. dendr/o _____

10. fibr/o _____

11. gli _____

12. gli/o _____

13. hem _____

14. immun/o _____

15. lei/o _____

16. leuk _____

17. leuk/o _____

18. lip/o _____

19. lymph _____

20. lymph/o _____

21. medull/o _____

22. melan _____

23. mening/i _____

24. mucos _____

25. myc/o _____

26. myel _____

27. my/o _____

28. capsul _____

29. nephr/o _____

30. neur/o _____

31. onc/o _____

32. oste/o _____

33. reticul/o _____

34. retin/o _____

35. rhabd/o _____

36. sarc _____

37. duct _____

38. semin _____

39. stom _____

40. terat _____

41. thym _____

42. tox _____

43. trism _____

## SUFFIXES

*Give the definitions of the following suffixes.*

1. -blast _____

2. -emia _____

3. -gen _____

4. -genes _____

5. -genic _____

6. -ia _____

7. -in _____

8. -itis _____

9. -oma _____

10. -ous _____

11. -plakia _____

12. -plasia _____

13. -plasm _____

14. -ate (d) _____

15. -therapy _____

16. -us _____

17. -al _____

18. -ar _____

19. -ion _____

20. -ive _____

21. -ant _____

22. -stasis _____

23. -oid _____

## Identifying Medical Terms

*In the spaces provided, write the medical terms for the following meanings.*

1. _____ Agent or substance that incites or produces cancer

2. _____ Cancerous tumor derived from cartilage cells

3. _____ Cancerous tumor of the brain

4. _____ Cancerous tumor of smooth muscle tissue

5. _____ Cancer of the blood-forming tissues

6. _____ Cancerous tumor of lymphoid tissue

7. _____ Cancerous black mole or tumor

8. _____ Cancerous tumor of muscle tissue

9. _____ Cancerous tumor composed of osseous tissue

10. _____ Cancerous tumor arising from connective tissue

## Matching

*Select the appropriate lettered meaning for each of the following words.*

_____ 1. Hodgkin's disease

_____ 2. exacerbation

_____ 3. differentiation

_____ 4. in situ

_____ 5. encapsulated

_____ 6. photodynamic therapy

_____ 7. fungating

_____ 8. hyperplasia

_____ 9. Kaposi's sarcoma

_____ 10. metastasis

a. Spreading process of cancer from one area of the body to another
b. Excessive formation and growth of normal cells
c. Enclosed within a sheath
d. Process by which normal cells have a distinct appearance and specialized function
e. Form of lymphoma that occurs in young adults
f. Type of laser therapy that involves the use of a special chemical that is injected into the bloodstream and absorbed by cells all over the body
g. Enclosed within a site
h. Malignant neoplasm that causes violaceous (purplish discoloration) vascular lesions and general lymphadenopathy
i. Process of increasing the severity of symptoms
j. Process of growing rapidly
k. Agent that causes a change in the genetic structure of an organism

## Abbreviations

*Place the correct word, phrase, or abbreviation in the space provided.*

1. adenocarcinoma _____

2. biopsy _____

3. CA _____

4. chemo _____

5. deoxyribonucleic acid _____

6. IRT _____

7. acute lymphocytic leukemia _____

8. ductal carcinoma in situ _____

9. BRCA _____

10. tumor, node, metastases _____

# PRACTICAL APPLICATION

## S O A P : Chart Note Analysis

*This exercise will make you aware of the information, abbreviations, and medical terminology typically found in an urology patient's chart.*

**Abbreviation Key**

| | | | | |
|---|---|---|---|---|
| **Abd** | abdomen | | **Ht** | height |
| **AFP** | alpha-fetoprotein | | **lb** | pound |
| **BP** | blood pressure | | **LDH** | lactate dehydrogenase |
| **CBC** | complete blood count | | **P** | pulse |
| **c/o** | complains of | | **R** | respiration |
| **CT** | computed tomography | | **R/O** | rule out |
| **CTA** | clear to auscultation | | **SOAP** | subjective, objective, assessment, plan |
| **CXR** | chest x-ray | | **T** | temperature |
| **DOB** | date of birth | | **Wt** | weight |
| **F** | Fahrenheit | | **y/o** | year(s) old |
| **HCG** | human chorionic gonadotropin | | | |

*Read the following chart note and then answer the questions that follow.*

**PATIENT:** Walker, Joseph                                                      **DATE:** 05/10/07

**DOB:** 03/29/78        **AGE:** 29        **SEX:** Male

**INSURANCE:** Best Care Insurance

**Vital Signs:**
   **T:** 98.8 F
   **P:** 84
   **R:** 22
   **BP:** 138/88
   **Ht:** 6'
   **Wt:** 201 lb

**Allergies:** Penicillin

**Chief Complaint:** Painless, hard lump, approximately pea sized in right testicle

**S** **Subjective:** 29 y/o male presents stating, "I was taking a shower and washing my genitals when I found a lump in my right testicle. It was about the size of a pea and hard as a rock. It doesn't hurt, but I remember hearing the news about Lance Armstrong having cancer of the testicle. I am here to have the doctor check me out. I sure don't want cancer, but I understand if it is caught early, there is a good chance for a cure."

**O** **Objective:**

**General Appearance:** Well-groomed, anxious male concerned with recent findings. No other obvious distress.

**Heart:** Regular rate and rhythm. No murmurs, gallops, or rubs.

**Lungs:** CTA.

**Abd:** Bowel sounds all 4 quadrants. No masses or tenderness.

**Male Genitalia**

Penis: Skin normal, without lesions or inflammation, urethral meatus is positioned centrally without discharge, hair distribution is consistent with age and without pest inhabitants. Shaft smooth, semifirm, and nontender.

Scrotum: Normal asymmetry noted with left scrotal half lower than right. Left testicle oval, smooth, firm and rubbery, and freely movable. Noted right testicle exhibiting proximal firm, nontender oval pea-sized mass that does not reduce with patient lying down. Unable to auscultate bowel sounds. Mass does not transilluminate. Bilaterally, testes slightly tender to moderate pressure. Epididymis discrete, softer than testis, smooth and nontender. Spermatic cord smooth and nontender.

Inguinal Lymph Nodes: Groin lymph nodes nonpalpable in horizontal chain inferior to the inguinal ligament and vertical chain along the upper inner thigh.

Hernia: Negative upon examination

**A** **Assessment:** Testicular cancer to be confirmed by orchidectomy and biopsy

**P** **Plan:**
1. Schedule for scrotal ultrasound.
2. Advised to go to the laboratory for CBC, complete urinalysis, and serum tests: HCG and LDH.
3. Schedule a CXR and CT scan of the abdomen to R/O potential metastasis to the lungs and abdomen.
4. Schedule for a radical inguinal orchidectomy, right testicle. A tissue biopsy will be performed following the removal of the right testicle.
5. Inform patient for additional information to call 1-800-CANCER, 1-800-422-6237, or 1-800-ACS-2345 or visit the following Web sites: www.cancer.gov or www.cancer.org.

**FYI:** An ultrasound can assist the physician in determining whether the mass is solid or fluid filled. The echoes from most tumors differ from those of normal tissue. If the mass is solid, it is most likely cancer. Certain blood tests such as HCG and LDH are helpful in diagnosing testicular tumors, which can secrete high levels of certain proteins, such as alpha-fetoprotein (AFP) and HCG. The tumors can also increase the levels of enzymes such as LDH. A radical inguinal orchidectomy is the removal of the entire testicle through an incision in the groin. The surgeon does not cut through the scrotum into the testicle because if cancer is present, it could spread into the scrotum and lymph nodes. A tissue sample is then viewed by a pathologist to check for cancer cells and if found, the cell type (seminoma or nonseminoma) is determined. This identification of type is important in planning the treatment.

## Chart Note Questions
*Place the correct answer in the space provided.*

1. Signs and symptoms of cancer in this patient included a painless, _____ lump in his right testicle.

2. How did the patient discover the lump? _____

3. What is the possible diagnosis for this patient? _____

4. Why is a scrotal ultrasound scheduled for Mr. Walker? _____

5. Certain blood tests such as _____ and LDH are helpful in diagnosing testicular tumors.

6. What two tests are done to R/O metastasis of CA to the lungs and abdomen? _____

7. What is a CBC? _____

8. A radical inguinal _____ is the removal of the entire testicle through an incision in the groin.

9. The surgeon does not cut through the scrotum into the testicle because if cancer is present it could spread into the _____ and lymph nodes.

10. Why is the identification of tissue type important? _____

# MULTIMEDIA PREVIEW

*Additional interactive resources and activities for this chapter can be found on the Companion Website. For videos, audio glossary, and review, access the accompanying CD-ROM in this book.*

 **CD-ROM HIGHLIGHTS**

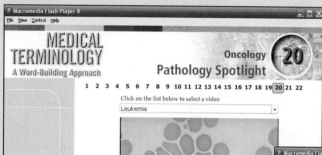

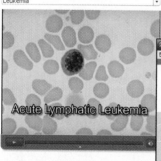

## PATHOLOGY SPOTLIGHT—LEUKEMIA

By viewing concepts in moving, living color, you'll get a fuller picture of the pathologies presented in this chapter. Earlier we discussed leukemia. Now click on this feature to watch a video that describes this condition in more detail.

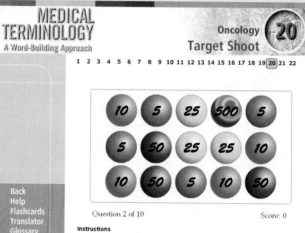

## TARGET SHOOTING

Here's a game that requires a quick mind and an even faster finger! As colored balls flash on your screen, click on the highest point values to reveal a question. A correct answer earns the points. How high can you score?

**WEBSITE HIGHLIGHTS—www.prenhall.com/rice**

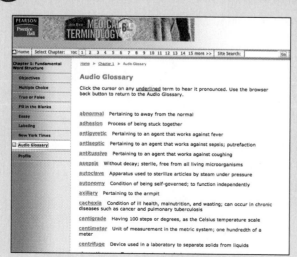

## AUDIO GLOSSARY

Click here and take advantage of the free-access on-line study guide that accompanies your textbook. You'll find an audio glossary with definitions and audio pronunciations for every term in the book. By clicking on this URL you'll also access a variety of quizzes with instant feedback, links to download mp3 audio reviews, and current news articles.

# Radiology and Nuclear Medicine

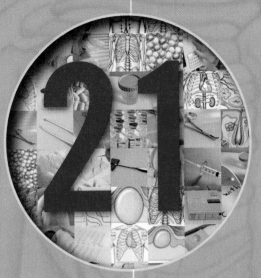

**21**

## ◼ OUTLINE

## ◼ OBJECTIVES

*On completion of this chapter, you will be able to:*

- Define *radiology.*
- Describe dangers and safety precautions associated with x-rays.
- Describe the positions used in radiography.
- Describe diagnostic imaging.
- Describe nuclear medicine.
- Describe interventional radiology.
- Analyze, build, spell, and pronounce medical words.
- Identify and define selected abbreviations.
- Describe each of the techniques presented in Radiology & Nuclear Medicine Spotlights.
- Review the Medical Vocabulary Checkpoint.
- Complete the Study and Review section and the Chart Note Analysis.

# Overview of Radiology and Nuclear Medicine

## RADIOLOGY

**Radiology** is the science of high-energy radiation; its sources; and the chemical, physical, and biologic effects of such radiation. It is the scientific discipline of medical imaging using radionuclides, ionizing radiation, nuclear magnetic resonance, and ultrasound. This medical specialty was developed after the discovery of an unknown ray in 1895 by Wilhelm Konrad Roentgen, a German physicist, who called his discovery *x-ray*. An **x-ray** is produced by the collision of a stream of electrons against a target (usually an anode of one of the heavy metals) contained within a vacuum tube. This collision produces electromagnetic rays of short wavelengths and high energy. The physician who specializes in radiology, roentgen diagnosis, and roentgen therapy is called a **radiologist.**

### Characteristics of X-Rays

The following are the characteristics of x-rays applicable to its medical use.

1. X-rays are an invisible form of radiant energy with short wavelengths traveling at 186,000 miles per second. They are able to penetrate different substances to varying degrees.

2. X-rays cause **ionization** of the substances through which they pass. Ionization is a process resulting in the gain or loss of one or more electrons in neutral atoms. The gain of an electron creates a negative electrical charge, whereas the loss of an electron results in a positively charged particle. These negatively or positively charged particles are called *ions*.

3. X-rays cause fluorescence of certain substances, thus allowing for the process known as **fluoroscopy** (see Figure 21–1 ▼), the examination of the tissues and deep structures of the body by x-ray, using the **fluoroscope,** a device that projects x-ray images in a movielike sequence onto a screen monitor. This process allows the physician to visual-

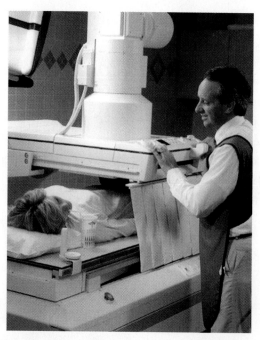

▶ **FIGURE 21–1** Advantx™ radiography/ fluoroscopy system. (Courtesy of GE Medical Systems)

ize internal structures that are in motion and to make permanent records of the examination for future study.

4. X-rays travel in a straight line, thus allowing the x-ray beam to be directed at a specific site during radiotherapy or to produce high-quality shadow images on **film** (radiographs).

5. X-rays are able to penetrate substances of different densities. In the body, x-rays pass through air in the lungs, fluids such as blood and lymph, and fat around muscles. Such substances are said to be **radiolucent.** Substances that obstruct the passage of radiant energy, in other words absorb radiant energy, such as calcium in bones, lead, or barium (Ba), are called **radiopaque.** Control of the voltage and amperage applied to the x-ray tube plus the duration of the exposure allows images of body structures of varying densities. A contrast medium can be introduced into the body to enhance certain x-ray images. This characteristic allows x-rays to be used as a diagnostic tool.

6. X-rays can destroy body cells. Radiation can be used to treat malignant tumors. In these cases, the x-ray voltage is administered by a radiotherapist using radiotherapy machines such as a linear accelerator or betatron. Care must be exercised in administering radiotherapy because x-rays can destroy healthy as well as abnormal tissue.

## Dangers and Safety Precautions

Because x-rays are invisible and produce no sound or smell, those working around and with them need to take certain precautions to avoid unnecessary exposure. Following are some of the dangers known to be associated with x-rays and the safety precautions designed to prevent unnecessary exposure.

### Prolonged Exposure

Prolonged and continued exposure to x-rays can cause damage to the gonads (testes or ovaries) and/or depress the hematopoietic system, which can cause leukopenia and/or leukemia. Personnel involved with radiation therapy should spend the minimal amount of time necessary when caring for patients receiving internal radiation therapy. The farther away an individual is from the source of radiation, the less the degree of exposure.

### Secondary Radiation

X-rays can scatter or be diverted from their normal straight paths when they strike radiopaque objects. This scatter or secondary radiation tends to add unwanted density to the image; therefore, a device known as a **grid** is positioned between the x-ray machine and the patient to absorb scatter before it reaches the x-ray film.

### Safety Precautions

Not all scatter or secondary radiation is absorbed by a grid; therefore, those working in areas adjacent to x-ray equipment risk unintentional exposure from this source unless proper safety precautions are observed. Generally, these safety precautions include the five described below.

Film Badge.    A **film badge,** usually pinned to a medical worker's clothing, is a device that is sensitive to ionizing radiation and monitors exposure to beta and gamma rays. A periodic analysis of the film badge reveals the amount of radiation the individual has received.

Lead Barrier.    Persons who operate x-ray machines do so from behind barriers equipped with a lead-treated window for viewing the patient.

Lead-Lined Room.    X-ray equipment should be housed in an area featuring lead-lined walls, floors, and doors to prevent the escape of radiation from the room.

Protective Clothing.    People who hold or position patients for x-ray examination should wear lead-lined gloves and aprons, especially if they hold a patient, such as a child, while an x-ray is being taken.

Gonad Shield.    The reproductive organs are radiosensitive and must be protected by a lead shield while x-rays are being taken. X-rays can cause damage to the genetic material within the reproductive organs, which could lead to birth defects or cancer.

## Positions Used in Radiography

### Anteroposterior Position

In the **anteroposterior** (AP) **position,** the patient is placed with the anterior (front) part of the body facing the x-ray tube and the posterior (back) of the body facing the film. X-rays pass through the body from the front to the back in reaching the film.

### Posteroanterior Position

In the **posteroanterior** (PA) **position,** the patient is placed with the posterior (back) portion of the body facing the x-ray tube and the anterior (front) of the body facing the film. The x-rays pass through the body from the back to the front to reach the film.

### Lateral Position

In the **lateral** (lat) **position,** the x-ray beam passes from one side of the patient's body to the opposite side to reach the film. Placing the patient's right side next to the film and passing x-rays through the body from left to right is known as the *right lateral position*. Placing the patient's left side next to the film and passing x-rays through the body from right to left is known as the *left lateral position*.

### Supine Position

In the **supine position,** the patient rests on the back, face upward, allowing the x-rays to pass through the body from the front to the back.

### Prone Position

In the **prone position,** the patient is placed lying face down with the head turned to one side. The x-rays pass from the back to the front side of the body.

### Oblique Position

In the **oblique position,** the patient is placed so that the body or body part to be imaged is at an angle to the x-ray beam.

## Diagnostic Imaging

**Diagnostic imaging** involves the use of x-rays, ultrasound, radiopharmaceuticals, radiopaque media, and computers to provide the radiologist images of internal body organs and processes. These images are used to identify and locate tumors, fractures, hematomas, disease processes, and other abnormalities within the body. In recent years, advances in the field of electronics have produced a variety of computer-assisted x-ray machines to enhance the images obtained by the radiologist. These sophisticated machines now make possible noninvasive procedures for the visualization of organs and processes that were previously not accessible or that required exploratory surgical procedures for examination.

Pregnant health care practitioners are permitted to work in and around certain diagnostic imaging machines. Acceptable activities include, but are not limited to, positioning patients, scanning, archiving, injecting contrast, and entering the scan room in response to an emergency. Pregnant practitioners are requested not to remain within the room during the actual data acquisition or scanning. Pregnant patients can be accepted to undergo certain scanning if, in the determination of a designated attending radiologist, the risk-benefit ratio for the patient warrants that the study be performed. The radiologist should confer with the referring physician and document that the data is needed and the physician does not believe that it is prudent to wait until the patient is no longer pregnant.

### Computed Tomography

**Computed tomography** (CT) is sometimes referred to as a **CAT scan** (computerized axial tomography). It combines an advanced x-ray scanning system with a powerful mini-computer and has vastly improved imaging quality while making it possible to view parts of the body and abnormalities not previously open to radiography. The CT scanner combines tomography, the process of imaging structures by focusing on a specific body plane and blurring all details from other planes, with a microprocessor that provides high-speed analysis of the tissue variances scanned (see Figure 21–2 ▼).

CT scans reveal both bone and soft tissues, including organs, muscles, and tumors (see Figure 21–3 ▶). Image tones can be adjusted to highlight tissues of similar density, and, through graphics software, the data from multiple cross-sections can be assembled into 3-D images. CT aids diagnosis, surgery, and treatment, including radiation therapy, in which effective dosage depends highly on the precise density, size, and location of a tumor.

A person having a CT scan is asked to refrain from eating or drinking for 4 hours before the scan. All jewelry and metal objects that could interfere with the exam need to be removed beforehand. Women are asked if they are pregnant. A person having a CT scan needs to undress and put on an exam gown.

Next, the person lies on a narrow table that slides through the opening in a machine that is shaped like a doughnut with a hole in its center. The opening is called the *gantry*. While in the gantry, an x-ray tube travels around the individual, creating computer-generated x-ray images. Some types of exams require the patient to receive an intravenous injection of iodinated contrast, which is a dye that makes some tissues show up better. Scans of the intestines sometimes call for the person to drink diluted iodinated contrast solution prior to the exam. After the exam, the technologist views the pictures. If they are adequate, the person is free to leave.

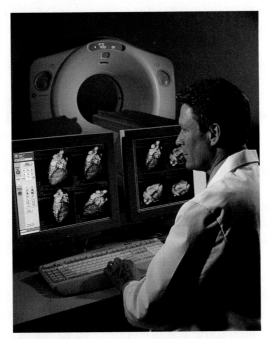

▶ **FIGURE 21–2**  LightSpeed[16]™ computed tomography system. (Courtesy of GE Medical Systems)

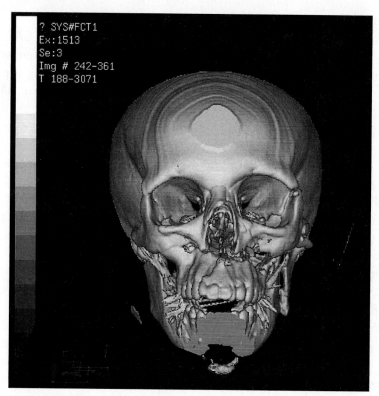

? SYS#FCT1
Ex:1513
Se:3
Img # 242-361
T 188-3071

▶ **FIGURE 21–3**   3D CT scan, multiple facial fractures. (Courtesy of Teresa Resch)

### Magnetic Resonance Imaging

**Magnetic resonance imaging** (MRI) is a noninvasive imaging technique. The MRI machine is used to view organs, bone, and other internal body structures. The imaged body part is exposed to radio waves while in a magnetic field. The picture is produced by energy emitted from hydrogen atoms in the human body. The patient is not exposed to radiation during this test.

MRI can be used for a variety of purposes. A physician can order an MRI of the brain, known as a *cranial MRI*, to evaluate a person's tumor, seizure disorder, or headache symptoms. See Figure 21–4 ▶. An MRI of the spine examines a disc problem in a person's spine. If an individual has sustained injury to the shoulder or knee, an MRI is frequently used to study these large joints. Disease of the heart, chest, abdomen, and pelvis are also commonly evaluated with MRI.

Before the test, the physician assesses the patient for any drug or food allergies (especially shellfish or foods with added iodine such as table salt) and whether the person has experienced claustrophobia, or anxiety in enclosed spaces. If this is a problem, mild sedating medication may be given. A woman is asked if she is pregnant.

The person is asked to remove all metal objects such as belts, jewelry, and any pieces of removable dental work. Internal metal objects that cannot be removed can distort the final images so the person should inform the MRI technologist about any previous surgery that required placement of metal in the body, such as a hip pinning. Because the magnetic field can damage watches and credit cards, these objects are not taken into the MRI scanner.

Typically, the person having the test does not need to restrict food or fluids before an MRI scan. Certain tests, such as an MRI-guided biopsy, do require certain food and fluid restrictions. The person should consult the health care provider for instructions prior to the MRI.

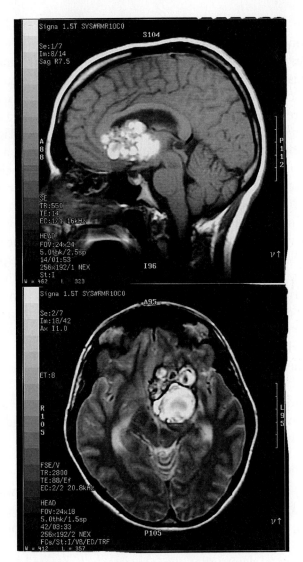

▶ **FIGURE 21–4** MRI head showing large hemorrhagic lesion. (Courtesy of Teresa Resch)

As the test begins, the person lying on his or her back slides into the **bore** (horizontal tube running through the magnet from front to back) on a special table. To prevent image distortion on the final images, the person must lie very still for the duration of the test. Commonly, a special substance called a *contrast agent* is administered prior to or during the test. The contrast agent is used to enhance internal structures and improve image quality. Typically, this material is injected into a vein in the arm.

The scanning process is painless. However, the part of the body being imaged can feel a bit warm. This sensation is harmless and normal. The person hears loud banging and knocking noises during many stages of the exam. Earplugs are provided for people who find the noises disturbing.

A radiologist analyzes the MRI images. Frequently, the MRI helps to better evaluate a disease or disorder affecting organs and blood vessels. MRI is particularly useful in evaluating the size and location of tumors as well as bleeding at various clotting stages. The health care provider and the radiologist use this information to help guide the next course of action for the individual's condition.

### Ultrasound

**Ultrasound** literally means *beyond sound*. It is sound whose frequency is beyond the range of human hearing. Ultrasound is widely used in diagnostic imaging to evaluate a patient's internal organs. Its energy is transmitted into the patient and, because various internal organs and structures reflect and scatter sound differently, returning echoes can be used to form an image of a particular structure. These ultrasonic echoes are then recorded as a composite picture of the internal organ and/or structure. See Figures 21–11 and 21–12 on page 725.

**Ultrasonography** is the process of using ultrasound to produce a record of ultrasonic echoes as they strike tissues of different densities. The record produced by this process is called a **sonogram** or **echogram.** An adaptation of ultrasound technology is **Doppler echocardiography.** It is a noninvasive technique for determining the blood flow velocity in different locations in the heart. This same technique can be used to determine the uterine artery blood flow velocity during pregnancy as well as the fetal heart rate.

The test is done in the ultrasound or radiology department. The patient lies down for the procedure. A clear, water-based conducting gel is applied to the skin over the area being examined to help with the transmission of the sound waves. A handheld probe called a *transducer* is then moved over the area being examined. The patient can be asked to change position so that other areas can be examined.

Preparation for the procedure depends on the body region being examined. Ultrasound procedures generally cause little discomfort, although the conducting gel can feel slightly cold and wet.

Results are considered normal if the organs and structures in the area being examined are normal in appearance. The significance of abnormal results depends on the body region being examined and the nature of the symptom.

### Other Imaging Techniques

Other diagnostic imaging techniques being used include **thermography,** in which detailed images of body parts are developed from data showing the degree of heat and cold present in areas being studied, and **scintigraphy,** which involves the production of two-dimensional images of tissue areas from the scintillations emitted by an internally administered radiopharmaceutical device that concentrates on a targeted site.

## NUCLEAR MEDICINE

**Nuclear medicine** is a subspecialty within the field of radiology that uses radioactive substances to produce images of body anatomy and function. The images are developed based on the detection of energy emitted from the radioactive substance given to the patient either intravenously (IV) or by mouth (PO). These images are used to diagnose disease processes and evaluate organ functioning. Some of the general uses of nuclear medicine follow:

- Image blood flow and heart function.
- Scan lungs.
- Evaluate kidney function.
- Identify blockage of the gallbladder.
- Evaluate bones for fracture, infection, arthritis, tumors.
- Identify bleeding into the colon.
- Locate an infection site.
- Measure thyroid function for hyperactivity or hypoactivity.

Certain imaging procedures, including PET scanning, employ radionuclides to provide real-time visuals of biochemical processes. One device, a nuclear imaging machine, employs a scintillation camera that can rotate around the body to pick up radiation emitted by an injected substance, such as radioactive iodine, which localizes in the thyroid, or radioactive thallium, which localizes in the heart. Through computerization, a digitized image of a particular organ is produced.

### Positron Emission Tomography

**Positron emission tomography** (PET), commonly called a **PET scan,** is a diagnostic procedure that involves the development of biologic images based on the detection of radiation from the emission of positrons. **Positrons** are tiny particles emitted from a radioactive substance that has been administered to the patient. The subsequent images or views of the human body developed with this technique are used to aid diagnosis and evaluate a range of diseases.

## INTERVENTIONAL RADIOLOGY

**Interventional radiology** (IR) is a branch of medicine in which certain diseases are treated nonoperatively. An **interventional radiologist** is a physician who has had special training in imaging and who specializes in treating diseases percutaneously. An interventional radiologist uses radiologic imaging to guide catheters, balloons, stents, filters, and other tiny instruments through the body's vascular system and/or other systems.

The procedures and/or surgeries are performed in an interventional suite, generally on an outpatient basis. General anesthesia is usually unnecessary, and conscious sedation and/or local anesthesia is more commonly used. These procedures are cost effective and are increasingly replacing traditional surgery for certain conditions and procedures as described in the following table.

### Some Interventional Procedures

| | |
|---|---|
| Angiography | X-ray exam of the arteries using an injected contrast agent (radiopaque substance) to make the artery visible on x-ray and a catheter to enter the artery |
| Balloon angioplasty | Opens blocked or narrowed blood vessels |
| Chemoembolization | Delivers cancer-fighting agents directly to the tumor site |
| Embolization | Delivers clotting agents directly to an area that is bleeding or to block blood flow to a problem area, such as a fibroid tumor |
| Fallopian tube catheterization | Opens blocked fallopian tubes, a cause of infertility in women |
| Needle biopsy | Diagnostic test for breast or other cancers; an alternative to surgical biopsy |
| Stent-graft placement | Reinforces a ruptured or ballooning section of an artery with a fabric-wrapped stent, a small cagelike tube that serves to patch the vessel |
| Thrombolysis | Dissolves blood clots |
| Transjugular intrahepatic portosystemic shunt (TIPS) | Improves blood flow for patients with severe liver dysfunction |
| Varicocele occlusion | Treats varicose veins in the testicles, a cause of infertility in men |
| Vena cava filters | Prevents blood clots from reaching the heart |

### Radiation Therapy

The treatment of disease by ionizing radiation is called **radiotherapy, x-ray therapy, cobalt treatment,** or simply **radiation therapy.** In all cases, this treatment seeks to deliver a precise, calculated dose of radiation to diseased tissue, such as a tumor, while causing the least possible damage to surrounding normal tissue. See Chapter 20, Oncology, on page 676 for more information about radiation therapy.

# LIFE SPAN CONSIDERATIONS

## ■ THE CHILD

Nuclear medicine can be used in the diagnostic workup of childhood disorders that are congenital or acquired later. Such disorders include urinary blockage involving the kidneys, bone infection and trauma, gastrointestinal bleeding, and various tumors. Most procedures involve an intravenous injection of a radiopharmaceutical (radiotracer) based on body weight. If the child is younger than 4 years of age, sedation is usually necessary.

During the procedure, the child lies on a scanning table. The previously administered radiopharmaceutical (radiotracer) gives off gamma rays that the gamma camera detects. The gamma camera, which works in conjunction with a computer to develop an image, moves slowly along or around the child to obtain images of the part of the body being examined. Scanning time varies from 20 to 45 minutes. The child is exposed to a small dose of radiation, but there are no known long-term adverse effects from such low-dose tests.

The nuclear medicine physician interprets the images and forwards a report to the referring physician. This process usually takes one to three days.

## ■ THE OLDER ADULT

About 170,000 people in the United States are diagnosed with lung cancer each year. Most are diagnosed when their disease is advanced, and nearly 90% die within two years. Identifying lung cancer early while surgery is a treatment option improves survival rates; 70% of patients who are diagnosed early survive at least 5 years.

A new study from the National Cancer Institute (NCI) shows that screening for lung cancer with chest x-rays can detect early lung cancer but can also produce false-positive test results, causing needless extra tests. Between 1993 and 2001 the prostate, lung, colorectal, and ovarian (PLCO) investigators enrolled 154,942 men and women, 55 to 74 years of age, in a study. These participants included current and former smokers as well as individuals who never smoked.

Of the cancers detected by the trial study, 44% were Stage I, meaning those patients were good candidates for surgery. Another NCI-supported study, the National Lung Screening Trial (NLST), is comparing 2 ways to detect lung cancer: spiral computed tomography (CT) and standard chest x-ray. Both of these tests have been used to find lung cancer in its early stage. So far, neither chest x-rays nor spiral CT scans have been shown to reduce a person's chance of dying from lung cancer. One of the long-term goals of the PLCO trial is to determine whether chest x-rays can reduce lung cancer mortality in men and women 55 to 74 years of age. The current analysis confirmed that smoking vastly increases the risk for lung cancer.

# BUILDING YOUR MEDICAL VOCABULARY

This section provides the foundation for learning medical terminology. Review the following alphabetized word list. Note how common prefixes and suffixes are repeatedly applied to word roots and combining forms to create different meanings.

| | |
|---|---|
| **P** | Prefix |
| **R** | Root |
| **CF** | Combining form |
| **S** | Suffix |

| | |
|---|---|
| Pink words | Terms not built from word parts. |
| **\*** | Indicates words covered in the Pathology Spotlights section. |
| | Check the CD-ROM for more information. |

| MEDICAL WORD | WORD PARTS (WHEN APPLICABLE) | | | DEFINITION |
|---|---|---|---|---|
| | **Part** | **Type** | **Meaning** | |
| **angiocardiogram** (ăn″ jĭ-ō-kăr′ dĭ-ō-grăm) | angi/o cardi/o -gram | CF CF S | vessel heart record | X-ray record of the heart and great vessels made visible through the use of a radiopaque contrast medium |
| **angiogram** (ăn′ jĭ-ō-grăm) | angi/o -gram | CF S | vessel record | X-ray record of the blood vessels made visible through the use of an injected radiopaque contrast medium |
| **angiography** (ăn″ jĭ-ŏg′ ră-fē) | angi/o -graphy | CF S | vessel recording | Process of making an x-ray record of blood vessels |
| **aplastic anemia** (ă-plăs′ tĭk ăn-nē′ mĭ-ă) | | | | Type of anemia with aplasia or destruction of the bone marrow; can be caused by chemotherapeutic agents, x-rays, or other sources of ionizing radiation |
| **arteriography** (ăr″ tē-rĭ-ŏg′ ră-fē) | arteri/o -graphy | CF S | artery recording | Process of making an x-ray record of the arteries |
| **arthrography** (ăr-thrŏg′ ră-fē) | arthr/o -graphy | CF S | joint recording | Process of making an x-ray record of a joint |
| **barium (Ba) sulfate** (bā′ rĭ-ŭm sŭl′ fāt) | | | | Radiopaque barium compound used as a contrast medium in x-ray examination of the digestive tract; may be administered orally or via a barium enema (BE) |
| **beam** | | | | Ray of light; in radiology and nuclear medicine, radiant energy emitted by a group of atomic particles traveling a parallel course |
| **bronchogram** (brŏng′ kō-grăm) | bronch/o -gram | CF S | bronchi record | X-ray record of the bronchial tree made visible through the use of a radiopaque contrast medium |
| **cassette** | | | | Light-proof case or holder for x-ray film |

| MEDICAL WORD | WORD PARTS (WHEN APPLICABLE) | | | DEFINITION |
|---|---|---|---|---|
| | **Part** | **Type** | **Meaning** | |
| **cathode** (kăth′ ōd) | | | | Negative pole of an electrical current |
| **cholangiogram** (kō-lăn′ jĭ-ō-grăm) | chol | R | gall, bile | X-ray record of the bile ducts made visible through the use of a radiopaque contrast medium |
| | angi/o | CF | vessel | |
| | -gram | S | record | |
| **cholecystogram** (kō″ lē-sĭs′ tō-grăm) | chole | R | gall | X-ray record of the gallbladder made visible through the use of a radiopaque contrast medium |
| | cyst/o | CF | bladder | |
| | -gram | S | record | |
| **cinematoradiography** (sĭn″ ĭ-măt″ ō-rā′ dĭ-ŏg′ ră-fē) | cinemat/o | CF | motion | Process of making an x-ray record of an organ in motion |
| | radi/o | CF | x-ray | |
| | -graphy | S | recording | |
| **cineradiography** (sĭn″ ē-rā″ dē-ŏg′ ră-fē) | cine | R | motion | Process of making a motion picture record of successive x-ray images appearing on a fluoroscopic screen |
| | radi/o | CF | x-ray | |
| | -graphy | S | recording | |
| **cobalt-60** (kō′ balt) | | | | Radionuclide that serves as the radioactive substance in teletherapy machines; also used for implantation (interstitial) in the treatment of some malignancies |
| **contrast medium** (kŏn′ trăst mēd′ ĭ-ūm) | | | | Radiopaque substance used in certain x-ray procedures to permit visualization of organs or structures |
| **curie (Ci)** (kūr′ e) | | | | Unit of radioactivity |
| **digital subtraction angiography** (dĭj′ ĭ-tăl sŭb-trăk′ shŭn ăn″ jĭ-ŏg′ ră-fē) | digit | R | finger | Method by which a computer performs instantaneous subtraction of x-ray images, giving high-quality x-ray images of blood vessels with less x-ray dye. *Note: In this instance, digital refers to an Arabic number from 0 to 9, so named from counting on the fingers.* |
| | -al | S | pertaining to | |
| | sub- | P | below | |
| | tract | R | to draw | |
| | -ion | S | process | |
| | angi/o | CF | vessel | |
| | -graphy | S | recording | |
| **dose** | | | | Amount of medication or radiation to be administered |
| **echoencephalography** (ĕk″ ō-ĕn-sĕf″ ă-lŏg′ ră-fē) | ech/o | CF | echo | Process of using ultrasound to study intracranial structures of the brain. Useful for diagnosing conditions that cause a shift in the midline structures of the brain. |
| | encephal/o | CF | brain | |
| | -graphy | S | recording | |
| **echography** (ĕk-ŏg′ ră-fē) | ech/o | CF | echo | Process of using ultrasound as a diagnostic tool by making a record of the echo produced when sound waves are reflected back through tissues of different density |
| | -graphy | S | recording | |
| **film** | | | | Thin, cellulose-coated, light-sensitive sheet or slip of material used in taking pictures |

| MEDICAL WORD | WORD PARTS (WHEN APPLICABLE) | | | DEFINITION |
|---|---|---|---|---|
| | Part | Type | Meaning | |
| **film badge** | | | | Device that is sensitive to ionizing radiation worn by a person who works with x-rays to monitor the degree of exposure to beta and gamma rays. See Figure 21–5 ▼. |
| **fluorescence**<br>(floo″ ō-rĕs′ ĕnts) | | | | Property of certain substances to emit light as a result of exposure to and absorption of radiant energy |
| **fluoroscopy**<br>(floo-răs′ kə-pē) | fluor/o<br><br>-scopy | CF<br><br>S | fluorescence, luminous<br>visual examination, to view, examine | Process of examining internal structures by viewing the shadows cast on a fluorescent screen after the x-ray has passed through the body |
| **hysterosalpingo-<br>gram**<br>(hĭs″ tĕr-ō-săl-pĭn′ gō-grăm) | hyster/o<br>salping/o<br>-gram | CF<br>CF<br>S | uterus<br>fallopian tube<br>record | X-ray record of the uterus and fallopian tubes that is made visible through the use of a radiopaque contrast medium |
| **intravenous<br>pyelogram**<br>(ĭn″ tră-vē′ nŭs<br>pī′ ĕ-lō-grăm) | intra-<br>ven<br>-ous<br>pyel/o<br>-gram | P<br>R<br>S<br>CF<br>S | within<br>vein<br>pertaining to<br>renal pelvis<br>record | X-ray record of the kidney and renal pelvis made visible through the use of an injected radiopaque contrast medium |
| **ion**<br>(ī-ŏn) | | | | Atomic particle consisting of an atom or a group of atoms that carry an electrical charge, either negative or positive |
| **ionization**<br>(ī″ ŏn-ĭ-zā′ shŭn) | | | | Process of breaking up molecules into their component parts |
| **ionizing<br>radiation**<br>(ī′ ŏn-ī-zĭng<br>rā″ dĭ-ā′ shŭn) | | | | Powerful invisible energy capable of producing ions |
| **ionometer**<br>(ĭŏn′ ō-mē-tĕr) | ion/o<br>-meter | CF<br>S | ion<br>instrument to measure | Instrument used to measure the amount of radiation used by x-rays or radioactive substances |
| **ionotherapy**<br>(ī″ ŏn-ō-thĕr′ ă-pē) | ion/o<br>-therapy | CF<br>S | ion<br>treatment | Treatment by introducing ions into the body |

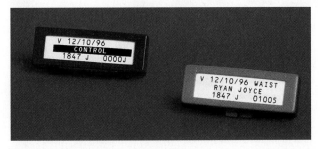

▶ **FIGURE 21–5** Types of radiation badges to be worn by all staff around x-ray equipment.

| MEDICAL WORD | WORD PARTS (WHEN APPLICABLE) | | | DEFINITION |
|---|---|---|---|---|
| | Part | Type | Meaning | |
| **iontoradiometer**<br>(ī-ŏn″ tō-rā″ dĭ-ŏm′ ĭ-tĕr) | iont/o<br>radi/o<br>-meter | CF<br>CF<br>S | ion<br>x-ray<br>instrument to<br>measure | Instrument used to measure the amount and intensity of x-rays |
| **irradiation**<br>(i-rā″ dē-ā′ shŭn) | ir (in)-<br>radiat<br>-ion | P<br>R<br>S | into<br>radiant<br>process | Process of using x-rays, radium rays, ultraviolet rays, gamma rays, or infrared rays in the diagnosis or therapeutic treatment of a patient |
| **isotope**<br>(ī′ sō-tōp) | | | | One of a series of nuclides that are chemically identical yet differ in atomic weight and electrical charge. Radioactive isotopes are composed of unstable atoms, and most are artificially produced. For example, cobalt-60 is a radioactive isotope artificially produced from naturally occurring cobalt-59. |
| **lead (Pb)**<br>(lĕd) | | | | Soft, heavy, inelastic, malleable, ductile, bluish-gray metallic element used in its metallic form as a protective shielding against x-rays. See Figure 21–6 ▼. |
| **lymphangiogram**<br>(lĭm-făn″ jē-ō-grăm) | lymph<br>angi/o<br>-gram | R<br>CF<br>S | lymph<br>vessel<br>record | X-ray record of the lymph vessels made visible with radiopaque contrast medium |
| **lymphangiography**<br>(lĭm-făn″ jē-ŏg′ ră-fē) | lymph<br>angi/o<br>-graphy | R<br>CF<br>S | lymph<br>vessel<br>recording | Process of making an x-ray record of the lymph vessels |

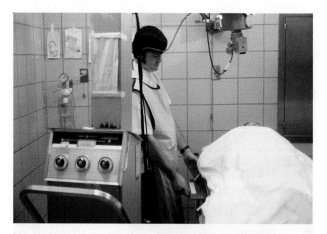

▶ **FIGURE 21–6** X-ray technician in a lead apron positions a photographic plate beneath a patient undergoing an x-ray procedure. This apron is a protective shield of lead and rubber worn by a patient or those taking x-rays to protect the genitals and other vital organs from excessive exposure to x-rays.

| MEDICAL WORD | WORD PARTS (WHEN APPLICABLE) | | | DEFINITION |
|---|---|---|---|---|
| | **Part** | **Type** | **Meaning** | |
| **mammography**<br>(măm-ŏg′ ră-fē)<br>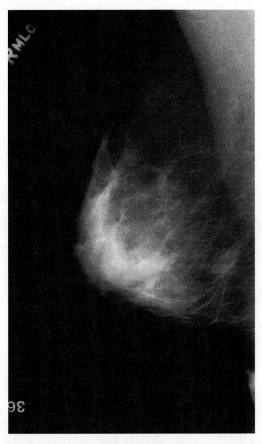 | mamm/o<br>-graphy | CF<br>S | breast<br>recording | Process of obtaining images of the breast with x-rays See Figure 21–7 ▼. ✳ See Radiology and Nuclear Medicine Spotlight: Mammography on page 728. |
| **millicurie (mCi)**<br>(mĭl″ ĭ-kū′ rē) | milli-<br>curie | P<br>R | one-thousandth<br>curie | 0.001 Ci |
| **myelogram**<br>(mī′ ĕ-lō-grăm) | myel/o<br>-gram | CF<br>S | spinal cord<br>record | X-ray record of the spinal cord made visible with a radiopaque contrast medium |
| **oscilloscope**<br>(ŏ-sĭl′ ō-skōp) | oscill/o<br>-scope | CF<br>S | to swing<br>instrument for examining | Instrument used to record an electrical wave visually on a fluorescent screen of a cathode-ray tube |
| **photofluorogram**<br>(fō″ tō-floo′ ĕr-ō-grăm) | phot/o<br>fluor/o<br>-gram | CF<br>CF<br>S | light<br>fluorescence<br>record | X-ray record of images seen during fluoroscopic examination |
| **physicist**<br>(fīz′ ĭ-sĭst) | physic<br>-ist | R<br>S | nature<br>one who specializes | Person who specializes in the science of physics |

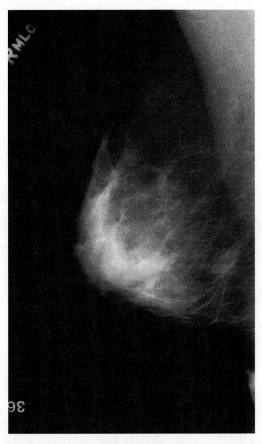

▶ **FIGURE 21–7**  Normal mammogram obtained through the process of mammography. (Courtesy of Teresa Resch)

| MEDICAL WORD | WORD PARTS (WHEN APPLICABLE) | | | DEFINITION |
|---|---|---|---|---|
| | Part | Type | Meaning | |
| **rad**<br>(răd) | | | | Amount of radiation absorbed; the letters stand for **r**adiation **a**bsorbed **d**ose |
| **radiation**<br>(rā-dĭ-ā′ shŭn) | radiat<br>-ion | R<br>S | radiant<br>process | Process by which radiant energy is propagated through space or matter |
| **radioactive**<br>(rā″ dĭ-ō-ăk′ tĭv) | radi/o<br>act<br>-ive | CF<br>R<br>S | ray, x-ray<br>acting<br>nature of | Characterized by emitting radiant energy |
| **radiodermatitis**<br>(rā″ dĭ-ō-dur′ mă-tī′ tĭs) | radi/o<br>dermat<br>-itis | CF<br>R<br>S | ray, x-ray<br>skin<br>inflammation | Inflammation of the skin caused by exposure to x-rays or radioactive substances |
| **radiograph**<br>(rā′ dĭ-ō-grăf) | radi/o<br>-graph | CF<br>S | ray, x-ray<br>instrument for recording | Picture produced on a sensitized film or plate by rays; an *x-ray record* |
| **radiographer**<br>(rā″ dĭ-ŏg′ ră-fĕr) | radi/o<br>-graph<br><br>-er | CF<br>S<br><br>S | ray, x-ray<br>instrument for recording<br>one who | Person skilled in making x-ray records |
| **radiography**<br>(rā″ dĭ-ŏg′ ră-fē) | radi/o<br>-graphy | CF<br>S | ray, x-ray<br>recording | Process of making an x-ray record |
| **radiologist**<br>(rā″ dĭ-ŏl′ ō-jĭst) | radi/o<br>log<br>-ist | CF<br>R<br>S | ray, x-ray<br>study of<br>one who specializes | Physician who specializes in radiology. See Figure 21–8 ▼. |
| **radiology**<br>(rā″ dĭ-ŏl′ ō-jē) | radi/o<br>-logy | CF<br>S | ray, x-ray<br>study of | Study of x-rays, radioactive substances, radioactive isotopes, and ionizing radiation |

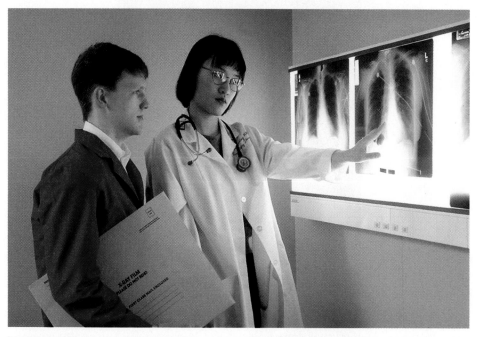

▶ **FIGURE 21–8**   Radiologist examines an x-ray of the chest.

| MEDICAL WORD | WORD PARTS (WHEN APPLICABLE) | | | DEFINITION |
|---|---|---|---|---|
| | Part | Type | Meaning | |
| **radiolucent** (rā″ dĭ-ō-lū′ sĕnt) | radi/o lucent | CF R | ray, x-ray to shine | Pertaining to property of permitting the passage of radiant energy |
| **radionuclide** (rā″ dĭ-ō-nū′ klĭd) | radi/o nucl -ide | CF R S | ray, x-ray nucleus having a particular quality | Radioactive species of an atomic nucleus identified by its atomic number, mass, and energy state |
| **radiopaque** (rā″ dĭ-ō-pāk′) | radi/o paque | CF R | ray, x-ray dark | Pertaining to property of obstructing the passage of radiant energy |
| **radioscopy** (rā″ dĭ-ŏs′ kō-pē) | radi/o -scopy | CF S | ray, x-ray visual examination, to view, examine | Process of viewing and examining the inner structures of the body through the process of x-rays |
| **radiotherapy** (rā″ dĭ-ō-thĕr′ ă-pē) | radi/o -therapy | CF S | ray, x-ray treatment | Treatment of disease by the use of x-rays, radium, and other radioactive substances |
| **radium (Ra)** (rā′ dĭ-ŭm) | | | | Radioactive isotope used to treat certain malignant diseases |
| **roentgen (R)** (rĕnt′ gĕn) | | | | International unit for describing exposure dose of x-ray or γ-radiation |
| **roentgenology** (rĕnt″ gĕn-ŏl′ ō-jē) | roent gen/o -logy | R CF S | roentgen kind study of | Study of roentgen rays for diagnostic and therapeutic purposes |
| **scan** | | | | Process of using a moving device or a sweeping beam of radiation to produce images of organs or structures of the body. See Figure 21–9 ▶ and Figure 21–10 ▶. ✳ See Radiology and Nuclear Medicine Spotlight: Bone Scan on page 727 and Figure 21–14. |
| **shield** | | | | Protective structure used to prevent or reduce the passage of particles or radiation |
| **sialography** (sī″ ă-lŏg′ ră-fē) | sial/o -graphy | CF S | salivary recording | Process of making an x-ray record of the salivary ducts and glands |
| **sonogram** (sōn′ ō-grăm) | son/o -gram | CF S | sound record | Record produced by ultrasonography. See Figure 21–11 ▶. |
| **tagging** | | | | Process of tracing a radioactive isotope that has become involved in metabolic or chemical actions |
| **thermography** (thĕr-mŏg′ ră-fē) | therm/o -graphy | CF S | heat recording | Process of recording heat patterns of the body's surface; useful in the detection of breast cancer |
| **tomography** (tō-mŏg′ ră-fē) | tom/o -graphy | CF S | to cut recording | Process of cutting across and producing images of single tissue planes |

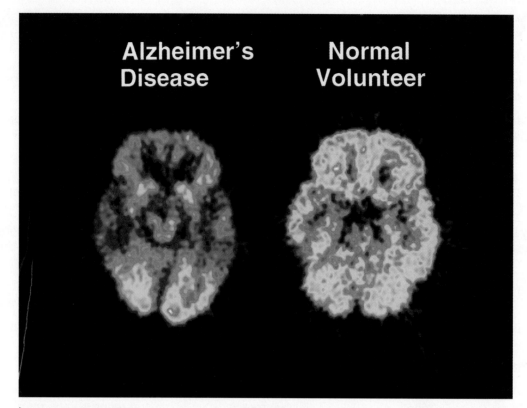

▶ **FIGURE 21–9**   PET scan comparing the metabolic activity levels of a normal brain and the brain of an Alzheimer's sufferer. Red and yellow colors indicate high activity levels; blue colors represent low activity levels.

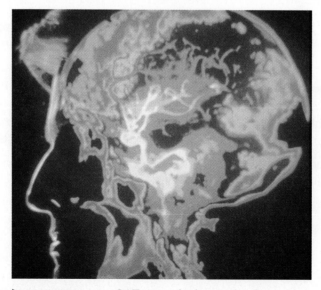

▶ **FIGURE 21–10**   CAT scan of a human head in profile.

| MEDICAL WORD | WORD PARTS (WHEN APPLICABLE) | | | DEFINITION |
|---|---|---|---|---|
| | Part | Type | Meaning | |
| **ultrasonic**<br>(ŭl″ tră-sŏn′ ĭk) | ultra-<br>son<br>-ic | P<br>R<br>S | beyond<br>sound<br>pertaining to | Pertaining to sounds beyond 20,000 cycles/sec |
| **ultrasonography**<br>(ŭl″ tră-sŏn-ŏg′ ră-fē) | ultra-<br>son/o<br>-graphy | P<br>CF<br>S | beyond<br>sound<br>recording | Process of using ultrasound to produce a record of ultrasonic echoes as they strike tissues of different densities. See Figure 21–12 ▼. |
| **venography**<br>(vē-nŏg′ ră-fē) | ven/o<br>-graphy | CF<br>S | vein<br>recording | Process of making an x-ray record of veins |

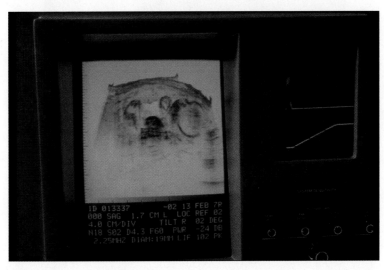

▶ **FIGURE 21–11**    Human fetus image called a sonogram is displayed on an ultrasound monitor.

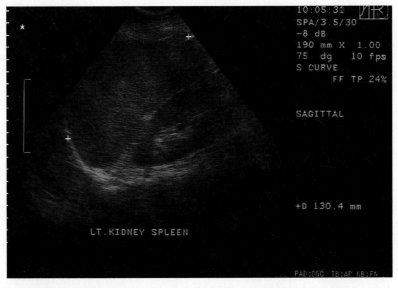

▶ **FIGURE 21–12**    Ultrasound, left kidney, and spleen. (Courtesy of Teresa Resch)

| MEDICAL WORD | WORD PARTS (WHEN APPLICABLE) | | | DEFINITION |
|---|---|---|---|---|
| | Part | Type | Meaning | |
| x-ray | | | | Electromagnetic wave of high energy produced by the collision of a beam of electrons with a target in a vacuum tube (x-ray tube). See Figure 21–13 ▼. |

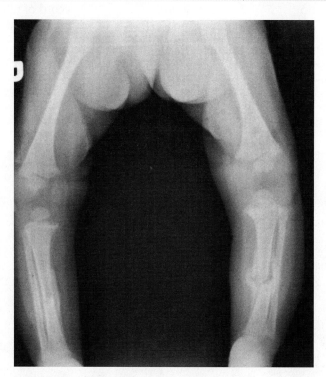

▶ FIGURE 21–13  X-ray of a child's lower legs showing fractures in the right tibia, heel, and left tibia.

## ABBREVIATIONS

| ABBREVIATION | MEANING | ABBREVIATION | MEANING |
|---|---|---|---|
| AP | anteroposterior | NCI | National Cancer Institute |
| Ba | barium | NLST | National Lung Screening Trial |
| BE | barium enema | PA | posteroanterior |
| BSE | breast self-examination | Pb | lead |
| CAT | computerized axial tomography | PET | positron emission tomography |
| Ci | curie | PLCO | prostate, lung, colorectal, and |
| CT | computed tomography | | ovarian (Study) |
| DEXA | dual-energy x-ray absorptiometry | PO | orally; by mouth |
| | | R | roentgen |
| IR | interventional radiology | Ra | radium |
| IV | intravenous | rad | radiation absorbed dose |
| lat | lateral | TIPS | transjugular intrahepatic |
| mCi | millicurie | | portosystemic shunt |
| MRI | magnetic resonance imaging | | |

# RADIOLOGY AND NUCLEAR MEDICINE SPOTLIGHTS

## ✶ Bone Densitometry

**Bone densitometry** is an enhanced form of x-ray technology called *dual-energy x-ray absorptiometry* (DEXA). It is a noninvasive procedure used to diagnose osteoporosis and to assess the risk of developing fractures. It is also effective in monitoring the effects of treatment for osteoporosis. This test is recommended for postmenopausal women; individuals with a history of hip fracture; people prone to fractures; smokers; men who have clinical conditions associated with bone loss; and patients with Type 1 diabetes, liver disease, kidney disease, a family history of osteoporosis, and hyperthyroidism.

The two types of DEXA equipment are the central device and the peripheral device. The central device measures bone density in the hip and spine. The peripheral device measures it in the wrist, heel, or finger. The test takes from 10 to 30 minutes, depending on the equipment used and the parts of the body being examined. A radiologist interprets the bone density exam and sends the results to the referring physician. The test results are in the form of two scores:

**T Score.**  This number shows the amount of bone a person has as compared with a young adult of the same gender with peak bone mass. A score above −1 is considered normal. A score between −1 and −2.5 indicates the first stage of bone loss (osteopenia). A score below −2.5 indicates osteoporosis.

**Z Score.**  This number reflects the amount of bone a person has compared with other people in the same age group and of the same size and gender. If it is unusually high or low, further evaluation could be recommended.

## ✶ Bone Scan

A **bone scan** is a test used to find cancer, infection, fractures, or injuries in the bone and to check a person's response to treatment for certain bone conditions, such as Paget's disease, a condition that destroys bone. See Figure 21–14 ▶.

A bone scan takes about an hour, not including prescan waiting time. A radioactive substance is injected into a vein in the arm of the person having the scan. The test usually begins after a wait of 2 to 3 hours.

Before the test, the person undresses completely and puts on an exam gown. All jewelry and metal objects, including body-piercing jewelry, must be removed so they will not interfere with the exam. A woman is asked if she is pregnant. When the test starts, the person lies flat on his or her back on a table. A special camera is positioned so the entire body can be scanned. Rays from the radioactive substance previously injected into the person are detected by the camera, which sends pictures to a computer.

This test can do the following:

- Show specific areas of irregular bone metabolism, which can suggest certain diseases based on the pattern of abnormality.
- Detect abnormal blood flow to a particular bony region.
- Help evaluate metabolic diseases that affect bones, such as certain thyroid conditions.
- Detect the spread of cancer to the bones and help the physician evaluate results of cancer treatment.

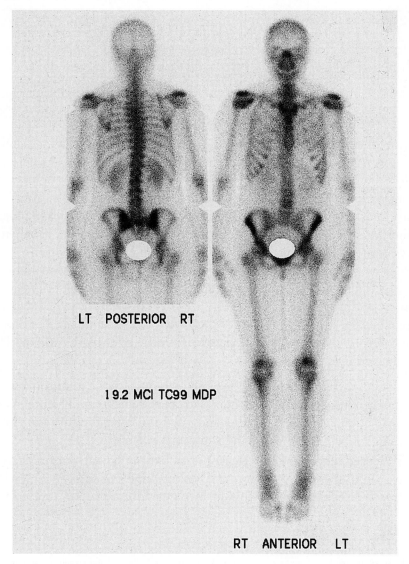

LT   POSTERIOR   RT

1 9.2 MCI TC99 MDP

RT   ANTERIOR   LT

▶ **FIGURE 21–14**   Nuclear medicine bone scan. (Courtesy of Teresa Resch)

- Provide information for the physician to diagnose bone changes from a condition called *reflex sympathetic dystrophy*, a disorder of nerves that causes pain, usually in the hands or feet.

 ★ **Mammography**

**Mammography** is a specific type of imaging that uses a low dose x-ray system for examination of the breasts. A mammography exam is called a *mammogram*. See Figure 21–15 ▶.

The two types of mammograms are *screening*, which is generally used to detect breast cancer or other changes in the breast tissue in women who do not have symptoms, and *diagnostic*, which can be ordered when a screening mammogram shows something abnormal in the breast. A diagnostic mammogram can also be ordered if the woman has symptoms that suggest breast cancer, such as the following:

- Discharge from the nipple other than breast milk.
- Lump or swelling in the breast or underarm area.
- Nipple pain.
- Redness or scaliness of the nipple or breast skin.

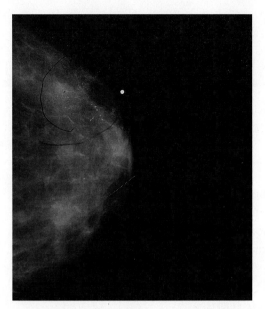

▶ **FIGURE 21–15**   Mammogram showing cancer with microcalcifications. (Courtesy of Teresa Resch)

- Retraction, or turning inward, of the nipple.
- Skin irritation or dimpling.

The American Cancer Society and the National Cancer Institute endorse the following breast cancer screening guidelines:

- Practice monthly breast self-examination (BSE).
- Between the ages of 40 and 49, have breasts examined by a health professional every year and get a mammogram every 1 or 2 years.
- After age 49, have a mammogram (along with a manual breast examination) every year.

Breast cancer screening with mammograms has reduced deaths from breast cancer in women 40 to 69 years of age. A mammogram can detect changes in the breast, such as cancer, often before a lump can be felt. It can also show calcifications, or mineral deposits, cysts, or fluid-filled masses, leaking breast implants, and noncancerous tumors or growths. See Figure 21–15.

During a screening mammography, the woman undresses to the waist and puts on a gown that opens from the front. The technologist places one breast on an x-ray film **cassette,** which resembles a metal shelf. The woman, usually in a standing position, rests her breast on the film cassette. A plastic paddle briefly squeezes the breast from above to flatten it out, allowing a clearer x-ray to be taken. Two views are usually taken of each breast for a screening mammogram. A diagnostic mammogram requires more views and more detail than the screening exam. Modern mammography equipment used specifically for breast x-rays use very low levels of radiation.

Approximately 1,300 men a year are diagnosed with breast cancer. A male who is scheduled for a mammogram may be embarrassed because he could believe that breast cancer is strictly a female disease. The male breast generally does not contain as much adipose tissue as the female breast, so it can be difficult to place the man's breast onto the film holder and obtain the proper amount of compression.

# ✓MEDICAL VOCABULARY CHECKPOINT

*Following is a list of the medical vocabulary that you have seen in the chapter. Review this checklist to make sure that you are familiar with the meaning of each term.*

## Diagnostic Imaging

- ❏ angiocardiogram
- ❏ angiogram
- ❏ angiography
- ❏ arteriography
- ❏ arthrography
- ❏ bronchogram
- ❏ cholangiogram
- ❏ cholecystogram
- ❏ cinematoradiography
- ❏ cineradiography
- ❏ digital subtraction angiography
- ❏ echoencephalography
- ❏ echography
- ❏ fluoroscopy
- ❏ hysterosalpingogram
- ❏ intravenous pyelogram
- ❏ lymphangiogram
- ❏ lymphangiography
- ❏ mammography
- ❏ myelogram
- ❏ radiography
- ❏ scan
- ❏ sialography
- ❏ sonogram

- ❏ thermography
- ❏ tomography
- ❏ ultrasonography
- ❏ venography
- ❏ x-ray

## Associated Terms

- ❏ aplastic anemia
- ❏ barium sulfate
- ❏ barium enema
- ❏ beam
- ❏ cassette
- ❏ cathode
- ❏ cobalt-60
- ❏ contrast medium
- ❏ curie
- ❏ dose
- ❏ film
- ❏ film badge
- ❏ fluorescence
- ❏ ion
- ❏ ionization
- ❏ ionization radiation
- ❏ ionometer
- ❏ ionotherapy
- ❏ ionoradiometer

- ❏ irradiation
- ❏ isotope
- ❏ lead
- ❏ millicurie
- ❏ oscilloscope
- ❏ physicist
- ❏ rad
- ❏ radiation
- ❏ radioactive
- ❏ radiodermatitis
- ❏ radiograph
- ❏ radiographer
- ❏ radiologist
- ❏ radiology
- ❏ radiolucent
- ❏ radionuclide
- ❏ radiopaque
- ❏ radioscopy
- ❏ radium
- ❏ roentgen
- ❏ roentgenology
- ❏ shield
- ❏ tagging
- ❏ ultrasonic

# STUDY AND REVIEW

## Overview of Radiology and Nuclear Medicine

*Write your answers to the following questions. Do not refer to the text.*

1. Define *radiology.* _____

   _____

2. Name three characteristics of x-rays.

   a. _____    b. _____

   c. _____

3. Name two dangers of x-rays.

   a. _____    b. _____

4. List five safety precautions designed to prevent unnecessary exposure to x-rays.

   a. _____    b. _____

   c. _____    d. _____

   e. _____

5. Name five techniques used in diagnostic imaging.

   a. _____    b. _____

   c. _____    d. _____

   e. _____

## Word Parts

1. In the spaces provided, write the definition of these prefixes, roots, combining forms, and suffixes. Do not refer to the listings of medical words. Leave blank those words you cannot define.

2. After completing as many as you can, refer to the medical word listings to check your work. For each word missed or left blank, write the word and its definition several times on the margins of these pages or on a separate sheet of paper.

3. To maximize the learning process, it is to your advantage to do the following exercises as directed. To refer to the word-building section before completing these exercises invalidates the learning process.

## PREFIXES

*Give the definitions of the following prefixes.*

1. sub- _____

2. intra- _____

3. milli- _____

4. ultra- _____

5. ir- (in-) _____

## ROOTS AND COMBINING FORMS

*Give the definitions of the following roots and combining forms.*

1. act _____

2. angi/o _____

3. digit _____

4. arteri/o _____

5. arthr/o _____

6. bronch/o _____

7. cardi/o _____

8. chol _____

9. chole _____

10. cine _____

11. cinemat/o _____

12. tract _____

13. curie _____

14. cyst/o _____

15. dermat _____

16. ech/o _____

17. encephal/o _____

18. fluor/o _____

19. gen/o _____

20. hyster/o _____

21. ion/o _____

22. iont/o _____

23. nucl _____

24. log _____

25. lucent _____

26. lymph _____

27. mamm/o _____

28. myel/o _____

29. oscill/o _____

30. paque _____

31. phot/o _____

32. physic _____

33. pyel/o _____

34. radiat _____

35. radi/o _____

36. roent _____

37. salping/o _____

38. sial/o _____

39. son _____

40. son/o _____

41. therm/o _____

42. tom/o _____

43. ven _____

44. ven/o _____

## SUFFIXES

*Give the definitions of the following suffixes.*

1. -er _____

2. -genic _____

3. -al _____

4. -gram _____

5. -graph _____

6. -graphy _____

7. -ic _____

8. -ion _____

9. -ist _____

10. -itis _____

11. -ive _____

12. -logy _____

13. -meter _____

14. -ous _____

15. -scope _____

16. -scopy _____

17. -therapy _____

18. -ide _____

## Identifying Medical Terms

*In the spaces provided, write the medical terms for the following meanings.*

1. _____ Process of making an x-ray record of blood vessels

2. _____ Process of making an x-ray record of a joint

3. _____ X-ray record of the gallbladder made visible through the use of a radiopaque contrast medium

4. _____ Treatment by introducing ions into the body

5. _____ Process of obtaining x-ray pictures of the breast

6. _____ 0.001 Ci

7. _____ Person who specializes in the science of physics

8. _____ Process whereby radiant energy is propagated through space or matter

9. _____ Caused or produced by radioactivity

10. _____ Person skilled in making x-ray records

11. _____ Pertaining to property of permitting the passage of radiant energy

12. _____ Pertaining to property of obstructing the passage of radiant energy

13. _____ Record produced by ultrasonography

## Spelling

*In the spaces provided, write the correct spelling of these misspelled words.*

1. hystersalpingram _____
2. echgraphy _____
3. lymphangography _____
4. myleogram _____
5. casette _____
6. radiactive _____
7. radigraphy _____
8. silography _____
9. tomgraphy _____
10. vengraphy _____

## Matching

*Select the appropriate lettered meaning for each of the following words.*

_____ 1. betatron

_____ 2. cathode

_____ 3. beam

_____ 4. cassette

_____ 5. rad

_____ 6. lead

_____ 7. radium

_____ 8. scan

_____ 9. shield

_____ 10. tagging

a. Protective structure used to prevent or reduce the passage of particles or radiation
b. Radioactive isotope used to treat certain malignant diseases
c. Ray of light
d. Megavoltage machine used to administer external radiation therapy
e. Negative pole of an electrical current
f. Loss of energy
g. Light-proof case or holder for x-ray film
h. Process of tracing a radioactive isotope that has become involved in metabolic or chemical reactions
i. Process of using a moving device or sweeping beam of radiation to produce images of organs or structures of the body
j. Amount of radiation absorbed
k. Metallic chemical element

## Abbreviations

*Place the correct word, phrase, or abbreviation in the space provided.*

1. anteroposterior _____
2. barium _____
3. computed tomography _____
4. IR _____
5. lat _____
6. Ra _____
7. magnetic resonance imaging _____
8. PA _____
9. curie _____
10. PET _____

# PRACTICAL APPLICATION

## SOAP: Chart Note Analysis

*This exercise will make you aware of the information, abbreviations, and medical terminology typically found in a family practice patient's chart.*

### Abbreviation Key

| | | | |
|---|---|---|---|
| **Abd** | abdomen | **lb** | pound |
| **BP** | blood pressure | **P** | pulse |
| **BSE** | breast self-exam | **R** | respiration |
| **cm** | centimeter | **ROM** | range of motion |
| **CTA** | clear to auscultation | **SOAP** | subjective, objective, assessment, plan |
| **DCIS** | ductal carcinoma in situ | **T** | temperature |
| **DOB** | date of birth | **UOQ** | upper outer quadrant |
| **F** | Fahrenheit | **Wt** | weight |
| **Ht** | height | **y/o** | year(s) old |

*Read the following chart note and then answer the questions that follow.*

**PATIENT:** Calloway, Susan                                    **DATE:** 07/12/2007

**DOB:** 02/28/70        **AGE:** 37        **SEX:** Female

**INSURANCE:** Physicare Health Insurance

**Vital Signs:**

   **T:** 98.4 F

   **P:** 74

   **R:** 20

   **BP:** 138/84

   **Ht:** 5' 6''

   **Wt:** 147 lb

**Allergies:** Penicillin

**Chief Complaint:** Painless mass in left breast, located in the upper outer quadrant

**S** | **Subjective:** 37 y/o white female presents stating, "I was doing my monthly breast exam, you know, just after my period, and I felt this lump in my left breast." Also explaining, "It doesn't hurt, but I am afraid that it might be cancer. There is no history of breast cancer in my immediate family, but I don't know about my aunts. Our family has never been close."

**O** | **Objective:**

**General Appearance:** Apprehensive female with no obvious physical distress. Posture stiff, voice trembling.

**Head:** Normocephalic, no lumps, no lesions, no tenderness.

**Neck:** Supple with full ROM. No pain. Symmetric, no lymphadenopathy or masses noted. Trachea midline, thyroid not palpable.

**Heart:** Regular rate and rhythm. No mumurs, gallops, or rubs.

**Lungs:** CTA.

**Abd:** Bowel sounds in all 4 quadrants. No masses or tenderness noted.

**Breast Exam:**

**Visual inspection:** Bilaterally symmetrical, nipples everted. No lesions, dimpling, retractions, erythema, nipple scaling, or fixation. Axillary and supraclavicular regions without bulging, discoloration, or edema.

**Palpation:** Right breast firm without mass, tenderness or discharge upon expression. Left breast firm with one mass noted in UOQ adjacent to areola at 1 o'clock position. At 3 o'clock position noted another mass. No tenderness or discharge noted upon expression. Both lumps round, firm with smooth discrete borders, and moveable. No axillary lymphadenopathy bilaterally.

**A**　**Assessment:** Ductal carcinoma in situ (DCIS)

**P**　**Plan:** After receiving the results of the mammogram and a fine needle aspiration biopsy, the diagnosis was confirmed.

1. Schedule visit with a general surgeon. Would like Ms. Calloway to be considered for a breast-conserving lumpectomy (left breast), with no axillary dissection. To notify this office of surgery plans.
2. Discuss radiation therapy and explain its benefits.
3. Give the patient a list of radiation oncologists located within driving distance of her home.
4. Review breast self-exam (BSE) techniques with patient and stress the importance of continuing routine exams each month, the week following menses. Explain that this routine allows for familiarity of her breast, which makes changes easier to detect.
5. Educate patient that 70% of breast cancer patients have no family history. Risk increases with 1st or 2nd degree relatives—maternal or paternal: mother, daughter, sister, aunt, grandmother. Risk increases with increased number of incidence.
6. Explain that a mammogram will be scheduled in six months, and she will be notified by letter of the date and time.
7. Schedule a return visit for four weeks to evaluate patient's progress.

**FYI:** Ms. Calloway's mammogram revealed microcalcification clusters in the left breast, one noted in the upper outer quadrant adjacent to the areola measuring 1.5 × 2 cm, and the other lesion in the 3 o'clock position measuring a total of 1.5 × 1.5 cm. A fine needle aspiration biopsy further confirmed the diagnosis by removing a sample of cells examined by a pathologist. DCIS must be removed with clean margins to lower the risk of developing invasive cancer.

*Note:* Radiation therapy is recommended to follow surgery to reduce the risk of regrowth of cancer cells.

## Chart Note Questions

*Place the correct answer in the space provided.*

1. Signs and symptoms of breast cancer in this patient included a painless _____ in her left breast.

2. The diagnosis was determined by a mammogram and confirmed by _____.

3. Where was the mass in the UOQ of the left breast located? _____

4. How did the patient discover the lump? _____

5. What type of surgery was recommended for this patient?

_____

6. What does the abbreviation DCIS mean? _____

7. When and how often does a BSE need to be performed? _____

8. What percentage of breast cancer patients have no family history of breast cancer? _____

9. During the palpation of the right breast, the physician noted that it was _____.

10. Why is radiation therapy recommended for this patient?_____

# MULTIMEDIA PREVIEW

*Additional interactive resources and activities for this chapter can be found on the Companion Website. For videos, audio glossary, and review, access the accompanying CD-ROM in this book.*

 **CD-ROM HIGHLIGHTS**

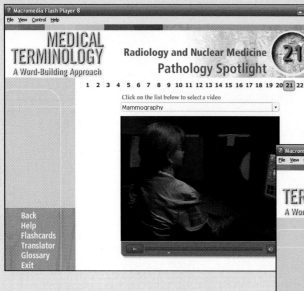

## PATHOLOGY SPOTLIGHT— MAMMOGRAPHY

By viewing concepts in moving, living color, you'll get a fuller picture of the pathologies presented in this chapter. Earlier we discussed mammography. Now click on this feature to watch a video that describes this procedure in more detail.

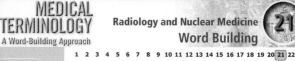

## WORD BUILDING

Are you ready to master the technique of constructing terms using word parts? Put it all together by clicking and dragging the right prefixes, suffixes, roots, and combining forms together to match the definitions provided.

 **WEBSITE HIGHLIGHTS—www.prenhall.com/rice**

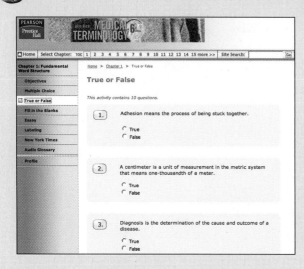

## TRUE/FALSE QUIZ

Take advantage of the free-access on-line study guide that accompanies your textbook. You'll find a true/false quiz that provides instant feedback, allowing you to check your score and see what you got right or wrong. By clicking on this URL you'll also access links to download mp3 audio reviews, current news articles, and an audio glossary.

# Mental Health

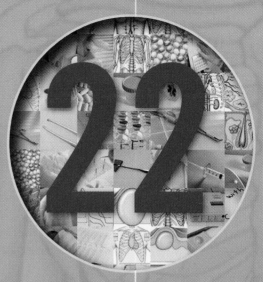

## ■ OUTLINE

## ■ OBJECTIVES

*On completion of this chapter, you will be able to:*

- Define *mental health.*
- Describe mental illness.
- List the six contributing factors that can be part of the cause of mental illness.
- Give the general symptoms that can suggest a mental disorder as seen in adults, adolescents, and younger children.
- Describe the purpose of the *Diagnostic and Statistical Manual of Mental Disorders,* 4th ed. (Text Revision).
- Describe tests used to evaluate a patient's mental health and intelligence.
- Define *psychotherapy,* and describe the various types.
- Describe depression as seen in the child and the older adult.
- Analyze, build, spell, and pronounce medical words.
- Comprehend the drugs highlighted in this chapter.
- Identify and define selected abbreviations.
- Describe each of the conditions presented in the Pathology Spotlights.
- Review the Pathology Checkpoint.
- Complete the Study and Review section and the Chart Note Analysis.

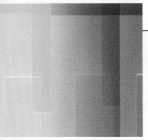

# Overview of Mental Health and Mental Illness

The World Health Organization (WHO) defines **health** as a state of complete physical, mental, and social well-being, not merely the absence of disease or infirmity. It defines **mental health** as a state of well-being in which an individual realizes his or her own abilities, can cope with the normal stresses of life, can work productively and fruitfully, and is able to make a contribution to his or her community.

**Mental illness** is an abnormal condition of the brain or mind. It affects the way a person thinks, feels, behaves, and relates to others and to his or her surroundings. In most cases, the exact cause of mental illness is not known. Contributing factors include genetics, the environment, chemical changes occurring in the brain, use of certain drugs, and psychological, social, and cultural conditions. Most mental health disorders are caused by a combination of factors, such as biologic, psychologic, environmental, and social. See Figure 22–1 ▼. These disorders can be severe, seriously interfere with a person's life, and even cause a person to become disabled.

Many different conditions are classified as mental illnesses. The more common types include mood disorders (depression and bipolar disorder), anxiety disorders, attention-deficit/hyperactivity disorder (AD/HD), eating disorders, schizophrenia, impulse control and addiction disorders, and personality disorders. Other, less common types of mental illnesses include adjustment disorder, dissociative disorders, factitious disorders, sexual and

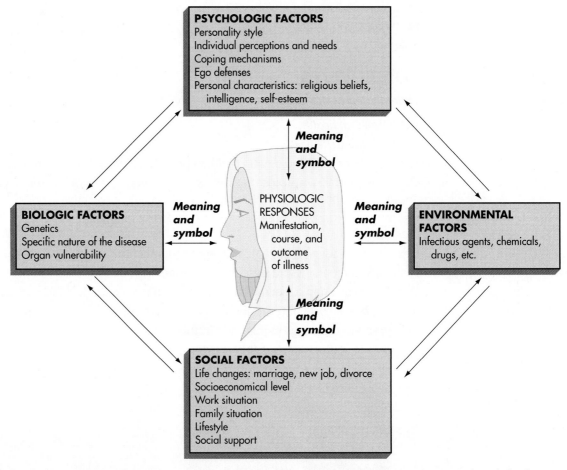

▶ **FIGURE 22–1** Multicausational concept of the illness process. The phrase *meaning and symbol* refers to the fact that a patient interprets all experiences in a highly individual manner according to his or her specific meaning and the broader meaning in the patient's culture.

gender disorders, somatoform disorders, and tic disorders. Various sleep-related problems and some forms of dementia, including Alzheimer's disease (see Chapter 14 on page 478 for information about Alzheimer's disease and dementia), can be classified as mental illnesses because they involve the brain.

According to the U.S. Surgeon General, during a given year, an estimated 44 million adults and about 20% of American children suffer from a mental disorder. About 5 million American adults and more than 5 million children and adolescents suffer from a serious mental condition. Major depression, bipolar disorder, and schizophrenia are among the top ten leading causes of disability in the United States.

# SYMPTOMS OF A MENTAL DISORDER

Symptoms of a mental disorder vary according to the type and severity of the condition and the age of the individual. General symptoms for each age group suggest a mental disorder.

In an adult, these are the following:

- Confused thinking.
- Long-lasting sadness or irritability.
- Extreme highs and lows in mood.
- Excessive fear, worry, or anxiety.
- Social withdrawal.
- Dramatic changes in eating or sleeping patterns.
- Strong feelings of anger.
- Delusion or hallucinations.
- Increasing inability to cope with daily problems and activities.
- Thoughts of suicide.
- Denial of obvious problems.
- Many unexplained physical problems.
- Abuse of drugs and/or alcohol.

In an adolescent, general symptoms that can suggest a mental disorder include these:

- Abuse of drugs and/or alcohol.
- Inability to cope with daily problems and activities.
- Changes in eating or sleeping patterns.
- Excessive complaints of physical problems.
- Defying authority, skipping school, stealing, or damaging property.
- Intense fear of gaining weight.
- Long-lasting negative mood.
- Thoughts of death.
- Frequent outbursts of anger.

In younger children, general symptoms that can suggest a mental disorder include the following:

- Changes in school performance.
- Poor grades despite strong efforts.
- Excessive worry or anxiety.

- Hyperactivity.
- Persistent nightmares.
- Continual disobedience and/or aggressive behavior.
- Frequent temper tantrums.

## DIAGNOSIS OF MENTAL ILLNESS

The standard manual used by experts for the diagnosis of recognized mental illness in the United States is the *Diagnostic and Statistical Manual of Mental Disorders*, 4th ed. (Text Revision (DSM-IV-TR). This official manual of mental health disorders is compiled by the American Psychiatric Association (APA) and identifies categories of adult mental illness. Psychiatrists, psychologists, social workers, and other health care providers use it to understand and diagnose mental health disorders. Insurance companies and health care providers also use it to classify and code mental health disorders for reimbursment of services rendered.

**Psychiatry** is the branch of medicine that deals with the diagnosis, treatment, and prevention of mental illness. A person who specializes in this field of medicine is a **psychiatrist** who is a medical doctor (MD) with specialized training in **psychotherapy** and drug therapy. The psychiatrist can further specialize in the treatment of children (child psychiatry) or in the legal aspects of psychiatry, such as the determination of mental competence in criminal cases (forensic psychiatry). **Psychoanalysts** are psychiatrists with specialized training in **psychoanalysis,** a method of obtaining a detailed account of past and present mental and emotional experiences and repressions.

**Psychology** is the study of the mind. A **psychologist** is a person who is not a medical doctor but has a master's degree or doctor of philosophy (PhD) degree in a specific field of psychology, such as clinical, experimental, or social.

Clinical psychologists are patient-oriented and can use various methods of psychotherapy to treat patients but cannot prescribe medications or electroconvulsive therapy (ECT). They are trained in the use of tests to evaluate various aspects of a patient's mental health and intelligence. Examples are **intelligence quotient** (IQ) tests such as the **Stanford-Binet Intelligence Scale** and the **Wechsler Adult Intelligence Scale** (WAIS). Other tests used are the **Rorschach Inkblot Test** and the **Thematic Apperception Test** (TAT), in which pictures are used as stimuli for the patient to create stories. The **Minnesota Multiphasic Personality Inventory** (MMPI) consists of true-false questions that can reveal aspects of personality, such as dominance, sense of duty or responsibility, and ability to relate to others; it is used as an objective measure of psychological disorders in adolescents and adults. A patient's responses to the questions can be compared with responses made by individuals with diagnoses of schizophrenia, depression, and many other mental disorders.

Psychiatrists and psychologists also use specially designed interview and assessment tools to evaluate a person for a mental illness. The therapist bases the diagnosis on the person's report of symptoms, including any social or functional problems caused by the symptoms. The therapist then determines whether the person's symptoms and degree of disability indicate a diagnosis of a specific disorder.

## TREATMENTS FOR MENTAL ILLNESS

The three basic forms of treatment for mental illness are **drug therapy, psychotherapy,** and **electroconvulsive therapy.**

## Drug Therapy

Drugs that are generally used to treat mental disorders include anti-anxiety agents, antidepressant agents, antimanic agents, and antipsychotic agents. Drugs used for attention-deficit/hyperactivity disorder include stimulants. See Drug Highlights on page 756 for more information on drug therapy for mental disorders.

## Psychotherapy

*Psychotherapy* is a method of treating mental disorders using psychological techniques instead of physical methods. It involves talking, interpreting, listening, rewarding, and role-playing. Psychotherapy should be performed by a trained mental health professional, such as a psychiatrist, psychologist, social worker, or counselor.

Types of psychotherapy include cognitive-behavioral therapy, family therapy, group therapy, play therapy, art therapy, hypnosis, and psychoanalysis.

- **Cognitive-behavioral therapy** (CBT) has two components. The cognitive component helps people change thinking patterns that keep them from overcoming their fears. The behavioral component seeks to change people's reactions to anxiety-provoking situations. A key element of this component is exposure, in which people confront the things they fear. Research has shown that CBT is an effective form of psychotherapy for several anxiety disorders, particularly panic disorder and social phobia.
- **Family therapy** involves an entire family. The focus is on resolving and understanding conflicts and problems as a *family* situation, not just as an individual member's problem.
- **Group therapy** involves small groups of people with similar problems attending meetings together. There are discussions and interactions between group participants; a therapist helps to focus and guide the therapy sessions.
- **Play therapy** involves a child using toys, such as dolls and puppets, to express thoughts, feelings, fantasies, and conflicts. Because most emotionally disturbed children will not talk about their problems, play therapy provides an alternative method to encourage children to open up about what is troubling them. Children reveal themselves when they play with toys provided by the therapist and often act out their problems (see Figure 22–2 ▼).

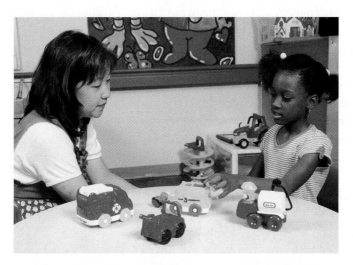

▶ **FIGURE 22–2** Psychologist using play therapy to help Cassandra reenact her car crash. This helps her gain control over the event so that it is not so frightening.

- **Art therapy** can be used to encourage a child to portray his or her feelings in drawings. When asked to draw the family or a picture of himself or herself, information about the child, the family, and their interactions can be revealed.

- **Hypnosis** is a state of altered consciousness, usually artificially induced, used in treating mental illness by lessening the mind's unconscious defenses and allowing some patients to be able to recall and even re-experience important childhood events that have long been forgotten or repressed. Historically, Dr. Sigmund Freud, a noted Austrian neurologist and psychoanalyst, developed the theory of the unconscious as a result of his experiments with a hypnotized patient.

- **Psychoanalysis** is a method of obtaining a detailed account of past and present mental and emotional experiences and repressions. It also was developed by Dr. Freud. Psychoanalysis attempts, through free association and dream interpretation, to reveal and resolve the unconscious conflicts that are considered to be at the root of some mental illnesses. It is believed that these conflicts have been repressed since childhood and after being brought to the conscious level can be resolved.

## Electroconvulsive Therapy

**Electroconvulsive therapy** (ECT) is the use of an electric shock to produce convulsions. It is useful for individuals whose depression is severe or life threatening, particularly for those who cannot take antidepressant medication. In recent years, ECT has been much improved. A muscle relaxant is given to the patient before treatment, which is performed under brief anesthesia. Electrodes are placed at precise locations on the head to deliver electrical impulses. The stimulation causes a brief (about 30-second) seizure within the brain. The person receiving ECT does not consciously experience the electrical stimulus. For full therapeutic benefit, at least several sessions of ECT, typically given at the rate of three per week, are required.

# LIFE SPAN CONSIDERATIONS

## ■ THE CHILD

Only in the past two decades has **depression** in children been taken very seriously. The depressed child can pretend to be sick, refuse to go to school, cling to a parent, or worry that the parent could die. Older children sulk; get into trouble at school; and are negative, grouchy, and feel misunderstood. Because normal behaviors vary from one childhood stage to another, it can be difficult to tell whether a child is just going through a temporary phase or suffering from depression. Sometimes the parents become worried about how the child's behavior has changed, or a teacher comments, "Jason doesn't seem to be himself." If a visit to the child's pediatrician rules out physical causes, the doctor is likely to suggest that a psychiatrist who specializes in the treatment of children evaluate the child.

## Symptoms of Depression in the Child

Symptoms in different age groups follow.

**Toddlers.** Sadness, inactivity, complaints of stomachaches, and, in rare cases, self-destructive behavior.

**Elementary-school-age children.** Unhappiness, poor school performance, irritability, refusal to take part in activities he or she used to enjoy, and occasional thoughts of suicide.

**Adolescents.** Sadness, withdrawal, feelings of hopelessness or guilt, changes in sleeping or eating habits, and frequent thoughts of suicide.

A child does not understand feelings of stress, anxiety, or depression and does not know how to ask for help, so when a child exhibits dramatic mood or behavior shifts, a physician should be consulted immediately. The physician could recommend psychotherapy or prescribe an antidepressant for children who are at least five years of age or older.

The National Institute of Mental Health (NIMH) has identified the use of medications for depression in children as an important area for research. The NIMH-supported Research Units on Pediatric Psychopharmacology (RUPPs) form a network of seven research sites where clinical studies on the effects of medications for mental disorders can be conducted on children and adolescents. Among the medications being studied are antidepressants, some of which have been found to be effective in treating children with depression if properly monitored by the child's physician.

## ■ THE OLDER ADULT

Older Americans are disproportionately likely to die by suicide. Although individuals age 65 and older compose only 13% of the U.S. population, they accounted for 18% of all suicide deaths in 2000. Among the highest rates (when categorized by gender and race) were white men age 85 and older: 59 deaths per 100,000 persons in 2000, more than five times the national rate of 10.6 per 100,000. Of those who commit suicide, 90% suffer from depression or a diagnosable mental or substance abuse disorder. Clearly, depression is a serious problem in the elderly.

Of the nearly 35 million Americans age 65 and older, an estimated 2 million have a depressive illness (major depression; dysthymia, which is moderate but long-term; chronic depression; or bipolar disorder), and another 5 million may have **subsyndromal depression,** or depressive symptoms that fall short of meeting full diagnostic criteria for a depressive illness. Subsyndromal depression is especially common among older persons and is associated with an increased risk of developing major depression.

In any of these forms, however, depressive symptoms are *not* a normal part of aging. In contrast to the normal emotional experiences of sadness, grief, loss, or passing mood states, some depressive symptoms tend to be persistent and to interfere significantly with an individual's ability to function. A loss of interest in food, sex, work, family, friends, and hobbies should be noted in an older person.

Depression often co-occurs with other serious illnesses such as heart disease, stroke, diabetes, cancer, and Parkinson's disease. Because many older adults face these illnesses as well as various social and economic difficulties, health care professionals often mistakenly conclude that depression is a normal consequence of these problems—an attitude often shared by patients themselves. These factors together contribute to the underdiagnosis and undertreatment of depressive disorders in older people. See Figure 22–3 ▶. Depression can and should be treated when it co-occurs with other illnesses because untreated depression can delay recovery from or worsen the outcome of other illnesses.

If a diagnosis of depression is made, treatment with medication and/or psychotherapy will help the depressed person return to a happier, more fulfilling life. Recent research suggests that brief **psychotherapy** is effective in reducing symptoms in short-term depression in older persons who are medically ill. Psychotherapy is also useful in older patients who cannot or will not take medication. Improved recognition and treatment of depression in later life will make those years more enjoyable and fulfilling for the depressed older person, the family, and caregivers.

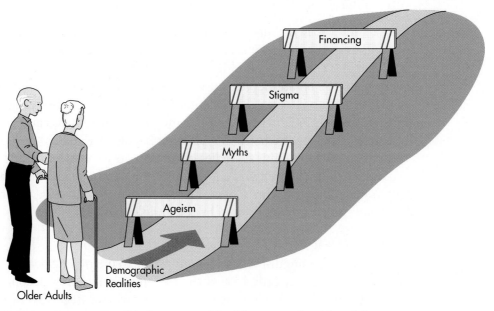

Mental health services

**FIGURE 22–3**   Roadblocks to mental health services for older adults.

# BUILDING YOUR MEDICAL VOCABULARY

This section provides the foundation for learning medical terminology. Review the following alphabetized word list. Note how common prefixes and suffixes are repeatedly applied to word roots and combining forms to create different meanings.

| | | | | |
|---|---|---|---|---|
| **P** | Prefix | | Pink words | Terms not built from word parts. |
| **R** | Root | | ✳ | Indicates words covered in the Pathology Spotlights section. |
| **CF** | Combining form | | | |
| **S** | Suffix | | 💿 | Check the CD-ROM for more information. |

| MEDICAL WORD | WORD PARTS (WHEN APPLICABLE) | | | DEFINITION |
|---|---|---|---|---|
| | **Part** | **Type** | **Meaning** | |
| **affect**<br>(ăf'fěkt) | | | | In psychology, observable evidence of an individual's emotional reaction associated with an experience |
| **affective disorder**<br>(ă f-fěk'tīv dĭs-ōr' děr) | | | | Characterized by a disturbance of mood accompanied by a manic or depressive syndrome; this syndrome is not caused by any other physical or mental disorder |
| **agoraphobia**<br>(ăg" ō-ră-fō' bĭ ă) | agor/a<br>-phobia | CF<br>S | marketplace<br>fear | Abnormal fear of being in public places; fear of leaving the safety of home; an anxiety syndrome and panic disorder |

| MEDICAL WORD | WORD PARTS (WHEN APPLICABLE) | | | DEFINITION |
|---|---|---|---|---|
| | **Part** | **Type** | **Meaning** | |
| **anorexia nervosa**<br>(ăn"ō-rĕk-sē-ă nĕr-vō-să) | an-<br>-orexia | P<br>S | lack of, without<br>appetite | Complex psychological disorder in which the individual refuses to eat or has an abnormally limited eating pattern. People with eating disorders may engage in self-induced vomiting and abuse of laxatives, diuretics, or prolonged exercise to control their weight. The condition could lead them to become excessively thin or even emaciated. In severe cases, this condition can be life threatening. See Figure 22–4 ▼. |
| **anxiety**<br>(ăng-zī'ĕ-tē) | | | | Feeling of uneasiness, apprehension, worry, or dread; involuntary or reflex reaction of the body to stress |
| **anxiety disorders**<br>(ăng-zī'ĕ-tē) | | | | Serious mental illnesses that affect approximately 19 million American adults. Anxiety disorders share the common theme of excessive, irrational fear and dread and are chronic, growing progressively worse if not treated. See Figure 22–5 ▼ for physiologic responses in anxiety disorders. ✱ See Pathology Spotlights for information on panic |

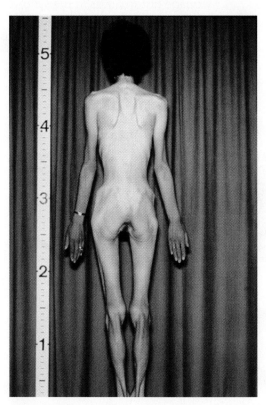

▶ **FIGURE 22–4**   Emaciated young woman with anorexia nervosa. (Source: Custom Medical Stock Photo, Inc.)

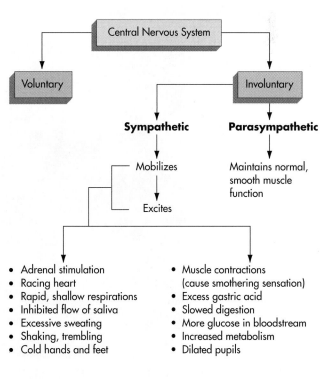

▶ **FIGURE 22–5**   Physiologic responses in anxiety disorders.

| MEDICAL WORD | WORD PARTS (WHEN APPLICABLE) | | | DEFINITION |
|---|---|---|---|---|
| | Part | Type | Meaning | |
| | | | | disorder (page 761), obsessive-compulsive disorder (page 761), post-traumatic stress disorder (page 762), social phobia (page 763), and generalized anxiety disorder (page 760). |
| **apathy** (ăp′ă-thē) | | | | Condition in which a person lacks feelings and emotions and is indifferent |
| **apperception** (ăp″ĕr-sĕp′shŭn) | | | | Comprehension or assimilation of the meaning and significance of a particular sensory stimulus as modified by an individual's own experiences, knowledge, thoughts, and emotions |
| **attention-deficit/ hyperactivity disorder (AD/HD)** | | | | Chronic condition marked by inattention, impulsivity, and hyperactivity. It is the most commonly diagnosed behavioral disorder among children and adolescents and often continues into adulthood. ✳ See Pathology Spotlight: Attention-Deficit/Hyperactivity Disorder on page 758. |
| **autism** (ŏ′tĭzm) | aut -ism | R S | self condition | Mental disorder in which the individual may be self-absorbed, inaccessible, unable to relate to others, and has language disturbances. It is a syndrome usually beginning in infancy and becoming apparent in the first or second year of life. See Figure 22–6 ▼. |

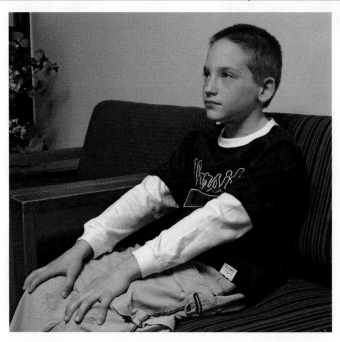

▶ **FIGURE 22–6**   This child with autism sits stiffly in the chair. He has a disengaged look and does not readily interact with other children or adults who are in his environment.

| MEDICAL WORD | WORD PARTS (WHEN APPLICABLE) | | | DEFINITION |
|---|---|---|---|---|
| | Part | Type | Meaning | |
| **bipolar disorder**<br>(bī-pōl'ăr dĭs-ōr' dĕr) | | | | Brain disorder also known as *manic-depressive illness* that causes unusual shifts in a person's mood, energy, and ability to function. ✶ See Pathology Spotlight: Bipolar Disorder on page 759. |
| **compulsion**<br>(kŏm-pŭl'ŭn) | | | | Uncontrollable, recurrent, and distressing urge to perform an act in order to relieve fear connected with obsession. Common compulsions involve excessive handwashing, touching objects, and continual counting and checking. ✶ See Pathology Spotlight: Obsessive-Compulsive Disorder on page 761. |
| **cyclothymic disorder**<br>(sī"klŏ-thī'mĭk dĭs-ōr' dĕr) | cycl/o<br>thym<br>-ic | CF<br>R<br>S | circle, cycle<br>mind, emotion<br>pertaining to | Mood disorder characterized by alternating moods of elation and depression, similar to bipolar disorder but of milder intensity |
| **delirium**<br>(dē-lĭr' ĭ-ŭm) | | | | State of mental confusion marked by illusions, hallucinations, excitement, restlessness, delusions, and speech incoherence |
| **delusion**<br>(dē-loo'zhŭn) | delus<br>-ion | R<br>S | to cheat<br>process | Occurrence of bizarre thoughts that have no basis in reality; a fixed, false belief or abnormal perception held by a person despite evidence to the contrary |
| **dementia**<br>(dē-mĕn' shē-ă) | | | | Problem in the brain that makes it difficult for a person to remember, learn and communicate and eventually to take care of himself or herself; can also affect a person's mood and personality. Dementia of the Alzheimer's type is the most common form. See Chapter 14 on page 478 for more information about this condition. |
| **depression**<br>(dē-prĕsh'ŭn) | | | | Mental disorder marked by altered mood and loss of interest in things that are usually pleasurable such as food, sex, work, friends, hobbies, or entertainment. See Figure 22–7 ▶. ✶ See Pathology Spotlight: Depression on page 760. |
| **dissociation**<br>(dĭs-sō"sē-ā'shun) | | | | Defense mechanism in which a group of mental processes become separated from normal consciousness and, thus separated, function as a unitary whole. In *dissociative disorder* there is a severe disturbance or trauma that causes changes in memory, consciousness, identity, and general awareness of oneself and one's environment. There are four primary types of dissociative |

| MEDICAL WORD | WORD PARTS (WHEN APPLICABLE) | | | DEFINITION |
|---|---|---|---|---|
| | Part | Type | Meaning | |
| | | | | disorders: **psychogenic amnesia, psychogenic fugue, multiple personality disorder**, and **depersonalization disorder**. |
| **eating disorder** | | | | Health condition characterized by a preoccupation with weight that results in severe disturbances in eating behavior; *anorexia nervosa* and *bulimia* are the most common types. According to the APA, between 0.5% and 3.7% of females experience anorexia nervosa, and between 1.1% and 4.2% of females experience bulimia in their lifetime. |
| **egocentric** (ē″ gō-sĕn′ trĭk) | ego centr -ic | CF R S | I, self center pertaining to | Pertaining to being self-centered |
| **factitious disorder** (făk-tĭsh′ŭs dĭs-ōr′dĕr) | | | | Disorder that is not real, genuine, or natural. The physical and psychological symptoms are produced by the person to place himself or herself or another in the role of a patient or someone in need of help. These patients have a severe personality disturbance. **Munchausen's syndrome** is a chronic factitious disorder in which a healthy person habitually seeks medical treatment; in the rare **Munchausen by proxy syndrome** (MBPS), a parent (usually the mother) or other caregiver is the deliberate cause of a child's illness (by poisoning, for instance) to gain sympathy or attention. |

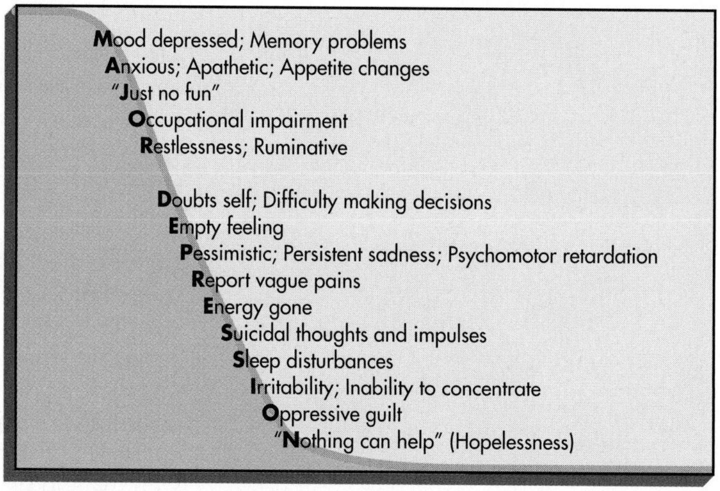

**M**ood depressed; Memory problems
**A**nxious; Apathetic; Appetite changes
"**J**ust no fun"
**O**ccupational impairment
**R**estlessness; Ruminative

**D**oubts self; Difficulty making decisions
**E**mpty feeling
**P**essimistic; Persistent sadness; Psychomotor retardation
**R**eport vague pains
**E**nergy gone
**S**uicidal thoughts and impulses
**S**leep disturbances
**I**rritability; Inability to concentrate
**O**ppressive guilt
"**N**othing can help" (Hopelessness)

▶ **FIGURE 22–7** Characteristics of major depression.

| MEDICAL WORD | WORD PARTS (WHEN APPLICABLE) | | | DEFINITION |
|---|---|---|---|---|
| | **Part** | **Type** | **Meaning** | |
| **fugue**<br>(fūg) | | | | Dissociative disorder in which amnesia is accompanied by physical flight from customary surroundings. In psychogenic fugue, there is sudden, unexpected travel away from an individual's home or place of work with inability to recall the past. The individual can assume a partial or completely new identity. This condition is usually of short duration but can last for months. Following recovery, the person does not recall anything that happened during the fugue. |
| **generalized anxiety disorder (GAD)** | | | | Characterized by much higher levels of anxiety than people normally experience day to day. It is chronic and fills a person's day with exaggerated worry and tension. Having this disorder means always anticipating disaster, often worrying excessively about health, money, family, or work. ✳ See Pathology Spotlight: Generalized Anxiety Disorder on page 760. |
| **hallucination**<br>(hă-loo-sĭ-nā′shŭn) | hallucinat<br>-ion | R<br>S | to wander in mind<br>process | Process of experiencing sensations that have no source. Some examples of hallucinations include hearing nonexistent voices, seeing nonexistent things, and experiencing burning or pain sensations with no physical cause. |
| **hypomania**<br>(hī″pō-mā′nē-ă) | hypo-<br>-mania | P<br>S | deficient, below<br>madness | Abnormal mood of mild mania characterized by hyperactivity, inflated self-esteem, talkativeness, heightened sexual interest, quickness to anger, irritability, and a decreased need for sleep. ✳ See Pathology Spotlight: Bipolar Disorder on page 759. |
| **impulse control disorder** | | | | Mental condition in which the person is unable to resist urges or impulses to perform acts that could be harmful to himself, herself, or others. **Pyromania** (starting fires), **kleptomania** (stealing), and compulsive gambling are examples of impulse control disorders. |
| **mania**<br>(mă′nē-ă) | | | | Mental disorder characterized by excessive excitement; literally means *madness* |
| **mood** | | | | Pervasive and sustained emotion that plays a key role in an individual's perception of the world. Examples include depression, joy, elation, anger, and anxiety. |

| MEDICAL WORD | WORD PARTS (WHEN APPLICABLE) | | | DEFINITION |
|---|---|---|---|---|
| | **Part** | **Type** | **Meaning** | |
| **neurotic**<br>(nŭ-rōt′ĭk) | neur/o<br>-tic | CF<br>S | nerve<br>pertaining to | Pertaining to one who has an abnormal emotional or mental disorder |
| **norepinephrine**<br>(nor-ĕpĭ-nĕf′rīn) | | | | Hormone produced by the adrenal medulla that acts as a neurotransmitter. It is believed that disturbances in its metabolism at important brain sites can be implicated in affective disorders. |
| **obsession** | | | | Neurotic state in which an individual has a recurrent, persistent thought, image, or impulse that is unwanted and distressing and comes involuntarily to mind despite attempts to resist. ✱ See Pathology Spotlight: Obsessive-Compulsive Disorder on page 761. |
| **paranoia**<br>(păr″ ă-noy′ ă) | para-<br>-noia | P<br>S | beside, abnormal<br>mind | Mental disorder characterized by highly exaggerated or unwarranted mistrust or suspiciousness; generally classified into 3 categories: *paranoid personality disorder, delusional (paranoid) disorder,* and *paranoid schizophrenia.* Delusional (paranoid) disorder is characterized by persistent delusions of persecution or grandeur, or a combination of the two. |
| **personality disorder** | | | | Mental disorder characterized by inflexible and maladaptive personality traits that are distressing to the person and/or cause problems in work, school or social relationships. In addition, the person's pattern of thinking and behavior significantly differ from the expectations of society and are so rigid that he or she does not function well. Examples include **antisocial personality disorder, narcissistic personality disorder, obsessive-compulsive disorder, paranoid disorder,** and **schizoid personality disorder.** |
| **phobia**<br>(fō′ bē-ă) | | | | Morbid and persistent fear of a specific object, activity, or situation that results in a compelling desire to avoid the feared stimulus. Examples include **claustrophobia** (fear of enclosed places), **acrophobia** (fear of heights), **photophobia** (fear of light), **arachnophobia** (fear of spiders), **nyctophobia** (fear of darkness/night), and **hematophobia** or **hemophobia** (fear of blood/bleeding). |

| MEDICAL WORD | WORD PARTS (WHEN APPLICABLE) | | | DEFINITION |
|---|---|---|---|---|
| | Part | Type | Meaning | |
| **post-traumatic stress disorder (PTSD)** | | | | Debilitating mental and emotional condition that can develop following a terrifying event. ✳ See Pathology Spotlight: Post-traumatic Stress Disorder on page 762. |
| **psychiatrist** (sī-kī′ ă-trĭst) | psych iatr -ist | R R S | mind treatment one who specializes | Physician who specializes in the study, treatment, and prevention of mental disorders |
| **psychoanalysis** (sī″ kō-ă-năl′ĭ-sĭs) | | | | Method of investigating the mental processes of an individual using the techniques of free association, interpretation, and dream analysis |
| **psychologist** (sī-kŏl′ ō-jĭst) | psych/o log -ist | CF R S | mind study of one who specializes | Person who specializes in the study of the mind |
| **psychology** (sī-kŏl′ ō-jē) | psych/o -logy | CF S | mind study of | Study of the mind |
| **psychopath** (sī′ kō-păth) | psych/o path | CF R | mind disease | Mentally ill individual with an antisocial personality disorder; also called *sociopath* |
| **psychosis** (sī-kō′ sĭs) | psych -osis | R S | mind condition (usually abnormal) | Serious, abnormal mental condition in which the individual's mental capacity to recognize reality and communicate with and relate to others is impaired; the person can experience delusions and hallucinations |
| **psychosomatic** (si″ kō-sō-măt′ ĭk) | psych/o somat -ic | CF R S | mind body pertaining to | Pertaining to the interrelationship of the mind and the body |
| **psychotherapy** (sī′ kō-thěr′ă-pē) | psych/o -therapy | CF S | mind treatment | Method of treating mental disorders by using psychological techniques instead of physical methods; may involve talking, interpreting, listening, rewarding, and role-playing |
| **psychotropic** (sī′kō-trŏ″ĭk) | | | | Drug that affects psychic function, behavior, or experience |
| **pyromania** (pī″ rō-mā′(nĭ-ă) | pyro- -mania | P S | fire madness | Impulsive disorder consisting of a compulsion to set fires or to watch fires; literally means a *madness for fire*; person suffering from this disorder (pyromaniac) receives pleasure and emotional relief from these activities |
| **schizophrenia** (skĭz″ō-frěn′ē-ă) | schiz/o phren -ia | CF R S | to divide mind condition | Mental disorder characterized by *positive* and *negative* symptoms. Positive (psychotic), symptoms include delusions, hallucinations, and disordered thinking (apparent from a person's fragmented, disconnected, and sometimes nonsensical speech). Negative symptoms |

| MEDICAL WORD | WORD PARTS (WHEN APPLICABLE) | | | DEFINITION |
|---|---|---|---|---|
| | Part | Type | Meaning | |
| | | | | include social withdrawal, extreme apathy, diminished motivation, and blunted emotional expression. ✳ See Pathology Spotlight: Schizophrenia on page 762. |
| **seasonal affective disorder (SAD)** | | | | Form of depression that appears related to fluctuations in a person's exposure to natural light; usually strikes during autumn and often continues through the winter when natural light is reduced. Researchers have found that people who have SAD can be helped if they spend blocks of time bathed in light from a special full-spectrum light source called a *light box.* |
| **serotonin** (sĕr″ō-tōn′ĭn) | | | | Chemical present in gastrointestinal mucosa, platelets, mast cells, and carcinoid tumors; a vasoconstrictor and a neurotransmitter in the central nervous system (CNS); and affects sleep and sensory perception |
| **sexual disorders** | | | | Disorders that affect sexual desire, performance, and behavior. **Sexual dysfunction, gender identity disorder** (characterized by a persistent discomfort concerning one's anatomic sexual makeup and the desire to live as a member of the opposite sex), and **paraphilias** are examples. In paraphilia, sexual arousal requires unusual or bizarre fantasies or acts involving nonhuman objects, sexual activity with humans in which real or simulated suffering or humiliation occurs, or sexual activity with nonconsenting partners. Included in this disorder are **bestiality, fetishism, transvestism, zoophilia, pedophilia, exhibitionism, voyeurism, sexual masochism,** and **sexual sadism.** |
| **somatoform disorder** (sŏ-măt′ō-fŏrm dĭs-ōr′ dĕr) | somat/o -form | CF S | body shape | Mental disorder, previously known as *psychosomatic disorder,* in which the person experiences physical symptoms of an illness that are not explained by medical condition or medication. Included in this disorder are **body dysmorphic disorder** (BDD), which involves a disturbed body image; **hypochondriasis,** which is a preoccupation with fears of having or the belief that one has a serious disease based on misinterpretation of bodily |

| MEDICAL WORD | WORD PARTS (WHEN APPLICABLE) | | | DEFINITION |
|---|---|---|---|---|
| | Part | Type | Meaning | |
| | | | | symptoms; **somatization disorder,** a chronic condition in which there are numerous physical complaints; **conversion disorder,** in which emotional distress or unconscious conflicts are expressed through physical symptoms; and **somatoform pain disorder,** in which persistent and chronic pain is experienced by a person in the absence of physiologic causes. |
| **substance abuse** | | | | Misuse of medications, alcohol, or illegal substances |
| **suicide** | | | | Willfully ending one's own life. Suicide is the 8th leading cause of death in the United States, claiming about 30,000 lives a year, and suicide attempts are among the leading causes of hospital admissions in persons under 35. Of persons who commit or attempt suicide, 90% have depression or another diagnosable mental or substance abuse disorder. |
| **tic disorder** (tĭk dĭs-ōr′ dĕr) | | | | Characterized by spasmodic muscular contractions most commonly involving the face, mouth, eyes, head, neck, or shoulder muscles. People with tic disorders make sounds or display body movements that are repeated, quick, sudden, and/or uncontrollable. In general, tics are of psychological origin. |

# DRUG HIGHLIGHTS

| | |
|---|---|
| **Antianxiety agents** | Chemical substances that relieve anxiety and muscle tension are indicated when anxiety interferes with a person's ability to function properly. |
| Benzodiazepines | The *benzodiazepines* are a group of drugs with similar chemical structures and pharmaceutical activities. They are the most widely prescribed drugs for the treatment of anxiety. |
| | *Examples: Xanax (alprazolam), Klonopin (clonazepam), Tranxene (clorazepate), Librium (chlordiazepoxide HCl), Valium (diazepam), Ativan (lorazepam), and Serax (oxazepam)* |
| Azipirones | Antianxiety medication used to treat generalized anxiety disorder (GAD). Possible side effects include dizziness, headaches, and nausea. Unlike the benzodiazepines, buspirone must be taken consistently for at least two weeks to achieve an antianxiety effect. |
| | *Example: BuSpar (buspirone)* |
| **Antidepressant agents** | Chemical substances that relieve the symptoms of depression are indicated when depression interferes with a person's ability to function properly. Antidepressant agents can be grouped as SSRIs, SNRIs, TCAs, or MAOIs. |
| Selective serotonin reuptake inhibitor (SSRIs) | Drugs in this group specifically block reabsorption of serotonin. |
| | *Examples: Prozac (fluoxetine), Zoloft (sertraline), Paxil (paroxetine), and Luvox (fluvoxamine)* |
| Serotonin-norepinephrine reuptake inhibitor (SNRIs) | Drugs in this group block the reabsorption of serotonin and norepinephrine. |
| | *Example: Effexor (venlafaxine).* |
| Tricyclic antidepressants (TCAs) | Drugs in this group raise the level of norepinephrine and serotonin in the brain by slowing the rate at which they are reabsorbed by nerve cells. |
| | *Examples: Tofranil (imipramine), Pamelor (nortriptyline), and Asendin (amoxapine)* |
| Monoamine oxidase inhibitors (MAOIs) | Drugs in this group work by blocking the breakdown of two potent neurotransmitters—norepinephrine and serotonin—and by allowing them to bathe the nerve endings for an extended length of time. |
| | *Examples: Nardil (phenelzine) and Parnate (tranylcypromine).* |
| **Lithium carbonate** | Although not a group of drugs, various lithium medications control mood disorders by directly affecting internal nerve cell processes in all of the neurotransmitter systems. Lithium is best known as an antimanic drug used in the treatment of bipolar disorder. |
| | *Example: Eskalith (lithium carbonate).* |
| **Miscellaneous drugs** | Many newly created drugs treat depression. Some of these drugs are used for other illnesses and are being tested for treating depression; others do not fit into any of the described groups. |
| | *Examples: Mirapex (pramipexole), Serzone (nefazodone), Wellbutrin (bupropion), and Remeron (mirtazapine).* |
| **Antipsychotic agents** | Called *neuroleptics*, these agents modify psychotic behavior. Many antipsychotic agents are derivatives of phenothiazine (an organic compound used in the manufacture of certain of these drugs). These agents are used in the treatment of acute and chronic schizophrenia, organic psychoses, the manic phase of bipolar disorder, and psychotic disorders. |
| | *Example: Thorazine (chlorpromazine HCl). Some antipsychotic agents are not actually phenothiazines but resemble them in action. Others resemble tricyclic antidepressants, while some are miscellaneous compounds.* |
| | *Examples: Clozaril (clozapine), Zyprexa (olanzapine), Loxitane (loxapine), and Orap (pimozide).* |

| | |
|---|---|
| **Atypical antipsychotics** | Drugs in this group affect serotonin and dopamine. *Examples: Risperdal (risperidone), Clozaril (clozapine), and Syprexa (olanzapine).* |
| **Stimulants** | These drugs stimulate the central nervous system (CNS) and are generally prescribed for attention-deficit/hyperactivity disorder. Patients using these drugs must take care to avoid abuse and excessive CNS stimulation by overdose. Many of these drugs are Schedule II agents with very high potential for abuse. *Examples: Dexedrine (dextroamphetamine sulfate), Ritalin (methylphenidate HCl), and Adderall, which is a combination of amphetamine salts.* |

# ABBREVIATIONS

| ABBREVIATION | MEANING | ABBREVIATION | MEANING |
|---|---|---|---|
| AD/HD | attention-deficit/hyperactivity disorder | NIH | National Institutes of Health |
| APA | American Psychiatric Association | NIMH | National Institute of Mental Health |
| BDD | body dysmorphic disorder | OCD | obsessive-compulsive disorder |
| CBT | cognitive-behavioral therapy | PhD | doctor of philosophy (also doctor of pharmacy) |
| CNS | central nervous system | PTSD | post-traumatic stress disorder |
| DSM-IV-TR | *Diagnostic and Statistical Manual of Mental Disorders,* 4th ed. (Text Revision) | RUPPs | Research Units on Pediatric Psychopharmacology |
| ECT | electroconvulsive therapy | SAD | seasonal affective disorder |
| GAD | generalized anxiety disorder | SNRI | serotonin-norepinephrine reuptake inhibitor |
| HHS | Department of Health and Human Services | SSRIs | selective serotonin reuptake inhibitors |
| IQ | intelligence quotient | | |
| MAOIs | monoamine oxidase inhibitor | TAT | Thematic Apperception Test |
| MD | medical doctor | TCAs | tricyclic antidepressants |
| MMPI | Minnesota Multiphasic Personality Inventory | WAIS | Wechster Adult Intelligence Scale |
| MBPS | Munchausen by proxy syndrome | WHO | World Health Organization |

# PATHOLOGY SPOTLIGHTS

*Please note that the following information on mental disorders has been adapted from the National Institute of Mental Health (NIMH), which is a component of the National Institutes of Health (NIH), a part of the U.S. Department of Health and Human Services (HHS).*

## ✴ Attention-Deficit/Hyperactivity Disorder

Children with **attention-deficit/hyperactivity disorder** (AD/HD), one of the most common of the psychiatric disorders that appear in childhood, cannot stay focused on a task, cannot sit still, act without thinking, and rarely finish anything. AD/HD affects an estimated 4.1% of youths ages 9 to 17, and about 2 to 3 times more boys than girls are affected. AD/HD often co-occurs with other problems, such as depressive and anxiety disorders, conduct disorder, drug abuse, or antisocial behavior. Children with untreated AD/HD have higher than normal rates of injury, and the disorder can have long-term effects on a child's ability to make friends or do well at school or work. Over time, children with AD/HD can develop depression, poor self-esteem, and other emotional problems. The disorder frequently persists into adolescence and affects between 2% to 4% of adults. More than 50% of those who took medication for AD/HD as children still need medication as adults.

The three different types of attention-deficit/hyperactivity disorder are inattentive, hyperactive-impulsive, and combined attention-deficit/hyperactivity disorder. The most common type is combined attention-deficit/hyperactivity disorder, which, as the name implies, is a combination of the inattentive and the hyperactive-impulsive types. Children with combined attention-deficit/hyperactivity disorder can

Have short attention spans.

Not pay attention to details.

Make many mistakes.

Fail to finish things.

Have trouble remembering things.

Not seem to listen.

Not be able to stay organized.

Fidget and squirm.

Be unable to stay seated or play quietly.

Be distracted easily.

Run or climb too much or when they should not.

Talk too much or when they should not.

Blurt out answers before questions are completed.

Have trouble taking turns.

Interrupt others.

A diagnosis of attention-deficit/hyperactivity disorder usually is made when a child has several of these symptoms that begin before age 7 and last at least 6 months. Generally, symptoms have to be observed in at least two different settings, such as home and school, before a diagnosis is made. A comprehensive medical evaluation of the child must be conducted to establish a correct diagnosis of AD/HD and to rule out other potential causes of the symptoms. Ideally, a health care practitioner making a diagnosis should include input from both parents and teachers.

Many types of medications have been used to treat AD/HD. The most widely used drugs are stimulants, which increase activity in parts of the brain that appear to be underactive in children and adolescents with this disorder. Experts believe that this is why stimulants improve attention and reduce impulsive, hyperactive, or aggressive behavior. For some children and adolescents, certain antidepressants also help alleviate symptoms of the disorder. Care must be taken when prescribing and monitoring all medications. Ritalin (methylphenidate HCl), the most common drug prescribed for AD/HD, is classified as a

Schedule II drug under the Federal Control Substances Act with a high potential for abuse. Like most medications, those used to treat AD/HD have side effects; some are severe.

Another treatment approach, called *behavior therapy*, involves using techniques and strategies to modify the behavior of children with the disorder. Behavior therapy includes the following:

- Instruction for parents and teachers on how to manage and modify the child's behavior, such as rewarding good behavior.
- Use of daily report cards to link efforts between home and school; parents reward the child for good school performance and behavior.
- Attendance at special classes that use intensive behavior modification.
- Use of specially trained aides in the classroom.

While a combination of stimulants and behavior therapy is believed to be helpful, it is not clear how long the benefits from this approach last. The NIMH is supporting research on the long-term benefits of various treatments, and to determine whether medication and behavior treatment are more effective when combined. Ongoing research efforts also are aimed at identifying new medicines and treatments.

## ∗ Bipolar Disorder

A type of depressive disorder, **bipolar disorder,** also called *manic-depressive illness*, is a brain disorder that causes unusual shifts in a person's mood, energy, and ability to function. More than 2 million American adults, or about 1% of the population age 18 and older in any given year, have the illness. Bipolar disorder is characterized by cycling mood changes: severe highs (**mania**) and lows (**depression**). Sometimes the mood switches are dramatic and rapid, but most often they are gradual. When in the depressed cycle, an individual can have any or all of the symptoms of depression (see Pathology Spotlight: Depression on page 760 for a list of symptoms of depression). Mania, left untreated, may worsen to a psychotic state. Symptoms of mania include the following:

- Abnormal or excessive elation.
- Unusual irritability.
- Decreased need for sleep.
- Grandiose notions.
- Increased talking.

- Racing thoughts.
- Increased sexual desire.
- Markedly increased energy.
- Poor judgment.
- Inappropriate social behavior.

Bipolar disorder typically develops in late adolescence or early adulthood, although some people have their first symptoms during childhood, and some have them late in life. These symptoms often are not recognized as an illness, and people suffer for years before it is properly diagnosed and treated. Sometimes, severe episodes of mania or depression include symptoms of **psychosis** (psychotic symptoms) such as **hallucinations** and **delusions.** People with bipolar disorder who have these symptoms are sometimes incorrectly diagnosed as having schizophrenia. Without treatment, people who have bipolar disorder often go through devastating life events such as marital breakups, job loss, substance abuse, and suicide.

A mild to moderate level of mania is called **hypomania,** which can feel good to the person who experiences it and can even be associated with good functioning and enhanced productivity. Thus, even when family and friends learn to recognize the mood swings as possible bipolar disorder, the person could deny that anything is wrong. Without proper treatment, however, hypomania can become severe mania in some people or can cycle into depression.

In some cases, symptoms of mania and depression occur together in what is called a **mixed bipolar state.** Symptoms often include agitation, trouble sleeping, significant changes in appetite, psychosis, and suicidal thinking. A person can have a very sad, hopeless mood while at the same time feel extremely energized.

Of people who have bipolar disorder, 80% to 90% can be treated effectively with medication and psychotherapy. Self-help groups can offer emotional support and assistance in recognizing signs of relapse to avert a full-blown episode of bipolar disorder. The most commonly prescribed medications to treat bipolar disorder are three mood stabilizers: lithium (Eskalith), carbamazepine (Tegretol), and valproate (Depakote).

## * Depression

**Depression** varies in intensity, severity, persistence, and number of symptoms. **Major depression** is characterized by a combination of symptoms that interfere with the ability to work, study, sleep, eat, and enjoy once pleasurable activities. Symptoms can be so severe that the person literally is unable to drag himself or herself out of bed. Such a disabling episode of depression can occur only once but more commonly occurs several times in a lifetime. A less severe type of depression, **dysthymia,** involves long-term, chronic symptoms that do not disable but keep an individual from functioning well or feeling good. Many people with dysthymia also experience major depressive episodes at some time in their lives.

Not everyone who is depressed experiences every symptom. Some people experience a few symptoms, some many. Severity of symptoms varies with individuals and over time. Symptoms of depression include these:

- Persistent sad, anxious, or *empty* mood.
- Feelings of hopelessness, pessimism.
- Feelings of guilt, worthlessness, helplessness.
- Loss of interest or pleasure in hobbies and activities including sex.
- Decreased energy, fatigue, feeling slowed down.
- Difficulty concentrating, remembering, making decisions.
- Insomnia, early-morning awakening, or oversleeping.
- Appetite and/or weight loss or overeating and weight gain.
- Restlessness, irritability.
- Persistent physical symptoms that do not respond to treatment, such as headaches, digestive disorders, and chronic pain.
- Thoughts of death or suicide; suicide attempts.

A diagnosis of depression is made when four or more of the previously described symptoms have been present continually or most of the time for more than 2 weeks. The term *clinical depression* means the episode of depression is serious enough to require treatment.

Four major types of medication are used to treat depression: tricyclic antidepressants (TCAs); selective serotonin reuptake inhibitors (SSRIs), serotonin-norepinephrine reuptake inhibitor (SNRIs) and monoamine oxidase inhibitors (MAOIs). Electroconvulsive therapy (ECT) is useful, particularly for individuals whose depression is severe or life threatening or who cannot take antidepressant medication.

## * Generalized Anxiety Disorder

**Generalized anxiety disorder** (GAD) is much more than the normal anxiety people experience. It is chronic and fills a person's life with exaggerated worry and tension. Having this disorder means always anticipating disaster and worrying excessively about health, money, family, or work. Sometimes, though, the source of the worry is difficult to pinpoint. Simply the thought of getting through the day provokes anxiety.

People with GAD seem unable to shake their concerns, even though they usually realize that their anxiety is more intense than the situation warrants. Their worries are accompanied by physical symptoms, especially fatigue, headaches, muscle tension, muscle aches, difficulty swallowing, nausea, trembling, twitching, lightheadedness, irritability, sweating, hot flashes, and trouble sleeping.

GAD affects about 4 million adult Americans and about twice as many women as men. The disorder comes on gradually and can begin across the life cycle, although the risk is highest between childhood and middle age. It is diagnosed when someone spends at least 6 months worrying excessively about a number of everyday problems. There is evidence that genes play a modest role in GAD. BuSpar (buspirone) is an antianxiety medication that is used to treat generalized anxiety disorder.

## ✶ Obsessive-Compulsive Disorder

**Obsessive-compulsive disorder** (OCD) involves persistent, unwelcome thoughts or images or the urgent need to engage in certain rituals that the person cannot control. For example, individuals can exhibit the following:

- Obsession with germs or dirt and wash their hands over and over.
- Doubt and the need to check things repeatedly.
- Frequent thoughts of violence and the fear that they will harm someone close to them.
- Long periods of touching or counting things or being preoccupied with order or symmetry.
- Persistent thoughts of performing repulsive sexual acts.
- Thoughts against their religious beliefs.

The disturbing thoughts or images are called **obsessions,** and the rituals performed to try to prevent or get rid of them are called **compulsions.** The person experiences only temporary relief not pleasure in carrying out the rituals, caused by the anxiety that increases when they are not performed.

OCD afflicts about 3.3 million adult Americans. It strikes men and women in approximately equal numbers and usually first appears in childhood, adolescence, or early adulthood. One-third of adults with OCD report having experienced their first symptoms as children. The course of the disease is variable; symptoms can come and go, can ease over time, or can become progressively worse. Research evidence suggests that OCD could run in families. Benzodiazepines are the class of drugs most often prescribed for this anxiety disorder.

## ✶ Panic Disorder

People with **panic disorder,** a form of anxiety disorder often called *panic attacks*, have feelings of terror that strike suddenly and repeatedly with no warning. They cannot predict when an attack will occur, and many develop intense anxiety between episodes, worrying about when and where the next one will strike. Panic disorder affects about 2.4 million adult Americans and is twice as common in women as in men. It most often begins during late adolescence or early adulthood. Risk of developing panic disorder appears to be inherited.

When having a panic attack, a person feels sweaty, flushed or chilled, weak, faint, or dizzy. The hands can tingle or feel numb. There can be nausea, chest pain or a smothering sensation, a sense of unreality, or fear of impending doom or loss of control. The individual can genuinely believe that he or she is having a heart attack, losing his or her mind, or on the verge of death.

Some people's lives become so restricted that they avoid normal, everyday activities and become housebound. When this happens, in about one-third of people with panic disorder, the condition is called **agoraphobia.** Benzodiazepines are the class of drugs most often prescribed for panic disorder.

## ✳ Post-Traumatic Stress Disorder

**Post-traumatic stress disorder** (PTSD), one of the anxiety disorders, is a debilitating condition that can develop following a terrifying event. Often, people with PTSD have persistent frightening thoughts and memories of their ordeals and feel emotionally numb, especially with people to whom they were once close. PTSD was first brought to public attention by war veterans, but it can result from any number of traumatic incidents, such as a mugging, rape, or torture; being kidnapped or held captive; child abuse; serious accidents such as car or train wrecks; and natural disasters such as floods and earthquakes. The event that triggers PTSD can be something that threatened the person's life or the life of someone close to the person. It also could be something witnessed, such as massive death and destruction after a building is bombed or a plane crashes.

Whatever the source of the problem, some people with PTSD repeatedly relive the trauma in the form of nightmares and disturbing recollections during the day. They can also experience other sleep problems, feel detached or numb, or be easily startled. They can lose interest in things they used to enjoy and have trouble feeling affectionate. They can feel irritable, more aggressive than before, even violent. Things that remind them of the traumas can be very distressing, which could lead them to avoid certain places or situations that bring back those memories. Anniversaries of the traumatic event are often very difficult.

PTSD affects about 5.2 million adult Americans. Women are more likely than men to develop PTSD. It can occur at any age, including childhood, and there is some evidence that susceptibility to PTSD runs in families. The disorder is often accompanied by depression, substance abuse, or one or more other anxiety disorders. In severe cases, the person has trouble working or socializing.

Not every traumatized person experiences full-blown PTSD or PTSD at all. PTSD is diagnosed only if the symptoms last more than a month. In those who do develop PTSD, symptoms usually begin within 3 months of the trauma, and the course of the illness varies. Some people recover within 6 months, others have symptoms that last much longer. In some cases, the condition is chronic. Occasionally, the illness does not develop until years after the traumatic event. As with the other anxiety disorders, benzodiazepines are the class of drugs most often prescribed for this disorder.

## ✳ Schizophrenia

**Schizophrenia,** which generally begins in late adolescence or early adulthood, is a mental disorder characterized by *positive* and *negative* symptoms. Positive (psychotic) symptoms include delusions, hallucinations, and disordered thinking. Negative symptoms include social withdrawal, extreme apathy, diminished motivation, and blunted emotional expression. Negative symptoms are sometimes mistaken for laziness or depression, hindering diagnosis. Cognitive symptoms (or cognitive deficits), such as problems with attention and certain types of memory, and the functional ability to plan and organize can also be present. These can be difficult to recognize as part of the disorder but often are the most destructive in terms of leading a normal life.

Schizophrenia is one of the most disabling and puzzling mental disorders. Researchers now consider schizophrenia to be a group of mental disorders rather than a single illness.

The causes of schizophrenia are unknown, but the disease affects perception, memory, attention, cognition, and emotion—some of the most highly evolved functions in humans. Recent research suggests that heredity (a child who has one parent with schizophrenia has about a 10% chance of developing the illness versus a 1% chance if neither parent has schizophrenia), events during fetal development that affect the brain (such as viral infections in the mother during pregnancy), environmental stressors (such as exposure to pollutants or toxins), and psychological stress are interactive factors that can produce schizophrenia. Abnormalities in both the brain's structure and biochemical activities also seem to be implicated in the illness.

People who have schizophrenia often require medication to control the most troubling symptoms. Antipsychotic medications help bring biochemical imbalances closer to normal, and some may be effective for symptoms such as social withdrawal, extreme apathy, and blunted emotional expression. Psychotherapy and electroconvulsive therapy can be part of a treatment regimen for certain patients.

According to The National Alliance on Mental Illness, treatment of schizophrenia is successful in 60% of patients. After the symptoms are controlled, psychotherapy and self-help groups can assist people who have schizophrenia learn to develop social skills, cope with stress, identify early warning signs of relapse, and prolong periods of remission. In addition, support groups and family therapy can give the patient's loved ones a better understanding of the illness and help them provide the compassion and support that play an important role in recovery.

## ✶ Social Phobia (Social Anxiety Disorder)

**Social phobia,** also called **social anxiety disorder,** involves overwhelming anxiety and excessive self-consciousness in everyday social situations. People with social phobia have a persistent, intense, and chronic fear of being watched and judged by others and being embarrassed or humiliated by their own actions. Their fear can be so severe that it interferes with work, school, and other ordinary activities.

Social phobia can be limited to only one type of situation, such as the fear of speaking in formal or informal situations or eating, drinking, or writing in front of others, or, in its most severe form, can be so broad that people experience symptoms almost anytime they are around other people.

Physical symptoms often accompany the intense anxiety of social phobia and include blushing, profuse sweating, trembling, nausea, and difficulty talking. People with social phobia are aware that their feelings are irrational.

Social phobia affects about 5.3 million adult Americans. Women and men are equally likely to develop social phobia. The disorder usually begins in childhood or early adolescence, and some evidence suggests that genetic factors are involved. Benzodiazepines are the class of drugs most often prescribed for social phobia, an anxiety disorder.

## ✶ Suicidal Feelings

Anyone who is thinking about committing suicide needs immediate attention. Anyone who talks about suicide should be taken seriously. Risk for **suicide** appears to be highest in those with mental illnesses such as depression and bipolar disorder.

Signs and symptoms that can accompany suicidal feelings include these:

- Talking about feeling suicidal or wanting to die.
- Feeling hopeless, that nothing will ever change or get better.
- Feeling helpless, that nothing the person does makes any difference.
- Feeling like a burden to family and friends.

- Abusing alcohol or drugs.
- Putting affairs in order (organizing finances or giving away possessions).
- Writing a suicide note.
- Putting oneself in harm's way or in situations that involve a danger of being killed.

# ✔ PATHOLOGY CHECKPOINT

*Following is a concise list of the pathology-related terms that you have seen in the chapter. Review this checklist to make sure that you are familiar with the meaning of each term before moving to the next section.*

## Conditions and Symptoms

- ❏ affective disorder
- ❏ agoraphobia
- ❏ anorexia nervosa
- ❏ anxiety
- ❏ anxiety disorders
- ❏ apathy
- ❏ attention-deficit/hyperactivity disorder
- ❏ autism
- ❏ bipolar disorder
- ❏ bulimia nervosa
- ❏ compulsion
- ❏ cyclothymic disorder
- ❏ delirium
- ❏ delusion
- ❏ dementia
- ❏ depressive disorders
- ❏ dissociation
- ❏ dysthymia
- ❏ eating disorder
- ❏ factitious disorder
- ❏ fugue
- ❏ generalized anxiety disorder

- ❏ hallucination
- ❏ hypomania
- ❏ impulse control disorder
- ❏ mania
- ❏ Munchausen by proxy syndrome
- ❏ Munchausen's syndrome
- ❏ neurotic
- ❏ obsessive-compulsive disorder
- ❏ paranoia
- ❏ personality disorder
- ❏ phobia
- ❏ post-traumatic distress disorder
- ❏ psychosis
- ❏ pyromania
- ❏ schizophrenia
- ❏ seasonal affective disorder
- ❏ sexual disorders
- ❏ social phobia
- ❏ social anxiety disorder
- ❏ somatoform disorder
- ❏ substance abuse

- ❏ subsyndromal depression
- ❏ suicidal feelings
- ❏ tic disorder

## Diagnosis and Treatment

- ❏ art therapy
- ❏ cognitive-behavioral therapy
- ❏ drug therapy
- ❏ electroconvulsive therapy
- ❏ family therapy
- ❏ group therapy
- ❏ hypnosis
- ❏ intelligence quotient (IQ) test
- ❏ Minnesota Multiphasic Personality Inventory
- ❏ play therapy
- ❏ psychoanalysis
- ❏ psychotherapy
- ❏ Rorschach Inkblot Test
- ❏ Stanford-Binet Intelligence Scale
- ❏ Thematic Apperception Test
- ❏ Wechsler Adult Intelligence Scale

# STUDY AND REVIEW

## Overview: Mental Health and Mental Illness

*Write your answers to the following questions. Do not refer to the text.*

1. _____ is an abnormal condition of the brain.

2. List the three mental disorders that are listed among the top ten causes of disability in the United States.

   a. _____

   b. _____

   c. _____

3. _____ is the branch of medicine that deals with the diagnosis, treatment, and prevention of mental illness.

4. Give the three basic forms of treatment for mental illness.

   a. _____

   b. _____

   c. _____

5. _____ is a method of obtaining a detailed account of past and present mental and emotional experiences and repressions.

## Word Parts

1. In the spaces provided, write the definitions of these prefixes, roots, combining forms, and suffixes. Do not refer to the listings of medical words. Leave blank those words you cannot define.

2. After completing as many as you can, refer to the medical word listings to check your work. For each word missed or left blank, write the word and its definition several times on the margins of these pages or on a separate sheet of paper.

3. To maximize the learning process, it is to your advantage to do the following exercises as directed. To refer to the word-building section before completing these exercises invalidates the learning process.

## PREFIXES

*Give the definitions of the following prefixes.*

1. an- _____    2. hypo- _____

3. para- _____    4. pyro- _____

## ROOTS AND COMBINING FORMS

*Give the definitions of the following roots and combining forms.*

1. agor/a _____

2. aut _____

3. centr _____

4. cycl/o _____

5. delus _____

6. ego _____

7. hallucinat _____

8. iatr _____

9. log _____

10. neur/o _____

11. path _____

12. phren _____

13. psych _____

14. psych/o _____

15. schiz/o _____

16. somat _____

17. somat/o _____

18. thym _____

## SUFFIXES

*Give the definitions of the following suffixes.*

1. -form _____

2. -ia _____

3. -ic _____

4. -ion _____

5. -ism _____

6. -ist _____

7. -logy _____

8. -mania _____

9. -noia _____

10. -orexia _____

11. -osis _____

12. -phobia _____

13. -therapy _____

14. -tic _____

## Identifying Medical Terms

*In the spaces provided, write the medical terms for the following meanings.*

1. _____ Abnormal fear of being alone in public places

2. _____ Mental condition in which a person lacks feelings and emotions

3. _____ Fixed, false belief or abnormal perception

4. _____ Mental disorder marked by altered mood

5. _____ Pertaining to being self-centered

6. _____ Mental disorder characterized by excessive excitement

7. _____ Morbid and persistent fear of a specific object, activity, or situation that results in a compelling desire to avoid the feared stimulus

8. _____ Physician who specializes in the study, treatment and prevention of mental disorders

9. _____ Method of treating mental disorders by using psychological techniques instead of physical methods

10. _____ Madness for fire

## Spelling

*In the spaces provided, write the correct spelling of these misspelled words.*

1. anxeity _____

2. autesm _____

3. bulemia _____

4. dementea _____

5. factious _____

6. halluciation _____

7. parnoia _____

8. psychomatic _____

9. schizphrenia _____

10. somatform _____

## Matching

*Select the appropriate lettered meaning for each of the following words.*

_____ 1. dysthymia

_____ 2. seasonal affective disorder

_____ 3. bipolar disorder

_____ 4. schizophrenia

_____ 5. delusions

_____ 6. hallucinations

_____ 7. obsessive-compulsive disorder

_____ 8. post-traumatic stress disorder

_____ 9. generalized anxiety disorder

_____ 10. attention-deficit/hyperactivity disorder

a. Characterized by positive, negative, and cognitive symptoms

b. Characterized hearing nonexistent voices, seeing nonexistent things, and experiencing burning or pain sensations with no physical cause

c. Characterized by unusual shifts in a person's mood, energy, and ability to function

d. Less severe type of depression involving long-term, chronic symptoms that do not disable but keep the person from functioning well or from feeling good

e. Debilitating condition that can develop following a terrifying event

f. Characterized by bizarre thoughts that have no basis in reality

g. Form of depression associated with changes in the amount of available daylight that one receives

h. Chronic condition that fills the person's day with exaggerated worry and tension

i. Characterized by anxious thoughts or rituals that the person feels compelled to perform and cannot control

j. One of the most common psychiatric conditions that appears in childhood

k. Anxiety syndrome and panic disorder

## Abbreviations

*Place the correct word, phrase, or abbreviation in the space provided.*

1. cognitive-behavioral therapy _____

2. *Diagnostic and Statistical Manual of Mental Disorders,* 4th ed. (Text Revision)

   _____

3. ECT _____

4. MMPI _____

5. National Institute of Mental Health _____

6. OCD _____

7. post-traumatic stress disorder _____

8. SAD _____

9. TAT _____

10. World Health Organization _____

# PRACTICAL APPLICATION

## S O A P : Chart Note Analysis

*This exercise will make you aware of information, abbreviations, and medical terminology found in a patient's chart at an internal medicine office.*

### Abbreviation Key

| | | | | |
|---|---|---|---|---|
| **bid** | twice a day | | **P** | pulse |
| **BP** | blood pressure | | **PE** | physical examination |
| **c/o** | complains of | | **R** | respiration |
| **CTA** | clear to auscultation | | **R/O** | rule out |
| **DOB** | date of birth | | **SOAP** | subjective, objective, assessment, plan |
| **F** | Fahrenheit | | **T** | temperature |
| **Ht** | height | | **TCA** | tricyclic antidepressant |
| **lb** | pound | | **Wt** | weight |
| **Mg** | milligram | | **y/o** | year(s) old |
| **NKDA** | no known drug allergies | | | |

*Read the following chart note and then answer the questions that follow.*

**PATIENT:** O'Leary, Catherine                                    **DATE:** 07/10/07

**DOB:** 05/01/40        **AGE:** 67        **SEX:** Female

**INSURANCE:** Excel Healthcare

**Vital Signs:**
  T: 98.6 F
  P: 72
  R: 20
  BP: 138/86
  Ht: 5' 6"
  Wt: 166 lb

**Allergies:** NKDA

**Chief Complaint:** Persistent sadness, loss of interest, decreased energy, difficulty concentrating and remembering, loss of appetite, and feelings of guilt.

**S** | **Subjective:** 67 y/o white female c/o sadness. She describes loss of interest in eating, social activities, sex, and even talking with friends. She states that she finds herself "crying for no apparent reason" and doesn't really enjoy doing "much of anything." She has no energy and feels guilty about not feeling good. She has difficulty concentrating and adding figures. "I have felt like nothing for the past 2 months."

**O** | **Objective:**

**General Appearance:** Older female with cheerless, rundown appearance and poor eye contact. Spoke in soft, low voice with little spontaneity.

**Lungs:** CTA

**Heart:** Normal rate and rhythm. No murmurs, gallops or rubs.

**Abd:** Bowel sounds in all 4 quadrants. No masses or tenderness.

**MS:** Osteoarthritis noted in thumb and first digit of right hand.

**Neuro:** Alert and oriented x 3. Reflexes intact.

**Skin:** Warm and dry to touch.

**A** | **Assessment:** Depression

**P** | **Plan:** To rule out any physical cause for her symptoms, a medical history was taken and a PE was performed. A physical cause of depression was ruled out.

1. Asendin (amoxapine) 25 mg, bid for six months.
2. Inform of medication regimen. Advise that this medicine could impair mental or physical abilities or both. Instruct not to mix with alcohol, as an additive effect could occur. Instruct to not arise suddenly because dizziness and orthostatic hypotension (low blood pressure due to sudden change in position) can happen. Advise to be aware of possible side effects such as flushing, diaphoresis, blurred vision, constipation, or urinary retention and if persist, to notify the office.
3. Counsel about lifestyle changes that could help her during this period of depression.
4. Schedule a follow-up visit for six weeks. *Note:* If patient has not improved, will recommend referral to a psychiatrist.

**FYI:** Ascendin is classified as a TCA and prescribed to elevate patient's mood, increase physical activity and mental alertness, and improve appetite and sleep.

**Recommended Lifestyle Changes for Improving Depression**
- Rejoin social activities as soon as possible.
- Go out to eat with family and friends.
- Eat a healthy diet that is low in fat, high in fiber, and rich in vitamins and minerals.
- Specific dietary factors that can be beneficial in depression are the B-complex vitamins found in whole grains and omega-3 fatty acids found in cold water fish, fish oil, and flax seeds.
- Take up a new hobby or engage in a new activity.
- Exercise on a regular basis.
- Set goals that are attainable.
- List things that need to be done. Break large tasks into smaller ones and set priorities.
- Be patient with yourself.
- Increase social and spiritual support.
- Reduce stress by getting adequate sleep, rest, and recreation.
- Postpone important decisions until depression has lifted.

## Chart Note Questions
*Place the correct answer in the space provided.*

1. Some of the signs and symptoms of depression are loss of interest in _____, social activities, sex, and even talking with friends.

2. How did the physician rule out a physical cause of depression? _____

3. Give the definition for the abbreviation TCA. _____

4. The prescribed medicine should elevate Ms. O'Leary's mood, increase her physical activity and mental alertness, and improve her _____ and sleep.

5. Which two dietary factors mentioned could be beneficial in depression? _____

6. What is the medical term for profuse sweating? _____

7. Ascendin should not be mixed with _____?

8. Define *orthostatic hypotension.* _____

9. Possible side effects of Ascendin include flushing, diaphoresis, _____, constipation, or urinary retention

10. During the physical exam, Ms. O'Leary appeared _____, rundown, and had poor eye contact.

# MULTIMEDIA PREVIEW

*Additional interactive resources and activities for this chapter can be found on the Companion Website. For videos, audio glossary, and review, access the accompanying CD-ROM in this book.*

 **CD-ROM HIGHLIGHTS**

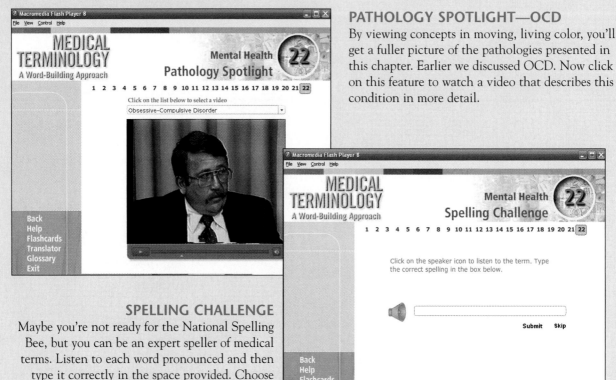

## PATHOLOGY SPOTLIGHT—OCD

By viewing concepts in moving, living color, you'll get a fuller picture of the pathologies presented in this chapter. Earlier we discussed OCD. Now click on this feature to watch a video that describes this condition in more detail.

## SPELLING CHALLENGE

Maybe you're not ready for the National Spelling Bee, but you can be an expert speller of medical terms. Listen to each word pronounced and then type it correctly in the space provided. Choose your letters carefully!

 **WEBSITE HIGHLIGHTS—www.prenhall.com/rice**

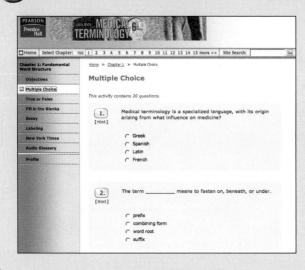

## MULTIPLE CHOICE QUIZ

Take advantage of the free-access on-line study guide that accompanies your textbook. You'll find a multiple choice quiz that provides instant feedback, allowing you to check your score and see what you got right or wrong. By clicking on this URL you'll also access links to download mp3 audio reviews, current news articles, and an audio glossary.

## Appendix I

### ■ CHAPTER 1

#### WORD PARTS

##### Prefixes

1. without
2. away from
3. against
4. self
5. bad
6. one hundred, one hundredth
7. through
8. different
9. bad
10. small
11. one thousandth
12. many, much
13. new
14. beside
15. before
16. together
17. apart
18. upon
19. out
20. in, into

##### Roots and Combining Forms

1. stuck to
2. armpit
3. center
4. chemical
5. a shaping
6. formation, produce
7. a thousand
8. large
9. death
10. law
11. rule
12. tumor
13. organ
14. fever
15. heat, fire
16. ray, x-ray
17. to examine
18. putrefaction
19. hot, heat
20. place
21. cough
22. to infect
23. people
24. cause
25. to cut
26. bad kind
27. greatest
28. least
29. palm
30. guarding

##### Suffixes

1. pertaining to
2. pertaining to
3. surgical puncture
4. a course
5. shape
6. to flee
7. formation, produce
8. knowledge
9. a step
10. a weight
11. recording
12. condition
13. pertaining to
14. process
15. condition
16. nature of, quality of
17. liter
18. study of
19. instrument to measure
20. condition (usually abnormal)
21. pertaining to
22. disease
23. to carry
24. instrument for examining
25. decay
26. treatment
27. pertaining to
28. condition

#### IDENTIFYING MEDICAL TERMS

1. adhesion
2. asepsis
3. axillary
4. chemotherapy
5. heterogeneous
6. malformation
7. microscope
8. multiform
9. neopathy
10. oncology

#### SPELLING

1. antiseptic
2. autonomy
3. centimeter
4. diaphoresis
5. milligram
6. necrosis
7. paracentesis
8. radiology

#### MATCHING

1. f      3. j
2. d      4. g

5. a      8. i
6. k      9. c
7. b      10. e

**ABBREVIATIONS**

1. abnormal
2. axillary
3. Bx
4. cardiovascular
5. neurology
6. ENT
7. FP
8. g
9. gynecology
10. pediatrics

## ■ CHAPTER 2

**IDENTIFYING SUFFIXES**

1. cardi<u>ac</u>
2. cephal<u>ad</u>
3. enur<u>esis</u>
4. obstet<u>rician</u>
5. bronchi<u>ole</u>
6. pust<u>ule</u>
7. dent<u>algia</u>
8. dia<u>betes</u>
9. hyper<u>emesis</u>
10. hem<u>optysis</u>

**DEFINING SUFFIXES**

1. weakness
2. process
3. inflammation
4. softening
5. enlargement, large
6. disease
7. deficiency
8. to digest
9. fear
10. rupture
11. pertaining to
12. pertaining to
13. use, action
14. condition
15. to make
16. resemble

17. one who
18. pertaining to
19. pertaining to
20. nourishment
21. tissue, structure

**SPELLING**

1. auricle
2. bronchiole
3. cardiologist
4. cephalad
5. cyanotic
6. embolism
7. podiatry
8. pustule

**USING SUFFIXES TO BUILD MEDICAL WORDS**

1. hyperhidrosis
2. muscular
3. macula
4. alopecia
5. ventricle
6. decubitus
7. integumentary
8. penile
9. congenital
10. anterior

**IDENTIFYING MEDICAL TERMS**

1. abrasion
2. anesthetize
3. arousal
4. asymmetry
5. asystole
6. comatose
7. dyarthria
8. grandiose
9. gynecoid
10. palpate

## ■ CHAPTER 3

**IDENTIFYING PREFIXES**

1. <u>a</u>pnea
2. <u>brady</u>pnea
3. <u>dys</u>pnea
4. <u>eu</u>pnea

5. <u>hyper</u>pnea
6. <u>hypo</u>pnea
7. <u>tachy</u>pnea
8. <u>bi</u>nary
9. <u>con</u>centration
10. <u>extra</u>ocular

**DEFINING PREFIXES**

1. against
2. short
3. through
4. different
5. similar, same
6. water
7. micro, small
8. scanty, little
9. all
10. false
11. without
12. without
13. two
14. twice
15. with, together
16. down, away from
17. outside
18. excessive
19. under
20. not
21. between
22. many
23. beside
24. around
25. many
26. before
27. again, backward
28. below
29. upper, above
30. not

**SPELLING**

1. binary
2. concentration
3. occlusion
4. parasternal
5. pericardial
6. latent

7. patent
8. unconscious

## USING PREFIXES TO BUILD MEDICAL WORDS

1. anicteric
2. hyperactive
3. multifocal
4. decompensation
5. intermediary
6. bifurcate
7. polydactyly
8. hypoplasia
9. subacute
10. uncoscious

## IDENTIFYING MEDICAL TERMS

1. afebrile
2. extraocular
3. insomnia
4. arrest
5. enucleate
6. lumen
7. patent
8. react
9. sign
10. symptom

## ■ CHAPTER 4

### ANATOMY AND PHYSIOLOGY

1. body . . . cells . . . sustain
2. cell membrane
3. cell membrane . . . cytoplasm . . . nucleus
4. metabolism . . . growth . . . reproduction
5. embryonic cell
6. a. protection
   b. absorption
   c. secretion
   d. excretion
7. Connective
8. a. striated (voluntary)
   b. cardiac
   c. smooth (involuntary)
9. excitability . . . conductivity

10. tissue serving a common purpose
11. group of organs functioning together for a common purpose
12. a. integumentary
    b. skeletal
    c. muscular
    d. digestive
    e. cardiovascular
    f. blood and lymphatic
    g. respiratory
    h. urinary
    i. endocrine
    j. nervous
    k. reproductive
13. a. above, in an upward direction
    b. in front of, before
    c. toward the back
    d. pertaining to the head
    e. nearest the midline or middle
    f. to the side, away from the middle
    g. nearest the point of attachment
    h. away from the point of attachment
14. midsagittal plane
15. transverse or horizontal
16. coronal or frontal
17. a. thoracic
    b. abdominal
    c. pelvic
18. a. cranial
    b. spinal

## WORD PARTS

### Prefixes

1. both
2. up, apart
3. two
4. color
5. down, away from
6. apart
7. outside
8. within

9. similar, same
10. middle
11. through
12. first
13. one
14. upper, above

### Roots and Combining Forms

1. fat
2. man
3. life
4. tail
5. cell
6. cell
7. to pour
8. tissue
9. water
10. cell's nucleus
11. side
12. disease
13. nature
14. to drink
15. body
16. place
17. a turning
18. body organs
19. toward the front
20. cranium
21. away from the point of origin
22. backward
23. to strain through
24. horizon
25. below
26. groin
27. within
28. side
29. toward the middle
30. organ
31. to show
32. behind, toward the back
33. near the point of origin
34. near the surface
35. a composite whole
36. near the belly side

### Suffixes

1. pertaining to

2. use, action
3. formation, produce
4. pertaining to
5. process
6. study of
7. form, shape
8. resemble
9. pertaining to
10. a thing formed, plasma
11. body
12. control, stop, stand still
13. incision
14. pertaining to
15. pertaining to
16. type

## IDENTIFYING MEDICAL TERMS

1. android
2. bilateral
3. cytology
4. ectomorph
5. karyogenesis
6. somatotrophic
7. unilateral

## SPELLING

1. adipose
2. caudal
3. cytology
4. diffusion
5. histology
6. mesomorph
7. perfusion
8. proximal
9. somatotrophic
10. unilateral

## MATCHING

1. c        6. i
2. d        7. g
3. e        8. h
4. f        9. j
5. a        10. b

## ABBREVIATIONS

1. abd
2. anatomy and physiology
3. central nervous system
4. CV

5. GI
6. lateral
7. respiratory
8. endoplasmic reticulum
9. anteroposterior
10. posteroanterior

## MEDICAL RECORD EXERCISE

1. written transcript of information about a patient and his or her health care
2. Health Insurance Portability and Accountability Act of 1996
3. a. patient information form
   b. medical history
   c. physical examination
   d. consent form
   e. informed consent form
   f. physician's orders
   g. nurse's notes
   h. physician's progress notes
   i. consultation report
   j. ancillary/miscellaneous reports
   k. diagnostic tests/laboratory reports
   l. operative report
   m. anesthesiology report
   n. pathology report
   o. discharge summary
4. a. subjective
   b. objective
   c. assessment
   d. plan
5. diagnosis
6. plan

## ■ CHAPTER 5

## ANATOMY AND PHYSIOLOGY

1. skin
2. a. hair
   b. nails
   c. sebaceous glands
   d. sweat glands
3. a. protection
   b. regulation

   c. sensory reception
   d. secretion
4. epidermis . . . dermis
5. a. stratum corneum
   b. stratum lucidum
   c. stratum granulosum
   d. stratum germinativum
6. Keratin
7. Melanin
8. dermis
9. a. papillary layer
   b. reticular layer
10. lunula

## WORD PARTS

### Prefixes

1. without, lack of
2. self
3. out
4. down
5. out
6. excessive
7. under
8. within
9. around
10. below

### Roots and Combining Forms

1. extremity
2. ray
3. gland
4. white
5. cancer
6. heat
7. juice
8. corium
9. skin
10. skin
11. skin
12. skin
13. skin
14. skin
15. fox mange
16. red
17. sweat
18. jaundice
19. tumor
20. horn

21. white
22. study of
23. black
24. black
25. fungus
26. nail
27. little cell
28. nail
29. thick
30. a louse
31. cord
32. wrinkle
33. hard
34. oil
35. old
36. hot, heat
37. to pull
38. hair
39. nail
40. yellow
41. dry
42. to lie
43. little bag
44. a covering
45. yellow
46. plate
47. millet (tiny)
48. itching
49. end, distant
50. vessel

### Suffixes

1. pertaining to
2. pain
3. pertaining to
4. pertaining to
5. skin
6. pertaining to
7. sensation
8. pencil, grafting knife
9. condition
10. pertaining to
11. process
12. condition
13. one who specializes
14. inflammation
15. study of

16. dilatation
17. resemble
18. tumor
19. condition (usually abnormal)
20. pertaining to
21. surgical repair
22. flow, discharge
23. instrument to cut

### IDENTIFYING MEDICAL TERMS

1. actinic dermatitis
2. cutaneous
3. dermatitis
4. dermatology
5. pruritus
6. hyperhidrosis
7. hypodermic
8. icteric
9. onychitis
10. pachyderma
11. thermanesthesia
12. xanthoderma

### SPELLING

1. causalgia
2. dermomycosis
3. ecchymosis
4. excoriation
5. hyperhidrosis
6. melanoma
7. onychomycosis
8. rhytidoplasty
9. scleroderma
10. seborrhea

### MATCHING

1. d    6. i
2. f    7. b
3. e    8. g
4. h    9. a
5. j    10. c

### ABBREVIATIONS

1. FUO
2. TIMs
3. history
4. I & D
5. SG
6. intradermal

7. T
8. UV
9. foreign body
10. psoralen-ultraviolet light

### DIAGNOSTIC AND LABORATORY TESTS

1. c
2. d
3. a
4. b
5. a

### CHART NOTE EXERCISE

1. bid
2. pruritus
3. vesicles
4. contact dermatitis
5. antihistamine
6. avoid poison ivy; wear clothing that covers arms and legs; wash skin with soap and water within 15 minutes of exposure; know how to recognize poison ivy and where it is found
7. erythroderma
8. edema
9. tub soaks with colloidal oatmeal (Aveeno); apply cold, wet compress tid or qid × 20 minutes; apply Calamine lotion to affected area
10. 6 months

### ■ CHAPTER 6

### ANATOMY AND PHYSIOLOGY

1. 206
2. a. axial
   b. appendicular
3. a. flat . . . ribs, scapula, parts of the pelvic girdle, bones of the skull
   b. long . . . tibia, femur, humerus, radius
   c. short . . . carpal, tarsal
   d. irregular . . . vertebrae, ossicles of the ear
   e. sesamoid . . . patella
*Optional answer to question 3:

f. sutural or wormian . . . between the flat bones of the skull

4. a. shape, support
   b. protection
   c. storage
   d. formation of blood cells
   e. attachment of skeletal muscles
   f. movement through articulation

5. a. ends of a developing bone
   b. shaft of a long bone
   c. membrane that forms the covering of bones except at their articular surfaces
   d. dense, hard layer of bone tissue
   e. narrow space or cavity throughout the length of the diaphysis
   f. tough connective tissue membrane lining the medullary canal and containing the bone marrow
   g. reticular tissue that makes up most of the volume of bone

6. Matching answers:
   1. f
   2. k
   3. d
   4. m
   5. h
   6. j
   7. i
   8. n
   9. a
   10. l
   11. b
   12. c
   13. g
   14. e

7. a. synarthrosis
   b. amphiarthrosis
   c. diarthrosis

8. Abduction

9. moving a body part toward the midline
10. Circumduction
11. bending a body part backward
12. Eversion
13. straightening a flexed limb
14. Flexion
15. turning inward
16. Pronation
17. moving a body part forward
18. Retraction
19. moving a body part around a central axis
20. Supination

## WORD PARTS

### Prefixes

1. without
2. apart
3. water
4. between
5. beyond
6. around
7. many, much
8. under, beneath
9. together
10. back

### Roots and Combing Forms

1. acetabulum, hip socket
2. gristle
3. extremity, point
4. extremity
5. stiffening, crooked
6. joint
7. joint
8. a pouch
9. heel bone
10. to place
11. cancer
12. wrist
13. wrist
14. cartilage
15. cartilage
16. clavicle, collarbone
17. fastened
18. coccyx, tail bone

19. coccyx, tail bone
20. glue
21. to lead
22. to bind together
23. rib
24. rib
25. crescent
26. light
27. skull
28. skull
29. finger or toe
30. finger or toe
31. femur
32. carrying
33. fibula
34. x-ray
35. humerus
36. ilium
37. ilium
38. ischium
39. a hump
40. lamina (thin plate)
41. bending, curve, swayback
42. loin, lower back
43. loin
44. lower jawbone
45. jawbone
46. jaw
47. bone marrow
48. bone marrow
49. discharge
50. elbow
51. bone
52. kneecap
53. to draw
54. foot
55. phalanges (finger/toe bones)
56. a passage
57. spine
58. radius
59. sacrum
60. flesh
61. shoulder blade
62. curvature
63. curvature
64. spine

65. vertebra
66. sternum, breastbone
67. sternum, breastbone
68. tendon
69. tibia
70. ulna, elbow
71. ulna, elbow
72. vertebra
73. vertebra
74. sword

### Suffixes

1. pertaining to
2. pertaining to
3. pain
4. pertaining to
5. pertaining to
6. immature cell, germ cell
7. surgical puncture
8. related to
9. process
10. pain
11. excision
12. swelling
13. formation, produce
14. formation, produce
15. mark, record
16. instrument for recording
17. pertaining to
18. inflammation
19. nature of
20. instrument for examining
21. softening
22. structure
23. resemble
24. tumor
25. shoulder
26. condition (usually abnormal)
27. deficiency
28. growth
29. formation
30. surgical repair
31. formation
32. instrument to cut
33. incision
34. structure, tissue

### IDENTIFYING MEDICAL TERMS

1. acroarthritis
2. ankylosis
3. arthritis
4. calcaneal
5. chondral
6. coccygodynia
7. costal
8. craniectomy
9. dactylic
10. hydrarthrosis
11. intercostal
12. ischialgia
13. lumbar
14. myeloma
15. osteoarthritis
16. osteomyelitis or myelitis
17. osteopenia
18. pedal
19. xiphoid

### SPELLING

1. acromion
2. arthroscope
3. bursitis
4. chrondroblast
5. connective
6. cranioplasty
7. dislocation
8. ischial
9. myelitis
10. osteochondritis
11. phosphorus
12. patellar
13. phalangeal
14. rachigraph
15. scoliosis
16. spondylitis
17. symphysis
18. tenonitis
19. ulnocarpal
20. vertebral

### MATCHING

1. i     4. c
2. j     5. b
3. e     6. h
7. g     9. d
8. a     10. f

### ABBREVIATIONS

1. CDH
2. DJD
3. long leg cast
4. osteoarthritis
5. PEMFs
6. rheumatoid arthritis
7. SPECT
8. thoracic vertebra, first
9. temporomandibular joint
10. Tx

### DIAGNOSTIC AND LABORATORY TESTS

1. c
2. d
3. c
4. b
5. b

### CHART NOTE EXERCISE

1. kyphosis
2. one 5mg Tab daily
3. vitamin A
4. vitamin C
5. calcium
6. measure bone density, confirm diagnosis, predict future risks, evaluate treatment
7. 1.0 inches to 1.5 inches
8. compression
9. family history; lack of exercise; thin, small frame; never been pregnant; early menopause; tendency to fractures; loss of height in the past few years; avoidance of dairy products as a child; smoking; drinking alcoholic beverages; diet high in salt, caffeine, or fat, and insufficient intake of vitamin D
10. evaluate effectiveness of treatment

# ■ CHAPTER 7

## ANATOMY AND PHYSIOLOGY

1. a. skeletal
   b. smooth
   c. cardiac
2. 42
3. a. nutrition
   b. oxygen
4. a. origin
   b. insertion
5. voluntary or striated
6. aponeurosis
7. a. body
   b. origin
   c. insertion
8. a. muscle that counteracts the action of another muscle
   b. muscle that is primary in a given movement produced by its contraction
   c. muscle that acts with another muscle to produce movement
9. involuntary, visceral, or unstriated
10. a. digestive tract
    b. respiratory tract
    c. urinary tract
    d. eye
    e. skin
11. Cardiac
12. a. movement
    b. maintain posture
    c. produce heat

## WORD PARTS

### Prefixes

1. lack of
2. away from
3. toward
4. against
5. two
6. slow
7. with
8. through
9. difficult
10. into
11. within
12. water
13. four
14. with, together
15. three

### Roots and Combining Forms

1. agony
2. arm
3. clavicle
4. to cut through
5. neck
6. finger or toe
7. to lead
8. work
9. a band
10. skin
11. discharge
12. fiber
13. fiber
14. equal
15. a rind
16. lifter
17. an addition
18. breast
19. hot, heat
20. to measure
21. muscle
22. muscle
23. muscle
24. muscle
25. nerve
26. disease
27. to loosen
28. rod
29. to turn
30. a turning
31. flesh
32. hardening
33. to gain
34. convulsive
35. sternum
36. tendon
37. tone, tension
38. twisted
39. to draw
40. will
41. synovial membrane
42. twisted

### Suffixes

1. pain
2. pertaining to
3. pertaining to
4. weakness
5. immature cell, germ cell
6. head
7. binding
8. pain
9. chemical
10. treatment
11. instrument for recording
12. condition
13. pertaining to
14. process
15. agent
16. inflammation
17. condition
18. motion
19. motion
20. study of
21. process
22. softening
23. resemble
24. tumor
25. a doer
26. condition (usually abnormal)
27. weakness
28. disease
29. a fence
30. surgical repair
31. stroke, paralysis
32. suture
33. pertaining to
34. tension, spasm
35. order
36. instrument to cut
37. incision
38. nourishment, development
39. condition
40. condition

## IDENTIFYING MEDICAL TERMS

1. atonic
2. bradykinesia

3. dactylospasm
4. dystrophy
5. intramuscular
6. levator
7. myasthenia
8. myology
9. myoparesis
10. myoplasty
11. myosarcoma
12. myotomy
13. polyplegia
14. tenodesis
15. synergetic
16. triceps

## SPELLING

1. fascia
2. myokinesis
3. dermatomyositis
4. rhabdomyoma
5. sarcolemma
6. sternocleidomastoid
7. dystrophin
8. torticollis

## MATCHING

| | | | |
|---|---|---|---|
| 1. | d | 6. | a |
| 2. | i | 7. | h |
| 3. | g | 8. | c |
| 4. | e | 9. | b |
| 5. | j | 10. | f |

## ABBREVIATIONS

1. above elbow
2. aspartate aminotransferase
3. Ca
4. EMG
5. full range of motion
6. musculoskeletal
7. ROM
8. sh
9. total body weight
10. triceps jerk

## DIAGNOSTIC AND LABORATORY TESTS

| | | | |
|---|---|---|---|
| 1. | b | 4. | c |
| 2. | d | 5. | a |
| 3. | b | | |

## CHART NOTE EXERCISE

1. waddling
2. electromyography
3. minimize deformities; preserve mobility
4. muscle weakness in the legs
5. creatine kinase
6. electromyography
7. help delay permanent muscular contracture
8. penicillin
9. yes
10. no

# ■ CHAPTER 8

## ANATOMY AND PHYSIOLOGY

1. a. mouth
   b. pharynx
   c. esophagus
   d. stomach
   e. small intestine
   f. large intestine
2. a. salivary glands
   b. liver
   c. gallbladder
   d. pancreas
3. a. digestion
   b. absorption
   c. elimination
4. small mass of masticated food ready to be swallowed
5. series of wavelike muscular contractions that are involuntary
6. hydrochloric acid and gastric juices
7. duodenum
8. chyme
9. circulatory system
10. cecum, colon, rectum, and anal canal
11. liver
12. stores and concentrates bile
13. produces digestive enzymes

14. a. plays an important role in metabolism
    b. manufactures bile
    c. stores iron, vitamins $B_{12}$, A, D, E, and K
15. small intestine
16. parotid, sublingual, submandibular
17. a. insulin
    b. glucagon

## WORD PARTS

### Prefixes

1. lack of
2. difficult
3. above
4. excessive, above
5. deficient, below
6. bad
7. around
8. after
9. through
10. below

### Roots and Combining Forms

1. to suck in
2. gland
3. starch
4. a building up
5. a casting down
6. orange-yellow
7. appendix
8. appendix
9. gall, bile
10. cheek
11. abdomen, belly
12. lip
13. gall, bile
14. common bile duct
15. colon
16. colon
17. colon
18. colon
19. bladder
20. tooth
21. to press together
22. diverticula
23. duodenum

24. small intestine
25. to remove dregs
26. esophagus
27. stomach
28. stomach
29. gums
30. tongue
31. sweet, sugar
32. blood
33. liver
34. liver
35. hernia
36. ileum
37. ileum
38. lip
39. abdomen
40. to loosen
41. tongue
42. fat
43. study of
44. middle
45. pancreas
46. to digest
47. pharynx
48. meal
49. to vomit
50. anus and rectum
51. pylorus, gatekeeper
52. rectum
53. saliva
54. sigmoid
55. spleen
56. mouth
57. poison
58. a breaking out
59. worm
60. breath
61. vein liable to bleed
62. nourishment
63. to chew
64. to disable; paralysis
65. hair
66. nest
67. to roll
68. tooth

## Suffixes

1. pertaining to
2. pertaining to
3. pain, ache
4. pertaining to
5. enzyme
6. hernia
7. resemble
8. condition of
9. surgical excision
10. vomiting
11. shape
12. formation, produce
13. pertaining to
14. pertaining to
15. process
16. condition
17. one who specializes
18. inflammation
19. nature of, quality of
20. study of
21. destruction, to separate
22. enlargement, large
23. tumor
24. appetite
25. condition (usually abnormal)
26. flow
27. to digest
28. pertaining to
29. to eat, to swallow
30. instrument for examining
31. visual examination, to view, examine
32. contraction
33. new opening
34. incision
35. pertaining to
36. suture

## IDENTIFYING MEDICAL TERMS

1. amylase
2. anabolism
3. anorexia
4. appendectomy
5. appendicitis
6. biliary
7. celiac
8. dysphagia
9. hepatitis
10. herniorrhaphy
11. postprandial
12. splenomegaly
13. sigmoidoscope

## SPELLING

1. biliary
2. colonoscopy
3. enteroclysis
4. gastroenterology
5. hepatotoxin
6. laxative
7. peristalsis
8. sialadenitis
9. vagotomy
10. vermiform

## MATCHING

1. e        6. h
2. f        7. j
3. d        8. a
4. b        9. g
5. i        10. c

## ABBREVIATIONS

1. ac
2. bowel movement
3. bowel sounds
4. cholesterol
5. GB
6. HAV
7. nasogastric
8. nothing by mouth
9. pc
10. TPN

## DIAGNOSTIC AND LABORATORY TESTS

1. a
2. c
3. d
4. c
5. c

## CHART NOTE EXERCISE

1. epigastric

2. culture

3. bleeding, obstruction, perforation

4. antibiotics

5. smoking

6. hypertension

7. heartburn

8. can stimulate the stomach to produce more acid and digestive juices

9. gastroinomas

10. patients' failure to adhere to regimen

## ■ CHAPTER 9

### ANATOMY AND PHYSIOLOGY

1. a. heart

   b. arteries

   c. veins

   d. capillaries

2. a. endocardium

   b. myocardium

   c. pericardium

3. 300

4. atria . . . interatrial

5. ventricles . . . interventricular

6. a. superior and inferior vena cavae

   b. right atrium

   c. tricuspid valve

   d. right ventricle

   e. pulmonary semilunar valve

   f. left and right pulmonary arteries

   g. lungs

   h. left and right pulmonary veins

   i. left atrium

   j. bicuspid or mitral valve

   k. left ventricle

   l. aortic valve

   m. aorta

   n. capillaries

7. autonomic nervous system

8. sinoatrial node

9. Purkinje system

10. a. radial . . . on the radial side of the wrist

    b. brachial . . . in the antecubital space of the elbow

    c. carotid . . . in the neck

11. a. pressure exerted by the blood on the walls of the vessels

    b. difference between the systolic and diastolic readings

12. man's fist . . . 60 to 100

13. 100 and 140 . . . 60 and 90

14. transport blood from the right and left ventricles of the heart to all body parts

15. transport blood from peripheral tissues to the heart

### WORD PARTS

#### Prefixes

1. lack of

2. two

3. slow

4. together

5. within

6. within

7. outside

8. excessive, above

9. deficient, below

10. around

11. difficult, abnormal

12. half

13. fast

14. three

#### Roots and Combining Forms

1. vessel

2. to choke

3. vessel

4. opening

5. aorta

6. artery

7. artery

8. artery

9. fatty substance, porridge

10. fatty substance, porridge

11. atrium

12. atrium

13. heart

14. heart

15. heart

16. dark blue

17. listen to

18. to widen

19. electricity

20. a throwing in

21. sweet, sugar

22. blood

23. to hold back

24. bile

25. study of

26. moon

27. thin

28. mitral valve

29. muscle

30. circular

31. sour, sharp, acid

32. vein

33. vein

34. sound

35. lung

36. rhythm

37. hardening

38. a curve

39. pulse

40. narrowing

41. chest

42. to draw, to bind

43. to limp

44. pressure

45. clot of blood

46. small vessel

47. vessel

48. reflected sound

49. vein

50. body

51. ventricle

52. fibrils (small fibers)

53. blood

54. power

55. infarct (necrosis of an area)

56. to shut up

57. oxygen
58. throbbing
59. a partition
60. end
61. clot of blood
62. solid (fat)
63. chest
64. fat

**Suffixes**

1. pertaining to
2. pertaining to
3. pertaining to
4. record
5. surgical puncture
6. point
7. measurement
8. dilatation
9. surgical excision
10. blood condition
11. relating to
12. formation, produce
13. instrument for recording
14. recording
15. condition
16. pertaining to
17. having a particular quality
18. process
19. condition
20. one who specializes
21. inflammation
22. nature of, quality of
23. study of
24. softening
25. enlargement, large
26. instrument to measure
27. tumor
28. one who
29. condition (usually abnormal)
30. disease
31. surgical repair
32. to pierce
33. instrument for examining
34. contraction, spasm
35. incision

36. tissue
37. pertaining to

**IDENTIFYING MEDICAL TERMS**

1. angioma
2. angioblast
3. angioplasty
4. angiostenosis
5. arteriotomy
6. arteritis
7. bicuspid
8. cardiologist
9. cardiomegaly
10. cardiopulmonary
11. constriction
12. embolism
13. phlebitis
14. tachycardia
15. vasodilator

**SPELLING**

1. anastomosis
2. atherosclerosis
3. atrioventricular
4. endocarditis
5. extracorporeal
6. ischemia
7. myocardial
8. oxygen
9. phlebitis
10. palpitation

**MATCHING**

1. d        6. c
2. e        7. a
3. f        8. i
4. g        9. j
5. b       10. h

**ABBREVIATIONS**

1. AMI
2. A-V, AV
3. blood pressure
4. coronary artery disease
5. CC
6. electrocardiogram
7. high-density lipoprotein
8. H & L

9. myocardial infarction
10. tissue plasminogen activator

**DIAGNOSTIC AND LABORATORY TESTS**

1. c
2. a
3. b
4. c
5. b

**CHART NOTE EXERCISE**

1. dyspnea
2. blood enzyme
3. sublingual
4. prn
5. immediately
6. 15
7. oxygenated
8. electrocardiogram
9. coronary vasodilator
10. abnormal breath

## ■ CHAPTER 10

**ANATOMY AND PHYSIOLOGY**

1. a. erythrocytes
   b. thrombocytes
   c. leukocytes
2. transport oxygen and carbon dioxide
3. 5
4. 80 to 120 days
5. body's main defense against the invasion of pathogens
6. 8000
7. a. neutrophils
   b. eosinophils
   c. basophils
   d. lymphocytes
   e. monocytes
8. play an important role in the clotting process
9. 200,000 to 500,000
10. a. A
    b. B
    c. AB
    d. O

11. a. transports proteins and fluids
    b. protects the body against pathogens
    c. serves as a pathway for the absorption of fats
12. a. spleen
    b. tonsils
    c. thymus

## WORD PARTS

### Prefixes

1. lack of
2. against
3. self
4. up
5. beyond
6. excessive
7. deficient
8. one
9. all
10. many
11. before
12. across
13. deficient

## ROOTS AND COMBINING FORMS

1. gland
2. gland
3. clumping
4. other
5. vessel
6. unequal
7. base
8. lime, calcium
9. color
10. to pour
11. clots, to clot
12. flesh, creatine
13. cell
14. blood
15. cell
16. rose-colored
17. red
18. globe
19. little grain, granular
20. blood

21. blood
22. blood
23. white
24. white
25. fat
26. study of
27. lymph
28. lymph
29. large
30. neither
31. kernel, nucleus
32. eat, engulf
33. a thing formed, plasma
34. net
35. putrefying
36. whey, serum
37. iron
38. fiber
39. spleen
40. sea
41. clot
42. clot
43. thymus
44. fiber
45. tonsil
46. formation
47. immunity
48. vessel
49. whey
50. a developing
51. vessel
52. small vessel

### Suffixes

1. capable
2. forming
3. immature cell, germ cell
4. body
5. swelling
6. to separate
7. cultivation
8. cell
9. surgical excision
10. blood condition
11. work
12. formation, produce

13. protection
14. protein
15. tissue
16. pertaining to
17. chemical
18. process
19. one who specializes
20. inflammation
21. study of
22. destruction
23. enlargement
24. tumor
25. condition (usually abnormal)
26. lack of
27. removal
28. attraction
29. attraction
30. formation
31. bursting forth
32. control, stop, stand still
33. incision
34. condition
35. oxygen

## IDENTIFYING MEDICAL TERMS

1. agglutination
2. allergy
3. antibody
4. anticoagulant
5. antigen
6. basocyte
7. coagulable
8. creatinemia
9. eosinophil
10. granulocyte
11. hematologist
12. hemoglobin
13. hyperglycemia
14. hyperlipemia
15. leukocyte
16. lymphostasis
17. mononucleosis
18. prothrombin
19. splenopexy
20. thrombocyte

## SPELLING

1. allergy
2. creatinemia
3. extravasation
4. erythrocytosis
5. thromboplastin
6. hematocrit
7. hemorrhage
8. leukemia
9. lymphadenotomy
10. anaphylaxis

## MATCHING

1. h
2. d
3. e
4. g
5. f
6. c
7. b
8. a
9. j
10. i

## ABBREVIATIONS

1. AIDS
2. BSI
3. chronic myelogenous leukemia
4. Hb, Hgb
5. hematocrit
6. HIV
7. *Pneumocystis carinii* pneumonia
8. prothrombin time
9. red blood cell (count)
10. RIA

## DIAGNOSTIC AND LABORATORY TESTS

1. d
2. c
3. c
4. b
5. a

## CHART NOTE EXERCISE

1. diarrhea
2. positive
3. Norvir (ritonavir)
4. hypertension
5. headache
6. not concerned about pregnancy
7. risk of becoming infected due to compromised immune system

8. twice a day
9. yes
10. handwashing

## ■ CHAPTER 11

### ANATOMY AND PHYSIOLOGY

1. a. nose
   b. pharynx
   c. larynx
   d. trachea
   e. bronchi
   f. lungs
2. to furnish oxygen for use by individual cells and to take away their gaseous waste product, carbon dioxide
3. process in which the lungs are ventilated and oxygen and carbon dioxide are exchanged between the air in the lungs and the blood within capillaries of the alveoli
4. process in which oxygen and carbon dioxide are exchanged between the bloodstream and the cells of the body
5. a. serves as an air passageway
   b. warms and moistens inhaled air
   c. its cilia and mucous membrane trap dust, pollen, bacteria, and foreign matter
   d. contains olfactory receptors that sort out odors
   e. aids in phonation and the quality of voice
6. a. nasopharynx
   b. oropharynx
   c. laryngopharynx
7. a. serves as a passageway for air
   b. serves as a passageway for food
   c. aids in phonation by changing its shape
8. acts as a lid to prevent aspiration of food into the trachea
9. narrow slit at the opening between the true vocal folds

10. production of vocal sounds
11. serves as a passageway for air
12. right bronchus . . . left bronchus
13. provide a passageway for air to and from the lungs
14. cone-shaped, spongy organs of respiration lying on either side of the heart
15. serous membrane composed of several layers
16. diaphragm
17. mediastinum
18. 3 . . . 2
19. alveoli
20. to bring air into intimate contact with blood so that oxygen and carbon dioxide can be exchanged in the alveoli
21. temperature, pulse, respiration, and blood pressure
22. a. amount of air in a single inspiration and expiration
    b. amount of air remaining in the lungs after maximal expiration
    c. volume of air that can be exhaled after a maximal inspiration
23. medulla oblongata . . . pons
24. 30 to 80
25. 15 to 20

### WORD PARTS

#### Prefixes

1. lack of
2. upon
3. difficult
4. within
5. good
6. out
7. below, deficient
8. excessive
9. in
10. fast

#### Roots and Combining Forms

1. to draw in
2. small, hollow air sac

3. coal
4. imperfect
5. bronchi
6. bronchi
7. bronchiole
8. bronchi
9. dust
10. dark blue
11. breathe
12. blood
13. larynx, voice box
14. larynx, voice box
15. larynx, voice box
16. lobe
17. sac
18. fiber
19. nose
20. straight
21. middle
22. a little swelling
23. palate
24. breast, chest
25. pharynx, throat
26. pharynx, throat
27. nipple
28. partition
29. pleura
30. pleura
31. pleura
32. lung, air
33. lung, air
34. lung
35. lung
36. pus
37. nose
38. a curve, hollow
39. breath
40. breathing
41. chest
42. to air
43. almond, tonsil
44. trachea, windpipe
45. trachea, windpipe
46. snore
47. flesh
48. diaphragm, partition

## Suffixes

1. pertaining to
2. pain
3. hernia, tumor, swelling
4. surgical puncture
5. pain
6. dilation
7. surgical excision
8. pertaining to
9. condition
10. process
11. inflammation
12. instrument to measure
13. condition (usually abnormal)
14. tumor
15. dripping
16. surgical repair
17. a doer
18. breathing
19. to spit
20. flow, discharge
21. instrument for examining
22. new opening
23. incision
24. pertaining to

## IDENTIFYING MEDICAL TERMS

1. alveolus
2. bronchiectasis
3. bronchitis
4. dysphonia
5. eupnea
6. hemoptysis
7. inhalation
8. laryngitis
9. pneumothorax
10. rhinoplasty
11. rhinorrhea
12. sinusitis

## SPELLING

1. bronchoscope
2. diaphragmatocele
3. expectoration
4. laryngeal
5. orthopnea
6. pleuritis

7. pulmonectomy
8. rhoncus
9. tachypnea
10. tracheal

## MATCHING

| | | | |
|---|---|---|---|
| 1. h | | 6. b | |
| 2. i | | 7. d | |
| 3. k | | 8. a | |
| 4. f | | 9. e | |
| 5. c | | 10. g | |

## ABBREVIATIONS

1. AFB
2. cystic fibrosis
3. CXR
4. COLD
5. endotracheal
6. postnasal drip, paroxysmal nocturnal dyspnea
7. R
8. sudden infant death syndrome
9. SOB
10. tuberculosis

## DIAGNOSTIC AND LABORATORY TESTS

1. b
2. c
3. c
4. d
5. a

## CHART NOTE EXERCISE

1. sputum culture
2. warm
3. Rales
4. ethambutal
5. multidrug-resistant tuberculosis
6. 6 months
7. positive to negative
8. directly observed therapy
9. airborne droplets
10. treatment

## ■ CHAPTER 12

### ANATOMY AND PHYSIOLOGY

1. a.   kidneys

b. ureters

c. bladder

d. urethra

2. extraction of certain wastes from the bloodstream, conversion of these materials to urine, and transport of the urine from the kidney, via the ureters, to the bladder for elimination

3. a. true capsule

b. perirenal fat

c. renal fascia

4. a notch

5. saclike collecting portion of the kidney

6. arteries, veins, convoluted tubules, and glomerular capsules

7. inner

8. structural and functional unit of the kidney

9. renal corpuscle . . . tubule

10. glomerulus . . . Bowman's capsule

11. to remove the waste products of metabolism from the blood plasma

12. filtration . . . reabsorption

13. 95 . . . 5

14. 1000 to 1500

15. narrow, muscular tubes that transport urine from the kidneys to the bladder

16. muscular, membranous sac that serves as a reservoir for urine

17. small, triangular area near the base of the bladder

18. convey urine and semen

19. convey urine

20. urinary meatus

21. physical, chemical, and microscopic examination of urine

22. a. yellow to amber

b. clear

c. 4.6 to 8.0

d. 1.003 to 1.030

e. aromatic

f. 1000 to 1500 mL/day

23. a. renal

b. transitional

c. squamous

24. diabetes mellitus

25. renal disease, acute glomerulonephritis, pyelonephritis

## WORD PARTS
### Prefixes

1. without

2. against

3. complete, through

4. complete, through

5. difficult, painful

6. within

7. water

8. outside, beyond

9. not

10. scanty

11. through

12. beyond

13. excessive

### Roots and Combining Forms

1. sifted out

2. protein

3. bacteria

4. bile

5. calcium

6. colon

7. to hold

8. bladder

9. body

10. bladder

11. skin

12. glomerulus, little ball

13. glomerulus, little ball

14. glucose, sugar

15. blood

16. ketone

17. stone

18. study of

19. blood

20. passage

21. to urinate

22. kidney

23. kidney

24. night

25. peritoneum

26. perineum

27. sound

28. to tighten, contraction

29. pus

30. renal pelvis

31. kidney

32. hardening

33. trigone

34. urine

35. urine

36. ureter

37. urethra

38. urethra

39. urine

40. urine

41. urine

42. urination

### Suffixes

1. pertaining to

2. pain

3. pertaining to

4. hernia

5. pain

6. pertaining to

7. pertaining to

8. surgical excision

9. blood condition

10. a mark, record

11. pertaining to

12. chemical

13. process

14. one who specializes

15. inflammation

16. stone

17. study of

18. separation, loosening, dissolution

19. crushing

20. process

21. instrument to measure

22. tumor

23. condition (usually abnormal)

24. disease

25. surgical repair

26. instrument for examining
27. condition
28. new opening
29. incision
30. urine

## IDENTIFYING MEDICAL TERMS

1. antidiuretic
2. cystectomy
3. cystitis
4. dysuria
5. glomerulitis
6. hypercalciuria
7. micturition
8. nephrolith
9. periurethral
10. pyuria
11. ureteropathy
12. urethralgia
13. urologist

## SPELLING

1. excretory
2. enuresis
3. glycosuria
4. hematuria
5. incontinence
6. nephrocystitis
7. nocturia
8. ureteroplasty
9. urinalysis
10. urobilin

## MATCHING

1. d        6. g
2. e        7. j
3. b        8. c
4. f        9. h
5. a       10. i

## ABBREVIATIONS

1. ARF
2. blood urea nitrogen
3. CRF
4. cystoscopy
5. genitourinary
6. hemodialysis
7. IVP

8. peritoneal dialysis
9. hydrogen ion concentration
10. UA

## DIAGNOSTIC AND LABORATORY TESTS

1. c
2. c
3. b
4. c
5. b

## CHART NOTE EXERCISE

1. increased
2. urinalysis
3. Bactrim DS
4. the short length of the urethra, which promotes the transmission of bacteria from the skin and genitals to the bladder
5. *Escherichia coli (E. coli)*
6. wipe from front to back
7. sexual transmission of bacteria during intercourse
8. pain
9. irritation
10. people can be sensitive to burns and photosensitivity while taking sulfonamides

## ■ CHAPTER 13

### ANATOMY AND PHYSIOLOGY

1. a. pituitary
   b. pineal
   c. thyroid
   d. parathyroid
   e. islets of Langerhans
   f. adrenals
   g. ovaries
   h. testes
2. a. thymus
   b. placenta during pregnancy
   c. gastrointestinal mucosa
3. involves the production and regulation of chemical substances (hormones) that play an essential role in maintaining homeostasis
4. chemical transmitter that is released in small amounts and transported via the bloodstream to a targeted organ or other cells
5. synthesizes and secretes releasing hormones, releasing factors, release-inhibiting hormones, and release inhibiting factors
6. because of its regulatory effects on the other endocrine glands
7. a. growth hormone (GH)
   b. adrenocorticotropin (ACTH)
   c. thyroid-stimulating hormone (TSH)
   d. follicle-stimulating hormone (FSH)
   e. luteinizing hormone (LH)
   f. prolactin (PRL)
   g. melanocyte-stimulating hormone (MSH)
8. a. antidiuretic hormone (ADH)
   b. oxytocin
9. melatonin . . . serotonin
10. plays a vital role in metabolism and regulates the body's metabolic processes
11. a. thyroxine (T4)
    b. triiodothyronine (T3)
    c. calcitonin
12. serum calcium . . . phosphorus
13. blood sugar
14. glucocorticoids, mineralocorticoids, and the androgens
15. a. regulates carbohydrate, protein, and fat metabolism
    b. stimulates output of glucose from the liver (gluconeogenesis)
    c. increases the blood sugar level
    d. regulates other physiologic body processes

*Optional answers to question 15:

   e. promotes the transport of amino acids into extracellular tissue

   f. influences the effectiveness of catecholamines such as dopamine, epinephrine, and norepinephrine

   g. has an anti-inflammatory effect

   h. helps the body cope during times of stress

16. a. use of carbohydrates
   b. absorption of glucose
   c. gluconeogenesis
   d. potassium and sodium metabolism

17. Aldosterone

18. substance or hormone that promotes the development of male characteristics

19. a. dopamine
   b. epinephrine
   c. norepinephrine

20. a. elevates the systolic blood pressure
   b. increases the heart rate and cardiac output
   c. Increases glycogenolysis, thereby hastening release of glucose from the liver. This action elevates the blood sugar level and provides the body with a spurt of energy.

*Optional answers to question 20:

   d. dilates the bronchial tubes
   e. dilates the pupils

21. estrogen . . . progesterone

22. testosterone

23. a. thymosin
   b. thymopoietin

24. a. gastrin
   b. secretin
   c. pancreozymincholecystokinin
   d. enterogastrone

## WORD PARTS

### Prefixes

1. through
2. within
3. good, normal
4. out, away from
5. out, away from
6. excessive
7. deficient, under
8. beside
9. before
10. upon
11. water

### Roots and Combining Forms

1. acid
2. extremity
3. gland
4. gland
5. cortex
6. flesh
7. cretin
8. man
9. to secrete
10. to secrete
11. small
12. milk
13. old age
14. giant
15. little acorn
16. sweet, sugar
17. seed
18. hairy
19. insulin
20. cortex
21. insulin
22. potassium
23. drowsiness
24. study of
25. mucus
26. eye
27. pine cone
28. kidney
29. pituitary gland
30. kidney
31. kidney
32. mad desire
33. thymus
34. to bear
35. thyroid, shield
36. thyroid, shield
37. poison
38. nourishment
39. masculine
40. body
41. testicle
42. solid
43. thyroid, shield
44. vessel
45. to press
46. adrenal gland
47. adrenal gland
48. pancreas

### Suffixes

1. pertaining to
2. formation, produce
3. pertaining to
4. to go
5. surgical excision
6. swelling
7. blood condition
8. formation, produce
9. condition
10. pertaining to
11. condition
12. one who specializes
13. inflammation
14. study of
15. hormone
16. enlargement, large
17. resemble
18. tumor
19. condition (usually abnormal)
20. disease
21. substance
22. growth
23. chemical
24. flow, discharge
25. pertaining to

## IDENTIFYING MEDICAL TERMS

1. adenosis
2. cretinism
3. diabetes
4. endocrinology
5. euthyroid

6. exocrine
7. gigantism
8. glucocorticoid
9. hyperkalemia
10. hypogonadism
11. lethargic
12. thymitis

**SPELLING**

1. catecholamines
2. cretinism
3. exophthalmic
4. hypothyroidism
5. myxedema
6. pineal
7. pituitary
8. thyroid
9. oxytocin
10. virilism

**MATCHING**

1. e       6. i
2. f       7. c
3. b       8. j
4. g       9. d
5. h      10. a

**ABBREVIATIONS**

1. BMR
2. DM
3. fasting blood sugar
4. glucose tolerance tests
5. PBI
6. parathyroid hormone (parathormone)
7. radioimmunoassay
8. STH
9. thyroid function studies
10. vasopressin

**DIAGNOSTIC AND LABORATORY TESTS**

1. a
2. c
3. c
4. b
5. c

**CHART NOTE EXERCISE**

1. polydipsia

2. glucose
3. diet
4. polydipsia
5. polyuria
6. polyphagia
7. fatigue
8. excessive adipose tissue
9. glucose tolerance test
10. 25

# ■ CHAPTER 14

**ANATOMY AND PHYSIOLOGY**

1. a. central
   b. peripheral
2. Neurons
3. a. cause contractions in muscles
   b. cause secretions from glands and organs
   c. inhibit the actions of glands and organs
4. long process reaching from the cell body to the area to be activated
5. resembles the branches of a tree and has short, unsheathed processes that transmit impulses to the cell body
6. sensory nerves transmit impulses to the central nervous system
7. interneurons
8. a. single elongated process
   b. bundle of nerve fibers
   c. groups of nerve fibers
9. brain . . . spinal cord
10. a. receives impulses
    b. processes information
    c. responds with appropriate action
11. a. dura mater
    b. arachnoid
    c. pia mater
12. a. cerebrum
    b. diencephalon
    c. midbrain
    d. cerebellum

   e. pons
   f. medulla oblongata
   g. reticular formation
13. frontal lobe
14. somesthetic area
15. auditory . . . language
16. vision
17. a. relay center for all sensory impulses
    b. relays motor impulses from the cerebellum to the cortex
18. a. is a regulator
    b. produces neurosecretions
    c. produces hormones
19. sensory perception and motor output
20. a. regulates and controls breathing
    b. regulates and controls swallowing
    c. regulates and controls coughing
    d. regulates and controls sneezing
    e. regulates and controls vomiting
21. a. conducts sensory impulses
    b. conducts motor impulses
    c. is a reflex center
22. 120 . . . 150
23. a. olfactory
    b. optic
    c. oculomotor
    d. trochlear
    e. trigeminal
    f. abducens
    g. facial
    h. acoustic
    i. glossopharyngeal
    j. vagus
    k. accessory
    l. hypoglossal
24. a. controls sweating
    b. controls the secretions of glands
    c. controls arterial blood pressure

d. controls smooth muscle tissue

25. a. sympathetic
    b. parasympathetic

## WORD PARTS

### Prefixes

1. lack of
2. lack of
3. star-shaped
4. slow
5. down
6. difficult
7. upon
8. half
9. water
10. excessive
11. within
12. small
13. little
14. beside
15. beside
16. many
17. four
18. below

### Roots and Combining Forms

1. to walk
2. dura, hard
3. head
4. side
5. little brain
6. cerebrum
7. color
8. shaken violently
9. skull
10. skull
11. cell
12. tree
13. a disk
14. dura, hard
15. electricity
16. brain
17. brain
18. feeling
19. numbness, sleep, stupor
20. knot
21. glue

22. sleep
23. globus pallidus
24. thin plate
25. lobe
26. study of
27. membrane, meninges
28. membrane, meninges
29. membrane, meninges
30. mind
31. memory
32. spinal cord
33. spinal cord
34. muscle
35. nerve
36. nerve
37. nerve
38. papilla
39. dusky
40. gray
41. hardening
42. a thorn
43. vertebra
44. sleep
45. sympathy
46. vagus, wandering
47. little belly

### Suffixes

1. pertaining to
2. condition of pain
3. pain
4. pertaining to
5. weakness
6. germ cell
7. hernia
8. cell
9. binding
10. surgical excision
11. swelling
12. feeling
13. glue
14. mark, record
15. instrument for recording
16. recording
17. condition
18. pertaining to
19. process

20. condition
21. one who specializes
22. inflammation
23. motion, movement
24. motion
25. seizure
26. a sheath, husk
27. diction, word, phrase
28. study of
29. nourishment, development
30. measurement
31. visual examination, to view, examine
32. tumor
33. condition (usually abnormal)
34. weakness
35. disease
36. to eat, swallow
37. speak, speech
38. action
39. nourishment
40. order, coordination
41. incision
42. pertaining to
43. condition

## IDENTIFYING MEDICAL TERMS

1. amnesia
2. analgesia
3. aphagia
4. ataxia
5. cephalalgia
6. cerebellar
7. craniectomy
8. dyslexia
9. encephalitis
10. epidural
11. hemiparesis
12. meningitis
13. neuralgia
14. neuritis
15. neurocyte
16. neurology
17. neuroma
18. palsy
19. polyneuritis
20. somnambulism

21. vagotomy
22. ventriculometry

## SPELLING

1. anesthesia
2. bradykinesia
3. cerebrospinal
4. craniotomy
5. epilepsy
6. meningioma
7. meningomyelocele
8. neuropathy
9. poliomyelitis
10. ventriculometry

## MATCHING

1. g      6. h
2. d      7. j
3. c      8. f
4. b      9. a
5. e      10. i

## ABBREVIATIONS

1. AD
2. ALS
3. central nervous system
4. cerebral palsy
5. CT
6. HDS
7. intracranial pressure
8. lumbar puncture
9. multiple sclerosis
10. PET

## DIAGNOSTIC AND LABORATORY TESTS

1. a      4.  d
2. b      5.  c
3. c

## CHART NOTE EXERCISE

1. memory
2. osteoarthritis
3. l
4. electroencephalogram
5. to assist in the confirming of the diagnosis
6. cholinesterase inhibitor
7. cognitive
8. no known drug allergies

9. XI
10. 50

## ■ CHAPTER 15

### ANATOMY AND PHYSIOLOGY

1. hearing . . . equilibrium
2. external . . . middle. . . inner
3. auricle, external acoustic meatus, tympanic membrane
4. auricle
5. a. lubrication
   b. protection
6. a. malleus
   b. incus
   c. stapes
7. to transmit sound vibrations
8. a. transmitting sound vibrations
   b. equalizing air pressure
   c. control of loud sounds
9. cochlea, vestibule, and the semicircular canals
10. a. cochlear duct
    b. semicircular ducts
    c. utricle and saccule
11. organ of Corti
12. vestibule
13. eighth cranial nerve
14. the position of the ear
15. a. endolymph
    b. perilymph

### WORD PARTS

#### Prefixes

1. within
2. within
3. around
4. twice
5. one

#### Roots and Combining Forms

1. hearing
2. to hear
3. to hear
4. hearing
5. the ear
6. gall, bile

7. land snail
8. electricity
9. maze, inner ear
10. maze, inner ear
11. larynx, voice box
12. study of
13. mastoid process, breast-shaped
14. fungus
15. eardrum, tympanic membrane
16. eardrum, tympanic membrane
17. nerve
18. ear
19. ear
20. pharynx
21. voice
22. old
23. pus
24. nose
25. hardening
26. stapes, stirrup
27. fat
28. drum
29. ear
30. window
31. middle
32. eardrum, tympanic membrane

#### Suffixes

1. pertaining to
2. pain
3. hearing
4. pain
5. surgical excision
6. a mark, record
7. recording
8. pertaining to
9. one who specializes
10. inflammation
11. stone
12. study of
13. serum, clear fluid
14. instrument to measure
15. measurement
16. resemble
17. tumor
18. condition (usually abnormal)
19. surgical repair

20. flow
21. instrument for examining
22. instrument to cut
23. incision
24. pertaining to
25. small
26. process
27. condition

## IDENTIFYING MEDICAL TERMS

1. audiologist
2. audiometry
3. auditory
4. endaural
5. labyrinthitis
6. myringoplasty
7. myringotome
8. otodynia
9. otolaryngology
10. otopharyngeal
11. otoscope
12. perilymph
13. stapedectomy
14. tympanectomy
15. tinnitus

## SPELLING

1. acoustic
2. audiology
3. cholesteatoma
4. electrocochleography
5. labyrinthitis
6. myringoplasty
7. otomycosis
8. otosclerosis
9. tympanic
10. tympanitis

## MATCHING

1. h    6. b
2. e    7. j
3. i    8. c
4. a    9. d
5. g    10. f

## ABBREVIATIONS

1. AC
2. BC
3. decibel
4. ENG
5. ear, nose, throat
6. HD
7. OM

## DIAGNOSTIC AND LABORATORY TESTS

1. a
2. b
3. c
4. d
5. b

## CHART NOTE EXERCISE

1. night awakening
2. pain in the ear, earache
3. otoscopy
4. acute otitis media
5. analgesic/antipyretic, pain, fever
6. antibiotic, infection
7. allergic one
8. breathing
9. acid
10. eustachian tube

# ■ CHAPTER 16

## ANATOMY AND PHYSIOLOGY

1. orbit, muscles, eyelids, conjunctiva, and the lacrimal apparatus
2. fatty tissue
3. optic nerve . . . ophthalmic artery
4. a. support
   b. rotary movement
5. intense light, foreign particles, . . . impact
6. mucous membrane that acts as a protective covering for the exposed surface of the eyeball
7. structures that produce, store, and remove the tears that cleanse and lubricate the eye
8. eyeball, its structures, and the nerve fibers
9. vision
10. optic disk
11. process of sharpening the focus of light on the retina
12. Matching answers:
    1. c
    2. e
    3. b
    4. a
    5. f
    6. d
    7. h
    8. i
    9. j
    10. g

## WORD PARTS

### Prefixes

1. lack of, without
2. two
3. in
4. in
5. inward
6. beyond
7. within
8. three
9. out
10. half
11. lack of
12. behind

### Roots and Combining Forms

1. dull
2. to join together, conjunctiva
3. unequal
4. eyelid
5. eyelid
6. choroid
7. cold
8. pupil
9. cornea
10. ciliary body
11. ciliary body
12. to remove the kernel of
13. tear, lacrimal duct, tear duct
14. less, smaller
15. electricity
16. focus

17. angle
18. iris
19. iris
20. cornea
21. cornea
22. tear
23. study of
24. measure
25. to shut
26. muscle
27. night
28. eye
29. eye
30. eye
31. eye
32. eye
33. lens
34. lentil, lens
35. light
36. old
37. pupil
38. retina
39. retina
40. sclera
41. point
42. tone
43. turn
44. uvea
45. foreign material
46. dry
47. dilation, widen
48. straight
49. disintegrate
50. to clot
51. radiating out from a center
52. lens
53. fiber
54. a squinting
55. hair

**Suffixes**

1. pertaining to
2. pertaining to
3. pertaining to
4. germ cell
5. condition

6. surgical excision
7. mark, record
8. recording
9. condition
10. pertaining to
11. process
12. condition
13. one who specializes
14. inflammation
15. study of
16. destruction, to separate
17. formation
18. instrument to measure
19. tumor
20. sight, vision
21. condition (usually abnormal)
22. disease
23. fear
24. surgical repair
25. stroke, paralysis
26. prolapse, drooping
27. instrument for examining
28. pertaining to
29. incision
30. structure

**IDENTIFYING MEDICAL TERMS**

1. amblyopia
2. bifocal
3. blepharoptosis
4. corneal
5. dacryoma
6. diplopia
7. emmetropia
8. intraocular
9. keratitis
10. keratoplasty
11. lacrimal
12. ocular
13. photophobia

**SPELLING**

1. astigmatism
2. cycloplegia
3. iridectomy
4. ophthalmologist
5. phacosclerosis

6. pupillary
7. retinoblastoma
8. scleritis
9. tonometer
10. uveal

**MATCHING**

| | | | |
|---|---|---|---|
| 1. e | | 6. d | |
| 2. f | | 7. g | |
| 3. j | | 8. b | |
| 4. h | | 9. a | |
| 5. c | | 10. i | |

**ABBREVIATIONS**

1. Acc
2. emmetropia
3. hypermetropia (hyperopia)
4. IOL
5. ST
6. myopia
7. visual acuity
8. intraocular pressure
9. VF
10. exotropia

**DIAGNOSTIC AND LABORATORY TESTS**

1. c
2. b
3. c
4. d
5. d

**CHART NOTE EXERCISE**

1. blurred vision
2. ophthalmologist
3. ultrasound
4. 20/70
5. pupils equal, round, react to light and accommodation
6. transparent
7. gray
8. photophobia
9. sleeping
10. AOL

## ■ CHAPTER 17

**ANATOMY AND PHYSIOLOGY**

1. a. ovaries

b. fallopian tubes

c. uterus

d. vagina

e. vulva

f. breasts

2. to perpetuate the species through sexual or germ cell reproduction

3. anteflexion

4. rounded portion of the uterine body superior to the attachment of the fallopian tube

5. a. broad ligaments

b. round ligaments

c. uterosacral ligaments

d. ligaments that attach to the bladder

6. a. perimetrium

b. myometrium

c. endometrium

7. a. organ of uterine cyclic changes that occur in the structure of the endometrium

b. provides a place for the protection and nourishment of the fetus during pregnancy

c. contracts rhythmically and powerfully during labor to expel the fetus from the uterus

8. a. bent backward at an angle with the cervix usually unchanged from its normal position

b. fundus forward toward the pubis with the cervix tilted up toward the sacrum

c. bent backward with the cervix pointing forward toward the symphysis pubis

9. uterine tubes or oviducts

10. a. serosa

b. muscular

c. mucosa

11. fingerlike structures that work to propel the discharged ovum into the fallopian tube

12. fertilization

13. a. serve as ducts to convey the ovum from the ovary to the uterus

b. serve as ducts to convey spermatozoa from the uterus toward each ovary

14. almond-shaped organs attached to the uterus by the ovarian ligament

15. a. primary

b. growing

c. graafian

16. pituitary gland (anterior lobe)

17. a. production of ova

b. production of hormones

18. musculomembranous . . . vestibule

19. a. female organ of copulation

b. passageway for discharge of menstruation

c. passageway for birth of the fetus

20. a. mons pubis

b. labia major

c. labia minora

d. vestibule

e. clitoris

21. mammary glands

22. areola . . . nipple

23. a. prolactin

b. insulin

c. glucocorticoids

24. thin yellowish secretion containing mainly serum and white blood cells; the "first milk"

25. a. follicular phase

b. ovulation

c. luteal phase

26. condition that affects certain women and can cause distressful symptoms such as nausea, constipation, diarrhea, anorexia, headache, appetite cravings, backache, muscular aches, edema, insomnia, clumsiness, malaise, irritability, indecisiveness, mental confusion, and depression

## WORD PARTS

### Prefixes

1. lack of

2. against

3. difficult, painful

4. within

5. within

6. scanty

7. around

8. after

9. backward

### Roots and Combining Forms

1. Bartholin's glands

2. receive

3. cervix

4. a coming together

5. vagina

6. cul-de-sac

7. bladder

8. fibrous tissue

9. belonging to birth

10. female

11. life

12. hymen

13. womb, uterus

14. womb, uterus

15. study of

16. breast

17. breast

18. month, menses, menstruation

19. month, menses, menstruation

20. womb, uterus

21. uterus

22. muscle

23. ovum, egg

24. ovary

25. ovary

26. to bear

27. cessation

28. rectum

29. fallopian tube

30. fallopian tube

31. formation, produce

32. uterus

33. vagina

34. sexual intercourse

35. turning
36. lump
37. lying beside, sexual intercourse

**Suffixes**

1. pertaining to
2. beginning
3. hernia
4. surgical puncture
5. surgical excision
6. formation, produce
7. condition
8. pertaining to
9. process
10. one who specializes
11. inflammation
12. tumor
13. condition (usually abnormal)
14. surgical repair
15. to burst forth
16. flow
17. instrument for examining
18. pertaining to
19. resemble
20. pertaining to

**IDENTIFYING MEDICAL TERMS**

1. cervicitis
2. dysmenorrhea
3. fibroma
4. gynecology
5. hymenectomy
6. mammoplasty
7. menorrhea
8. oogenesis
9. dyspareunia
10. genitalia

**SPELLING**

1. bartholinitis
2. hysterotomy
3. menorrhagia
4. oophoritis
5. salpingitis
6. vaginitis
7. venereal
8. menarche
9. oligomenorrhea

10. postcoital

**MATCHING**

1. e       6. h.
2. b       7. j.
3. a       8. g
4. c       9. i.
5. d      10. f

**ABBREVIATIONS**

1. abdominal hysterectomy
2. diethylstilbestrol
3. BCP
4. IUD
5. PID
6. CIN
7. dysfunctional uterine bleeding
8. premenstrual syndrome
9. D&C
10. TSS

**DIAGNOSTIC AND LABORATORY TESTS**

1. a
2. c
3. d
4. b
5. d.

**CHART NOTE EXERCISE**

1. GYN
2. hot flashes
3. hot flashes
4. yes
5. rule out
6. dyspareunia
7. soybeans
8. JVD
9. normal
10. rule out uterine fibroid tumor

## ■ CHAPTER 18

**AN OVERVIEW OF OBSTETRICS**

1. Obstetrics
2. Fertilization
3. zygote
4. yolk sac and amniotic cavity

5. placenta
6. a. time period from conception to onset of labor
   b. last phase of pregnancy to the time of delivery
   c. act of giving birth, also known as *childbirth* or *delivery*
   d. the 6 weeks following childbirth and expulsion of the placenta
7. a. signs experienced by the expectant mother that suggest pregnancy but are not positive signs
   b. signs that are observable by the examiner
   c. presence of fetal heart activity, fetal movements felt by an examiner, and visualization of the fetus with ultrasound
8. a. determines blood type
   b. determine risk for maternal-fetal blood incompatibility
   c. check for infection, renal disease, or diabetes
   d. screen for gestational diabetes
   e. diagnostic test that examines blood from the fetus to detect fetal abnormalities
   f. determine chromosomal abnormalities and biochemical disorders
   g. determine chromosomal abnormalities and biochemical disorders
   h. to screen for vaginal strep B infection
9. a. begins from the onset of true labor and lasts until the cervix is fully dilated to 10 cm
   b. continues after the cervix is dilated to 10 cm until the delivery of the baby
   c. delivery of the placenta
10. epidural block

## WORD PARTS

### Prefixes

1. before
2. through
3. difficult, painful
4. out
5. excessive
6. new
7. around
8. excessive
9. before
10. first
11. false
12. three
13. beyond

### Roots and Combining Forms

1. to miscarry
2. amniotic fluid
3. cord
4. displaces
5. knowledge
6. pregnancy
7. pregnancy
8. water
9. to shine
10. month
11. birth
12. birth
13. to bear
14. pelvis
15. external genitals
16. second
17. substituted
18. birth

### Suffixes

1. pertaining to
2. use
3. surgical puncture
4. pregnancy
5. vomiting
6. condition
7. pertaining to
8. pertaining to
9. process
10. study of
11. measurement
12. sound
13. tissue

## IDENTIFYING MEDICAL TERMS

1. abortion
2. antepartum
3. chloasma
4. cordocentesis
5. dystocia
6. linea nigra
7. neonatal
8. placenta previa
9. prenatal
10. primigravida
11. primipara
12. pseudocyesis
13. pudendal
14. secundines
15. trimester

## SPELLING

1. aminocentesis
2. cerclage
3. chloasma
4. dystocia
5. eclampsia
6. lochia
7. polyhydramnios
8. primigravida
9. pudendal
10. secundines

## MATCHING

1. d
2. j
3. f
4. h
5. g
6. b
7. i
8. a
9. c
10. e

## ABBREVIATIONS

1. alpha-fetoprotein
2. artificial rupture of membranes
3. cesarean section
4. CVS
5. electronic fetal monitor
6. estimated date of delivery
7. GBS
8. obstetrics
9. spontaneous abortion
10. UC

## DIAGNOSTIC AND LABORATORY TESTS

1. c
2. a
3. d
4. b
5. c

## CHART NOTE EXERCISE

1. hemorrhage
2. transabdominal ultrasound
3. allow the fetus to mature
4. hemoglobin and hematocrit
5. if severe or life-threatening hemorrhage occurs or fetal distress is apparent
6. multiparity
7. external
8. because of the potential for hemorrhage
9. if hemorrhage persists or becomes more severe, and results of blood test indicate the need for a transfusion
10. multiparity, increasing age (over 35 y/o), prior cesarean birth, smoking, recent spontaneous or induced abortion, ineffective development of blood vessels in the decidua, and large placenta

## ■ CHAPTER 19

## ANATOMY AND PHYSIOLOGY

1. a. testes
   b. various ducts
   c. urethra
   d. bulbourethral gland
   e. prostate gland
   f. seminal vesicles

2. a. scrotum

   b. penis

3. provide the sperm cells necessary to fertilize the ovum, thereby perpetuating the species

4. pouchlike structure located behind the penis

5. corpora cavernosa penis and the corpus spongiosum

6. 15 to 20

7. glans penis

8. loose skin folds that cover the penis

9. lubricating fluid

10. a. male organ of copulation

    b. site of the orifice for the elimination of urine and semen from the body

11. two ovoid-shaped organs located in the scrotum; each testis is about 4 cm long and 2.5 cm wide

12. seminiferous tubules

13. a. responsible for the development of secondary male characteristics during puberty

    b. essential for normal growth and development of the male accessory sex organs

    c. plays a vital role in the erection process of the penis.

    d. affects the growth of hair on the face

    e. affects muscular development and vocal timbre

14. rete testis

15. coiled tube lying on the posterior aspect of the testis

16. a. storage site for sperm

    b. duct for the passage of sperm

17. vas deferens or ductus deferens

18. a. vas deferens or ductus deferens

    b. arteries

    c. veins

    d. lymphatic vessels

    e. nerves

19. production of a slightly alkaline fluid

20. about 4 cm wide and weighs about 20 g; composed of glandular, connective, and muscular tissues and lies behind the urinary bladder

21. enlargement of the prostate that can occur in older men

22. bulbourethral . . . Cowper's

23. a. prostatic

    b. membranous

    c. penile

24. transmits urine and semen out of the body

25. 20

## WORD PARTS

### Prefixes

1. lack of
2. lack of
3. around
4. upon
5. water
6. under
7. scanty
8. beside
9. into
10. good
11. different
12. similar, same
13. three

### Roots and Combining Forms

1. glans
2. to cut
3. hidden
4. not natural
5. testis
6. to pour
7. testicle
8. testicle
9. testicle
10. a muzzle
11. prostate
12. to prune
13. a rent (opening)
14. seed
15. seed, semen
16. seed, sperm
17. seed, sperm
18. testicle
19. twisted vein
20. vessel
21. vesicle
22. animal
23. life
24. to throw out
25. genitals
26. female
27. breast
28. sex
29. thread
30. body

### Suffixes

1. pertaining to
2. pertaining to
3. immature cell, germ cell
4. hernia, swelling, tumor
5. to kill
6. surgical excision
7. formation, produce
8. condition
9. process
10. condition
11. inflammation
12. use
13. condition (usually abnormal)
14. formation, produce
15. flow
16. incision
17. pertaining to

## IDENTIFYING MEDICAL TERMS

1. balanitis
2. epididymectomy
3. orchidectomy
4. prepuce
5. hydrocele
6. condyloma
7. spermatoblast
8. spermatozoon
9. spermicide
10. testicular

## SPELLING

1. cryptorchidism

2. hypospadias
3. orchidotomy
4. eugenics
5. trisomy

## MATCHING

1. e
6. i
2. c
7. h
3. f
8. k
4. b
9. a
5. g
10. d

## ABBREVIATIONS

1. BPH
2. gonorrhea
3. HPV
4. herpes simplex virus-2
5. sexually transmitted diseases
6. ED
7. transurethral resection of the prostate
8. nongonococcal urethritis
9. VD
10. PSA

## DIAGNOSTIC AND LABORATORY TESTS

1. c
2. a
3. b
4. c
5. c

## CHART NOTE EXERCISE

1. urgency
2. digital rectal exam
3. Proscar
4. PSA
5. impotence
6. 5.5
7. 1.5
8. dihydrotestosterone (DHT)
9. reduce
10. 6

## ■ CHAPTER 20

## AN OVERVIEW OF CANCER

1. a. carcinomas

b. sarcomas
c. mixed cancers
2. process in which normal cells have a distinct appearance and specialized function
3. process in which normal cells lose their specialization and become malignant
4. a. active migration
b. direct extension
c. metastasis
5. a. Change in bowel or bladder habits
b. Sore that does not heal
c. Unusual bleeding or discharge
d. Thickening or lump in breast or elsewhere
e. Indigestion or difficulty in swallowing
f. Obvious change in a wart or mole
g. Nagging cough or hoarseness
6. a. surgery
b. chemotherapy
c. radiation therapy
d. immunotherapy

## SPELLING

1. anaplasia
2. fibrosarcoma
3. lymphosarcoma
4. myeloma
5. oncogenic
6. seminoma

## WORD PARTS

### Prefixes

1. up, apart, backward
2. star-shaped
3. excessive
4. new
5. little
6. before
7. in
8. in
9. beyond
10. short

### Roots and Combining Forms

1. gland
2. vessel
3. cancer, crab
4. cancer
5. cancer
6. cartilage
7. chorion
8. cell
9. tree
10. fiber
11. glue
12. glue
13. blood
14. safe
15. smooth
16. white
17. white
18. fat
19. lymph
20. lymph
21. marrow
22. black
23. meninges, membrane
24. mucus
25. fungus
26. bone marrow
27. muscle
28. a little box
29. kidney
30. nerve
31. tumor
32. bone
33. net
34. retina
35. rod
36. flesh
37. to lead
38. seed
39. mouth
40. monster
41. thymus
42. poison
43. grating

### Suffixes

1. immature cell

2. blood condition
3. formation, produce
4. formation, produce
5. formation, produce
6. condition
7. substance
8. inflammation
9. tumor
10. pertaining to
11. plate
12. formation
13. a thing formed
14. use, action
15. treatment
16. pertaining to
17. pertaining to
18. pertaining to
19. process
20. nature of
21. forming
22. control
23. resemble

## IDENTIFYING MEDICAL TERMS

1. carcinogen
2. chondrosarcoma
3. glioma
4. leiomyosarcoma
5. leukemia
6. lymphoma
7. melanoma
8. myosarcoma
9. osteogenic sarcoma
10. sarcoma

## MATCHING

1. e      6. f
2. i      7. j
3. d      8. b
4. g      9. h
5. c      10. a

## ABBREVIATIONS

1. Adeno-CA
2. Bx
3. cancer
4. chemotherapy

5. DNA
6. internal radiation therapy
7. ALL
8. DCIS
9. breast cancer gene
10. TNM

## CHART NOTE EXERCISE

1. hard
2. testicular self-examination (TSE)
3. testicular cancer to be confirmed by orchidectomy and biopsy
4. determine whether the mass is solid or fluid filled
5. HCG
6. CXR and CT
7. complete blood count
8. orchidectomy
9. scrotum
10. Identification of cell type (seminoma or nonseminoma) is important in planning the treatment.

## ■ CHAPTER 21

### AN OVERVIEW OF RADIOLOGY AND NUCLEAR MEDICINE

1. study of x-rays, radioactive substances, radioactive isotopes, and ionizing radiation
2. a. invisible
   b. cause ionization
   c. cause fluorescence
*Alternate characteristics to those listed:
   d. travel in a straight line
   e. able to penetrate substances
   f. destroy cells
3. a. can depress the hematopoietic system, cause leukopenia, leukemia
   b. can damage the gonads
4. a. wearing a film badge
   b. lead screens
   c. lead-lined room

   d. protective clothing
   e. gonad shield
5. a. computed tomography
   b. magnetic resonance imaging
   c. ultrasound
   d. thermography
   e. scintigraphy

## WORD PARTS

### Prefixes

1. below
2. within
3. one-thousandth
4. beyond
5. into

### Roots and Combining Forms

1. acting
2. vessel
3. finger
4. artery
5. joint
6. bronchi
7. heart
8. gall, bile
9. gall
10. motion
11. motion
12. to draw
13. curie
14. bladder
15. skin
16. echo
17. brain
18. fluorescence
19. kind
20. uterus
21. ion
22. ion
23. nucleus
24. study of
25. to shine
26. lymph
27. breast
28. spinal cord
29. to swing
30. dark

31. light
32. nature
33. renal pelvis
34. radiant
35. x-ray
36. roentgen
37. fallopian tube
38. salivary
39. sound
40. sound
41. heat
42. to cut
43. vein
44. vein

*Suffixes*

1. one who
2. formation, produce
3. pertaining to
4. record
5. instrument for recording
6. recording
7. pertaining to
8. process
9. one who specializes
10. inflammation
11. nature of
12. study of
13. instrument to measure
14. pertaining to
15. instrument for examining
16. visual examination, to view, examine
17. treatment
18. having a particular quality

## IDENTIFYING MEDICAL TERMS

1. angiography
2. arthrography
3. cholecystogram
4. ionotherapy
5. mammography
6. millicurie
7. physicist
8. radiation
9. radioactive
10. radiographer

11. radiolucent
12. radiopaque
13. sonogram

## SPELLING

1. hysterosalpingogram
2. echography
3. lymphangiography
4. myelogram
5. cassette
6. radioactive
7. radiography
8. sialography
9. tomography
10. venography

## MATCHING

1. d          6. k
2. e          7. b
3. c          8. i
4. g          9. a
5. j         10. h

## ABBREVIATIONS

1. AP
2. Ba
3. CT
4. interventional radiology
5. lateral
6. radium
7. MRI
8. posteroanterior
9. Ci
10. positron emission tomography

## CHART NOTE EXERCISE

1. lump
2. fine needle aspiration biopsy
3. adjacent to areola at 1 o'clock
4. monthly BSE
5. lumpectomy
6. ductal carcinoma in situ
7. each month, the week following menses
8. 70%
9. firm without mass
10. reduce the risk of regrowth of cancer cells

## ■ CHAPTER 22

### AN OVERVIEW: MENTAL HEALTH AND MENTAL ILLNESS

1. Mental illness
2. a. major depression
   b. bipolar disorder
   c. schizophrenia
3. Psychiatry
4. a. drug therapy
   b. psychotherapy
   c. electroconvulsive therapy
5. Psychoanalysis

### WORD PARTS

*Prefixes*

1. lack of, without
2. deficient, below
3. beside, abnormal
4. fire

*Roots and Combining Forms*

1. marketplace
2. self
3. center
4. circle, cycle
5. to cheat
6. I, self
7. to wander in mind
8. treatment
9. study of
10. nerve
11. disease
12. mind
13. mind
14. mind
15. to divide
16. body
17. body
18. mind, emotion

*Suffixes*

1. shape
2. condition
3. pertaining to
4. process
5. condition
6. one who specializes
7. study of

8. madness

9. mind

10. appetite

11. condition (usually abnormal)

12. fear

13. treatment

14. pertaining to

**IDENTIFYING MEDICAL TERMS**

1. agoraphobia

2. apathy

3. delusion

4. depression

5. egocentric

6. mania

7. phobia

8. psychiatrist

9. psychotherapy

10. pyromania

**SPELLING**

1. anxiety

2. autism

3. bulimia

4. dementia

5. factitious

6. hallucination

7. paranoia

8. psychosomatic

9. schizophrenia

10. somatoform

**MATCHING**

1. d        6. b

2. g        7. i

3. c        8. e

4. a        9. h

5. f       10. j

**ABBREVIATIONS**

1. CBT

2. DSM-IV-TR

3. electroconvulsive therapy

4. Minnesota Multiphasic Personality Inventory

5. NIMH

6. obsessive-compulsive disorder

7. PTSD

8. seasonal affective disorder

9. Thematic Apperception Test

10. WHO

**CHART NOTE EXERCISE**

1. eating

2. by medical history and physical examination

3. tricyclic antidepressant

4. appetite

5. B-complex vitamins and omega-3 fatty acids

6. diaphoresis

7. alcohol

8. low blood pressure due to sudden change in position

9. blurred vision

10. cheerless

# GLOSSARY OF WORD PARTS

## APPENDIX II

### PREFIXES

| | |
|---|---|
| a- | no, not, without, lack of, apart |
| ab- | away from |
| ad- | toward, near |
| ambi- | both, both sides, around, about |
| an- | no, not, without, lack of |
| ana- | up, apart, backward, again, anew |
| ant- | against |
| ante- | before, forward |
| anti- | against |
| apo- | separation |
| astro- | star-shaped |
| auto- | self |
| bi- | two, double |
| bin- | twice, two |
| brachy- | short |
| brady- | slow |
| cac- | bad |
| centi- | one hundred, one hundredth |
| chromo- | color |
| circum- | around |
| con- | with, together |
| contra- | against, opposite |
| de- | down, away from |
| deca- | ten |
| di- | two, double |
| di (a)- | through, between, complete |

| | |
|---|---|
| dia- | through, between, complete |
| dif- | apart, free from, separate |
| di(s)- | two, apart |
| dis- | apart |
| dys- | bad, difficult, painful, abnormal |
| ec- | out, outside, outer |
| ecto- | out, outside, outer |
| em- | in |
| en- | in, within |
| end- | within, inner |
| endo- | within, inner |
| ep- | upon, over, above |
| epi- | upon, over, above |
| eso- | inward |
| eu- | good, normal |
| ex- | out, away from |
| exo- | out, away from |
| extra- | outside, beyond |
| hemi- | half |
| heter- | different |
| hetero- | different |
| homo- | similar, same |
| homeo- | similar, same, likeness, constant |
| hydr- | water |
| hydro- | water |
| hyp- | below, deficient |
| hyper- | above, beyond, excessive |

| | |
|---|---|
| hypo- | below, under, deficient |
| in- | in, into, not |
| infer- | below |
| inter- | between |
| intra- | within |
| ir- | not |
| macro- | large |
| mal- | bad |
| mega- | large, great |
| meso- | middle |
| meta- | beyond, over, between, change |
| micro- | small |
| milli- | one-thousandth |
| mon (o)- | one |
| mono- | one |
| multi- | many, much |
| neo- | new |
| nulli- | none |
| olig- | little, scanty |
| oligo- | little, scanty |
| pan- | all |
| par- | around, beside |
| para- | beside, alongside, abnormal |
| per- | through |
| peri- | around |
| poly- | many, much, excessive |
| post- | after, behind |
| pre- | before, in front of |

A-33

| | |
|---|---|
| primi- | first |
| pro- | before, in front of |
| proto- | first |
| pseudo- | false |
| pyro- | fire |
| quadri- | four |
| re- | back, backward, again |
| retro- | backward |
| semi- | half |
| sub- | below, under, beneath |
| supra- | above, beyond, superior |
| super- | upper, above, |
| sym- | together, with |
| syn- | together, with |
| tachy- | fast |
| trans- | across |
| tri- | three |
| ultra- | beyond |
| un- | back, reversal, not, annulment |
| uni- | one |

## WORD ROOTS/COMBINING FORMS

| | |
|---|---|
| abdomin | abdomen |
| abort | to miscarry |
| absorpt | to suck in |
| acanth | thorn |
| acetabul | acetabulum, hip socket |
| acid | acid |
| acoust | hearing |
| acr | extremity, point |
| acr/o | extremity, point |
| act | acting, act |
| actin | ray |
| acute | sharp |
| aden | gland |
| aden/o | gland |
| adhes | stuck to |
| adip | fat |
| adren | adrenal gland |

| | |
|---|---|
| adren/o | adrenal gland |
| agglutinat | clumping |
| agon | agony |
| agor/a | market place |
| albin | white |
| albumin | protein |
| alimentat | nourishment |
| all | other |
| alveol | small, hollow air sac |
| ambyl | dull |
| ambul | to walk |
| amni/o | amniotic fluid |
| ampere | ampere |
| amputat | to cut though |
| amyl | starch |
| anabol | building up |
| anastom | opening |
| andr | man |
| andr/o | man |
| ang | vessel |
| ang/i | vessel |
| angin | to choke |
| angi/o | vessel |
| anis/o | unequal |
| ankyl | stiffening, crooked |
| an/o | anus |
| anter | toward the front |
| anthrac | coal |
| aort | aorta |
| aort/o | aorta |
| append | appendix |
| arachn | spider |
| arous | alertness, to rise |
| arche | beginning |
| arter | artery |
| arter/i | artery |
| arteri/o | artery |
| arthr | joint, to articulate |
| arthr/o | joint, to articulate |
| artific/i | not natural |
| aspirat | to draw in |
| atel | imperfect |
| atel/o | imperfect |

| | |
|---|---|
| ather | fatty substance, porridge |
| ather/o | fatty substance, porridge |
| atri | atrium |
| atri/o | atrium |
| aud/i | to hear |
| audi/o | to hear |
| auditor | hearing |
| aur | ear |
| aur/i | ear |
| auscultat | listen to |
| aut | self |
| axill | armpit |
| bacter/i | bacteria |
| balan | glans penis |
| bartholin | Bartholin's glands |
| bas/o | base |
| bil | bile, gall |
| bil/i | bile, gall |
| bi/o | life |
| blast/o | germ cell |
| blephar | eyelid |
| blephar/o | eyelid |
| brach/i | arm |
| bronch | bronchi |
| bronch/i | bronchi |
| bronchiol | bronchiole |
| bronch/o | bronchi |
| bucc | cheek |
| bucc/o | cheek |
| burs | pouch |
| calc | lime, calcium |
| calc/i | calcium |
| calcan/e | heel bone |
| cancer | crab, cancer |
| capn | smoke |
| capsul | little box |
| carcin | cancer |
| carcin/o | cancer |
| card | heart |
| card/i | heart |
| cardi/o | heart |

| | | | | | |
|---|---|---|---|---|---|
| carp | wrist | clavicul | clavicle, collar bone | crur | leg |
| carp/o | wrist | cleid/o | clavicle | cry/o | cold |
| cartil | gristle | coagul | to clot | crypt | hidden |
| castr | to prune | coagulat | to clot | cubit | elbow, to lie |
| catabol | casting down | coccyg/e | coccyx, tail bone | culd/o | cul-de-sac |
| caud | tail | coccyg/o | coccyx, tail bone | curie | curie |
| caus | heat | cochle/o | land snail | cutane | skin |
| cavit | cavity | coit | coming together | cutane/o | skin |
| celi | abdomen, belly | col | colon | cyan | dark blue |
| cellul | little cell | coll/a | glue | cycl | ciliary body of eye |
| centr | center | collis | neck | cycl/o | ciliary body of eye, |
| centrat | center | col/o | colon | | cycle, circle |
| centr/i | center | colon | colon | cyst | bladder, sac |
| cephal | head | colon/o | colon | cyst/o | bladder, sac |
| cept | receive | colp/o | vagina | cyt | cell |
| cerebell | little brain | comat | a deep sleep | cyth | cell |
| cerebell/o | little brain | compensat | to make good | cyt/o | cell |
| cerebr/o | cerebrum | concuss | shaken violently | dacry | tear, lacrimal duct, |
| cervic | cervix, neck | condyle | knuckle | | tear duct |
| cheil | lip | con/i | dust | dactyl | finger or toe |
| chem/o | chemical | conjunctiv | to join together, | dactyl/o | finger or toe |
| chir/o | hand | | conjunctiva | defecat | to remove dregs |
| chlor/o | green | connect | to bind together | delus | to cheat |
| chol | gall, bile | consci | aware | dem | people |
| chole | gall, bile | constipat | to press together | dendr/o | tree |
| chol/e | gall, bile | continence | to hold | dent | tooth |
| choledoch/o | common bile duct | cor | pupil | dent/i | tooth |
| chondr | cartilage | cord/o | cord | derm | skin |
| chondr/o | cartilage | coriat | corium | derm/a | skin |
| chord | cord | corne | cornea | dermat | skin |
| chori/o | chorion | corpor | body | dermat/o | skin |
| choroid | choroid | corpor/e | body | derm/o | skin |
| choroid/o | choroid | cortic | cortex | dextr/o | to the right |
| chromat | color | cortis | cortex | diaphragmat/o | diaphragm |
| chrom/o | color | cost | rib | didym | testis |
| chym | juice | cost/o | rib | digit | finger or toe |
| cine | motion | cox | hip | dilat | to widen |
| cinemat/o | motion | cran/i | skull | dipl/o | double |
| circulat | circular | crani/o | skull | disk | disk |
| cirrh | orange-yellow | creat | flesh | dist | away from the |
| cirrh/o | orange-yellow | creatin | flesh, creatine | | point of origin |
| cis | to cut | crine | to secrete | diverticul | diverticula |
| claudicat | to limp | crin/o | to secrete | dors | backward |

| dors/i | backward |
|---|---|
| duct | to lead |
| duoden | duodenum |
| dur | dura, hard |
| dur/o | dura, hard |
| dwarf | small |
| dynam | power |
| ech/o | echo |
| ectop | displaced |
| eg/o | I, self |
| ejaculat | to throw out |
| electr/o | electricity |
| eme | to vomit |
| embol | to cast, to throw |
| emulsificat | disintergrate |
| encephal | brain |
| encephal/o | brain |
| enchyma | to pour |
| enter/o | intestines (usually small intestine) |
| enucleat | to remove the kernel of |
| eosin/o | rose-colored |
| episi/o | vulva, pudenda |
| erget | work |
| erg/o | work |
| eructat | breaking out |
| erysi | red |
| erythr/o | red |
| esophag/e | esophagus |
| esophage/(o) | esophagus |
| esthesi/o | feeling, sensation |
| esthet | feeling, sensation |
| estr/o | mad desire |
| eti/o | cause |
| excretor | sifted out |
| fasc | band (fascia) |
| fasci/o | band (fascia) |
| febr | fever |
| femor | femur, thigh bone |
| femor/o | femur, thigh bone |
| fenestrat | window |
| fibr | fibrous tissue, fiber |
| fibrillat | fibrils (small fibers) |

| fibrin/o | fiber |
|---|---|
| fibr/o | fiber |
| fibul | fibula |
| filtrat | to strain through |
| fixat | fastened |
| flex | to bend |
| fluor/o | fluorescence, luminous |
| foc | focus |
| follicul | little bag |
| format | shaping |
| fungat | mushroom, fungus |
| furc | fork |
| fus | to pour |
| galact/o | milk |
| ganglion | knot |
| gastr | stomach |
| gastr/o | stomach |
| gen | formation, produce |
| gene | formation, produce |
| genet | formation, produce |
| genital | belonging to birth |
| gen/o | kind |
| ger | old age |
| gester | to bear |
| gigant | giant |
| gingiv | gums |
| glandul | little acorn |
| gli | glue |
| gli/o | glue |
| glob | globe |
| globin | globule |
| globul | globe |
| glomerul | glomerulus, little ball |
| glomerul/o | glomerulus, little ball |
| gloss/o | tongue |
| gluc/o | sweet, sugar |
| glyc | sweet, sugar |
| glyc/o | glucose, sweet, sugar |
| glycos | glucose, sugar |
| gnost | knowledge |
| gonad | seed |
| goni/o | angle |

| gon/o | genitals |
|---|---|
| grand/i | great |
| granul/o | little grain, granular |
| gravida | pregnancy |
| gravidar | pregnancy |
| gryp | curve |
| gurgitat | to flood |
| gynec/o | female |
| halat | breathe |
| hallucinat | to wander in mind |
| hallux | great (big) toe |
| hem | blood |
| hemat | blood |
| hemat/o | blood |
| hem/o | blood |
| hemorrh | vein liable to bleed |
| hepat | liver |
| hepat/o | liver |
| herni/o | hernia |
| hidr | sweat |
| hirsut | hairy |
| hist/o | tissue |
| hol/o | whole |
| horizont | horizon |
| humer | humerus |
| hydr | water |
| hymen | hymen |
| hypn | sleep |
| hyster | womb, uterus |
| hyster/o | womb, uterus |
| iatr | treatment |
| icter | jaundice |
| ile | ileum |
| ile/o | ileum |
| ili | ilium |
| ili/o | ilium |
| illus | foot |
| immun/o | safe, immunity |
| infarct | infarct (necrosis of an area) |
| infect | to infect |
| infer | below |

| | | | | | |
|---|---|---|---|---|---|
| inguin | groin | lingu | tongue | men | month, menses, menstruation |
| insul | insulin | lip | fat | mening | membrane, meninges |
| insulin/o | insulin | lipid | fat | mening/i | membrane, meninges |
| integument | covering | lip/o | fat | mening/o | membrane, meninges |
| intern | within | lith | stone | menise | crescent |
| ionizat | ion (going) | lith/o | stone | men/o | month, menses, menstruation |
| ion/o | ion | lob | lobe | menstru | to discharge the menses |
| iont/o | ion | lob/o | lobe | ment | mind |
| irid | iris | lobul | small lobe | mes | middle |
| irid/o | iris | locat | to place | mes/o | middle |
| isch | to hold back | log | study | mester | month |
| ischi | ischium | log/o | word | metr | to measure, womb, uterus |
| is/o | equal | lopec | fox mange | metr/i | womb, uterus |
| jaund | yellow | lord | bending, curve, swayback | micturit | to urinate |
| kal | potassium | lucent | to shine | miliar | millet (tiny) |
| kary/o | cell's nucleus | lumb | loin | minim | least |
| kel | tumor | lumb/o | loin, lower back | mi/o | less, smaller |
| kerat | horn, cornea | lump | lump | mit | thread |
| kerat/o | horn, cornea | lun | moon | mitr | mitral valve |
| keton | ketone | lymph | lymph, clear fluid | mnes | memory |
| kil/o | one thousand | lymph/o | lymph, clear fluid | mucos | mucus |
| kinet | motion | malign | bad kind | mucus | mucus |
| kyph | hump | mamm/o | breast | muscul | muscle |
| labi | lip | mandibul | lower jawbone | muscul/o | muscle |
| labyrinth | maze | man/o | thin | muta | to change |
| labyrinth/o | maze | mast | mastoid process, breast-shaped | mutat | to change |
| lacrim | tear | masticat | to chew | my | muscle |
| lamin | lamina, thin plate | mast/o | mastoid process, breast-shaped | myc | fungus |
| lamp (s) | to shine | mat | to ripen | myc/o | fungus |
| lapar/o | abdomen | maxill | jawbone | mydriat | dilation, widen |
| laryng | larynx, voice box | maxilla | jaw | myel | bone marrow, spinal cord |
| laryng/e | larynx, voice box | maxim | greatest | myel/o | bone marrow |
| laryng/o | larynx, voice box | meat | passage | my/o | muscle |
| later | side | meat/o | passage | my/o (s) | muscle |
| laxat | to loosen | med | middle | myring | eardrum, tympanic membrane |
| lei/o | smooth | medi | toward the middle | myring/o | eardrum, tympanic membrane |
| lemma | rind, sheath, husk | medull | marrow | | |
| lent | lens | medull/o | marrow | | |
| lept | seizure | melan | black | | |
| letharg | drowsiness | melan/o | black | | |
| leuk | white | | | | |
| leuk/o | white | | | | |
| levat | lifter | | | | |

| | | | | | |
|---|---|---|---|---|---|
| myx | mucus | oscill | to swing | phac/o | lens |
| narc/o | numbness, sleep, stupor | oscill/o | to swing | phag | to eat, engulf |
| | | oste | bone | phag/o | to eat, engulf |
| nas/o | nose | oste/o | bone | phak | lentil, lens |
| nat | birth | ot | ear | phalang/e | phalanges, finger/toe bones |
| nat/o | birth | ot/o | ear | | |
| necr | death | ovar | ovary | pharyng/o | pharynx, throat |
| necr/o | death | ovul | ovary | pharyng | pharynx, throat |
| nephr | kidney | ovulat | ovary | phas | speech |
| nephr/o | kidney | ox | oxygen | phen/o | to show |
| neur | nerve | ox/i | oxygen | phe/o | dusky |
| neur/i | nerve | oxy | sour, sharp, acid | phim | muzzle |
| neur/o | nerve | pachy | thick | phleb | vein |
| neutr/o | neither | palp | touch | phleb/o | vein |
| nid | nest | pancreat | pancreas | phon | voice |
| noct | night | paque | dark | phone | voice |
| nom | law | palat/o | palate | phon/o | sound |
| norm | rule | palliat | cloaked | phor | carrying |
| nucl | nucleus | pallid/o | globus, pallidus | phos | light |
| nucle | kernel, nucleus | palm | palm | phot/o | light |
| nyctal | night | palpitat | throbbing | phragm | partition |
| occlus | to shut up | papill | papilla | phras | speech |
| ocul | eye | para | to bear, bring forth | phren | mind |
| odont | tooth | paralyt | to disable, paralysis | physic | nature |
| olecran | elbow | pareun | lying beside, sexual intercourse | physi/o | nature |
| olecran/o | elbow | | | pil/o | hair |
| omphal/o | navel, umbilicus | partum | labor | pine | pine cone |
| onc/o | tumor | parturit | in labor | pineal | pineal body |
| onych | nail | patell | kneecap, patella | pin/o | to drink |
| onych/o | nail | path | disease | pituitar | pituitary gland |
| o/o | ovum, egg | path/o | disease | plak | plate |
| oophor | ovary | pause | cessation | plasma | thing formed, plasma |
| ophthalm | eye | pector | chest | plast | developing |
| ophthalm/o | eye | pectorat | breast, chest | pleur | pleura |
| opt | eye | ped | foot, child | pleura | pleura |
| opt/o | eye | ped/i | foot, child | pleur/o | pleura |
| or | mouth | pedicul | louse | plicat | to fold |
| orch | testicle | pelv/i | pelvis | pneum/o | lung, air |
| orchid | testicle | penile | penis | pneumon | lung |
| orchid/o | testicle | pept | to digest | pneumon/o | lung |
| organ | organ | perine | perineum | pod/o | foot |
| orth | straight | periton/e | peritoneum | poiet | formation |
| orth/o | straight | phac | lens | poli/o | gray |

| | | | | | | |
|---|---|---|---|---|---|---|
| pollex | thumb | regul | rule | sert | to gain |
| por | passage | relaxat | to loosen | sexu | sex |
| porphyr | purple | remiss | remit | sial | saliva |
| poster | behind, toward the back, back | ren | kidney | sial/o | salivary |
| | | ren/o | kidney | sider/o | iron |
| prand/i | meal | respirat | breathing | sigmoid | sigmoid |
| presby | old | reticul/o | net | sigmoid/o | sigmoid |
| press | to press | retin | retina | sin/o | curve |
| proct | anus and rectum | retin/o | retina | sinus | a hollow curve |
| proct/o | anus and rectum | rhabd/o | rod | situ | place |
| prophylact | guarding | rheumat | discharge | som | body |
| prostat | prostate | rheumat/o | discharge | somat | body |
| prosth/e | an addition | rhin/o | nose | somat/o | body |
| proxim | near the point of origin | rhonch | snore | somn | sleep |
| | | rhytid/o | wrinkle | son | sound |
| prurit | itching | roent | roentgen | son/o | sound |
| psych | mind | rotat | to turn | spadias | rent, opening |
| psych/o | mind | rrhyth | rhythm | spastic | convulsive |
| pudend | external genitals | rrhythm | rhythm | sperm | seed (sperm) |
| pulm/o | lung | rube/o | red | spermi | seed (sperm) |
| pulmon | lung | sacr | sacrum | spermat | seed (sperm) |
| pulmonar | lung | salping | tube, fallopian tube | spermat/o | seed (sperm) |
| pulmon/o | lung | salping/o | tube, fallopian tube | sphygm/o | pulse |
| pupill | pupil | salpinx | tube, fallopian tube | spin | spine, thorn |
| purpur | purple | sarc | flesh | spir/o | breath |
| py | pus | sarc/o | flesh | splen/o | spleen |
| pyel | renal pelvis | scapul | shoulder blade | spondyl | vertebra |
| pyel/o | renal pelvis | schiz/o | to divide | spondyl/o | vertebra |
| pylor | pylorus, gate keeper | scler | hardening | staped | stirrup |
| py/o | pus | scler/o | hardening | steat | fat |
| pyret | fever | scoli | curvature | sten | narrowing |
| pyr/o | heat, fire | scoli/o | curvature | ster | solid |
| rach | spine | scop | to examine | stern | sternum, breast bone |
| rachi | spine | seb/o | oil | stern/o | sternum, breast bone |
| radi | radius | secund | second | sterol | solid (fat) |
| rad/i | radiating out from a center | semin | seed, semen | steth | chest |
| | | seminat | seed, semen | steth/o | chest |
| radiat | radiant | senile | old | stigmat | point |
| radic/o | spinal nerve root | senil | old | stom | mouth |
| radicul | spinal nerve root | sept | putrefaction | stomat | mouth |
| radi/o | ray, x-ray | septic | putrefying | strabism | squinting |
| ras | to scrape off | ser (a) | whey, serum | strict | to tighten, contraction |
| rect/o | rectum | ser/o | whey, serum | | |

| | | | | | |
|---|---|---|---|---|---|
| superfic/i | near the surface | topic | place | vas | vessel |
| suppress | suppress | top/o | place | vascul | small vessel |
| surrog | substitute | tors | twisted | vas/o | vessel |
| sympath | sympathy | tort/i | twisted | vector | carrier |
| symmetric | symmetry | tox | poison | ven | vein |
| synov | synovial membrane | toxic | poison | venere | sexual intercourse |
| system | composite whole | trach/e | trachea | ven/i | vein |
| systol | contraction | trache/o | trachea | ven/o | vein |
| systole | contraction | tract | to draw | ventilat | to air |
| tars/o | ankle, tarsus | trephinat | bore | ventr | near or on the belly |
| tel | end, distant | trich | hair | | side of the body |
| tele | distant | trich/o | hair | ventricul | ventricle |
| tempor | temples | trigon | trigone | ventricul/o | little belly |
| tend/o | tendon | trism | grating | vermi | worm |
| tendin | tendon | trop | turning | vers | turning |
| ten/o | tendon | troph | a turning | vertebr | vertebra |
| tendon | tendon | tuber | bulge | vertebr/o | vertebra |
| tenos | tendon | tubercul | little swelling | vesic | bladder |
| tens | tension | turg | swelling | vesicul | seminal vesicle |
| tentori | tentorium, tent | tuss | cough | vir | virus (poison) |
| terat | monster | tympan | ear drum | viril | masculine |
| testicul | testicle | tympan/o | drum | viscer | body organs |
| test/o | testicle | uln | ulna, elbow | volt | volt |
| thalass | sea | uln/o | ulna, elbow | volunt | will |
| thel/i | nipple | umbilic | navel | volvul | to roll |
| therm | hot, heat | ungu | nail | vuls | to pull |
| therm/o | hot, heat | ur | urinate | watt | watt |
| thorac | chest | urea | urea | xanth/o | yellow |
| thorac/o | chest | uret | urine | xen | foreign material |
| thorax | chest | ureter | ureter | xer | dry |
| thromb | clot | ureter/o | ureter | xer/o | dry |
| thromb/o | clot | urethr | urethra | xiph | sword |
| thym | thymus, mind, | urethr/o | urethra | zo/o | animal |
| | emotion | urin | urine | zoon | life |
| thyr | thyroid, shield | urinat | urine | | |
| thyr/o | thyroid, shield | urin/o | urine | | |
| thyrox | thyroid, shield | ur/o | urination | **SUFFIXES** | |
| tibi | tibia | uter | uterus | -able | capable |
| toc | birth | uter/o | uterus | -ac | pertaining to |
| tom/o | to cut | uve | uvea | -act | to act |
| ton | tone, tension | vagin | vagina | -ad | pertaining to |
| ton/o | tone | vag/o | vagus, wandering | -age | related to |
| tonsill | tonsil, almond | varic/o | twisted vein | -al | pertaining to |

| | | | | | |
|---|---|---|---|---|---|
| -algesia | condition of pain | -ectomy | surgical excision, surgical removal, resection | -ism | condition |
| -algia | pain, ache | | | -ist | one who specializes, agent |
| -ant | forming | -edema | swelling | | |
| -ar | pertaining to | -emesis | vomiting | -itis | inflammation |
| -arche | beginning | -emia | blood condition | -ity | condition |
| -ary | pertaining to | -er | relating to, one who | -ive | nature of, quality of |
| -ase | enzyme | -ergy | work | -ize | to make, to treat or combine with |
| -asthenia | weakness | -esis | condition | | |
| -ate, -ate (d) | use, action, having the form of, possessing | -esthesia | feeling | -kinesia | motion, movement |
| | | -form | shape | -kinesis | motion, movement |
| | | -fuge | to flee | -lalia | to talk |
| -betes | to go | -gen | formation, produce | -lemma | sheath, rind |
| -blast | immature cell, germ cell, embryonic cell | -genes | produce | -lepsy | seizure |
| | | -genesis | formation, produce | -lexia | diction, word, phrase |
| | | -genic | formation, produce | -liter | liter |
| -body | body | -glia | glue | -lith | stone |
| -cele | hernia, tumor, swelling | -globin | protein | -logy | study of |
| | | -gnosis | knowledge | -lymph | clear fluid, serum, pale fluid |
| -centesis | surgical puncture | -grade | step | | |
| -ceps | head | -graft | pencil, grafting knife | -lysis | destruction, separation, breakdown, loosening, dissolution |
| -cide | to kill | -gram | weight, mark, record | | |
| -clasia | a breaking | -graph | to write, record, instrument for recording | | |
| -clasis | crushing, breaking up | | | -malacia | softening |
| -cle | small | | | -mania | madness |
| -clysis | injection | -graphy | recording | -megaly | enlargement, large |
| -cope | strike | -hexia | condition | -meter | instrument to measure |
| -crit | to separate | -ia | condition | | |
| -culture | cultivation | -iasis | condition | -metry | measurement |
| -cusis | hearing | -iatrics | treatment | -mnesia | memory |
| -cuspid | point | -iatry | treatment | -morph | form, shape |
| -cyesis | pregnancy | -ic | pertaining to | -noia | mind |
| -cyst | bladder, sac | -ician | specialist | -oid | resemble, like, similar |
| -cyte | cell | -ide | having a particular quality | -ole | opening, small |
| -derma | skin | | | -oma | tumor, mass, fluid collection |
| -dermis | skin | -ile | pertaining to | | |
| -desis | binding | -in | substance | -omion | shoulder |
| -dipsia | thirst | -ine | pertaining to, substance | -on | pertaining to |
| -drome | course | | | -one | hormone |
| -dynia | pain, ache | -ing | quality of | -opia | sight vision |
| -ectasia | dilatation | -ion | process | -opsia | sight, vision |
| -ectasis | dilatation, dilation, stretching, expansion | -ior | pertaining to | -opsy | to view |
| | | -is | pertaining to | -or | one who, doer |
| -ectasy | dilation | | | -orexia | appetite |

| | |
|---|---|
| -ose | pertaining to |
| -osis | condition (usually abnormal) |
| -ous | pertaining to |
| -oxia | oxygen |
| -paresis | weakness |
| -pathy | disease, emotion |
| -penia | lack of, deficiency, abnormal reduction |
| -pepsia | to digest |
| -pexy | surgical fixation |
| -phagia | to eat, to swallow |
| -phasia | to speak, speech |
| -pheresis | removal, remove |
| -phil | attraction |
| -philia | attraction |
| -phobia | fear |
| -phoresis | to carry |
| -phragm | fence |
| -phraxis | to obstruct |
| -phylaxis | protection |
| -physis | growth |
| -plakia | plate |
| -plasia | formation, produce |
| -plasm | thing formed, plasma |
| -plasty | surgical repair |
| -plegia | stroke, paralysis, palsy |

| | |
|---|---|
| -pnea | breathing |
| -poiesis | formation |
| -praxia | action |
| -ptosis | prolapse, drooping, sagging, falling down |
| -ptysis | to spit, spitting |
| -puncture | to pierce |
| -rrhage | to burst forth, bursting forth |
| -rrhagia | to burst forth, bursting forth |
| -rrhaphy | suture |
| -rrhea | flow, discharge |
| -rrhexis | rupture |
| -scope | instrument for examining |
| -scopy | to view, examine, visual examination |
| -sepsis | decay |
| -sis | state of, condition |
| -some | body |
| -sound | sound |
| -spasm | tension, spasm, contraction |
| -stalsis | contraction |
| -stasis | control, stop, stand still |

| | |
|---|---|
| -staxis | dripping, trickling |
| -sthenia | strength |
| -stomy | new opening |
| -systole | contraction |
| -taxia | order, coordination |
| -therapy | treatment |
| -thermy | heat |
| -tic | pertaining to |
| -tome | instrument to cut |
| -tomy | incision |
| -tone | tension |
| -tripsy | crushing |
| -troph(y) | nourishment, development |
| -trophy | nourishment, development |
| -type | type |
| -um | tissue, structure |
| -ure | process |
| -uria | urination, condition of urine |
| -us | pertaining to, structure |
| -y | condition, pertaining to, process |

# ABBREVIATIONS AND SYMBOLS

## APPENDIX III

### ABBREVIATIONS

#### A

| | |
|---|---|
| 17-KS | 17-ketosteroids |
| 17-OHCS | 17-hydroxycorticosteroids |
| a | ampere; anode; anterior; aqua; area; artery |
| aa | of each |
| A/G | albumin/globulin ratio |
| A&P | auscultation and percussion; anatomy and physiology |
| AB | abortion; abnormal |
| Ab | antibody |
| ABC | aspiration biopsy cytology |
| Abd | abdomen |
| ABGs | arterial blood gases |
| ABLB | alternate binaural loudness balance |
| ABMS | American Board of Medical Specialties |
| ABO | blood group |
| ABR | auditory brainstem response |
| AC | air conduction; anticoagulant |
| ac | before meals (ante cibum); acute |
| Acc | accommodation |
| ACE | angiotensin converting enzyme (inhibitor) |
| ACG | angiocardiography |
| ACh | acetylcholine |
| ACL | anterior cruciate ligament |
| ACOG | American College of Obstetrics and Gynecology |
| ACR | American College of Rheumatology |
| ACS | American Cancer Society |
| ACTH | adrenocorticotropic hormone |
| AD | Alzheimer's disease; advance directive |
| ad lib | as desired; freely |
| ADA | American Diabetes Association |
| adeno-CA | adenocarcinoma |
| ADH | antidiuretic hormone (vasopressin) |
| AD/HD | attention-deficit/hyperactivity disorder |
| ADL | activities of daily living |
| adm | admission |
| ADP | adenosine diphosphate |
| AE | above elbow |
| AED | automated external defibrillator |
| AF | atrial fibrillation |
| AFB | acid-fast bacilli |
| AFP | alpha-fetoprotein |
| Ag | antigen |
| AGN | acute glomerulonephritis |
| AH | abdominal hysterectomy |
| AHD | arteriosclerotic heart disease |
| AHF | antihemophilic factor VIII |
| AHG | antihemophillic globulin factor VIII |
| AI | artificial insemination; aortic insufficiency |
| AIDS | acquired immunodeficiency syndrome |
| AIH | artificial insemination homologous |
| AJ | ankle jerk |
| AK | above knee |
| AKA | above-knee amputation |
| alk phos | alkaline phosphatase |
| ALD | aldolase |
| ALL | acute lymphocytic leukemia |
| ALS | amyotrophic lateral sclerosis |
| ALT | argon laser trabeculoplasty; alanine aminotransferase |
| alt dieb | every other day |
| alt hor | every other hour |
| alt noc | every other night |
| AM, am | before noon (ante meridiem); morning |
| AMA | against medical advice; American Medical Association |
| Amb | ambulate; ambulatory |
| AMD | age-related macular degeneration |
| AMI | acute myocardial infarction |
| AML | acute myeloid leukemia |
| ANA | antinuclear antibodies |
| ANS | autonomic nervous system |
| ant | anterior |
| AOM | acute otitis media |
| AOP | acknowledgement of paternity |
| AP | anteroposterior |

| | |
|---|---|
| A-P | anterior-posterior |
| APA | American Psychiatric Association |
| approx | approximately |
| APTT | activated partial thromboplastin time |
| AQ, aq | water |
| ARD | acute respiratory disease |
| ARDS | acute respiratory distress syndrome |
| ARF | acute renal failure |
| ARMD | age-related macular degeneration |
| AROM | artificial rupture of membranes |
| AS | aortic stenosis |
| As, Ast, astigm | astigmatism |
| ASAP | as soon as possible |
| Ascus | atypical squamous cells of undetermined significance |
| ASD | atrial septal defect |
| ASH | asymmetrical septal hypertrophy |
| ASHD | arteriosclerotic heart disease |
| ASO | antistreptolysin O |
| AST | aspartate aminotransferase |
| ATN | acute tubular necrosis |
| ATP | adenosine triphosphate |
| A-V, AV | atrioventricular; arteriovenous |
| AVMs | arteriovenous malformations |
| AVR | aortic valve replacement |
| ax | axillary |
| AZT | zidovudine |

## B

| | |
|---|---|
| Ba | barium |
| BAC | blood alcohol concentration |
| BaE | barium enema |
| baso | basophil |
| BBB | bundle branch block |
| BBT | basal body temperature |
| BC | bone conduction |
| BCC | basal cell carcinoma |
| BCP | birth control pill |
| BDD | body dysmorphic disorder |
| BE | below elbow; barium enema |
| BG, bG | blood glucose |
| bid | twice a day |
| BIN, bin | twice a night |
| BK | below knee |
| BKA | below-knee amputation |
| BM | bowel movement |
| BMD | bone mineral density (test) |
| BMI | body mass index |
| BMR | basal metabolic rate |
| BNO | bladder neck obstruction |
| BP | blood pressure |

| | |
|---|---|
| BPH | benign prostatic hyperplasia (hypertrophy) |
| BRCA | breast cancer gene |
| BRP | bathroom privileges |
| BS | blood sugar; breath sounds; bowel sounds |
| BSE | breast self-examination |
| BSI | body systems isolation |
| BSP | bromsulphalein |
| BT | bleeding time |
| BUN | blood urea nitrogen |
| Bx | biopsy |

## C

| | |
|---|---|
| c̄ | with (cum) |
| C | centigrade, Celsius |
| C1, C2, etc. | first cervical vertebra; second cervical vertebra |
| C&S | culture and sensitivity |
| CA | cancer; carcinoembryonic antigen |
| CA-125 | cancer antigen 125 |
| Ca | calcium |
| CABG | coronary artery bypass graft |
| CAD | coronary artery disease |
| CAM | complementary and alternative medicines |
| cap | capsule |
| CAPD | continuous ambulatory peritoneal dialysis |
| CAT | computerized axial tomography |
| cath | catheterization; catheter |
| CBC | complete blood count |
| CBR | complete bed rest |
| CBS | chronic brain syndrome |
| CBT | cognitive-behavioral therapy |
| CC | cardiac catheterization; chief complaint; clean catch (urine) |
| CCU | coronary care unit |
| CDC | Centers for Disease Control and Prevention |
| CDH | congenital dislocation of hip |
| CEA | carcinoembryonic antigen |
| CF | cystic fibrosis |
| CGN | chronic glomerulonephritis |
| CHD | coronary heart disease |
| chemo | chemotherapy |
| CHF | congestive heart failure |
| CHO | carbohydrate |
| chol | cholesterol |
| CHT | congenital hypothyroidism |
| Ci | curie |

| | |
|---|---|
| Cib | food (cibus) |
| CIN | cervical intraepithelial neoplasia |
| CIS | carcinoma in situ |
| CK | creatine kinase |
| Cl | chlorine |
| CLI | critical limb ischemia |
| CLL | chronic lymphocytic leukemia |
| cm | centimeter |
| CMG | cystometrogram |
| CML | chronic myelocystic leukemia |
| CMP | cardiomyopathy |
| CMV | cytomegalovirus |
| CNS | central nervous system |
| c/o | complains of |
| CO | cardiac output |
| $CO_2$ | carbon dioxide |
| COLD | chronic obstructive lung disease |
| cont | continue |
| COPD | chronic obstructive pulmonary disease |
| CP | cerebral palsy |
| CPD | cephalopelvic disproportion |
| CPK | creatine phosphokinase |
| CPM | continuous passive motion |
| CPR | cardiopulmonary resuscitation |
| CPS | cycles per second |
| CR | computerized radiography |
| CRF | chronic renal failure; corticotropin-releasing factor |
| CS, C-section | cesarean section |
| CSF | cerebrospinal fluid |
| CT | computed tomography |
| CTA | clear to auscultation |
| CTS | carpal tunnel syndrome |
| CUC | chronic ulcerative colitis |
| CV | cardiovascular |
| CVA | cerebrovascular accident (stroke) |
| CVD | cardiovascular disease |
| CVP | central venous pressure |
| CVS | chorionic villus sampling |
| CWP | childbirth without pain |
| CXR | chest x-ray; chest radiograph |
| cysto | cystoscopic examination; cystoscopy |

**D**

| | |
|---|---|
| /d | per day |
| D | diopter (lens strength) |
| D&C | dilation (dilatation) and curettage |
| db, Db | decibel |
| DBS | deep brain stimulation |
| D&E | dilation and evacuation |

| | |
|---|---|
| DCIS | ductal carcinoma in situ |
| DDS | doctor of dental surgery; dorsal cord stimulation |
| decub | decubitus |
| Derm | dermatology |
| DES | diethylstilbestrol |
| DEXA | dual-energy x-ray absorptiometry |
| DHT | dihydrotestosterone |
| DI | diabetes insipidus; diagnostic imaging |
| diff | differential count (white blood cells) |
| dil | dilute; diluted |
| DJD | degenerative joint disease |
| DM | diabetes mellitus |
| DMARDs | disease-modifying antirheumatic drugs |
| DMD | Duchenne muscular dystrophy |
| DNA | deoxyribonucleic acid; does not apply |
| DNR | do not resuscitate |
| DNS | did not show |
| DO | doctor of osteopathy |
| DOA | dead on arrival |
| DOB | date of birth |
| DOT | directly observed therapy |
| Dr. | doctor |
| DRE | digital rectal examination |
| DRGs | diagnostic related groups |
| DS | double strength |
| DSA | digital subtraction angiography |
| DSM-IV-TR | *Diagnostic and Statistical Manual of Mental Disorders*, 4th ed. (Text Revision) |
| DTaP | diphtheria, tetanus, and pertussis (vaccine) |
| DTRs | deep tendon reflexes |
| DUB | dysfunctional uterine bleeding |
| DVA | distance visual acuity |
| DVT | deep vein thrombosis |
| D/W | dextrose in water |
| Dx | diagnosis |

**E**

| | |
|---|---|
| EBV | Epstein-Barr virus |
| ECC | extracorporeal circulation |
| ECCE | extracapsular cataract extraction |
| ECF | extracellular fluid; extended care facility |
| ECG, EKG | electrocardiogram |
| ECHO | echocardiogram |
| *E. coli* | *Escherichia coli* |
| ECSL | extracorporeal shockwave lithotriptor |
| ECT | electroconvulsive therapy |

| | |
|---|---|
| ED | erectile dysfunction |
| EDB | estimated date of birth |
| EDC | estimated date of confinement (delivery) |
| EDD | estimated date of delivery |
| EEG | electroencephalogram; electroencephalograph |
| EENT | eye, ear, nose, and throat |
| EFM | electronic fetal monitor |
| EGD | esophagogastroduodenoscopy |
| ELISA | enzyme-linked immunosorbent assay |
| EM | emmetropia |
| EMG | electromyography |
| ENG | electronystagmography |
| ENT | ear, nose, throat (otorhinolaryngology) |
| EOM | extraocular movement; extraocular muscles |
| eos, eosin | eosinophil |
| EPS | electrophysiology study (intracardiac) |
| ER | emergency room; endoplasmic reticulum |
| ERCP | endoscopic retrograde cholangiopancreatography |
| ERT | estrogen replacement therapy; external radiation therapy |
| ERV | expiratory reserve volume |
| ESL, ESWL | extracorporeal shock-wave lithotripsy |
| ESR | erythrocyte sedimentation rate |
| ESRD | end-stage renal disease |
| EST | electroshock therapy |
| ESWL | extracorporeal shockwave lithotripsy |
| ET | esotropia; endotracheal |
| Ex | examination |

**F**

| | |
|---|---|
| F | Fahrenheit; female |
| FACP | Fellow of the American College of Physicians |
| FACS | Fellow of the American College of Surgeons |
| FB | foreign body |
| FBG | fasting blood glucose |
| FBS | fasting blood sugar |
| FDA | Food and Drug Administration |
| FEF | forced expiratory flow |
| FEKG | fetal electrocardiogram |
| FEV | forced expiratory volume |
| FFA | free fatty acids |
| FH | family history |
| FHB | fetal heartbeat |
| FHR | fetal heart rate |

| | |
|---|---|
| FHS | fetal heart sound |
| FHT | fetal heart tone |
| FIV | forced inspiratory volume |
| FMS | fibromyalgia syndrome |
| FNA | fine needle aspiration |
| FP | family practice |
| FRC | forced residual capacity |
| FROM | full range of motion |
| FS | frozen section |
| FSH | follicle-stimulating hormone |
| FTA-ABS | fluorescent treponemal antibody absorption |
| FTND | full-term normal delivery |
| FUO | fever of undetermined origin |
| F-V loop | flow volume loop |
| FVC | forced vital capacity |
| Fx | fracture |

**G**

| | |
|---|---|
| g | gram |
| GAD | generalized anxiety disorder |
| GB | gallbladder |
| GBS | group B streptococcus |
| GC | gonorrhea |
| GCSF | granulocyte colony-stimulating factor |
| GERD | gastroesophageal reflux disease |
| GFR | glomerular filtration rate |
| GGT | gamma-glutamyl transferase |
| GH | growth hormone |
| GHRF | growth hormone-releasing factor |
| GI | gastrointestinal |
| GIFT | gamete intrafallopian transfer |
| GnRF | gonadotropin-releasing factor |
| GOT | glutamic oxaloacetic transaminase |
| Gpi | globus pallidus |
| GPT | glutamic pyruvic transaminase |
| grav I | pregnancy one |
| GTT | glucose tolerance test |
| GU | genitourinary |
| GYN | gynecology |

**H**

| | |
|---|---|
| $H_2O$ | water |
| H, hr | hour |
| H | hydrogen |
| H&L | heart & lungs |
| HAA | hepatitis-associated antigen |
| HAART | highly active antiretroviral therapy |
| HAV | hepatitis A virus |
| Hb, Hgb, HGB | hemoglobin |
| HBIG | hepatitis B immune globulin |

| | |
|---|---|
| HBOT | hyperbaric oxygen therapy |
| HBP | high blood pressure |
| HBV | hepatitis B virus |
| HCC | hepatocellular carcinoma |
| hCG, HCG | human chorionic gonadotropin |
| HCl | hydrochloric acid |
| HCO₃ | bicarbonate |
| Hct, HCT | hematocrit |
| HD | hip disarticulation; hearing distance; Hodgkin's disease; hemodialysis |
| HDL | high-density lipoprotein |
| HDN | hemolytic disease of the newborn |
| HDS | herniated disk syndrome |
| HEENT | head, eyes, ears, nose, throat |
| HER-2/neu | human epidermal growth factor receptor-2 |
| HF | heart failure |
| Hg | mercury |
| HHS | Health and Human Services (Department of) |
| HIPAA | Health Insurance Portability and Accountability Act of 1996 |
| HIV | human immunodeficiency virus |
| HLA | human leukocyte antigen |
| HMD | hyaline membrane disease |
| HNP | herniated nucleus pulposus (herniated disk) |
| Hpd | hematoporphyrin derivative |
| *H. pylori* | *Heliocobacter pylori* |
| HPV | human papillomavirus |
| HRT | hormone replacement therapy |
| HSG | hysterosalpingography |
| HSV | herpes simplex virus |
| HSV-2 | herpes simplex virus-2 |
| HT | hyperopia |
| Ht | height |
| HTLV | human T-cell leukemia-lymphoma virus |
| HTN | hypertension |
| Hx | history |
| hypo | hypodermic injection |

**I**

| | |
|---|---|
| I&D | incision and drainage |
| I&O | intake and output |
| IAS | interatrial septum |
| IBS | irritable bowel syndrome |
| IC | interstitial cystitis; inspiratory capacity |
| ICCE | intracapsular cataract cryoextraction |
| ICF | intracellular fluid |
| ICP | intracranial pressure |

| | |
|---|---|
| ICSH | interstitial cell-stimulating hormone |
| ICU | intensive care unit |
| ID | intradermal |
| IDDM | insulin-dependent diabetes mellitus |
| Ig | immunoglobulin |
| IH | infectious hepatitis |
| IHSS | idiopathic hypertropic subaortic stenosis |
| IL-2 | interleukin-2 |
| IM | intramuscular |
| inj | injection |
| IOL | intraocular lens |
| IOP | intraocular pressure |
| IPD | intermittent peritoneal dialysis |
| IPPB | intermittent positive-pressure breathing |
| IQ | intelligence quotient |
| IR | interventional radiology |
| IRDS | infant respiratory distress syndrome |
| IRT | internal radiation therapy |
| IRV | inspiratory reserve volume |
| IS | intercostal space |
| ITP | idiopathic thrombocytopenia purpura |
| IUD | intrauterine device |
| IUGR | intrauterine growth rate; intrauterine growth retardation |
| IV | intravenous |
| IVC | inferior vena cava; intravenous cholangiography; intraventricular catheter |
| IVF | in vitro fertilization |
| IVP | intravenous pyelogram |
| IVS | interventricular septum |
| IVU | intravenous urogram |

**J**

| | |
|---|---|
| J | joule |
| JNC | Joint National Committee |
| JRA | juvenile rheumatoid arthritis |
| jt | joint |
| JVD | jugular vein distention |

**K**

| | |
|---|---|
| K | potassium |
| KD | knee disarticulation |
| kg | kilogram |
| KJ | knee jerk |
| KS | Kaposi's sarcoma |
| KUB | kidney, ureter, and bladder |
| kV | kilovolt |

# L

| | |
|---|---|
| L1, L2, etc. | first lumbar vertebra, second lumbar vertebra, etc. |
| L | liter |
| L&A | light and accommodation |
| L&W | living and well |
| LA | left atrium |
| lab | laboratory |
| LAC | long arm cast |
| LAK | lymphokine-activated killer (cells) |
| LAT, lat | lateral |
| lb | pound |
| LB | large bowel |
| LBBB | left bundle branch block |
| LCIS | lobular carcinoma in situ |
| LD | lactate dehydrogenase |
| LDH | lactate dehydrogenase |
| LDL | low-density lipoprotein |
| LE | lupus erythematosus; lower extremity; left eye |
| LEDs | light-emitting diodes |
| LES | lower esophageal sphincter |
| LH | luteinizing hormone |
| LH-RH | luteinizing hormone-releasing hormone |
| lig | ligament |
| liq | liquid |
| LLC | long leg cast |
| LLCC | long leg cylinder cast |
| LLQ | left lower quadrant |
| LMP | last menstrual period |
| LOA | left occipitoanterior |
| LOC | level of consciousness |
| LOM | limitation or loss of motion |
| LP | lumbar puncture |
| LPI | laser peripheral iridotomy |
| LRQ | lower right quadrant |
| lt | left |
| LTH | lactogenic hormone |
| LUQ | left upper quadrant |
| LV | left ventricle |
| lymphs | lymphocytes |

# M

| | |
|---|---|
| M | molar; thousand; muscle; male |
| m | male; meter; minim |
| mA | milliampere |
| mAs | milliampere second |
| MALT | mucosal-associated-lymphoid type (lymphoma) |
| MAOIs | monoamine oxidase inhibitors |
| MBC | maximal breathing capacity |

| | |
|---|---|
| MBPS | Munchausen by proxy syndrome |
| mcg | microgram |
| MCH | mean corpuscular hemoglobin |
| MCHC | mean corpuscular hemoglobin concentration |
| mCi | millicurie |
| MCV | mean corpuscular volume |
| MD | medical doctor; muscular dystrophy |
| MDR TB | multidrug-resistant tuberculosis |
| mEq | milliequivalent |
| mets | metastases |
| MG | myasthenia gravis |
| mg | milligram (0.001 gram) |
| MH | marital history |
| MI | myocardial infarction; mitral insufficiency |
| MIF | melanocyte-stimulating hormone release-inhibiting factor |
| mix astig | mixed astigmatism |
| mL | milliliter (0.001 liter) |
| mm | millimeter (0.001 meter; 0.039 inch) |
| mMol | millimole |
| MMPI | Minnesota Multiphasic Personality Inventory |
| MMR | measles, mumps, and rubella (vaccine) |
| MMSE | Mini Mental State Examination |
| mol wt | molecular weight |
| mono | monocyte |
| MR | mental retardation |
| MRF | melanocyte-stimulating hormone-releasing factor |
| MRI | magnetic resonance imaging |
| MS | mitral stenosis; multiple sclerosis; musculoskeletal |
| MSH | melanocyte-stimulating hormone |
| MTD | right ear drum (membrana tympani dexter) |
| MTS | left ear drum (membrana tympani sinister) |
| MV | mitral valve; minute volume |
| mV | millivolt |
| MVP | mitral valve prolapse |
| MVV | maximal voluntary ventilation |
| MY | myopia |

# N

| | |
|---|---|
| n | nerve |
| Na | sodium |
| NaCl | sodium chloride |
| N&V | nausea & vomiting |
| NANBH | non-A, non-B hepatitis virus |

| | |
|---|---|
| NB | newborn |
| NCI | National Cancer Institute |
| nCi | nanocurie |
| NCV | nerve conduction velocity |
| neg | negative |
| Neuro | neurology |
| NG | nasogastric (tube) |
| ng | nanogram |
| NGU | nongonococcal urethritis |
| NH$_3$ | ammonia |
| NHLBI | National Heart, Lung and Blood Institute |
| NIDDM | noninsulin-dependent diabetes mellitus |
| NIH | National Institute of Health |
| NIMH | National Institute of Mental Health |
| NK | natural killer (cells) |
| NKDA | no known drug allergies |
| NLST | National Lung Screening Trial |
| NMR | nuclear magnetic resonance |
| NPH | nonprotein nitrogen |
| NPO, npo | nothing by mouth |
| NPT | nocturnal penile tumescence |
| NPUAP | National Pressure Ulcer Advisory Panel |
| NREM | no rapid eye movement (sleep) |
| NS | normal saline |
| NSAIDs | nonsteroidal anti-inflammatory drugs |
| NSSC | normal size, shape, and consistency |
| NST | nonstress test |
| NVA | near visual acuity |

**O**

| | |
|---|---|
| O | pint |
| O, O$_2$ | oxygen |
| O&P | ova and parasites |
| OA | osteoarthritis |
| OB | obstetrics |
| OB-GYN | obstetrics and gynecology |
| OC | oral contraceptive |
| OCD | obsessive-compulsive disorder |
| OCPs | oral contraceptive pills |
| OD | overdose |
| OHS | open heart surgery |
| OM | otitis media |
| OP | outpatient |
| OR | operating room |
| ORTH, ortho | orthopedics; orthopaedics |
| os | mouth opening; bone |
| OTC | over-the-counter |
| oto | otology |
| OV | office visit |
| oz | ounce |

**P**

| | |
|---|---|
| P | pulse; phosphorus |
| PA | posteroanterior; pernicious anemia |
| PAC | premature arterial contraction |
| PAD | peripheral artery disease |
| Pap | Papanicolaou (smear) |
| PAT | paroxysmal atrial tachycardia |
| Path | pathology |
| PBI | protein bound iodine |
| pc | after meals (post cibum) |
| PCL | posterior cruciate ligament |
| PCP | *Pneumocystis carinii* pneumonia |
| PCV | packed cell volume |
| PD | peritoneal dialysis |
| PDR | *Physicians' Desk Reference* |
| PE | physical examination; pulmonary embolism |
| Peds | pediatrics |
| PEEP | positive end-expiratory pressure |
| PEG | percutaneous endoscopic gastrostomy |
| PEMFs | pulsing electromagnetic fields |
| PERRLA | pupils equal, round, react to light and accommodation |
| PET | positron emission tomography |
| PE tube | polyethylene tube |
| PFT | pulmonary function test |
| pH | hydrogen ion concentration; degree of acidity |
| PH | past history |
| Ph.D. | doctor of philosophy, doctor of pharmacy |
| phaco | phacoemulsification |
| PHI | protected health information |
| PI | present illness |
| PID | pelvic inflammatory disease |
| PIF | prolactin release-inhibiting factor |
| PIH | pregnancy-induced hypertension |
| PIP | proximal interphalangeal |
| PKU | phenylketonuria |
| PLCO | Prostate, Lung, Colorectal and Ovarian (study) |
| PM | physical medicine |
| PM, pm | afternoon, evening |
| PMH | past medical history |
| PMI | point of maximal impulse |
| PMN | polymorphonuclear neutrophil |
| PMP | previous menstrual period |
| PMR | physical medicine and rehabilitation |
| PMS | premenstrual syndrome |
| PND | paroxysmal nocturnal dyspnea; postnasal drip |
| PNS | peripheral nervous system |
| PO | orally, by mouth |

| | | | | |
|---|---|---|---|---|
| poly | polymorphonuclear | | RBC | red blood cell; red blood cell (count) |
| PP | postprandial (after meals) | | RBCs | red blood cells |
| PPD | purified protein derivative (TB test); pack (s) per day | | RD | respiratory disease |
| | | | RDA | recommended dietary or daily allowance |
| PPI | proton pump inhibitor | | rDNA | recombinant deoxyribonucleic acid |
| pr | per rectum | | RDS | respiratory distress syndrome |
| PRF | prolactin-releasing factor | | RE | right eye |
| PRL | prolactin hormone | | REM | rapid eye movement (sleep) |
| PRN, prn | as necessary; as required; when necessary; as needed | | resp | respiratory |
| | | | RF | rheumatoid factor |
| PSA | prostate-specific antigen | | Rh | Rhesus blood factor (Rh+ or Rh−) |
| Psych | psychiatry, psychology | | RIA | radioimmunoassay |
| PT | physical therapy; prothrombin time | | RLF | retrolental fibroplasia |
| pt | patient; pint | | RLQ | right lower quadrant |
| PTC | percutaneous transhepatic cholangiography | | RNA | ribonucleic acid |
| | | | R/O | rule out |
| PTCA | percutaneous transluminal coronary angioplasty | | ROM | range of motion; read only memory |
| PTH | parathyroid hormone (parathormone) | | RP | retrograde pyelography |
| | | | RPE | retinal pigment epithelium |
| PTS | permanent threshold shift | | RPM | revolutions per minute |
| PTSD | post-traumatic stress disorder | | RQ | respiratory quotient |
| PTT | partial thromboplastin time | | RRR | regular rate and rhythm |
| PUBS | percutaneous umbilical blood sampling | | RSV | respiratory syncytial virus |
| | | | RT | radiation therapy |
| PUD | peptic ulcer disease | | RUPP | Research Units on Pediatric Psychopharmacology |
| PUL | percutaneous ultrasonic lithotropsy | | | |
| PUVA | psoralen-ultraviolet light | | RUQ | right upper quadrant |
| PVC | premature ventricular contraction | | RV | right ventricle; residual volume |
| PVD | peripheral vascular disease | | Rx | take thou; prescribe; treatment; therapy |
| PWB | partial weight bearing | | | |

**Q**

| | | | | |
|---|---|---|---|---|
| q | every (quaque) | | **S** | |
| qh | every hour | | s̄ | without |
| q2h | every 2 hours | | SA, S-A | sinoatrial (node) |
| q4h | every 4 hours | | SAB | spontaneous abortion |
| qid | four times a day | | SAC | short arm cast |
| qm | every morning (quaque mane) | | SAD | seasonal affective disorder |
| qns | quantity not sufficient | | SAH | subarachnoid hemorrhage |
| qs | quantity sufficient | | SALT | serum alanine aminotransferase |
| qt | quart | | SARS | severe acute respiratory syndrome |
| | | | SAST | serum aspartate aminotransferase |
| | | | SBFT | small-bowel followthrough |
| | | | SCA | sudden cardiac arrest |
| **R** | | | SCC | squamous cell carcinoma |
| R | respiration | | SCD | sudden cardiac death |
| R, rt | right | | SD | shoulder disarticulation; standard deviation |
| RA | right atrium; rheumatoid arthritis | | | |
| Ra | radium | | | |
| rad | radiation absorbed dose | | seg, poly | polymorphonuclear neutrophil |
| RAI | radioactive iodine | | segs | segmented (mature RBCs) |
| RAIU | radioactive iodine uptake | | SG | skin graft |

| | |
|---|---|
| SGOT | serum glutamic oxaloacetic transaminase |
| SGPT | serum glutamic pyruvic transaminase |
| SH | serum hepatitis |
| sh | shoulder |
| SIDS | sudden infant death syndrome |
| SK | streptokinase |
| SLC | short leg cast |
| SLE | systemic lupus erythematosus |
| SLT | selective laser trabeculoplasty |
| SMBG | self-monitoring of blood glucose |
| SNRI | serotonin-norepinephrine reuptake inhibitor |
| SOAP | subjective, objective, assessment, plan |
| SOB | shortness of breath |
| SOM | serous otitis media |
| sono | sonogram, sonography |
| SOP | standard operating procedure |
| SOS | if necessary (*si opus sit*) |
| SPECT | single photon emission computed tomography |
| sp. gr, SG | specific gravity |
| SPP | suprapubic prostatectomy |
| SR, sed rate | sedimentation rate |
| SS | Social Security |
| ss | one half |
| SSRIs | selective serotonin reuptake inhibitors |
| ST | esotropia |
| St | stage (of disease) |
| staph | staphylococcus |
| stat | immediately |
| STD | skin test done |
| STDs | sexually transmitted diseases |
| STH | somatotropin hormone |
| strep | streptococcus |
| STS | serologic test for syphilis |
| STSG | split thickness skin graft |
| Sub-Q, subQ | subcutaneous |
| SVC | superior vena cava |
| SVD | spontaneous vaginal delivery |
| Sx | symptom |
| syr | syrup |

**T**

| | |
|---|---|
| T1, T2, etc. | thoracic vertebrae first, thoracic vertebrae second, etc. |
| T3 | triiodothyronine |
| T3RU | triiodothyronine resin uptake |
| T3U | triiodothyronine uptake |
| T4 | thyroxine |

| | |
|---|---|
| T&A | tonsillectomy and adenoidectomy |
| T, temp | temperature |
| Tab, tab | tablet |
| TAH | total abdominal hysterectomy |
| TAT | Thematic Apperception Test |
| TB | tuberculosis |
| TBW | total body weight |
| TC | testicular cancer |
| TCAs | tricyclic antidepressants |
| TENS | transcutaneous electrical nerve stimulation |
| TFS | thyroid function studies |
| TH | thyroid hormone |
| THA | total hip arthroplasty |
| THR | total hip replacement |
| TIAs | transient ischemic attacks |
| tid | three times a day |
| TIMs | topical immunomodulators |
| TIPS | transjugular intrahepatic portosystemic shunt |
| TJ | triceps jerk |
| TKA | total knee arthroplasty |
| TKR | total knee replacement |
| TLC | tender loving care; total lung capacity |
| TM | tympanic membrane |
| TMJ | temporomandibular joint |
| TNF | tumor necrosis factor |
| TNM | tumor, node, metastasis |
| TNS | transcutaneous nerve stimulation |
| TOF | tetralogy of Fallot |
| top | topically |
| TPA | *Treponema pallidum* agglutination (test) |
| TPA, tPA | tissue plasminogen activator |
| TPE | Taxol, Platinol, and VePesid |
| TPN | total parenteral nutrition |
| TPR | temperature, pulse, respiration |
| tr, tinct | tincture |
| trans | transverse |
| TRH | thyrotropin-releasing hormone |
| TSE | testicular self-exam |
| TSH | thyroid-stimulating hormone |
| TSS | toxic shock syndrome |
| TTH | thyrotropic hormone |
| TUIP | transurethral incision of the prostate |
| TUMT | transurethral microwave thermotherapy |
| TUNA | transurethral needle ablation |
| TUR | transurethral resection |
| TURP | transurethral resection of the prostate |
| TV | tidal volume |
| Tx | traction; treatment; transplant |

## U

| | |
|---|---|
| UA | urinalysis |
| U&L, U/L | upper and lower |
| UC | uterine contractions |
| UCHD | usual childhood diseases |
| UG | urogenital |
| UGI | upper gastrointestinal |
| ULQ | upper left quadrant |
| ung | ointment |
| URI | upper respiratory infection |
| URQ | upper right quadrant |
| US | ultrasound |
| USP | United States Pharmacopeia |
| UTI | urinary tract infection |
| UV | ultraviolet |

## V

| | |
|---|---|
| v | vein |
| VA | visual acuity |
| VAD | vacuum-assisted needle biopsy device |
| VC | vital capacity |
| VCD | vacuum constriction device |
| VCG | vectorcardiogram |
| VCU, VCUG | voiding cystourethrogram |
| VD | venereal disease |
| VDRL | Venereal Disease Research Laboratory (syphilis test) |
| VF | visual field |
| VHD | ventricular heart disease |
| VLDL | very low-density lipoprotein |
| vol | volume |
| vol % | volume percent |
| VMA | vanillylmandelic acid |
| VP | vasopressin |
| VS, V/S | vital signs |
| VSD | ventricular septal defect |
| VT | ventricular tachycardia |

## W

| | |
|---|---|
| WAIS | Wechster Adult Intelligence Scale |
| WBC | white blood cell; white blood (cell) count |
| WDWN | well developed, well nourished |

| | |
|---|---|
| WF, BF | white female, black female |
| WHO | World Health Organization |
| WM, BM | white male, black male |
| WNL | within normal limits |
| Wt | weight |
| w/v | weight by volume |

## X

| | |
|---|---|
| XM | cross match for blood (type and cross match) |
| XP | xeroderma pigmentosum |
| XR | x-ray |
| XT | exotropia |
| XX | female sex chromosomes |
| XY | male sex chromosomes |

## Y

| | |
|---|---|
| YAG | yttrium-aluminum-garnet (laser) |
| y/o | year(s) old |
| YOB | year of birth |
| yr | year |

## Z

| | |
|---|---|
| z | atomic number |

## SYMBOLS

| | |
|---|---|
| $\times$ | times, power |
| $-$ | negative |
| $+$ | positive |
| $+/-$ | positive or negative |
| * | birth |
| † | death |
| % | percent |
| # | number; pound |
| = | equal |
| ? | question |
| ™ | trademark |
| © | copyright |
| ® | registered |
| ¶ | paragraph |

## APPENDIX IV

### ABBREVIATIONS USED IN REPORTING LABORATORY VALUES

| | |
|---|---|
| $cm^3$ | cubic centimeter |
| cu μ | cubic micron |
| dL | deciliter |
| fL | femtoliter |
| g | gram |
| g/dL | grams per deciliter |
| kg | kilogram |
| L | liter |
| mEq | milliequivalent |
| mg | milligram |
| mg/dL | milligram per deciliter |
| mm | millimeter |
| mmol | millimole |
| $mm^3$ | cubic millimeter |
| mm Hg | millimeter of mercury |
| mol (M) | mole |
| ng | nanogram |
| ng/dL | nanogram per deciliter |
| ng/mL | nanogram per milliliter |
| pg | picogram |
| mcg | microgram |

### HEMATOLOGY TESTS

| | Normal Ranges |
|---|---|
| Differential | |
| Neutrophils | 54–62 % |
| Lymphocytes | 20–40 % |
| Monocytes | 2–10 % |
| Eosinophils | 1–2 % |
| Basophils | 0–1 % |
| Erythrocytes—red blood cells (RBC) | |
| Females | 4.2–5.4 million/$mm^3$ |
| Males | 4.6–6.2 million/$mm^3$ |
| Children | 4.5–5.1 million/$mm^3$ |
| Hemoglobin (HGB, Hgb) | |
| Females | 12.0–14.0 g/dL |
| Males | 14.0–16.0 g/dL |

| | |
|---|---|
| Hematocrit (HCT) | 37.0–54 % |
| Females | 37–47 % |
| Males | 40–54 % |
| Leukocytes—white blood cells (WBC) | 4500–11,000/$mm^3$ |
| Thrombocytes—Platelets | 200,000– 400,000/ $mm^3$ |
| Mean corpuscular hemoglobin (MCH) | 27.0–31.2 pg |
| Mean corpuscular hemoglobin concentration (MCHC) | 31.8–37.4 g/dL |
| Mean corpuscular volume (MCV) | 80–97 fL |

### COAGULATION TESTS

| | |
|---|---|
| Bleeding time | 2.75–8.0 min |
| Coagulation time | 5–15 min |
| Prothrombin time (PT) | 12–14 sec |

### CHEMISTRIES

| | Normal Ranges |
|---|---|
| Sodium (Na) | 136–145 mEq/L |
| Potassium (K) | 3.5–5.0 mEq/L |
| Calcium (Ca) | 9.0–11.0 mg/dL |
| Chloride (Cl) | 100–108 mmol/L |
| $CO_2$ | 21–32 mmol/L |
| Phosphate ($PO_4$) | 3.0–4.5 mg/dL |
| Glucose (fasting) | 70–115 mg/dL |
| Blood urea nitrogen (BUN) | 8–20 mg/dL |
| Creatinine | 0.9–1.5 mg/dL |
| Creatine phosphokinase (CPK) | |
| Females | 30–135 U/L |
| Males | 55–170 U/L |
| Anion gap | 10–17 mEq/L |
| Alkaline phosphatase (ALP) | 20–90U/L |
| Alanine aminotransferase (ALT, SGPT) | 5–30 U/L |
| Albumin | 3.5–5.5 g/dL |
| Globulin | 1.4–4.8 g/dL |
| A/G ratio | 0.7–2.0 g/dL |

| | | | |
|---|---|---|---|
| Aspartate aminotransferase (AST, SGOT) | 10–30 U/L | | |
| Bilirubin | 0.3–1.1 mg/dL | | |
| Cholesterol | <200 mg/dL | | |
| High density lipoprotein (HDL) | >60 mg/dL | | |
| Low density lipoprotein (LDL) | <100 mg/dL | | |
| Triglycerides | <150 mg/dL | | |
| Uric acid | | | |
| Females | 1.5–7.0 mg/dL | | |
| Males | 2.5–8.0 mg/dL | | |
| Lactate dehydrogenase (LDH) | 100–190 U/L | | |
| Thyroxine (T4) | 4.4–9.9 µg/dL | | |
| Free T4 | 0.8–1.8 ng/dL | | |
| Thyroid stimulating hormone (TSH) | 0.5–6.0 uIU/mL | | |
| Prostate specific antigen (PSA) Male | 0.0–4.0 ng/mL | | |
| Testosterone | 241–827 ng/dL | | |

## URINALYSIS

| | Normal Ranges |
|---|---|
| Color | Yellow to amber |
| Turbidity (Appearance) | Clear |
| Specific gravity | 1.003–1.030 |
| Reaction (pH) | 4.6–8.0 |
| Odor | Faintly aromatic |
| Protein | Negative |
| Glucose | Negative |
| Ketones | Negative |
| Bilirubin | Negative |
| Blood | Negative |
| Urobilinogen | 0.1–1.0 |
| Nitrite | Negative |
| Leukocytes | Negative |